Sleep and Mental Illness

Sleep and Mental Illness

Edited by

S. R. Pandi-Perumal
Somnogen Inc.

Milton Kramer
University of Illinois, Chicago

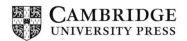

CAMBRIDGE UNIVERSITY PRESS
Cambridge, New York, Melbourne, Madrid, Cape Town, Singapore,
São Paulo, Delhi, Dubai, Tokyo

Cambridge University Press
The Edinburgh Building, Cambridge CB2 8RU, UK

Published in the United States of America by
Cambridge University Press, New York

www.cambridge.org
Information on this title: www.cambridge.org/9780521110501

First published 2010

Printed in the United Kingdom at the University Press, Cambridge

A catalog record for this publication is available from the British Library

Library of Congress Cataloging-in-Publication Data

Sleep and mental illness / edited by S. R. Pandi-Perumal, Milton Kramer.
  p.   cm.
  Includes bibliographical references and index.
  ISBN 978-0-521-11050-1 (hardback)
  1. Sleep disorders.   2. Mental illness–Complications.   I. Pandi-
Perumal, S. R.   II. Kramer, Milton, 1929–
  [DNLM: 1. Mental Disorders–complications.   2. Sleep Disorders–
complications. WM 140 S632 2010]
  RC547.S5177 2010
  616.8′498–dc22

                                                          2009050376

ISBN 978-0-521-11050-1 Hardback

To our families
who continue to support us selflessly and
unreservedly in this and
all our personal and professional endeavors.

Contents

Contributors

Joëlle Adrien, PhD
Faculté de Médecine Pierre et Marie Curie
Site Pitié-Salpêtrière
Paris, France

M. Y. Agargun, MD
Yuzuncu Yil University School of Medicine
Department of Psychiatry
Van, Turkey

Negar Ahmadi, BSc
Toronto Western Hospital
Psychiatry Department
Toronto, ON Canada

Imran M. Ahmed, MD
Sleep-Wake Disorders Center
Montefiore Medical Center and
Albert Einstein College of Medicine
Bronx, NY USA

J. Todd Arnedt, PhD
Clinical Assistant Professor of Psychiatry
Sleep and Chronophysiology Laboratory
University of Michigan
Department of Psychiatry
Ann Arbor, MI USA

Joseph Barbera, MD, FRCPC, DABSM
Department of Psychiatry
University of Toronto
Medical Director
The Youthdale Child and Adolescent Sleep Centre
Toronto, ON Canada

Simon Beaulieu-Bonneau, MPs
École de psychologie
Pavillon Félix-Antoine-Savard
Université Laval
Québec, Canada

Marie E. Beitinger, MSc
Max Planck Institute of Psychiatry
Munich, Germany

Francesco Benedetti, MD
Istituto Scientifico Universitario Ospedale San Raffaele
Dipartimento di Neuroscienze Cliniche
San Raffaele Turro
Milano, Italy

Glenn Berall, BSc, MD, FRCPC, MBA
Chief of Paediatrics
North York General
Assistant Professor Department of Paediatrics and
Department of Nutritional Sciences
University of Toronto
North York General Hospital
University of Toronto
SickKids Hospital Paediatric Suites
Toronto, ON Canada

Kirk J. Brower, MD
Professor of Psychiatry
Executive Director
University of Michigan
Addiction Treatment Services
University of Michigan
Department of Psychiatry
Ann Arbor, MI USA

Gregory M. Brown, MD, PhD, FRCPC, FRSC
Professor Emeritus
Department of Psychiatry
University of Toronto
Oakville, ON Canada

Kumaraswamy Budur, MD
Staff in Sleep Medicine/Psychiatry
Cleveland Clinic
Assistant Professor
Cleveland Clinic Lerner College of Medicine

Case Western Reserve University
Cleveland, OH USA

Daniel P. Cardinali, MD, PhD
Professor of Physiology
Superior Investigator CONICET
Department of Physiology
Faculty of Medicine
University of Buenos Aires, Paraguay
Buenos Aires, Argentina

Deirdre A. Conroy, PhD
Clinical Assistant Professor of Psychiatry
University of Michigan Addiction Treatment Services
University of Michigan
Department of Psychiatry
Ann Arbor, MI USA

Sara Dallaspezia, MD
Istituto Scientifico Universitario
Ospedale San Raffaele
Department of Clinical Neurosciences
San Raffaele Turro, Milan, Italy

José Manuel de la Fuente, MD, PhD
Professor of Psychiatry
CHS Lannemezan
Lannemezan, France

Paolo De Luca
Behavior and Sleep Research Lab
Douglas Research Institute
Verdun, QC Canada

Diana De Ronchi, MD, PhD
Full Professor
Institute of Psychiatry
University of Bologna
Bologna, Italy

Antonio Drago, MD
Assistant Professor
Institute of Psychiatry
University of Bologna
Bologna, Italy

Matthew R. Ebben, PhD
Assistant Professor of Psychology in Neurology
Center for Sleep Medicine
Weill Medical College of Cornell University
New York, USA

Irshaad Ebrahim, MBChB, MRCPsych
The London Sleep Centre
London, UK

Pingfu Feng, MD, PhD
Assistant Professor of Medicine and Psychiatry
Division of Pulmonary
Critical Care and Sleep Medicine
Department of Medicine and Department of Psychiatry
Director for Research
Center for Sleep Disorders Research
Case Western Reserve University/VA Med, USA

Peter B. Fenwick, DPM, BA, FRCPsych
The London Sleep Centre
London, UK

Lina Fine, MD
Center for Sleep Medicine
Weill Medical College of Cornell University
New York, USA

Jonathan Adrian Ewing Fleming, MB, BAO, BCh, FRCPC, DABPN, DABSM
Associate Professor
Department of Psychiatry UBC
Co-Director, Sleep Disorders Program
University Hospital
Vancouver, Canada
Sleep Program
University Hospital,
Vancouver, BC Canada

Paul A. Fredrickson, MD
Department of Psychiatry and Psychology
Mayo Clinic College of Medicine
Jacksonville, FL USA

Stephany Fulda, Dip.psych
Max-Planck-Institut für Psychiatrie
München, Germany

Lucile Garma, MD, PhD
Service du Pr Willer
Fédération des Pathologies du Sommeil
Hôpital Pitié-Salpêtrière
Paris, France

Roger Godbout, PhD
Professor of Psychiatry
Faculty of Medicine
Université de Montréal

Sleep Laboratory and Clinic
Hôpital Rivière-des-Prairies
Montréal, Québec, Canada

Reut Gruber, PhD
Clinical Psychologist
Assistant Professor
Department of Psychiatry
McGill University
Douglas Research Center
Verdun, Québec, Canada

J. Allan Hobson, PhD
Professor of Psychiatry Emeritus
Harvard Medical School Professor
Department of Psychiatry
Beth Israel Deaconess Medical Center
Laboratory of Neurophysiology
Massachusetts Mental Health Center
Harvard Medical School
Boston, MA USA

Andrea Iaboni, DPhil, MD
Centre for Sleep and Chronobiology
Toronto, ON Canada

Anna Ivanenko, MD, PhD
Assistant Professor
Clinical Psychiatry and Behavioral Science
Feinberg School of Medicine
Northwestern University
Division of Child and Adolescent Psychiatry
Children's Memorial Hospital
Chicago, IL USA

Mayumi Kimura, PhD
Neurogenetics of Sleep
Max Planck Institute of Psychiatry
Munich, Germany

Milton Kramer, MD
Clinical Professor of Psychiatry
University of Illinois at Chicago
Chicago, IL USA

Christoph J. Lauer, PhD
Professor of Psychology
Zentrum für psychische Gesundheit
Klinikum Ingolstadt
Ingolstadt, Germany

Remy Luthringer, PhD, CEO
Forenap Pharma and Forenap FRP
Rouffach, France

Luis Fernando Martínez, BA
Department of Psychiatry
University of California San Diego
La Jolla, CA USA

Sara Matteson-Rusby, PsyD, CBSM
Sleep and Neurophysiology Research Laboratory
Department of Psychiatry
University of Rochester
School of Medicine and Dentistry
Rochester, NY USA

Robert W. McCarley, MD
Head of the Harvard Department of Psychiatry,
and Head of the Laboratory of Neuroscience,
VA Boston Healthcare System
Brockton, MA USA

Charles J. Meliska, PhD
Project Scientist
Department of Psychiatry
University of California San Diego
La Jolla, CA USA

Harvey Moldofsky, MD, Dip.Psych, FRCPC
Centre for Sleep and Chronobiology
Toronto, ON Canada

Charles M. Morin, PhD
École de psychologie
Pavillon Félix-Antoine-Savard
Université Laval
Québec, Canada

Sricharan Moturi, MD, MPH
Division of Child and Adolescent Psychiatry
Children's Memorial Hospital
Chicago, IL USA

Marie-Christine Ouellet, PhD
Recherche en traumatologie et médecine d'urgence
Hôpital de l'Enfant-Jésus du CHA
Pavillon Notre-Dame, Québec, Canada

James F. Pagel, MS, MD
Associate Clinical Professor
University of Colorado School of Medicine
Director Rocky Mountain
Pueblo, CO USA

S. R. Pandi-Perumal, MSc
President and Chief Executive Officer
Somnogen Inc.
New York, USA

Barbara L. Parry, MD
Professor of Psychiatry
University of California San Diego
La Jolla, CA USA

Timo Partonen, MD, PhD
Docent of Psychiatry (University of Helsinki)
Academy Research Fellow (Academy of Finland)
National Public Health Institute
Department of Mental Health and Alcohol Research
Finland

Wilfred R. Pigeon, PhD, CBSM
Assistant Professor of Psychiatry
University of Rochester Medical Center
Sleep and Neurophysiology Research Laboratory
Rochester, NY USA

Thomas Pollmächer, MD
Professor of Psychiatry
Zentrum für psychische Gesundheit
Klinikum Ingolstadt
Germany

Nathalie Pross, PhD
Clinical Psychologist
Forenap Pharma
Rouffach, France

Elliott Richelson, MD
Neuropsychopharmacology Laboratory
Mayo Clinic College of Medicine
Jacksonville, FL USA

Naomi L. Rogers, PhD
Chronobiology and Sleep Group
Brain and Mind Research Institute
Camperdown, NSW Australia

Stefan Rupprecht-Mrozek, MD
Department of Psychiatry
Memory Clinic
Vivantes Hospital Berlin-Spandau
Berlin, Germany

Philip Saleh, BSc
Toronto Western Hospital
Department of Psychiatry
Toronto, ON Canada

Andreas Schuld, MD
Associate Professor of Psychiatry
Zentrum für psychische Gesundheit
Klinikum Ingolstadt, Germany

Alessandro Serretti, MD, PhD
Associate Professor
Institute of Psychiatry
University of Bologna
Bologna, Italy

Colin M. Shapiro, MBBCh, PhD, MRC Psych, FRCP(C)
Toronto Western Hospital
Psychiatry Department
Toronto, ON Canada

Christopher Michael Sinton, PhD
Department of Internal Medicine
University of Texas Southwestern Medical Center
Dallas, TX USA

Marcel G. Smits, MD, PhD
Department of Sleep-Wake Disorders
and Chronobiology
Hospital Gelderse Vallei
The Netherlands

D. Warren Spence, MA
Sleep and Alertness Clinic
University Health Network
Toronto, ON Canada

Jürgen Staedt, PhD
Head of the Department of Psychiatry
Memory Clinic
Vivantes Hospital Berlin-Spandau
Berlin, Germany

Corinne Staner, MD, CDO
Forenap Pharma
Rouffach, France

Luc Staner, MD,
Head of the Clinical Research Sleep Unit
Forenap FRP and Centre Hospitalier
Rouffach, France

Axel Steiger, MD
Research Group Leader
Endocrinology of Sleep
Senior Psychiatrist
Department of Psychiatry

Max Planck Institute of Psychiatry
Munich, Germany

Deborah Suchecki, PhD
Universidade Federal de São Paulo (UNIFESP)
Departamento de Psicobiologia
São Paulo, Brazil

Michael J. Thorpy, MD
Director
Sleep–Wake Disorders Center
Montefiore Medical Center and
Professor
The Saul R. Korey Department of Neurology
Division of Sleep Medicine and Chronobiology
Albert Einstein College of Medicine
Bronx, NY USA

Inna Voloh, MD, RPsgT
Toronto Western Hospital
Psychiatry Department
Toronto, ON Canada

Bradley G. Whitwell
Chronobiology and Sleep Group
Brain and Mind Research Institute
University of Sydney
Sydney, NSW Australia

Robert A. Zucker, PhD
Professor of Psychology in Psychiatry
and Psychology
Director
Substance Abuse Section
Department of Psychiatry
Director
University of Michigan
Addiction Research Center
Ann Arbor, MI USA

Foreword

Sleep as a model for mental illness

Sleep is a normal state that contains within it another normal state, dreaming. Dreaming shares with so-called "mental" illness the formal properties of psychosis (hallucinations and delusions) and is, by definition, a delirium (because it manifests visual hallucinations, disorientation, memory loss, and confabulation). So sleep is at the very least a model for mental illness. But sleep is certainly more than a model because it makes us think about what mental illness may really be. In so doing, it makes some of us realize that the term "mental illness" is really a misnomer. If we were more critical and more philosophical, we would substitute a definition like "diseases of the mind, the brain basis of which is not yet known."

Practically all of the so-called mental illnesses discussed in this book fit this cumbersome definition. They are diseases of the mind, the brain basis of which is not yet known. But dreaming, that normal model of mental illness, has a brain basis that is becoming increasingly well known. And as its brain basis is better and better detailed, its distinctive mental manifestations are increasingly ascribable to an equally distinctive brain physiology. Thus we might suggest, not altogether facetiously, that dreaming is a brain–mind state whose psychological features are a direct expression of altered brain physiology. In other words, dreaming is a state of mind, the brain basis of which is now, in part, known.

If this is true (and I will publicly debate with anyone who says it is not true), then there is no such thing as mental illness without an underlying brain illness. That being the case, such a term as mental illness is a misnomer. We had better refer to diseases (or if you prefer, disorders) of the mind whose brain basis is not yet known and turn our attention to the scientific investigation of the brain in those conditions.

One way to begin such an enterprise is to study sleep and mental illness. This is just what is done in this book. Since we know a great deal about the brain basis of sleep, we may be in a position to infer the brain basis of mental illness from observed changes in sleep. Let us look at several examples.

It is already clear that the aminergic neuromodulators mediate waking and, in order to go to sleep – and especially to dream – we need to be able to inhibit them powerfully. This is true of serotonin, norepinephrine, and histamine. The release of these neuromodulators throughout the brain decreases at sleep onset and is completely shut off in rapid eye movement (REM) sleep. That may be why dreaming, the psychological (or mental) concomitant of REM sleep, so faithfully simulates organic delirium. Organic delirium, after all, is commonly associated with toxic conditions that interfere with aminergic neuromodulation. I am referring to conditions such as delirium tremens, amphetamine psychosis, and other drug-induced states.

Major affective disorders similarly show aminergic abnormalities akin to REM sleep. In depression, we find reduced REM sleep latency and increased REM P1 intensity and duration. Most theories of depression postulate diminished aminergic synaptic efficacy and many drugs that are used to treat depression enhance aminergic synaptic efficacy. At the same time, and in keeping with the sleep as mental illness model, cholinergic mechanisms are enhanced, in both depressive and REM sleep. So why is the depressive affect seen so seldom in dreaming? Possibly because REM sleep only lasts minutes whereas depression lasts for weeks, months, and even years. The downstream effects of the similar neuromodulatory profiles may be quite different.

What about schizophrenia? It is phenomenologically even more different from dreaming than major affective disorder. The hallucinations are usually auditory and less commonly visual; the delusions are commonly paranoid, a feature that is very uncommon in dreaming. The flat effect that is so common in schizophrenia is never seen in dreaming. And the pathophysiology has little in common with dreaming. Most theories of schizophrenia focus on dopamine, an aminergic modulator that changes little in sleep. So, by the time we get to schizophrenia (usually at the top of everyone's list), we seem far away from dreaming.

But, wait. There is still the fact that both conditions represent mental aberrations. So we should not close the door on our analogy too quickly and we certainly should not slam it shut. Two caveats come to mind: (1) the role of dopamine in sleep has been less well studied than the roles of serotonin, norepinephrine, and histamine; and (2) the mechanism of action of atypical antipsychotics (such as clozapine) may be related to enhancing effects on the aminergic neuromodulators which are clearly sleep–wake efficacious.

The point of this foreword is to alert the reader to a strategic vantage point above the level of correlation appropriately taken by most of the chapters in this book. I am not saying that dreaming is a mental illness nor that mental illness does not exist. Instead, I am asserting that the proper scientific study of sleep considers it to be analogous to what we call mental illness, and those in sleep and dream science must strive to learn whatever we can about the brain's contribution to mental illness.

I am not arguing, either, for an eliminative materialism. That is to say, I recognize the contributions of problematical environmental surroundings to brain–mind health. And I certainly recognize the emotional salience of dreams, a salience that wise psychotherapists help their clients to appreciate. But I do seriously question what I consider to be the exaggerated emphasis on the psychogenic causation of dreaming posited by psychoanalysis. This is not the place to take up my cudgel again against Freudian theory, but its fate at the hands of neurobiology may be a warning of what is to come as we further explore the brain basis of so-called mental illness.

A major problem confronting us in our scientific quest is the absence of good animal models for the functional psychoses. Because all mammals have REM, our task is made considerably easier when we study the brain basis of dreaming. But we have no good animal models for major mental illness. What are we to do? One answer is to use the modern techniques for the study of the human brain for all that they are worth, and then some. Quantitative electroencephalography (EEG) and functional magnetic resonance imaging (fMRI) have already proven quite useful in discerning the brain underpinnings of such subtle mental states as lucid dreaming, which is distinctively different from both waking and dreaming (with both of which it shares features) so help may be on the way.

My introduction of the hybrid term brain–mind is meant to denote a step on the long road to a monism that never loses sight of the brain–mind nexus. In my crystal ball, brain is mind and mind is brain. They are two aspects of the same thing. Sleep, dreams, and what we now call mental illness are all functional states of the brain.

J. Allan Hobson
Professor of Psychiatry
Harvard Medical School

Preface

The idea for the first edition of this volume entitled *Sleep and Mental Illness* occurred to us when we published our earlier volume entitled *Sleep and Psychosomatic Medicine*. Mental disturbance is extremely common among those who suffer from sleep disorders. Despite the fact that a number of quality publications (including our own) exist on this increasingly popular research and clinical topic, each has certain gaps in coverage. We thus felt a need to address this deficiency by compiling one of the most comprehensive volumes ever published on sleep and mental illness. It has been an honor and privilege to edit this volume and to ensure that the necessary topics have been covered appropriately.

This volume is organized into three sections encompassing core topics in both sleep and mental illness as follows.

Section 1 provides up-to-date background information on the basic science of this area of investigation. The topics included in this section are the neuropharmacology of mental illness, the effects of antidepressants on gene expression, and the neurochemistry of sleep. Other topics include the neuropharmacology of depression and animal models of sleep and stress. Also covered are chapters dealing with the relation between depression and insomnia and associated changes on levels of orexin in the brain.

Section 2 covers the neuroendocrinological changes that are seen in pathophysiological states. These include the effects of disturbed sleep and depression on hormone secretion, sleep–endocrine relationships in depressed women across the reproductive cycle, and the relationship between melatonin and mental illness.

Finally, in **Section 3**, a series of clinical science topics relating to sleep and mental illness is presented. The range of clinical topics covered here represents the largest section of this volume. Starting with the International Classification of Sleep Disorders, this section addresses topics such as insomnia and the associated risk for developing psychiatric illness in the future, antidepressant-induced alterations in sleep EEG, long-term effects of antidepressants on sleep, sleep during antipsychotic treatment, sleep and substance use and abuse, cognitive effects of psychoactive medications, and sleep-related memory consolidation in mental illness. Other topics include fatigue and sleepiness in affective illness, sleep in attention-deficit/hyperactivity disorders, sleep in seasonal affective disorder, and sleep in traumatic brain injury. This section also covers sleep and borderline personality disorders, sleep and eating disorders, sleep in late-life depression, and forensic issues of sleep in psychiatric patients.

This is an exciting time for specialists in both sleep and psychiatry. We have many reasons to be optimistic that significant progress is being made in the understanding, prevention, and management of sleep disorders. Our growing understanding of the pathogenesis and pathophysiology of mental illness, coupled with the rapidly expanding field of sleep medicine, has also seen the growth of an increasing number of successful management strategies. It is our hope that this volume will have a positive effect on the care of patients, especially those who present with comorbid conditions in current clinical practice.

The advent of sleep medicine has brought with it new perspectives on mental illness, and in particular a growing awareness that problems with sleep can both exacerbate and portend the development of mental disturbance in the future. Additionally, the impairment of the role of dreaming in affect regulation may be central to understanding the mood changes in depression. What this has meant is that psychiatrists are now discarding some long-cherished prescribing practices such as an increasing trend toward prescribing sleeping aids in addition to antidepressants.

Multidisciplinary care and a team approach are the best foundations for the effective practice of sleep medicine. It seems that the best approach to comorbid sleep disorders is to involve a variety of experts in consultation as needed. This team approach should include consultations with psychiatrists, psychologists, behavioral sleep medicine professionals, and other sleep specialists. The management of comorbid insomnia symptoms in psychiatric patients can benefit greatly from the specialized knowledge of sleep professionals. It is the hope that advocacy of interdisciplinary care will promote excellence in the treatment of sleep disorders in mentally ill patients.

This volume is intended to be a resource for practitioners responsible for the care of sleep patients with mental illness and vice versa. That being said, this volume is appropriate for psychiatrists, psychologists, sleep specialists, and generalists alike. It can be useful for medical graduate students of biomedical and sleep medicine subspecialties. It will be also be of wide interest to others who want to get an overall grasp of sleep pharmacology and therapeutics and those physicians who evaluate and treat sleep disorders. In addition, the volume will be useful to clinicians of various disciplines who want to gain an overview of sleep psychiatry. This volume may serve as a reference work that will be of value to scientists and students alike. Since sleep disorders are almost

ubiquitous in clinical practice, we hope that you will find this material relevant and useful.

This volume includes contributions from a wide range of authors, many of whom are recognized internationally as authorities in their field. Overall, the reader may feel confident that the information presented is based on the old as well as most recent literature. Some of the information presented in this volume on older sedative hypnotics will be familiar to informed readers and will demonstrate to them how their previously acquired knowledge can be applied to the treatment of sleep disorders. Information about specific drugs may also be repeated in various chapters throughout this volume by very many authors. Inasmuch as repetition is the mother of learning, it is hoped that this redundancy will be construed as a benefit. The editors and authors would appreciate feedback on the contents of the volume with particular regard to any omissions or inaccuracies, which will be rectified in later editions. We also welcome your ideas, comments, and constructive criticisms, which are always appreciated.

S. R. Pandi-Perumal, New York, USA
Milton Kramer, Chicago, USA

Acknowledgments

The editors owe endless gratitude to, and wish to express their sincere appreciation to all of our distinguished contributors for their scholarly and diligent contributions that form the basis of this volume. Producing a volume such as this is a team effort and we acknowledge with gratitude the work of the editorial department of Cambridge University Press, England. We are especially indebted to Mr. Nicholas Dunton, commissioning editor of neurology, who was an enthusiastic and instrumental supporter from start to finish. Our profound gratitude is offered also to Ms. Katie James, editor, whose equally dedicated efforts promoted a smooth completion of this important project. Their commitment to excellence was a strong guiding force throughout the development of this volume. We were fortunate to experience warm, professional, and highly enthusiastic support from the wonderfully talented people at Cambridge University Press who made this project a pleasurable one.

There are many to thank for a book that has been based on contributions from so many different disciplines. To have found over 70 authors with a desire to contribute to the first edition could not have occurred without a tremendous concentration of effort and teamwork. Our publishing authors gracefully fulfilled our many requests, met our deadlines, and delivered their manuscripts accordingly, for which we are deeply grateful. We sincerely thank them for working with us through this long process. A number of individuals made outstanding contributions. A very special appreciation is also owed to several reviewers who made numerous helpful suggestions. Their candid comments and insights were invaluable.

Finally, we express our gratitude to our families for their patience and support. Their constant encouragement, understanding, and patience while the book was being developed are immeasurably appreciated.

S. R. Pandi-Perumal, New York, USA
Milton Kramer, Chicago, USA

1

Neuropharmacology of mental illness

Paul A. Fredrickson and Elliott Richelson

The interplay of mental illness and sleep is multifaceted. Most psychiatric disorders produce sleep complaints. Behavioral health clinicians routinely inquire about a patient's sleep during diagnostic assessment and to monitor treatment response. Mental illness treatment that does not address sleep problems may lead to relapse. Persistence of insomnia is a negative prognostic sign, particularly for depression.

Insomnia is the most common sleep complaint. Chronic insomnia is prevalent in about 10% of the United States' population. Only about one-fifth of these sufferers receive prescription hypnotics. Prescribing practices have changed in recent decades. From 1979 to 1999, survey data showed a decline in traditional hypnotics by 50%. Over that same span, the use of antidepressant drugs to treat insomnia increased more than two-fold [1].

Many people self-medicate for sleep problems. Over-the-counter remedies are primarily antihistaminic agents. Alcohol is also a common remedy, but, for reasons of limited efficacy and abuse potential, its use should be discouraged. Cognitive behavioral therapies, which are outside the scope of this chapter, are an effective alternative for many with chronic insomnia.

The focus of this chapter will be on the prescription drugs used to treat psychiatric disorders that either have beneficial or adverse effects on sleep. Some of these drugs are commonly prescribed off-label for insomnia. Others produce insomnia, excessive daytime sleepiness, or parasomnias.

Antidepressant therapies

Current treatments for depression are largely based on concepts arising from monoamine oxidase inhibitor (MAOI) and tricyclic antidepressant (TCA) drugs discovered decades ago. These drugs affect monoamines (serotonin, norepinephrine [NE], dopamine [DA]), particularly serotonin and norepinephrine reuptake. Monoamine transporter reuptake blockade is also the basis for newer, selective reuptake inhibitors that selectively either block the serotonin (e.g., serotonin specific reuptake inhibitors, or SSRIs, such as fluoxetine) or norepinephrine transporters (e.g., reboxetine). The major advantage of these drugs is they produce fewer side effects than older-generation antidepressants, largely by virtue of their weak or absent effects on many receptors for neurotransmitters. However, it is debatable whether the newer drugs are as effective as the older ones. Some new-generation antidepressants block both serotonin and NE transporters (venlafaxine, duloxetine). Dual (serotonin/NE) or triple (5-HT, NE, DA) transporter inhibitors may be more efficacious than single reuptake inhibitors, without the side effects of older-generation drugs [2, 3].

Non-therapeutic side effects of antidepressant medications arise when they affect additional neurotransmitter systems. For example, muscarinic receptor blockade causes dry mouth; histamine H_1 receptor blockade produces sedation; and α_1-adrenergic receptor blockade results in hypotension. Such adverse effects are more common with TCAs and MAOIs than newer, more selective agents [4–6].

Interestingly, many of the same systems targeted by psychiatric drugs are integral to control of sleep and wakefulness. Acetylcholine (ACh) projections from the basal forebrain; histamine from the tuberomammillary nucleus (TMN); norepinephrine from the locus coeruleus; dopamine from the substantia nigra/ventral tegmental area; and serotonin from the raphe nuclei promote wakefulness. Thus, it is not surprising that sleep disorders and affective syndromes coexist, or that treatment of depression may affect sleep. Blockade of these neurotransmitter effects may produce unwanted side effects such as sedation, but also have potential to treat insomnia complaints [7].

So-called "vegetative symptoms" of depression (sleep, appetite, libido) imply hypothalamic dysfunction. Although research on hypothalamic peptides and depression has not yet reached consensus, this is an intriguing area of study, particularly for the intersection of sleep and mental illness. Although a comprehensive review is beyond the scope of this chapter, one peptide of special interest is hypocretin (also known as orexin). Hypocretin is present in two forms: hypocretin 1 and 2 are 33 and 28 amino acid peptides respectively. Hypocretins are produced in the lateral hypothalamus, with projections to multiple brain areas. Loss of hypocretin neurons is found in narcolepsy. Its alerting effects are important in order to maintain a stable state of wakefulness and to prevent inadvertent switching between sleep and wake brain systems. Blockade of hypocretin effects has recently been explored as a treatment for insomnia. However, low activity of hypocretin neurons during rest means that hypocretin antagonists are likely to be most sedating during waking, active hours. This may limit utility for management of insomnia [8].

Antidepressant drugs to treat sleep disorders

Trazodone

The majority of depressed patients report difficulty initiating or maintaining sleep. Antidepressant drugs may help this symptom, make it worse, or have no effect. Stimulating antidepressants, such as bupropion and SSRIs, may produce insomnia or worsen a prior complaint. Trazodone is pharmacologically distinct from the SSRIs (see Figure 1.1). It is frequently prescribed to alleviate the sleep-disrupting effects of stimulating antidepressants. Effects on sleep are consistent with the drug's antagonism at α_1 and 5-HT$_2$ receptors (see Table 1.1). Several studies report subject improvement in sleep, and one double-blind crossover study showed increased sleep time, sleep efficiency, and slow-wave sleep in depressed insomnia patients treated with SSRIs [9].

A more controversial use for trazodone is as a hypnotic in patients without a diagnosis of depression.

Trazodone is now widely prescribed off-label for insomnia. Although risk vs. benefit has not been systematically assessed in general insomnia populations, its widespread use seems to derive in part from concerns regarding the safety and appropriateness of hypnotic drugs for long-term use.

Many patients recovering from alcohol or other addictions are prescribed trazodone because it is without abuse potential. Patients suffering from alcohol dependence often complain of insomnia during the initial weeks and months of abstinence. Concern about abuse potential of hypnotics may limit therapeutic intervention, thus running the risk of self-medication with alcohol. Not only do recovering alcoholic subjects report sleep initiation and maintenance problems, they also show objective evidence of lighter sleep. Polysomnographic studies show diminished slow-wave sleep. Because sleep architecture may not normalize for a year or more, long-term management of sleep problems is important. Trazodone seems promising in this population in that it promotes slow-wave sleep and improved sleep continuity, although its efficacy for this indication has not been rigorously studied [10].

Mirtazapine

Mirtazapine, a sedating antidepressant, is an antagonist (in order of its potency) of histamine H$_1$, 5-HT$_{2A}$, α_{2A}, and 5-HT$_3$ receptors. A recent report suggested mirtazapine may be effective for treatment of sleep apnea. However, a randomized placebo-controlled trial failed to confirm a beneficial effect on apnea [11]. Furthermore, because weight gain is common with mirtazapine, the drug should be prescribed with caution in this patient group. Similarly, off-label treatment of insomnia with mirtazapine should be approached with caution for this same reason.

Tricyclic antidepressants

The prototype drug in this class is amitriptyline. While no longer commonly prescribed as a first-line therapy for depression, many practitioners make use of amitriptyline for management of insomnia in preference to conventional hypnotic drugs. While safe from the standpoint of abuse potential, other adverse effects may limit tolerability and safety. Amitriptyline can produce unwanted daytime sedation, which may be a hazard when operating a motor vehicle. The majority of amitriptyline's sedative effects are due to its blockade of the histamine H$_1$ receptor.

Table 1.1 Receptor binding affinities of some psychotherapeutic drugs used to treat insomnia

Drug	Histamine H_1	Serotonin 5-HT_{2A}	Muscarinic acetylcholine	α_1-Adrenergic
Amitriptyline	91	3.4	5.6	3.7
Diphenhydramine	6.3	0.38	1.3	0.08
Doxepin	420	4.0	1.2	4.2
Mirtazapine	700	6.1	0.15	0.2
Quetiapine	5.2	3.2	0.1	12.3
Trazodone	0.29	13	0.00031	2.8

Notes: Affinity is $(1/K_d) \times 10^{-7}$, where K_d is the equilibrium dissociation constant in molarity. The higher the number, the more potent the binding. Data for antidepressants are from Richelson, Cusack, Richelson [4, 5, 21]; data for quetiapine are from Richelson [22], and data for diphenhydramine are from Mansbach [23].

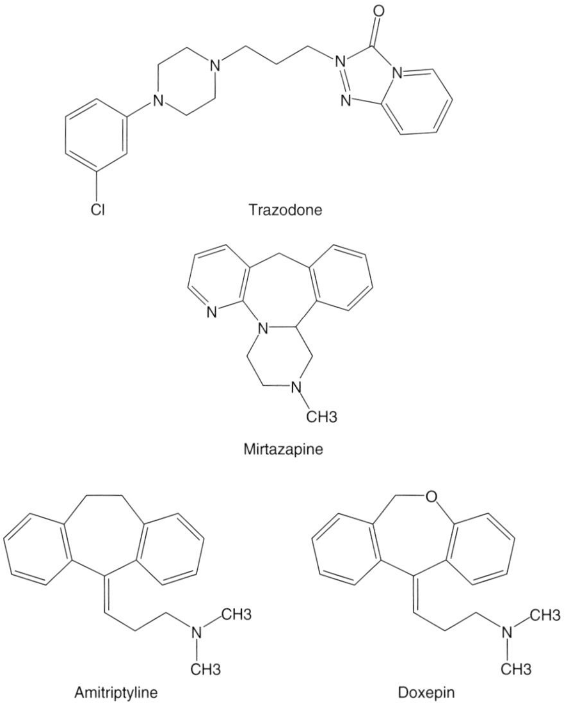

Figure 1.1 Structures of antidepressants used off-label as hypnotic drugs.

Doxepin is also sometimes prescribed for its sedating properties. It, too, is a potent H_1 receptor blocking drug. Due to its half-life of approximately 17 hours, daytime sedation may be a serious side effect. Dosing schedules for doxepin and the tricyclics as hypnotics have not been systematically reported in the literature. However, recent trials of very low dose doxepin (1 to 6 mg) show promise as a hypnotic [12]. Doxepin may be particularly effective for sleep-maintenance insomnia, a common problem in the elderly. Because brain histamine levels peak late in the night and in the morning hours, antihistaminic effects are apt to be most effective at those hours. Low doses in recent studies have not caused daytime sedation or weight gain.

Sleep disruption from antidepressant drugs

Insomnia: Many TCAs, MAOIs, most SSRIs, and bupropion can produce this complaint [13]. Patients with major depression have a high rate of insomnia. Antidepressant treatments, such as the SSRIs or bupropion, may initially worsen sleep, resulting in reduced compliance. Because sleep complaints are so commonly associated with depression, the impact of the drug on sleep may not be immediately recognized. However, if sleep complaints persist, or worsen, as other depressive symptoms improve, an adverse effect of the drug therapy may be inferred. Many clinicians choose trazodone as an adjunct, particularly with SSRIs and bupropion therapy.

Daytime sedation: This is an under-appreciated adverse effect in the opinion of the authors. Excessive daytime sleepiness, from any cause, is a source of motor vehicle accidents and may impair cognitive function in a variety of settings. Patients may not complain of this symptom, or may incorrectly attribute it to other causes such as normal aging. The clinician should remember that hypersomnia is a cardinal symptom of sleep apnea in snorers. Therefore, careful inquiry as to presence and course of this symptom is important. Any patient with intrusive daytime sleepiness merits close attention until the source is identified and resolved. The physician should discuss potential hazards of operating a motor vehicle while taking sedating medication.

Parasomnias: This is a category of "things that go bump in the night." Common examples are sleep walking and night terrors, which are more frequently encountered in children than adults. An important parasomnia in older adults is REM behavior disorder (RBD). This fascinating condition occurs as a result of the loss of normal skeletal muscle atonia during rapid eye movement (REM) sleep. As a result, patients may display complex movements during REM sleep that match dream imagery. One of the author's (PAF) elderly patients, dreaming she was a young girl swinging from tree branches, vaulted from bed and awoke on the floor. Injuries to the sleeper or bed partner make this a serious target of therapy. REM behavior disorder is most common in elderly males, and is often associated with Lewy body dementia, multiple system atrophy, Parkinson's, and other synucleinopathies. However, RBD may also be triggered by antidepressant therapy, particularly SSRIs [14]. A careful history will help determine whether antidepressant therapy needs to be modified. Some patients will benefit from consultation with a sleep medicine physician, and a full sleep study may be indicated. If the antidepressant regimen cannot easily be modified, a trial of clonazepam or melatonin may provide sufficient control of the parasomnia.

Circadian rhythms

Circadian rhythm disturbance has been inferred in depression from the clinical symptom of diurnal variation in mood. Many patients describe their lowest point of the day as morning, with some improvement occurring as the day progresses. Antidepressant gene expression abnormalities are a potential target for antidepressant drug therapy, but as yet, little clinical data exist. Agomelatine and other melatonin receptor agonists show antidepressant activity in animal models [15].

Circadian rhythm disorders are also relevant to sleep complaints. Adolescents frequently exhibit a phase delay (preferred bedtime and time of arising is much later than societal norms). The elderly often have phase advance. Their early morning awakening complaints mimic the sleep complaint of major depression, but they also have early bedtimes, consistent with their internal clock phase [16].

The atypical antipsychotics

Although developed for treatment of schizophrenia and other psychoses, new generation (also called atypical) antipsychotics are frequently prescribed as adjuncts for antidepressant therapy and for their anti-anxiety effects. Many clinicians prescribe these drugs for sleep complaints. Quetiapine appears to be a popular choice among this group. It has antagonistic effects at 5-HT_{2A} and histamine H_1 receptors that probably account for many of the benefits on sleep. Quetiapine has been reported as effective in primary insomnia, particularly sleep maintenance complaints [17]. However, definitive studies are lacking. Furthermore, potential adverse effects must be weighed against benefits. This is particularly true in the elderly demented.

Anti-anxiety and hypnotic agents: the GABAergic drugs

Just as antidepressant drug development has focused for decades on a narrow range of therapeutic targets, so, too, hypnotics, since the introduction of flurazepam, have primarily targeted GABA receptors, particularly the $GABA_A$ subtype. As for the 5-HT_3 receptors, $GABA_A$ receptors are pentameric ligand-gated ion channels (a pore is opened in the cell membrane when an agonist binds to the receptor, allowing flow of chloride ions into the cell). They comprise several types of subunits (alpha, beta, gamma) [18].

Prototype $GABA_A$ agonists are the benzodiazepines (BZDs). This class of drug has antianxiety, sedative, anticonvulsant, and muscle-relaxing properties. Although only a few BZDs are approved by the US Food and Drug Administration (FDA) as sedative – hypnotic drugs (temazepam, triazolam, estazolam, quazepam), the differences between "sedative" and "anxiolytic" BZDs has more to do with dosing and marketing than pharmacologic distinctions.

Benzodiazepines bind allosterically (i.e., away from the site where the native ligand GABA binds), and increase the affinity of the receptor for the open state [19]. Most $GABA_A$ receptors in the brain contain alpha 1, alpha 2, or alpha 3 subunits. $GABA_A$

receptors containing alpha 1 subunits are likely responsible for sedative actions of these drugs.

In the search for drugs with a more "pure" sedative effect, and less abuse potential, newer generation $GABA_A$ agonists have been developed (zolpidem, zaleplon, zopiclone, and eszopiclone). These drugs, particularly zolpidem and zaleplon, are specific in their affinity for $GABA_A$ receptors containing the alpha 1 subunit. They may, therefore, be less likely to have abuse potential and produce physical dependence. Indeed, experience in humans suggests they carry a low risk of physical dependence. In non-human primates, however, these drugs are self-administered, and discontinuation can lead to a withdrawal syndrome. Therefore, while they appear to be less likely to cause physical dependence, their suitability in populations susceptible to addiction is not established [20].

Summary

Clinical wisdom tells us psychotropic drugs are useful agents for the management of sleep complaints. We await confirmation from clinical trials for many of the compounds commonly used off-label to manage insomnia. A limited number of drugs are approved by the FDA in the United States for the management of insomnia, and most are GABAergic. New-generation GABAergic agents that are specific for the alpha 1 subunit do not have significant antianxiety effects as seen with the BZDs.

Concern about abuse potential has led many clinicians to question the suitability of BZD (and non-BZD GABAergic) hypnotics for long-term use, particularly in patients with a history of drug or alcohol problems. To some extent, prescribing practices reflect society's attitudes toward sleep problems vs. other complaints. Therefore, clinicians may feel more comfortable prescribing anxiolytic BZDs on a chronic basis for anxiety, but shy away from similar drugs for chronic insomnia complaints. Nevertheless, patients and clinicians require alternative therapies when traditional hypnotics fail, are not tolerated, or simply not preferred.

Psychotropic drugs may also have negative effects on sleep. Insomnia is common with SSRIs and bupropion. Less well appreciated is risk of RBD, thus far mostly reported with SSRIs.

Understanding the nature and source of the sleep complaint is key to successful therapy. Patients with anxiety contributing to difficulty falling asleep will benefit from anxiolytic drugs. Those with sleep maintenance complaints may do better with antidepressant or atypical antipsychotic therapy. Unfortunately, clinical trial data are sparse for effects of most psychotropic drugs on sleep complaints, particularly in patients with primary insomnia.

Further study of non-GABAergic drugs will broaden the therapeutic armamentarium for sleep complaints and help us understand the mechanisms of sleep complaints.

References
1. Roehrs T, Roth T. 'Hypnotic' prescription patterns in a large managed-care population. *Sleep Med.* 2004;5(5):463–6.

2. Berton O, Nestler EJ. New approaches to antidepressant drug discovery: beyond monoamines. *Nat Rev Neurosci.* 2006;7(2):137–51.

3. Liang Y, Shaw AM, Boules M, *et al.* Antidepressant-like pharmacological profile of a novel triple reuptake inhibitor, (1S,2S)-3-(methylamino)-2-(naphthalen-2-yl)-1-phenylpropan-1-ol (PRC200-SS). *J Pharmacol Exp Ther.* 2008;**327**(2): 573–83.

4. Richelson E, Nelson A. Antagonism by antidepressants of neurotransmitter receptors of normal human brain in vitro. *J Pharmacol Exp Ther.* 1984;**230**(1):94–102.

5. Cusack B, Nelson A, Richelson E. Binding of antidepressants to human brain receptors: focus on newer generation compounds. *Psychopharmacology (Berl).* 1994;**114**(4):559–65.

6. Richelson E. Pharmacology of antidepressants. *Mayo Clin Proc.* 2001;**76**(5):511–27.

7. McCarley RW. Neurobiology of REM and NREM sleep. *Sleep Med.* 2007;**8**(4):302–30.

8. Brisbare-Roch C, Dingemanse J, Koberstein R, *et al.* Promotion of sleep by targeting the orexin system in rats, dogs and humans. *Nat Med.* 2007;**13**(2):150–5.

9. Kaynak H, Kaynak D, Gozukirmizi E, Guilleminault C. The effects of trazodone on sleep in patients treated with stimulant antidepressants. *Sleep Med.* 2004;5(1):15–20.

10. Le Bon O, Murphy JR, Staner L, *et al.* Double-blind, placebo-controlled study of the efficacy of trazodone in alcohol post-withdrawal syndrome: polysomnographic and clinical evaluations. *J Clin Psychopharmacol.* 2003;23(4):377–83.

11. Marshall NS, Yee BJ, Desai AV, *et al.* Two randomized placebo-controlled trials to evaluate the efficacy and

tolerability of mirtazapine for the treatment of obstructive sleep apnea. *Sleep.* 2008;**31**(6):824–31.

12. Scharf M, Rogowski R, Hull S, *et al.* Efficacy and safety of doxepin 1 mg, 3 mg, and 6 mg in elderly patients with primary insomnia. *J Clin Psychiatry.* 2008;**69**(10):1557–64.

13. Mayers AG, Baldwin DS. Antidepressants and their effect on sleep. *Hum Psychopharmacol.* 2005;**20**(8):533–59.

14. Winkelman JW, James L. Serotonergic antidepressants are associated with REM sleep without atonia. *Sleep.* 2004;**27**(2):317–21.

15. Ghosh A, Hellewell JS. A review of the efficacy and tolerability of agomelatine in the treatment of major depression. *Expert Opin Investig Drugs.* 2007;**16**(12):1999–2004.

16. Barion A, Zee PC. A clinical approach to circadian rhythm sleep disorders. *Sleep Med.* 2007;**8**(6):566–77.

17. Wiegand MH, Landry F, Bruckner T, *et al.* Quetiapine in primary insomnia: a pilot study. *Psychopharmacology (Berl).* 2008;**196**(2):337–8.

18. Rudolph U, Mohler H. GABA-based therapeutic approaches: GABAA receptor subtype functions. *Curr Opin Pharmacol.* 2006;**6**(1):18–23.

19. Campo-Soria C, Chang Y, Weiss DS. Mechanism of action of benzodiazepines on GABAA receptors. *Br J Pharmacol.* 2006;**148**(7):984–90.

20. Licata SC, Rowlett JK. Abuse and dependence liability of benzodiazepine-type drugs: GABA(A) receptor modulation and beyond. *Pharmacol Biochem Behav.* 2008;**90**(1):74–89.

21. Richelson E. Interactions of antidepressants with neurotransmitter transporters and receptors and their clinical relevance. *J Clin Psychiatry.* 2003;**64**(Suppl 13):5–12.

22. Richelson E, Souder T. Binding of antipsychotic drugs to human brain receptors focus on newer generation compounds. *Life Sci.* 2000;**68**(1):29–39.

23. Mansbach R. In vitro pharmacological profile of doxepin, a sleep-promoting histamine H1 antagonist [abstract]. *Eur Neuropsychopharmacol.* 2008;**18**(S4): S357.

Effects of antidepressants on gene expression

Antonio Drago, Diana De Ronchi, and Alessandro Serretti

Introduction

Depressive disorder is a common disease that affects one out of six people during their lifetime in the United States [1], and 18.4 million people per year in Europe [2]. Core symptoms include psychological suffering (for example depressed mood, altered cognition) and neurovegetative symptoms (for example sleep disturbances, variations in food intake). Besides the psychological suffering and the economic burden [2], depressive disorder enhances the risk of mortality through higher suicide rates, higher risk of type 2 diabetes, and higher incidence of coronaropathy [3]. Moreover, it dramatically impacts the prognoses of hosts of other relevant diseases [4]. Despite this relevance, the impressive impact on the community and the efforts produced by the scientific community so far, the disrupted mechanisms related to depressive phenomenology have not been clarified. Knowledge of depressive pathophysiology is rudimentary compared to other relevant chronic diseases such as diabetes: this imbalance may be related to the etiopathogenesis of depressive disorder itself, which is thought to rely on functional neuronal networks that are poorly characterized so far and, thereby, difficult to investigate [5]. Moreover, the techniques used to investigate the brain suffer from a list of limitations that weaken their quality: post mortem studies rely on the treatment of cerebral tissues that enhances the variability of laboratory settings, and imaging studies detect changes in neuronal activity using indirect markers of activation [6]. Even though these techniques have provided useful insights helping the formulation of the most relevant theories of depression (neuronal circuitry imbalance; downregulation of monoamine tone; neurotrophins and neurogenesis, neuroendocrine and neuroimmune interactions), all

these models appear to be inadequate when facing the depressive phenotypes [5]. Finally, the incomplete knowledge of depressive disorder limits the characterization of its etiology to a description of risk factors [4, 7] impacted by the genetic background and reactivity by means that are poorly understood and inconsistently demonstrated [8], and the studies' designs rely on the definition of the disorder that is based on phenomenology and is constantly changing through years: there is a possibility that what is defined as depressive disorder in studies actually encompasses different pathophysiological processes still poorly understood. Consistently, the efficacy of antidepressant drug treatments, which are designed and based on the monaminergic theory of depression, is limited: up to 30% of depressed patients treated with antidepressant drugs do not reach remission [9]. More efforts are to be devoted in order to further investigate the field. One interesting and promising point of observation that could reveal some aspects of depressive disruptions and of the pharmacodynamics of antidepressant effects is the investigation of DNA reactivity to antidepressant treatment. While it is self-evident that this approach could give some interesting breakthroughs in pharmacodynamics, the boundary between antidepressant drug-triggered DNA reactivity and depressive phenotypes may be less obvious. Nevertheless, it must be underlined that antidepressants work in the majority of cases, and that even though their efficacy can vary greatly in one subject there are marginal differences between the different classes of antidepressants in large population samples. A common mechanism of action is to be hypothesized and it may – *ex adiuvantibus* – be related to the pathophysiology of depressive disorders. This accepted, the investigation of the DNA adaptations after antidepressant challenge may provide some more details to the still unresolved mosaic of evidence that focuses on the depressive phenotype. In the present chapter the most up-to-date knowledge on the impact of antidepressant treatments on transcription and translation events will be described.

The main role of human DNA is to store information and to perpetuate it through time. To achieve this result, DNA encodes sufficient information to form cells, tissues, and an organism, guaranteeing the molecular means for adaptation, viability, and reactivity of all of them. In order to adapt to the stimuli coming from the outside, DNA codes for, and is reactive to, a wide array of molecular feedback looped mechanisms, second messengers cascades, and complicated membrane–cytosol–nuclei crosstalking, which starts at the surfaces of cells and ends at the cores of the nuclei, and the other way round. Tissues are the tight orchestration of single cells influencing each other's DNA reactivity by the means of mechanisms that are still not completely known. Antidepressants impact DNA reactivity by acting as external stimuli. In the following discussion the most relevant theories related to the putative disruptions underlying depressive disorders will be commented on, along with antidepressant triggered modifications of the DNA expression profile.

Monoamines

The monoamine hypothesis of depression suggests that depressive disorder is caused by imbalanced monoaminergic tone in the brain. This hypothesis originates from early clinical observations [10, 11]. The first hints on which this theory was based came from two structurally unrelated drugs designed for other than psychiatric diseases that about 40 years ago turned out to have potent antidepressant effect in humans, and were later shown to enhance central serotonin and noradrenalin transmission. During the same period it was found that reserpine, which acts by depleting monoamine stores, determines a reduction in both blood pressure and depressive symptoms. Starting from this evidence, serotonin and noradrenalin were first identified as relevant putative candidates for the pathophysiological imbalances that underline depressive disorder. More recent antidepressant agents that show a more favorable therapeutic index still act on the reuptake of monoamines and are named upon this action: SSRIs

(selective serotonin reuptake inhibitors) and SNRIs (serotonin and noradrenalin reuptake inhibitors) are examples of drugs that have been designed on the basis of the monoaminergic theory of depressive disorder, and whose aim is to obtain an acute increase in monoaminergic tone in the synaptic cleft by inhibiting the reuptake of monoamines. These drugs are nowadays the first-line treatment for depressive disorder. Even though the monoamine-based agents are potent antidepressants [9], and alterations in central monoamine function might contribute marginally to genetic vulnerability to depressive disorder [12], it is not possible to define the cause of depressive disorder as simply being an imbalance in monoaminergic tone. In fact, the monoamine oxidase inhibitors and SSRIs produce immediate increases in monoamine transmission, which come before the effect on mood. Conversely, experimental depletion of monoamines can trigger a mild reduction in mood in unmedicated depressed patients, but does not alter mood in healthy controls [13]. With regard to the expression of genes triggered by antidepressant drugs designed on the monoaminergic theory, several lines of evidence report that antidepressants diminish the concentration of the noradrenalin or serotonin transporters on the surface of cells, but, interestingly, this event is not associated with altered mRNA expression of the genes that code for the serotonin transporter and for other serotonin receptors that have been put forward as possible mediators of the antidepressant effect (5-HT1A, 5-HT1B, 5-HT1C, and 5-HT2) [14–19]. The diminished concentration of serotonin transporter on the surface of cells is then to be associated with another event within the cell: this may be its inclusion into cytoplasmatic vesicles. The expression rate of the mRNA that codes for the VMAT2, an integral membrane protein that acts to transport monoamines – particularly neurotransmitters such as dopamine, norepinephrine, serotonin, and histamine – from cellular cytosol into synaptic vesicles, was reported to be diminished after short- and long-term treatment with fluoxetine [20], even though lack of effect on VMAT2 was detected after paroxetine or reserpine treatment [21]. The evidence so far is quite striking: the antidepressant treatment targeted on the serotonin system does not seem to play a major role in the genetic regulation of many of the most relevant mediators of serotonergic function. It must be said that at least one exception exists: tryptophan hydroxylase (TPH), which is the rate-limiting enzyme for the synthesis of serotonin. The expression level of the brain isoform of this enzyme was found to be affected by treatment with antidepressants [20, 22, 23]. Moreover, even though ineffective for these targets, antidepressants were found to affect the expression rates of the serotonin transporter, of serotonin receptor 2A and 1A mRNA in stressed animals and not in controls [23–26]: mRNA expression was enhanced in stressed animals before they were treated with antidepressants, but this difference was abolished after the treatment. This is a point of relevance: it could be derived that antidepressants are more effective, or at least act differently, on subjects prone to suffer anxiety or depressive episodes. Antidepressants could exert their activity within the brain in a different and specific way that is dependent on the background, both biological and psychological, of the subject. Beside this, there is evidence for a genetic regulation that is dependent on the serotonin system and that is mirrored by the expression rates of genes that do not code for strict serotonergic related products: monoaminergic receptors are not only expressed in cells that produce the mediator they are able to recognize, but they can be coded and exposed on the surface of cells that do not produce the corresponding ligand. In that case, the receptors are called heteroreceptors and their activity accounts for the complex net of interactions that bound the diverse monaminergic systems [27]. This may be related to the presence of altered mRNA expression of dopaminergic receptors after treatment with serotonergic drugs [28–31]. Finally, even though the expression level of some serotonergic receptors is not affected by the presence of antidepressants, the post-transcriptional events are actually impacted. In particular, the editing of the serotonin receptor 2C, which can be directed toward more or less functional isoforms of the receptor, is tuned toward the reduced function pole [32]. An impact on the editing of the AMPA/kainate receptors was found as well [33]. The evidence coming from these findings is still difficult to resolve into a consequential picture: the mutual relationships between the different neuronal nets and the relevance of specific sites of action of antidepressant within the central nervous system (CNS) tremendously increase the complexity of the field. Of note, the lack of association between antidepressants and the expression levels of serotonin-related receptor and transporter was detected when neurons were

investigated, while opposite findings were revealed in peripheral leukocytes, which showed lower baseline expression of the serotonin transporter gene. This difference was no more evident after treatment with antidepressants [34]. This opens the debate on how peripheral cells with specific differentiation may represent the biological reactions that pertain to the CNS. Even though some relevant variations of genes that belong to the serotonin system or to systems that are related to it have been shown to have their genetic expressive profile affected by antidepressant treatment, the monoaminergic theory of depression is probably not sufficient to cover the molecular disruptions that affect depressed individuals. There is some evidence that the most probable event that is related to the antidepressant efficacy of antidepressant treatments is based on neuroplastic changes that follow the acute effect of monoaminergic based antidepressants: this is more consistent with the time lag between therapy initiation and mood elevation that characterizes these drugs. Moreover, it is reasonable that the variation in the neuroplasticity of neurons, which is thought to be induced by antidepressants, takes some time to develop to an extent sufficient for a change in mood. Interestingly, the way antidepressants may achieve this goal is thought to be related to an impact on the transcriptional and translational activities within the CNS. Consistent with this, chronic treatment with antidepressants has been shown to upregulate the transcription factor CREB (cyclic-AMP-response element-binding protein), which is downstream of several serotonin and other stimulatory G-protein-coupled receptors, in the hippocampus, which is thought to be related to some aspects of the depressive phenotype, while the same cellular event is associated with depressive-like responses when triggered in the nucleus accumbens [3, 11, 35]. This further underlines the specificity of action of antidepressants in different parts of the brain. Consistent with this, the activity of a set of second messengers (protein kinase C (PKC)-delta, PKC-gamma, stress-activated protein kinase, cAMP-dependent protein kinase beta isoform, Janus protein kinase, and phosphofructokinase M) were all found to be downregulated after treatment with fluoxetine and citalopram in the whole brains of rats [36]. Moreover, treatment with citalopram and lithium (given separately) was found to be associated with an increased expression of the adenyl cyclase type 1 mRNA in the hippocampus, but not its corresponding protein, while GTP-associated adenyl cyclase activity was found to be increased after treatment: this may indicate that the antidepressant treatment caused an enhanced adenyl cyclase/G protein coupling [37].

Neurotrophins

Critical molecules regulating signaling and neuroplasticity as potential long-term mediators of mood stabilization have been identified and they may play a relevant role in the response to antidepressant treatments. Together, they act as neurotrophic agents and they concur to the neuroplasticity of cells defined as the sum of diverse processes of vital importance through which the brain perceives, adapts to, and responds to a variety of internal and external stimuli. In terms of biological structures, neuroplasticity includes alterations of dendritic function, synaptic remodeling, long-term potentiation, axonal sprouting, neurite extension, synaptogenesis, and even neurogenesis. Some of the most critical molecules that are involved in these processes are: CREB, BDNF, Bcl-2, p53, and MAP kinases. Neurotrophic factors (such as BDNF) promote cell survival largely by suppressing intrinsic, cellular apoptotic machinery, rather than by inducing cell survival pathways [38]. Two intracellular signal transduction pathways are crucial in promoting neuronal survival – the mitogen activated protein (MAP) kinase cascade and the phosphotidylinositol-3 kinase (PI-3K)/Akt pathway [39, 40]. The activation of the MAP kinase pathway can inhibit apoptosis by inducing the phosphorylation of Bad and increasing the expression of Bcl-2, the latter effect likely involving the cAMP response element binding protein (CREB) [41, 42]. Indeed, this mechanism was confirmed by recent analyses by Chen and colleagues who reported that fluoxetine can enhance the expression of bcl-2 [43]. Phosphorylation of Bad occurs via activation of a downstream target of the MAP kinase cascade, ribosomal S-6 kinase (Rsk). Ribosomal S-6 kinase phosphorylates Bad and thereby promotes its inactivation. Activation of Rsk also mediates the actions of the MAP kinase cascade and neurotrophic factors on the expression of Bcl-2. Ribosomal S-6 kinase can phosphorylate the cAMP response element binding protein (CREB) and this leads to induction of Bcl-2 gene expression. Not only the neuronal death that these mechanisms are organized to prevent, but also a lack of neurogenesis, may

represent mechanisms by which neuroresilience is dampened. Studies have demonstrated that the greatest density of new cell growth is observed in the subventricular zone and the subgranular layer of the hippocampus, and decreased neurogenesis occurs during stress – both acute and chronic. This effect appears to be mediated by glucocorticoid receptors [44]: chronic psychosocial stress or corticosterone administration caused apical dendritic atrophy of hippocampal CA3 pyramidal neurons, which may be mediated by activation of the hypothalamic–pituitary–adrenal (HPA) axis [45, 46]. This context opened the way to the formulation of drug designs based on the antagonism of glucocorticoid receptors. Intriguingly, antidepressant treatments can upregulate the brain-derived neurotrophic factor (BDNF) signaling cascade after chronic administration through their impact on the cAMP–CREB cascade, which regulates the BDNF [47, 48], and thereby produce an antidepressant effect by increasing the expression of neurotrophic factors in the hippocampus [49]. Consistently, animal studies suggested that the impairment of the BDNF/TrkB system exposes animals to a blunted antidepressant response more than to a higher risk of developing depressive-like phenotypes [50–52]. Interestingly, it has been demonstrated that localization is central to the effect of the presence or absence of the BDNF: the ablation of the BDNF in the forebrain including the hippocampus results in a lack of sensitivity to antidepressant treatment, while ablation in the reward pathway ameliorated the adverse effects of social defeat, and if the BDNF system is interrupted in the dentate gyrus and the CA1 regions, a lack of antidepressant effect (desipramine and citalopram) is to be expected [51, 53–55]. There are some more insights into this field. For example, there is one report of striking evidence: a non-correspondence between changes in BDNF mRNA and protein expression induced by the antidepressant treatments and lithium was revealed by Jacobsen and Mork [56], which may indicate that the means by which antidepressants exert their action on the neurotrophic elements of neurons act indirectly. Otherwise, a sort of editing process could be responsible for this lack of association: it has been reported that duloxetine increases the expression of certain exons of the BDNF coding sequence (namely exons V, I, and III but not exon IV). Indeed, not only is the BDNF upregulated, but a particular isoform of it is produced within neurons under the influence of antidepressant treatments [57]. On the other hand, by whatever means, it has been demonstrated that antidepressants modulate their neuroprotective effect on cells independently from the class they belong to (tricylic antidepressants, TCA; selective serotonin reuptake inhibitors, SSRI; or monoamine oxidase inhibitors, MAOI) while they do not share this faculty with molecules of other classes (antipsychotics or benzodiazepines for example) [58]: it has been proposed that a possible means by which this goal is achieved is the activity-regulated cytoskeletal-associated protein (Arc) gene. The Arc gene is an early gene implicated in long-term potentiation and other forms of neuroplasticity. There are two classes of early genes: transcription factors and effectors. The Arc gene belongs to the second class and may be relevant in this field as it has direct effects on cellular functions other than transcription factors. In particular, there is evidence of increased expression of Arc in neurons that had modified their function and structure after neuronal activity [59, 60]. Moreover, the expression of Arc is positively modulated by serotonin [61], and it was reported that paroxetine, venlafaxine, and desimipramine can increase the Arc mRNA concentration mostly in the hippocampus and cortex of animals, an effect that was found to be dependent on the antagonism on the serotonin receptor 1A and extended to reboxetine as well [62–64]. A set of 33 protein spots were isolated by Khawaja and colleagues [143] after a proteomic analysis of a rat hippocampus extract from animals exposed to chronic treatment with venlafaxine or fluoxetine. Wide analyses are at risk of false positive findings [65], but some interesting findings from that study were confirmed by further analysis. In particular, insulin-like growth factor 1 was found to have antidepressant-like effects on animals when administered chronically [66], comparable to those of BDNF [67], and this event was found to be regulated by serotonin [68, 69] and to be sensitive to lithium [70]. There are other candidates within the group of neurotrophic factors that are enhanced after antidepressant treatment: S100B, a cytokine with neurotrophic and neurite-extending activity [71], fibroblast growth factor 2 [72], CAM-L1 (cell adhesion molecule L1), and laminin (a protein of the external matrix) [73] are some examples. More evidence in this field must be collected before the complete picture of antidepressant-related neurotrophic factors is completed.

Neuroendocrine and neuroimmune interactions

There is a set of lines of evidence that suggest that depressive disorder is related to a disruption in the regulation of the immune system. One possible link between these two apparently different worlds (non-reactive chronically or recurrently depressed mood and inflammation of the tissues) is the role of cytokines (CK). Cytokines are small molecules that act as signaling molecules, like hormones and neurotransmitters. They are present in the organism at very low basal levels (picomolar concentration for IL-6 for example) but their concentration raises up to 1,000-fold during trauma or infections. One relevant characteristic of CK that differentiate them from hormones is that they are widely produced by cells of different embryonic origin in the organism. The most relevant and investigated cytokines are interleukins (IL-1 and IL-6 mainly) and tumor necrosis factor alpha (TNFα). Cytokines can impact on a cell function by autocrine, paracrine, and endocrine ways. That is, CK can influence the functions of neurons both when produced inside or outside the brain, and in all cases they can originate from peripheral immune cells and cross the blood–brain barrier [74, 75], or they can originate from neuronal and glial cells as well. Indeed, neuronal and glial cells are able to produce and recognize CK, and they are also able to produce an amplification of the CK signal, which in turn can have profound effect on neurotransmitters and on the release of the corticotrophin-releasing hormone (CRH) activating the neuroendocrine system [76]. This picture suggests that the biological reaction to stress, which includes an enhanced level of cortisol, a biologic mark of depressive disorder, along with the function of neuronal nets that relies on the fine tuning of the monoaminergic concentration, are imbalanced under conditions of high CK concentration: the question is whether this is a cause or an effect of depressive deregulation. In all events, some of the depressive symptoms (anhedonia, depressed mood, and diminished food intake) are commonly experienced by those suffering from influenza, which suggests that inflammation can mimic some aspects of depressive disorder but it still represents an independent pathophysiological mechanism. Moreover, there is not much evidence that addresses an antidepressant effect of anti-inflammatory drugs, and the production of CK is under the tonic control of the peripheral nervous system [77], and could then be imbalanced as a consequence of a primary, still unknown, CNS disruption. Despite these difficulties, there is some evidence to encourage this line of research. Inflammatory cytokines have been shown to alter monoamine turnover, decrease activity of presynaptic serotoninergic neurons, and activate serotonin reuptake from the synaptic cleft [78, 79]. These activities make them candidates for putative modulators of the depressive phenotype, and possible targets of the antidepressant activity of antidepressant drugs. The first step is to verify if peripheral activation of the immune system can impact on brain functioning: it has been demonstrated that the administration of interferon alpha to patients suffering from hepatitis C can enhance the level of IL-6 and monocyte chemoattractant protein-1 in the cerebrospinal fluid of patients while it does not impact the concentration of these mediators in the peripheral blood [80]. Interferons belong to the group of CK, they are produced by cells of the immune system in response to challenges by foreign agents and based on the just-mentioned evidence, it is understood that brain tissues are somehow specifically impacted by these peripheral challenges, and there is evidence that serotonin tone is impacted after administration of IFN-gamma and TNF-α decreases serotonin transporter function and expression [81]. The second point is to investigate whether the enhancement of these modulators can impact the function of neuronal nets. The evidence for this is provided by some hints on chronic stress: the brain reacts to stress by adapting its functions, basically neuromodulator balance and dendrite branching, in specific areas of the brain. The hippocampus and amygdala have been consistently demonstrated to be locations of high tissue remanagement during stress, this being biologically based on the presence of glucocorticoid receptors on the surface of neurons in these structures. The endocrine system, which is specifically activated during stress conditions, is closely linked to the immune and signalling system and especially glucocorticoids can modulate the immune response [82]. It is well known that the allostatic (i.e., adaptative) reactions to stress turn out to be maladaptative ("allostatic state") if prolonged through time, and this has been found to be associated with enhanced activation of the immunologic system [83]. Such a mechanism is thought to provide the basis for some aspects of post-traumatic stress disorder and depressive disorder [84]. The diminished viability of neuronal cells during chronic stress events has been shown to be related to a decreased production of BDNF [85], whose levels have been demonstrated to be impacted by the activity of autoreactive T cells [86], which also contribute to the protection and maintenance of injured CNS tissue [87, 88], provide maintenance of hippocampal neurogenesis [86], and are relevant to coping ability during stress [89, 90]. In accordance with this evidence, animal models with higher expression of IL-10 demonstrated a depressive-like phenotype (female rats) [91], and depressed patients showed significantly higher activation of the immune system compared to controls that could be partially abolished after treatment with fluoxetine [92]. This given, it can be said that an increase in the activation of the immune system, both centrally and peripherally, is associated with relevant changes in brain functions. There is now some consensus in extending the hypothesis related to the therapeutic effect of antidepressant treatments by attenuating brain expression or action of the inflammatory CK [93, 94], and these lines of evidence recently helped the design of a successful immunologic treatment of depressive disorder in one animal model based on immunization with a weak agonist of myelin-derived peptide [95]. Consistently with this, it has been reported that the administration of the TCA desipramine in rats resulted in a diminished concentration of TNF alpha [96, 97] and INT gamma induced production of IL-6 in microglial cells [98], while the intracerebroventricular microinfusion of TNF alpha counteracts the effect of desimipramine. Finally, TNF alpha antibody mimics the therapeutic effect of the antidepressant [99]. Interestingly, and consistent with these findings, antidepressants have been reported to be able to diminish peripheral inflammation as well [100, 101] and to reduce mortality in animal models of severe sepsis [102, 103]. This evidence suggests that the immune system is a target of antidepressant treatments. Furthermore, it has been reported that the IL-8 receptor is downregulated in schizophrenic patients after fluvoxamine is added to their antipsychotic treatment [104]. It has been recalled that the glucocorticoid system and the immune system are tightly bound and that their functions are highly orchestrated in order to best fit the response of the body to external stimuli. There is evidence that dysfunctions of the glucocorticoid receptors are involved in the hyperactivity of the HPA system in depressive disorder [105] and that this dysfunction is related to the phase of the depressive disorder [106, 107]. Interestingly, it has been reported that antidepressants can inhibit the expression of genes triggered by exposure to glucocorticoids in fibroblasts. Glucocorticoids bind to their receptors on the surface of cells and activate it to enter the nucleus and bind to a specific DNA sequence where they behave as a regulator of gene expression. This event is modulated by cyclic AMP protein kinase A (cyclic AMP/PKA), phospholipase C and protein kinase C (PLC/PKC), and the Ca^{++} calmodulin group (CAM)-mediated signal transduction pathway [108–110], whose activities are affected by antidepressant drugs [111–113]. Interestingly, a set of different antidepressants including imipramine, amitriptyline, desipramine, fluoxetine, tianeptine, mianserin, and moclobemide were found to be able to impact (diminish) the glucocorticoid-induced DNA activation in modified fibroblasts [114], while desimipramine and mirtazapine, but not maprotiline and imipramine, were found to decrease the expression of mRNA for the glucocorticoid receptors in monocytes, and mirtazapine upregulated the level of glucocorticoid receptors in a time-dependent manner.

Epigenetic mechanisms

There are several ways that external stimuli can produce long-lasting changes in protein availability and function: within them, epigenetic modifications have been highly investigated recently. Understanding epigenetic control of gene expression requires a rudimentary understanding of DNA and chromatin structure. Within eukaryotic cells, DNA is stored in the nucleus in a complex together with histone proteins, and during non-dividing cell phases it can be found as a compressed structure referred to as chromatin. Nucleosomes are the primary structural units of chromatin. Nucleosomes comprise a standard length of DNA (147 base pairs) wrapped around a histone octamer made up of four pairs of the basic histone proteins (H2A, H2B, H3 and H4). The methylation rate of DNA along with the structure of the chromatin, which can be highly compressed or otherwise slightly stuck, determines the availability of genes for transcription and is referred to as the epigenome. Cells with identical DNA can differentiate into very different types, building up one complex organism

through the fine orchestration of this mechanism. It was once thought that epigenetic mechanisms marked a cell's destiny early and definitively; it is now understood that epigenetic orchestration is at work during a set of adaptive processes throughout the life of a cell in adult organisms as well, and they are dynamically regulated in order to turn either on or off the expression of specific genes, giving rise to different proteomes during the cell's life turned on by environmental cues.

Epigenetic action can produce long-lasting modifications of DNA transcriptional activity that are largely independent from DNA mutations, by determining the accessibility of genes to the transcriptional machinery. This model may explain several aspects of depressive disorder including the discordance between monozygotic twins, the chronic relapsing of the disease, and the higher prevalence of depressive disorder in women. Moreover, epigenetic mechanisms offer a link between gene and environment, being the last one epigenetically decoded in order to best fit the DNA transcriptional activity toward environmental cues. Besides, the epigenetic modifications may explain the inconsistent findings of genetic association studies and provide the biological basis for the relevance of a set of stratification factors (for example education, marital status, socioeconomic level), which are thought to impact the depressive phenotype. There are at least three main ways by which DNA expression rate can be modified by epigenetic mechanisms: methylation (a covalent change to DNA), post-terminal modification of histones (acetylation), and non-transcriptional gene silencing mechanisms (microRNAs) [115]. Depressive disorder has been associated with two mechanisms of epigenetic modifications: DNA methylation of cytosine, which has been reported to be relevant to maternal behavior toward offspring, and histone acetylation, which seems to be the key to the antidepressant action. Methylation and histone acetylation are bound processes: the first step of methylation is the activation of methyl CpG binding proteins (MBD), which in turn activates another class of proteins able to deal with chromatin, the histone deacetylase (HDAC) that contributes to transcriptional repression or silencing, while histone acetylation occurs via histone acetyl transferases (HAT) that relax the tight coiling of DNA, decondense chromatin and determine transcriptional activation. The membrane-bound dipeptidase (MBD) enzymes related to the transcriptional repression in eukaryotic cells are MeCP2, MBD1, MBD2, and MBD3. In mammals, the methylation occurs almost exclusively within the context of a simple dinucleotide site – CpG. Roughly 70% of all CpG dinucleotides in the mammalian genome are methylated; the majority of these sites occur in repetitive DNA elements [116]. High levels of cytosine methylation are observed on the inactive X-chromosome and at imprinted loci [117]. The great part of the non-methylated CpG loci are found next to promoters and first exons regions [118, 119]. The mechanisms by which a part of the genome remains not methylated is a subject of controversy [120, 121], but the consequence is that the genome is divided into transcribed and non-transcribed by the activity of the MBD. The first member of the MBD family to be described at the molecular level was MeCP2 [122]. It is a multi-domain protein, [123] chromatin associated [124], and localizes to densely methylated regions of the genome in animals [125]. In MeCP2, only a small portion of the protein is devoted to selective recognition of methyl CpG. It also contains a transcriptional repression domain (TRD) that overlaps a nuclear localization signal [126]. MeCP2 is not essential in stem cells, but it is essential for embryonic development. MeCP2 gene mutations are the cause of some cases of Rett syndrome, a progressive neurologic developmental disorder and one of the most common causes of mental retardation in females. Relevant factors that bind the MeCP2 and impact its function are HDAC and Sin3 [127, 128]: it is thought that MeCP2 is recruited to methylated regions of the genome where its interactions with a protein complex containing Sin3 and histone deacetylases lead to the establishment and maintenance of repressive chromatin architecture [117]. Despite its relevance (276 articles on PubMed at the moment of writing), Sin3 was not investigated as a regulator of the antidepressant effect, while there are some details regarding HDAC as will be detailed hereafter. There are no specific known molecular characteristics of MBD1, MBD2, and MBD3 that may distinguish them from MeCP2 and account for an impact on antidepressant treatment [116]. On the other hand, there is some evidence of a role played by MeCP2, HAT, and HDAC in the response to drug treatment. One of the first and most interesting findings on animals in this field [129] reported that adult offspring born to poorly liking and grooming rat mothers showed increased anxiety and reduced expression of glucocorticoid receptors within the hippocampus compared with the offspring of mothers with higher rates of maternal sensitivity. The molecular way by which the expression of gluco-corticoid receptors in the hippocampus is decreased is the methylation of the promoter of the gene coding for the glucocorticoid receptors. In other words, the methylation of the promoter of the gene determines a decreased rate of genetic expression, and, by this, it concurs to induce a specific behavior (anxiety in the former example) that is reactive and somehow adaptative to the environment. Interestingly, this event occurs during the first weeks of development and it can be counteracted by the administration of tricho-statin A, a histone deacetylase inhibitor [129]. To determine the access of the transcriptional machinery to the DNA is to determine the cell fate, which is intuitively related to the functions of biological tissues. The brain does not represent an exception to this rule, as these mechanisms have been reported to be strongly related to relevant brain functions such as learning and memory: H3 acetylation rates in the hippocampus were found to be increased under conditions of fear-induced experiment in animals, and notable consequences on memory ability have been observed when the H3 acetylation process has been dampened [130, 131], and the blockage of the enzymes that inhibit the acetylation have been associated with enhanced memory. Consistently, acetylation has been reported to be a key factor for antidepressant activity: some aspects of social defeat were found to be responsive to imipramine treatment only under conditions of increased histone acetylation at the BDNF promoter [132], and histone deacetylase inhibitors have been reported to have antidepressant-like effect as the administration of sodium butyrate, which inhibits HDAC, produced an antidepressant effect in a behavioral despair model [133]. The relevance of these mechanisms prompted the design of antidepressant drugs based on the activity of specific histone deacetylases (HDAC5, class II HDAC) [134], even though this approach seems to be still in very early stages and it is still far from possible development into treatment modalities: there is conflicting evidence suggesting that the complete ablation of HDAC5 leads to a phenotype more vulnerable to depressed mood that is counterintuitive with respect to the findings of Tsankova [134, 135], and imipramine, which increases HDAC5 expression in the hippo-campus, showed the opposite effect in the nucleus accumbens [135] suggesting that things are quite complicated. Furthermore, it has been reported that the administration of antidepressants (fluoxetine) and of psychostimulants (cocaine) determines epigenetic changes by yet another way, which again seems to be contradictory to the findings of Tsankova [134], and works by increasing expression of the methyl CpG binding protein, the MeCP2 [136]. The activation of the MeCP2 would recruit HDAC and then inhibit gene expression by limiting the effects of the acetylation and not enhance gene expression as the imipramine does in the hippocampus. Besides these conflicting findings, a treatment on humans would still hold the risk of activating gene expression that is silenced in adulthood or in differentiated cells within or outside of the CNS, whose disrupted equilibrium after epigenetic manipulation would result in severe iatrogenic effect. This set of findings further emphasizes the regional specificity of stress-related events within the brain, and suggests that different brain regions express their plasticity and reactivity to the antidepressant treatment following paths, including epigenetics, that are dependent on the specific functional neuronal net under investigation. This point represents a major challenge to current research in biological psychiatry.

Interfering RNAs are small RNAs that are able to inhibit in a sequence-specific way gene expression at a post-transcriptional level, a phenomenon known as "RNA interference". Interfering RNAs produced by human cells are known as microRNAs (miRNAs). MicroRNAs are transcribed by intergene regions, introns, and even exons, either as polycistronic or as monocistronic transcripts [137–139], they are transported out of the nucleus by nuclear export factor 5 [140], and are further processed in the cytosol by the enzyme Dicer, a RNAse III endonuclease [141]. The processed miRNAs work in the cytosol, complexed to an association of molecules called RISC (RNA-induced silencing complex). Endowed in these complexes, miRNAs can bind and deactivate other mRNAs presenting with sequence homology. As a result, the bound mRNA is cleaved. The orchestration of this mechanism is able to tune and focus the mRNA expression of a cell. Its regulation is pivotal to define the proteome characteristics through time and its modulation allows the cell a mechanism of fine adjustment of its activity. Nevertheless, there is no intensive pharmacogenetic investigation focused on this field.

Conclusion

Depressive disorder is one of the most relevant diseases affecting the population worldwide. The incidence rates and the relevant burden in terms of concomitant diseases, the economic burden, and its chronic nature make it one of the most relevant medical challenges nowadays. Despite this relevance, there is poor knowledge of the pathophysiological mechanisms that unravel the disorder, and little is known about the mechanisms that rule the dynamics of antidepressant treatments. Since their first appearance in the treatment of depressive disorders, antidepressant drugs designed on the monoaminergic theory of depression have dominated the scene. According to this theory, depressive disorder is based on the imbalance of the monoamine tone within the CNS: the most relevant amines being serotonin and noradrenalin. Unfortunately, this theory cannot explain the biological disruptions that unravel depression: first of all, not all patients respond to drug treatment with serotonin or noradrenalin reuptake inhibitors, and the reasons why some individuals respond to a drug treatment and others do not are still poorly understood. Moreover, even in the best case when a good response is achieved, the elevation of mood follows treatment initiation by several days: this does not account for the immediate increase in the monoaminergic tone that is produced by the treatment, and suggests that other mechanisms are involved. One experimental way that can be used to obtain insights in this field is the identification of the genes for which expression is modified by the administration of antidepressants. Wide proteome investigations have been performed with interesting results [142, 143], but these analyses cannot be considered as definitive since a high rate of false positive findings is retrieved from them, and subsequent investigations are generally required before a good candidate that may widen the knowledge in the field is defined. Along the way, one of the most intriguing and replicated findings is the relevance of neurotrophic factors as modulators of the antidepressant response. The rationale of this relies on the hypothesis that neuroresilience is imbalanced in cases of depressive disorder, but the disrupted orchestration that dampens the viability of neurons can be healed after the administration of antidepressant treatments. The biological means by which this result is achieved rely on the function of neurotrophins, and BDNF among others seems to play a relevant role. Indeed, the increased expression of BDNF mRNA is one of the putative ways by which antidepressants are thought to act. Brain-derived neurotrophic factor is not the only neurotrophin likely involved in the process. Other candidates have entered the scene during the recent years of research and the involvement of some of them was replicated by independent analyses. Insulin-like growth factor and the Arc are good examples of gene products involved in the neuroresilience processes that are impacted by antidepressant treatments. The line of research that led to the definition of the neurotrophin hypothesis of depression started with the observation that the hippocampus of depressed patients was small compared to healthy subjects. This event was associated with the hypersecretion of glucocorticoids, receptors of which are widely expressed on the hippocampal cells. This evidence provides a relevant bound between depressive disorder and chronic stress, and suggests that the immune system may be involved in the pathophysiology of depressive disorders. The evidence that supports this hypothesis derives from the experience with interferons as therapeutic resources in the treatment of hepatitis. Nevertheless, anti-inflammatory drugs did not provide consistent evidence of their relevance as potential antidepressant devices, which may indicate that they are not involved in the causes of depressive disorders even if they may play a role in the cascade of events that characterize the disease. The epigenetic control of the expression rates of DNA is probably the future field in which new drugs will be developed. Methylation and acetylation control the rate of expression of genes in a specific way and through the fine tuning of the set of genes a cell expresses, specialization, viability, death, or recruitment of other cells into functional nets is achieved. Nonetheless, even though there is evidence that antidepressant drugs can modify this regulation, the design of antidepressant drugs acting specifically for this mechanism is still far from everyday practise.

In conclusion, antidepressants influence the expression of a large variety of genes in multiple pathways after their initial monoamine modulation. These are beginning to be known and are possible targets for new and more specific treatments. As we discussed, the whole picture is extremely complex as it is turning out to be a system where a large number of pathways are interacting in a dynamic way based on genetic predisposition and environmental influences.

References

1. Kessler RC, Chiu WT, Demler O, Merikangas KR, Walters EE. Prevalence, severity, and comorbidity of 12-month DSM-IV disorders in the National Comorbidity Survey Replication. *Arch Gen Psychiatry.* 2005;**62**(6):617–27.

2. Wittchen HU, Jacobi F. Size and burden of mental disorders in Europe – a critical review and appraisal of 27 studies. *Eur Neuropsychopharmacol.* 2005; **15**(4):357–76.

3. Nestler EJ, Barrot M, DiLeone RJ, *et al.* Neurobiology of depression. *Neuron.* 2002;**34**(1):13–25.

4. Evans DL, Charney DS, Lewis L, *et al.* Mood disorders in the medically ill: scientific review and recommendations. *Biol Psychiatry.* 2005;**58**(3):175–89.

5. Krishnan V, Nestler EJ. The molecular neurobiology of depression. *Nature.* 2008;**455**(7215):894–902.

6. Phelps EA, LeDoux JE. Contributions of the amygdala to emotion processing: from animal models to human behavior. *Neuron.* 2005;**48**(2):175–87.

7. Drevets WC. Neuroimaging and neuropathological studies of depression: implications for the cognitive-emotional features of mood disorders. *Curr Opin Neurobiol.* 2001;**11**(2):240–9.

8. López-León S, Janssens AC, González-Zuloeta Ladd AM, *et al.* Meta-analyses of genetic studies on major depressive disorder. *Mol Psychiatry.* 2008; **13**(8):772–85.

9. Trivedi MH, Rush AJ, Wisniewski SR, *et al.* Evaluation of outcomes with citalopram for depression using measurement-based care in STAR*D: implications for clinical practice. *Am J Psychiatry.* 2006;**163**(1):28–40.

10. Berton O, Nestler EJ. New approaches to antidepressant drug discovery: beyond monoamines. *Nat Rev Neurosci.* 2006;**7**(2):137–51.

11. Pittenger C, Duman RS. Stress, depression, and neuroplasticity: a convergence of mechanisms. *Neuropsychopharmacology.* 2008;**33**(1):88–109.

12. Ansorge MS, Hen R, Gingrich JA. Neurodevelopmental origins of depressive disorders. *Curr Opin Pharmacol.* 2007;**7**(1):8–17.

13. Ruhe HG, Mason NS, Schene AH. Mood is indirectly related to serotonin, norepinephrine and dopamine levels in humans: a meta-analysis of monoamine depletion studies. *Mol Psychiatry.* 2007;**12**(4):331–59.

14. Spurlock G, Buckland P, O'Donovan M, McGuffin P. Lack of effect of antidepressant drugs on the levels of mRNAs encoding serotonergic receptors, synthetic enzymes and 5HT transporter. *Neuropharmacology.* 1994;**33**(3–4):433–40.

15. Iceta R, Aramayona JJ, Mesonero JE, Alcalde AI. Regulation of the human serotonin transporter mediated by long-term action of serotonin in Caco-2 cells. *Acta Physiol (Oxf)*. 2008;**193**(1):57–65.

16. Arborelius L, Hawks BW, Owens MJ, Plotsky PM, Nemeroff CB. Increased responsiveness of presumed 5-HT cells to citalopram in adult rats subjected to prolonged maternal separation relative to brief separation. *Psychopharmacology (Berl)*. 2004; **176**(3–4):248–55.

17. Anthony JP, Sexton TJ, Neumaier JF. Antidepressant-induced regulation of 5-HT(1b) mRNA in rat dorsal raphe nucleus reverses rapidly after drug discontinuation. *J Neurosci Res*. 2000;**61**(1):82–7.

18. Benmansour S, Cecchi M, Morilak DA, *et al.* Effects of chronic antidepressant treatments on serotonin transporter function, density, and mRNA level. *J Neurosci*. 1999;**19**(23):10494–501.

19. Swan MC, Najlerahim AR, Bennett JP. Expression of serotonin transporter mRNA in rat brain: presence in neuronal and non-neuronal cells and effect of paroxetine. *J Chem Neuroanat*. 1997;**13**(2):71–6.

20. Di Lieto A, Leo D, Volpicelli F, di Porzio U, Colucci-D'Amato L. Fluoxetine modifies the expression of serotonergic markers in a differentiation-dependent fashion in the mesencephalic neural cell line A1 mes c-myc. *Brain Res*. 2007;**1143**:1–10.

21. Vilpoux C, Leroux-Nicollet I, Naudon L, Raisman-Vozari R, Costentin J. Reserpine or chronic paroxetine treatments do not modify the vesicular monoamine transporter 2 expression in serotonin-containing regions of the rat brain. *Neuropharmacology*. 2000;**39**(6):1075–82.

22. Abumaria N, Rygula R, Hiemke C, *et al.* Effect of chronic citalopram on serotonin-related and stress-regulated genes in the dorsal raphe nucleus of the rat. *Eur Neuropsychopharmacol*. 2007;**17**(6–7):417–29.

23. Shishkina GT, Kalinina TS, Dygalo NN. Up-regulation of tryptophan hydroxylase-2 mRNA in the rat brain by chronic fluoxetine treatment correlates with its antidepressant effect. *Neuroscience*. 2007;**150**(2):404–12.

24. Dygalo NN, Shishkina GT, Kalinina TS, Yudina AM, Ovchinnikova ES. Effect of repeated treatment with fluoxetine on tryptophan hydroxylase-2 gene expression in the rat brainstem. *Pharmacol Biochem Behav*. 2006;**85**(1):220–7.

25. Kitamura Y, Fujitani Y, Kitagawa K, *et al.* Effects of imipramine and bupropion on the duration of immobility of ACTH-treated rats in the forced swim test: involvement of the expression of 5-HT2A receptor mRNA. *Biol Pharm Bull*. 2008;**31**(2):246–9.

26. Morley-Fletcher S, Darnaudery M, Mocaer E, *et al.* Chronic treatment with imipramine reverses immobility behaviour, hippocampal corticosteroid receptors and cortical 5-HT(1A) receptor mRNA in prenatally stressed rats. *Neuropharmacology*. 2004;**47**(6):841–7.

27. Blier P. Crosstalk between the norepinephrine and serotonin systems and its role in the antidepressant response. *J Psychiatry Neurosci*. 2001;**26** Suppl:.S3–10.

28. Dziedzicka-Wasylewska M, Rogoz Z, Skuza G, Dlaboga D, Maj J. Effect of repeated treatment with tianeptine and fluoxetine on central dopamine D(2)/D(3) receptors. *Behav Pharmacol*. 2002;**13**(2):127–38.

29. Cyr M, Morissette M, Barden N, *et al.* Dopaminergic activity in transgenic mice underexpressing glucocorticoid receptors: effect of antidepressants. *Neuroscience*. 2001;**102**(1):151–8.

30. Lammers CH, Diaz J, Schwartz JC, Sokoloff P. Selective increase of dopamine D3 receptor gene expression as a common effect of chronic antidepressant treatments. *Mol Psychiatry*. 2000;**5**(4):378–88.

31. Ainsworth K, Smith SE, Zetterstrom TS, *et al.* Effect of antidepressant drugs on dopamine D1 and D2 receptor expression and dopamine release in the nucleus accumbens of the rat. *Psychopharmacology (Berl)*. 1998;**140**(4):470–7.

32. Drago A, Serretti A. Focus on HTR2C: A possible suggestion for genetic studies of complex disorders. *Am J Med Genet B Neuropsychiatr Genet*. 2009;**150B**(5):601–37.

33. Barbon A, Popoli M, La Via L, *et al.* Regulation of editing and expression of glutamate alpha-amino-propionic-acid (AMPA)/kainate receptors by antidepressant drugs. *Biol Psychiatry*. 2006;**59**(8):713–20.

34. Iga J, Ueno S, Yamauchi K, *et al.* Serotonin transporter mRNA expression in peripheral leukocytes of patients with major depression before and after treatment with paroxetine. *Neurosci Lett*. 2005;**389**(1):12–6.

35. Nestler EJ, Carlezon WA, Jr. The mesolimbic dopamine reward circuit in depression. *Biol Psychiatry*. 2006;**59**(12):1151–9.

36. Rausch JL, Gillespie CF, Fei Y, *et al.* Antidepressant effects on kinase gene expression patterns in rat brain. *Neurosci Lett*. 2002;**334**(2):91–4.

37. Prosperini E, Rizzi M, Fumagalli F, *et al.* Acute and chronic treatments with citalopram lower somatostatin levels in rat brain striatum through different mechanisms. *J Neurochem*. 1997;**69**(1):206–13.

38. Nibuya M, Takahashi M, Russell DS, Duman RS. Repeated stress increases catalytic TrkB mRNA in rat hippocampus. *Neurosci Lett*. 1999;**267**(2):81–4.

17

39. Tao X, Finkbeiner S, Arnold DB, Shaywitz AJ, Greenberg ME. Ca^{2+} influx regulates BDNF transcription by a CREB family transcription factor-dependent mechanism. *Neuron.* 1998;**20**(4):709–26.

40. Segal RA, Greenberg ME. Intracellular signaling pathways activated by neurotrophic factors. *Annu Rev Neurosci.* 1996;**19**:463–89.

41. Riccio A, Ahn S, Davenport CM, Blendy JA, Ginty DD. Mediation by a CREB family transcription factor of NGF-dependent survival of sympathetic neurons. *Science.* 1999;**286**(5448):2358–61.

42. Bonni A, Brunet A, West AE, *et al.* Cell survival promoted by the Ras-MAPK signaling pathway by transcription-dependent and -independent mechanisms. *Science.* 1999;**286**(5443):1358–62.

43. Chen SJ, Kao CL, Chang YL, *et al.* Antidepressant administration modulates neural stem cell survival and serotoninergic differentiation through bcl-2. *Curr Neurovasc Res.* 2007;**4**(1):19–29.

44. Gould E, Tanapat P. Stress and hippocampal neurogenesis. *Biol Psychiatry.* 1999;**46**(11):1472–9.

45. Sapolsky RM. Glucocorticoids and hippocampal atrophy in neuropsychiatric disorders. *Arch Gen Psychiatry.* 2000;**57**(10):925–35.

46. Magarinos AM, McEwen BS, Flugge G, Fuchs E. Chronic psychosocial stress causes apical dendritic atrophy of hippocampal CA3 pyramidal neurons in subordinate tree shrews. *J Neurosci.* 1996;**16**(10):3534–40.

47. Thome J, Sakai N, Shin K, *et al.* cAMP response element-mediated gene transcription is upregulated by chronic antidepressant treatment. *J Neurosci.* 2000;**20**(11):4030–6.

48. Shieh PB, Hu SC, Bobb K, Timmusk T, Ghosh A. Identification of a signaling pathway involved in calcium regulation of BDNF expression. *Neuron.* 1998;**20**(4):727–40.

49. Duman RS, Monteggia LM. A neurotrophic model for stress-related mood disorders. *Biol Psychiatry.* 2006;**59**(12):1116–27.

50. Saarelainen T, Hendolin P, Lucas G, *et al.* Activation of the TrkB neurotrophin receptor is induced by antidepressant drugs and is required for antidepressant-induced behavioral effects. *J Neurosci.* 2003;**23**(1):349–57.

51. Monteggia LM, Barrot M, Powell CM, *et al.* Essential role of brain-derived neurotrophic factor in adult hippocampal function. *Proc Natl Acad Sci USA.* 2004;**101**(29):10827–32.

52. Deltheil T, Guiard BP, Cerdan J, *et al.* Behavioral and serotonergic consequences of decreasing or increasing hippocampus brain-derived neurotrophic factor protein levels in mice. *Neuropharmacology.* 2008;**55**(6):1006–14.

53. Krishnan V, Han MH, Graham DL, *et al.* Molecular adaptations underlying susceptibility and resistance to social defeat in brain reward regions. *Cell.* 2007; **131**(2):391–404.

54. Berton O, McClung CA, Dileone RJ, *et al.* Essential role of BDNF in the mesolimbic dopamine pathway in social defeat stress. *Science.* 2006;**311**(5762):864–8.

55. Adachi M, Barrot M, Autry AE, Theobald D, Monteggia LM. Selective loss of brain-derived neurotrophic factor in the dentate gyrus attenuates antidepressant efficacy. *Biol Psychiatry.* 2008;**63**(7):642–9.

56. Jacobsen JP, Mork A. The effect of escitalopram, desipramine, electroconvulsive seizures and lithium on brain-derived neurotrophic factor mRNA and protein expression in the rat brain and the correlation to 5-HT and 5-HIAA levels. *Brain Res.* 2004;**1024**(1–2):183–92.

57. Calabrese F, Molteni R, Maj PF, *et al.* Chronic duloxetine treatment induces specific changes in the expression of BDNF transcripts and in the subcellular localization of the neurotrophin protein. *Neuropsychopharmacology.* 2007;**32**(11):2351–9.

58. Li YF, Liu YQ, Huang WC, Luo ZP. Cytoprotective effect is one of common action pathways for antidepressants. *Acta Pharmacol Sin.* 2003;**24**(10):996–1000.

59. Steward O, Worley PF. Selective targeting of newly synthesized Arc mRNA to active synapses requires NMDA receptor activation. *Neuron.* 2001;**30**(1):227–40.

60. Huang EP. Synaptic plasticity: regulated translation in dendrites. *Curr Biol.* 1999;**9**(5):R168–70.

61. Pei Q, Lewis L, Sprakes ME, *et al.* Serotonergic regulation of mRNA expression of Arc, an immediate early gene selectively localized at neuronal dendrites. *Neuropharmacology.* 2000;**39**(3):463–70.

62. Castro E, Tordera RM, Hughes ZA, Pei Q, Sharp T. Use of Arc expression as a molecular marker of increased postsynaptic 5-HT function after SSRI/5-HT1A receptor antagonist co-administration. *J Neurochem.* 2003;**85**(6):1480–7.

63. Tordera R, Pei Q, Newson M, *et al.* Effect of different 5-HT1A receptor antagonists in combination with paroxetine on expression of the immediate-early gene Arc in rat brain. *Neuropharmacology.* 2003;**44**(7):893–902.

64. De Foubert G, Carney SL, Robinson CS, *et al.* Fluoxetine-induced change in rat brain expression of brain-derived neurotrophic factor varies

depending on length of treatment. *Neuroscience.* 2004;**128**(3):597–604.

65. Binder EB, Holsboer F. Pharmacogenomics and antidepressant drugs. *Ann Med.* 2006;**38**(2):82–94.

66. Duman CH, Schlesinger L, Terwilliger R, *et al.* Peripheral insulin-like growth factor-I produces antidepressant-like behavior and contributes to the effect of exercise. *Behav Brain Res.* 2009;**198**(2):366–71.

67. Hoshaw BA, Malberg JE, Lucki I. Central administration of IGF-I and BDNF leads to long-lasting antidepressant-like effects. *Brain Res.* 2005;**1037**(1–2):204–8.

68. Hoshaw BA, Hill TI, Crowley JJ, *et al.* Antidepressant-like behavioral effects of IGF-I produced by enhanced serotonin transmission. *Eur J Pharmacol.* 2008;**594**(1–3):109–16.

69. Lambert HW, Lauder JM. Serotonin receptor agonists that increase cyclic AMP positively regulate IGF-I in mouse mandibular mesenchymal cells. *Dev Neurosci.* 1999;**21**(2):105–12.

70. Malberg JE, Platt B, Rizzo SJ, *et al.* Increasing the levels of insulin-like growth factor-I by an IGF binding protein inhibitor produces anxiolytic and antidepressant-like effects. *Neuropsychopharmacology.* 2007;**32**(11):2360–8.

71. Akhisaroglu M, Manev R, Akhisaroglu E, Uz T, Manev H. Both aging and chronic fluoxetine increase S100B content in the mouse hippocampus. *Neuroreport.* 2003;**14**(11):1471–3.

72. Maragnoli ME, Fumagalli F, Gennarelli M, Racagni G, Riva MA. Fluoxetine and olanzapine have synergistic effects in the modulation of fibroblast growth factor 2 expression within the rat brain. *Biol Psychiatry.* 2004;**55**(11):1095–102.

73. Laifenfeld D, Karry R, Grauer E, Klein E, Ben-Shachar D. Antidepressants and prolonged stress in rats modulate CAM-L1, laminin, and pCREB, implicated in neuronal plasticity. *Neurobiol Dis.* 2005;**20**(2):432–41.

74. Watkins LR, Maier SF, Goehler LE. Cytokine-to-brain communication: a review and analysis of alternative mechanisms. *Life Sci.* 1995;**57**(11):1011–26.

75. Banks WA, Kastin AJ. Relative contributions of peripheral and central sources to levels of IL-1 alpha in the cerebral cortex of mice: assessment with species-specific enzyme immunoassays. *J Neuroimmunol.* 1997;**79**(1):22–8.

76. Szelenyi J, Vizi ES. The catecholamine cytokine balance: interaction between the brain and the immune system. *Ann N Y Acad Sci.* 2007;**1113**:311–24.

77. Vizi ES. Receptor-mediated local fine-tuning by noradrenergic innervation of neuroendocrine and immune systems. *Ann N Y Acad Sci.* 1998;**851**:388–96.

78. Schiepers OJ, Wichers MC, Maes M. Cytokines and major depression. *Prog Neuropsychopharmacol Biol Psychiatry.* 2005;**29**(2):201–17.

79. Leonard BE. The immune system, depression and the action of antidepressants. *Prog Neuropsychopharmacol Biol Psychiatry.* 2001;**25**(4):767–80.

80. Raison CL, Borisov AS, Majer M, *et al.* Activation of central nervous system inflammatory pathways by interferon-alpha: relationship to monoamines and depression. *Biol Psychiatry.* 2009;**65**(4):296–303.

81. Foley KF, Pantano C, Ciolino A, Mawe GM. IFN-gamma and TNF-alpha decrease serotonin transporter function and expression in Caco2 cells. *Am J Physiol Gastrointest Liver Physiol.* 2007;**292**(3): G779–84.

82. Sperner-Unterweger B. Immunological aetiology of major psychiatric disorders: evidence and therapeutic implications. *Drugs.* 2005;**65**(11):1493–520.

83. Iga J, Ueno S, Ohmori T. Molecular assessment of depression from mRNAs in the peripheral leukocytes. *Ann Med.* 2008;**40**(5):336–42.

84. McEwen BS. Mood disorders and allostatic load. *Biol Psychiatry.* 2003;**54**(3):200–7.

85. Wang JW, Dranovsky A, Hen R. The when and where of BDNF and the antidepressant response. *Biol Psychiatry.* 2008;**63**(7):640–1.

86. Ziv Y, Ron N, Butovsky O, *et al.* Immune cells contribute to the maintenance of neurogenesis and spatial learning abilities in adulthood. *Nat Neurosci.* 2006;**9**(2):268–75.

87. Hauben E, Agranov E, Gothilf A, *et al.* Posttraumatic therapeutic vaccination with modified myelin self-antigen prevents complete paralysis while avoiding autoimmune disease. *J Clin Invest.* 2001;**108**(4):591–9.

88. Moalem G, Leibowitz-Amit R, Yoles E, *et al.* Autoimmune T cells protect neurons from secondary degeneration after central nervous system axotomy. *Nat Med.* 1999;**5**(1):49–55.

89. Lewitus GM, Cohen H, Schwartz M. Reducing post-traumatic anxiety by immunization. *Brain Behav Immun.* 2008;**22**(7):1108–14.

90. Cohen H, Ziv Y, Cardon M, Kaplan Z, *et al.* Maladaptation to mental stress mitigated by the adaptive immune system via depletion of naturally occurring regulatory CD4 + CD25 + cells. *J Neurobiol.* 2006;**66**(6):552–63.

91. Mesquita AR, Correia-Neves M, Roque S, *et al.* IL-10 modulates depressive-like behavior. *J Psychiatr Res.* 2008;**43**(2):89–97.

92. Tsao CW, Lin YS, Chen CC, Bai CH, Wu SR. Cytokines and serotonin transporter in patients with major depression. *Prog Neuropsychopharmacol Biol Psychiatry.* 2006;**30**(5):899–905.

93. Castanon N, Leonard BE, Neveu PJ, Yirmiya R. Effects of antidepressants on cytokine production and actions. *Brain Behav Immun.* 2002;**16**(5):569–74.

94. Licinio J, Wong ML. The role of inflammatory mediators in the biology of major depression: central nervous system cytokines modulate the biological substrate of depressive symptoms, regulate stress-responsive systems, and contribute to neurotoxicity and neuroprotection. *Mol Psychiatry.* 1999;**4**(4):317–27.

95. Lewitus GM, Wilf-Yarkoni A, Ziv Y, *et al*. Vaccination as a novel approach for treating depressive behavior. *Biol Psychiatry.* 2009;**65**(4):283–8.

96. Reynolds JL, Ignatowski TA, Sud R, Spengler RN. An antidepressant mechanism of desipramine is to decrease tumor necrosis factor-alpha production culminating in increases in noradrenergic neurotransmission. *Neuroscience.* 2005;**133**(2):519–31.

97. Ignatowski TA, Noble BK, Wright JR, *et al*. Neuronal-associated tumor necrosis factor (TNF alpha): its role in noradrenergic functioning and modification of its expression following antidepressant drug administration. *J Neuroimmunol.* 1997;**79**(1):84–90.

98. Hashioka S, Klegeris A, Monji A, *et al*. Antidepressants inhibit interferon-gamma-induced microglial production of IL-6 and nitric oxide. *Exp Neurol.* 2007;**206**(1):33–42.

99. Reynolds JL, Ignatowski TA, Sud R, Spengler RN. Brain-derived tumor necrosis factor-alpha and its involvement in noradrenergic neuron functioning involved in the mechanism of action of an antidepressant. *J Pharmacol Exp Ther.* 2004;**310**(3):1216–25.

100. Bianchi M, Sacerdote P, Panerai AE. Fluoxetine reduces inflammatory edema in the rat: involvement of the pituitary-adrenal axis. *Eur J Pharmacol.* 1994;**263**(1–2):81–4.

101. Bianchi M, Sacerdote P, Panerai AE. Chlomipramine differently affects inflammatory edema and pain in the rat. *Pharmacol Biochem Behav.* 1994;**48**(4):1037–40.

102. Roumestan C, Michel A, Bichon F, *et al*. Anti-inflammatory properties of desipramine and fluoxetine. *Respir Res.* 2007;**8**:35.

103. Brustolim D, Ribeiro-dos-Santos R, Kast RE, Altschuler EL, Soares MB. A new chapter opens in anti-inflammatory treatments: the antidepressant bupropion lowers production of tumor necrosis

104. Chertkow Y, Weinreb O, Youdim MB, Silver H. Gene expression changes in peripheral mononuclear cells from schizophrenic patients treated with a combination of antipsychotic with fluvoxamine. *Prog Neuropsychopharmacol Biol Psychiatry.* 2007;**31**(7):1356–62.

105. Arborelius L, Owens MJ, Plotsky PM, Nemeroff CB. The role of corticotropin-releasing factor in depression and anxiety disorders. *J Endocrinol.* 1999;**160**(1):1–12.

106. Holsboer F, Lauer CJ, Schreiber W, Krieg JC. Altered hypothalamic-pituitary-adrenocortical regulation in healthy subjects at high familial risk for affective disorders. *Neuroendocrinology.* 1995;**62**(4):340–7.

107. Ribeiro SC, Tandon R, Grunhaus L, Greden JF. The DST as a predictor of outcome in depression: a meta-analysis. *Am J Psychiatry.* 1993;**150**(11):1618–29.

108. Ning YM, Sanchez ER. Evidence for a functional interaction between calmodulin and the glucocorticoid receptor. *Biochem Biophys Res Commun.* 1995;**208**(1):48–54.

109. Moyer ML, Borror KC, Bona BJ, DeFranco DB, Nordeen SK. Modulation of cell signaling pathways can enhance or impair glucocorticoid-induced gene expression without altering the state of receptor phosphorylation. *J Biol Chem.* 1993;**268**(30):22933–40.

110. Maroder M, Farina AR, Vacca A, *et al*. Cell-specific bifunctional role of Jun oncogene family members on glucocorticoid receptor-dependent transcription. *Mol Endocrinol.* 1993;**7**(4):570–84.

111. Bouron A, Chatton JY. Acute application of the tricyclic antidepressant desipramine presynaptically stimulates the exocytosis of glutamate in the hippocampus. *Neuroscience.* 1999;**90**(3):729–36.

112. Mann CD, Vu TB, Hrdina PD. Protein kinase C in rat brain cortex and hippocampus: effect of repeated administration of fluoxetine and desipramine. *Br J Pharmacol.* 1995;**115**(4):595–600.

113. Nalepa I, Vetulani J. Involvement of protein kinase C in the mechanism of in vitro effects of imipramine on generation of second messengers by noradrenaline in cerebral cortical slices of the rat. *Neuroscience.* 1991;**44**(3):585–90.

114. Budziszewska B, Jaworska-Feil L, Kajta M, Lason W. Antidepressant drugs inhibit glucocorticoid receptor-mediated gene transcription – a possible mechanism. *Br J Pharmacol.* 2000;**130**(6):1385–93.

115. Tsankova N, Renthal W, Kumar A, Nestler EJ. Epigenetic regulation in psychiatric disorders. *Nat Rev Neurosci.* 2007;**8**(5):355–67.

116. Wade PA. Methyl CpG-binding proteins and transcriptional repression. *Bioessays.* 2001;**23**(12):1131–7.

117. Bird AP, Wolffe AP. Methylation-induced repression – belts, braces, and chromatin. *Cell.* 1999;**99**(5):451–4.

118. Lander ES, Linton LM, Birren B, *et al.* Initial sequencing and analysis of the human genome. *Nature.* 2001;**409**(6822):860–921.

119. Venter JC, Adams MD, Myers EW, *et al.* The sequence of the human genome. *Science.* 2001; **291**(5507):1304–51.

120. Bestor TH. The DNA methyltransferases of mammals. *Hum Mol Genet.* 2000;**9**(16):2395–402.

121. Robertson KD, Wolffe AP. DNA methylation in health and disease. *Nat Rev Genet.* 2000;**1**(1):11–9.

122. Lewis JD, Meehan RR, Henzel WJ, *et al.* Purification, sequence, and cellular localization of a novel chromosomal protein that binds to methylated DNA. *Cell.* 1992;**69**(6):905–14.

123. Nan X, Meehan RR, Bird A. Dissection of the methyl-CpG binding domain from the chromosomal protein MeCP2. *Nucleic Acids Res.* 1993;**21**(21):4886–92.

124. Meehan RR, Lewis JD, Bird AP. Characterization of MeCP2, a vertebrate DNA binding protein with affinity for methylated DNA. *Nucleic Acids Res.* 1992;**20**(19):5085–92.

125. Nan X, Tate P, Li E, Bird A. DNA methylation specifies chromosomal localization of MeCP2. *Mol Cell Biol.* 1996;**16**(1):414–21.

126. Nan X, Campoy FJ, Bird A. MeCP2 is a transcriptional repressor with abundant binding sites in genomic chromatin. *Cell.* 1997;**88**(4):471–81.

127. Meehan R, Lewis J, Cross S, *et al.* Transcriptional repression by methylation of CpG. *J Cell Sci Suppl.* 1992;**16**:9–14.

128. Nan X, Ng HH, Johnson CA, *et al.* Transcriptional repression by the methyl-CpG-binding protein MeCP2 involves a histone deacetylase complex. *Nature.* 1998;**393**(6683):386–9.

129. Weaver IC, Cervoni N, Champagne FA, *et al.* Epigenetic programming by maternal behavior. *Nat Neurosci.* 2004;**7**(8):847–54.

130. Levenson JM, Sweatt JD. Epigenetic mechanisms in memory formation. *Nat Rev Neurosci.* 2005;**6**(2):108–18.

131. Levenson JM, Sweatt JD. Epigenetic mechanisms: a common theme in vertebrate and invertebrate memory formation. *Cell Mol Life Sci.* 2006;**63**(9):1009–16.

132. Tsankova NM, Kumar A, Nestler EJ. Histone modifications at gene promoter regions in rat hippocampus after acute and chronic electroconvulsive seizures. *J Neurosci.* 2004;**24**(24):5603–10.

133. Schroeder FA, Lin CL, Crusio WE, Akbarian S. Antidepressant-like effects of the histone deacetylase inhibitor, sodium butyrate, in the mouse. *Biol Psychiatry.* 2007;**62**(1):55–64.

134. Tsankova NM, Berton O, Renthal W, *et al.* Sustained hippocampal chromatin regulation in a mouse model of depression and antidepressant action. *Nat Neurosci.* 2006;**9**(4):519–25.

135. Renthal W, Maze I, Krishnan V, *et al.* Histone deacetylase 5 epigenetically controls behavioral adaptations to chronic emotional stimuli. *Neuron.* 2007;**56**(3):517–29.

136. Cassel S, Carouge D, Gensburger C, *et al.* Fluoxetine and cocaine induce the epigenetic factors MeCP2 and MBD1 in adult rat brain. *Mol Pharmacol.* 2006;**70**(2):487–92.

137. Lagos-Quintana M, Rauhut R, Meyer J, Borkhardt A, Tuschl T. New microRNAs from mouse and human. *RNA.* 2003;**9**(2):175–9.

138. Lagos-Quintana M, Rauhut R, Lendeckel W, Tuschl T. Identification of novel genes coding for small expressed RNAs. *Science.* 2001;**294**(5543):853–8.

139. Lim LP, Glasner ME, Yekta S, Burge CB, Bartel DP. Vertebrate microRNA genes. *Science.* 2003;**299**(5612):1540.

140. Yi R, Qin Y, Macara IG, Cullen BR. Exportin-5 mediates the nuclear export of pre-microRNAs and short hairpin RNAs. *Genes Dev.* 2003;**17**(24):3011–6.

141. Hutvagner G, McLachlan J, Pasquinelli AE, *et al.* A cellular function for the RNA-interference enzyme Dicer in the maturation of the let-7 small temporal RNA. *Science.* 2001;**293**(5531):834–8.

142. Bisgaard CF, Jayatissa MN, Enghild JJ, *et al.* Proteomic investigation of the ventral rat hippocampus links DRP-2 to escitalopram treatment resistance and SNAP to stress resilience in the chronic mild stress model of depression. *J Mol Neurosci.* 2007;**32**(2):132–44.

143. Khawaja X, Xu J, Liang JJ, Barrett JE. Proteomic analysis of protein changes developing in rat hippocampus after chronic antidepressant treatment: Implications for depressive disorders and future therapies. *J Neurosci Res.* 2004;**75**(4):451–60.

Genetics of circadian rhythms in relation to mental illness

Sara Dallaspezia and Francesco Benedetti

Introduction

The accepted model for the molecular machinery that generates circadian rhythms involves a number of clock genes and their products. Clock genes function as transcriptional activators and regulate their own expression through a positive/negative feedback loop that cycles with a "free-running" period of approximately 24 hours. The genes CLOCK and BMAL1 form the positive regulator of the system while the genes PER 1–3, CRY 1–2, and REV-ERBα generate the negative feedback loop [1]. In this way, they allow the development of circadian and seasonal rhythms in lower organisms and in humans, with allelic variants influencing individual rhythms at a behavioral and cellular level [2, 3].

The control of circadian rhythms does not involve only clock genes, but it is a complex process implicating also environmental and physiological factors [4]. In mammals the circadian clock shows a hierarchical organization. The primary circadian pacemaker, the master clock, is located in the suprachiasmatic nuclei (SCN) of the anterior hypothalamus [5] and is synchronized to external 24-hour light/dark cycles by photic inputs coming from the retina through the retino-hypothalamic tract [6]. Light is a strong timing cue (zeitgeber), and the pacemaker's oscillation can be reset by light-induced phase shifts. The master pacemaker then communicates the timing information to peripheral oscillators present in the cells of most tissues. These signals include both direct (hormone secretion, sympathetic enervation) and indirect (body temperature, feeding intake) cues [7].

Clock genes variants as determinants of psychopathological features of mental illness

Genetic variability in clock genes has been associated with a number of phenotypic differences in circadian as well as sleep parameters, both in mouse models and in humans [8].

Moreover, clock genes are expressed in many brain structures other than in suprachiasmatic nuclei, including cingulate and parietal cortices [9]. Recent data suggested that they provide a mechanism for the control of circadian gene expression and of responsivity to stimuli at cellular level. Thus, they could play a role in yet unexploited brain functions [10]. For example, CLOCK gene expression was shown to be influenced by serotonergic agents [11] and to influence both dopaminergic neurotransmission and the behavioral effects of cocaine reward [12].

Clock gene variants could then bias some variables linked with psychiatric disorders (see Table 3.1).

Several human genetic studies have found a relationship between members of the molecular clock and psychiatric disorder. Few studies found an association of clock genes with schizophrenia and alcoholism. Spanagel and colleagues [13] found that the amount of alcohol consumption in alcoholic patients is related to haplotypes of the PER2 gene, while another group found that TIMELESS and PERIOD3 genes are involved in schizophrenia [14].

Most interesting results were found when considering mood disorders. Alteration of sleep–wake cycle and sleep structure are a core manifestation in

Table 3.1 Clock gene variants

Gene	Function	Polymorphisms	Condition	Implications
CLOCK	Activation of clock and clock-controlled gene (with BMAL1)	SNP	Healthy subjects	Influence on diurnal preference [40]
			Bipolar depression	Influence on diurnal activity [41, 42]
				Influence on sleep onset [41]
				Influence on the occurrence of insomnia both lifetime and during their depressive episodes [43, 44]
				Influence on neuropsychological performance and blood oxygen level dependent neural responses to a moral valence decision task [42]
		Gene knockout	Mania (animal model)	Transgenic mice showed a mania-like behavior which normalized: after chronic administration of lithium [50] by expressing a functional CLOCK protein [50]
GSK3-β	Essential element of Wnt/ beta-catenin pathway	SNP	Bipolar disorder	Influence on age at onset [35]
				Influence on response to lithium treatment [37]
			Bipolar depression	Influence on response to sleep deprivation treatment [36]
		Gene knockout	Animal model	Antagonist action on behavioral abnormalities induced by 5-HT deficiencies [38]
Period 3	Inhibition of CLOCK/ BMAL1-mediated transcription	VNTR	Bipolar disorder	Influence on age at onset [32]
		SNP	Schizophrenia	Association found [14]
		Haplotype that comprised six tagging SNPs	Bipolar disorder	Association found [30]
TIMELESS	Inhibition of CLOCK/ BMAL1-mediated transcription	SNP	Schizophrenia	Association found [14]
		SNP	Bipolar disorder	Association found [14]
Period 2	Inhibition of CLOCK/ BMAL1-mediated transcription	Haplotype that comprised four tagging SNPs	Alcoholism	Influence on alcohol consumption [13]
		SNP	Seasonal affective disorder	Association found [29]

Table 3.1 (cont.)

Gene	Function	Polymorphisms	Condition	Implications
BMAL1	Activation of clock and clock-controlled gene (with CLOCK)	SNP	Bipolar disorder	Association found [14]
Npas2	CLOCK homolog	SNP	Seasonal affective disorder	Association found [29]

major depression. Many other rhythms have been found to be disrupted in depressed patients, both unipolar and bipolar ones. These disrupted rhythms include the daily profiles of body temperature, cortisol, thyrotropin, prolactin, growth hormone, melatonin, and excretion of various metabolites in the urine [15, 16] and seem to return to normal with patient recovery. Moreover, patients affected by a major depressive episode often report an important variation in the intensity of perceived symptomatology during the day, and laboratory studies have revealed that mood, like physiological variables such as core body temperature, is regulated by a circadian clock interacting with the sleep homeostat [17]. Diurnal variations of mood are of great clinical relevance, because they have been shown to be a predictor of a good general clinical responsiveness both to antidepressant drugs [3] and to antidepressant sleep deprivation therapy [18]. Furthermore, some of the most rapid and powerful treatments that are currently used to treat mood disorder (total sleep deprivation, light therapy, sleep phase advance) are chronobiological interventions based on the manipulation of the sleep–wake and activity–rest rhythms [19, 20]. Finally, some of the neurotransmitters implicated in mood regulation, such as serotonin, norepinephrine and dopamine, and their receptors, show a circadian rhythm in their levels, release, and synthesis-related enzymes [21–24].

As clock genes play a pivotal role in maintaining circadian rhythms, abnormal function in them and their related pathways are hypothesized to contribute to the core pathophysiology of depression. In fact, polymorphisms in molecular clock genes not only show an association with affective disorder but also seem to influence symptomatology characteristics and response to treatment. Moreover, drugs used to treat mood disorder interact with clock genes. Chronic treatment with fluoxetine increases expression of

CLOCK and BMAL1 in the hippocampus [25], lithium salts inhibit GSK3-β expression [26] and lengthen the circadian period in several animal species and in humans [27], and valproate alters the expression of several circadian genes in the amygdala [28].

Preliminary association studies found positive results and suggested that seasonal affective disorder is associated with single nucleotide polymorphisms (SNPs) in Per2 and Npas2 [29]. An analysis of 46 SNPs in eight clock genes revealed a significant association of BMAL1 and TIM with bipolar disorder [14]. An independent study using haplotype analysis seems to confirm the association of bipolar disorder with BMAL1 and found a new association with PER3 [30].

Single gene polymorphims: PER3

The coding region of PER3 gene contains a variable-number tandem-repeat (VNTR) polymorphism in which a motif encoding 18 amino acids is repeated either four (Per3^4) or five times (Per3^5). These repeated units contain a cluster of putative phosphorylation sites, and this polymorphism can then influence Per3 function [31]. The polymorphism has been associated with diurnal preference, sleep structure, and sleep homeostasis in healthy subjects; while it influences age at onset in bipolar patients. An earlier age at onset in homozygote carriers of Per3^5 variant was found, while Per3^4 homozygotes showed a later age at onset and heterozygotes an intermediate one [32].

Single gene polymorphims: glycogen synthase kinase 3-β

Glycogen synthase kinase 3-β (GSK3-β) is an essential element of the Wnt/beta-catenin pathway, which is involved in the control of gene expression, cell behavior, cell adhesion, and cell polarity, and plays major roles in neurodevelopment and in the regulation of neuronal plasticity and cell survival. GSK3 is encoded in mammals by two isoforms: GSK3-α and GSK3-β. GSK3-β is the mammalian ortholog of the *Drosophila* gene SHAGGY, an enzyme that exerts a major role in the regulation of the molecular clock [33]. Human GSK3-β maps to 3q21.1 in the human genome, a region that was reported to be linked with bipolar disorder (HLOD in the range 1.2–1.9) [34]. An SNP (−50 T/C) falling in the effective promoter region (nt −171 to +29) of the gene coding for GSK3-β influences the age at onset of bipolar disorder, with homozygotes for the wild variant showing an earlier age at onset than carriers of the mutant allele [35]. Homozygotes for the mutant allele also showed better acute effects of total sleep deprivation treatment [36]. The same polymorphism was found to influence the response to lithium treatment: in a group of bipolar patients −50 C/T mutation improved the recurrence index following lithium administration [37]. Interestingly, in animal models GSK3-β knockout antagonized behavioral abnormalities induced by 5-HT deficiencies [38], thus suggesting the potentially great interest of these mechanisms as a target for antidepressant treatment.

Single gene polymorphisms: CLOCK

CLOCK is an essential positive regulator of the mammalian circadian feedback loop in the SCN. In the 3′ flanking region of the human CLOCK gene, a single nucleotide polymorphism (T to C nucleotide substitution in position 3,111 of the DNA sequence) was identified (rs1801260). Although a statistically significant association of rs1801260 with affective disorders has not been found [39], this polymorphism was shown to influence illness characteristics. The polymorphism influences diurnal preference both in healthy subjects and in depressed patients. Healthy carriers of the 3111C variant show a higher eveningness [40], and a significantly higher evening activity and a delayed sleep onset (mean 79 minutes later) were found in a group of bipolar depressed carriers of the same variant [41]. While C allele carriers increased their activity levels during the second part of the day, T/T homozygotes decreased them [42].

Among patients affected by mood disorders, carriers of the 3111C variant had an increased occurrence of insomnia both lifetime and during their depressive episodes, and showed the persistence of sleep complaints, but not of other symptoms, after successful antidepressant treatment [43, 44].

This effect was unrelated to diurnal mood fluctuations. Moreover, C/C homozygotes experienced a higher lifetime recurrence rate of illness episodes, possibly due to the triggering effect of sleep loss and phase delay on mood episodes [45].

The rs1801260 could also influence neuropsychological performance and blood oxygen level dependent neural responses to a moral valence decision task in patients affected by bipolar depression at functional magnetic resonance imaging (fMRI). During neuropsychological tests and fMRI scanning performed in the afternoon, latencies of response to emotional stimuli were shorter in C allele carriers than in T/T homozygotes, with no difference in response errors and severity of depression between the two groups. Maximal activations were detected in dorsal/posterior cingulate cortex; here C allele carriers showed higher neural responses for positive than negative stimuli, while T/T homozygotes showed an opposite pattern of responses [42]. The posterior cingulate areas where the interaction of genotype and moral valence of the stimuli were detected are known to be involved in moral judgment [46] and in assessment and encoding of self-relevant information [47]. Since in animal models CLOCK is expressed in the cingulate neurons, the differences observed between genotype groups could be due to a direct influence of CLOCK at this molecular level in neurons of the cingulate cortex; to an effect of CLOCK at the level of the SCN "master clock", influencing the reactivity to stimuli in other brain areas; to an effect of CLOCK on monoaminergic dopamine and serotonin projections to cingulate cortex; or to a combination of all these mechanisms. Interestingly, this latter study showed that CLOCK gene variants biased response to a moral valence decision task in the same areas that are influenced by variants of the promoter region of the serotonin transporter [48] and by depressive psychopathology [49], and thus supported the hypothesis that CLOCK genes could then bias "non-clock" functions, such as information processing and decision making, which are at the core of the cognitive dimension of depression and are a major target of antidepressant treatment.

Furthermore, transgenic mice carrying a mutation in the CLOCK gene showed a mania-like behavior, which normalized after chronic administration of lithium. These abnormal behaviors could be normalized by expressing a functional CLOCK protein via viral-mediated gene transfer specifically into the ventral tegmental area of mutant mice [50]. This

25

experiment further sustained the hypothesis of an involvement of CLOCK gene variants in genesis of mood disorders characteristics, and supported a major role for dopaminergic neurotransmission in mediating the effects of CLOCK on behavior. Interestingly, the behavioral effects of sleep deprivation in rodents provide an animal model of mania with face, construct, and predictive validity, with the behavioral activation following a dose–response curve based on length of treatment, and a time–response curve with progressive sensitization to the effects of repeated sleep deprivation [51], and, again, these effects are antagonized by lithium and antidopaminergic substances [52].

Altogether, these data then suggest that clock genes exert their role on human psychopathology by closely interacting with the rhythmic activity of brain neurotransmitter systems.

Future developments: the clock machinery as a target for the treatment of mental illness

The biological master clock in the SCN and the control of biological rhythms are emerging targets for antidepressant drug treatment [53]. Given that monoaminergic input is able to influence the circadian functioning of the molecular machinery of the clock, and that the very scarce evidence available sustains the hypothesis that existing antidepressant drugs can modify its functioning as well [54], it is possible that modifications of the biological rhythms could be a yet unexplored and only partially exploited component of the mechanism of action of many active treatments for depression [20].

The term of "psychiatric chronotherapeutics" has been introduced to indicate the controlled exposure to environmental stimuli that act on biological rhythms in order to achieve therapeutic effects in the treatment of psychiatric conditions [19]. It refers to non-pharmacological and biologically based clinical interventions including sleep deprivation or wake therapy, sleep phase advance, light and dark therapy [20], which evolved both from empirical observation of impressive clinical changes following random exposure to environmental stimuli and from neurobiological models of behavior and are now part of the state-of-the-art treatment options for mood disorders [55]. Sleep deprivation directly targets the sleep–wake

rhythm and can influence SCN function by modifying vigilance state transitions and sleep states [56], is clinically synergistic with the administration of light therapy in the morning, which is the main environmental synchronizer of the internal clock [57], and could then have these effects as part of its mechanism of action. The only clinical study on this topic reported a correlation between positive antidepressant response to sleep deprivation and actimetric advance of the activity–rest circadian cycle [58]. Very interestingly, a preclinical study showed that fluoxetine produced robust phase advances of unit firing of SCN neurons maintained in slice culture [54], thus suggesting that effective chronotherapeutic and pharmacological antidepressant interventions could share similar effects on the biological clock.

The main hypothesis is that internal timing could be a key to mental health, but sound basic research is still needed to get a full mechanistic account of the clock's role in mental health [59]. Very interesting recent technical advances allow us to quantitate alterations in the period length of the endogenous human circadian oscillator by studying cultured fibroblast cells [2]. These pivotal studies showed (1) that the individual behavioral phenotypes result from interactions between the clock gene machinery and cellular components that affect period length, amplitude, and phase of the circadian oscillator, and (2) that the molecular basis of the individual chronotype and rhythms of activity can be studied and described with the methods of molecular biology. This approach, which has been exploited in normal subjects only, will probably be able to provide a molecular basis for the proposed link between sleep, temperature, hormone and mood changes in depression, and disturbances in circadian-related processes, thus leading to the identification of new therapeutic targets and new effective treatments [60].

References

1. Lowrey PL, Takahashi JS. Genetics of the mammalian circadian system: photic entrainment, circadian pacemaker mechanisms, and posttranslational regulation. *Annu Rev Genet.* 2000;**34**:533–62.

2. Brown SA, Kunz D, Dumas A, *et al.* Molecular insights into human daily behavior. *Proc Natl Acad Sci USA.* 2008;**105**(5):1602–7.

3. Fahndrich E. Biological predictors of success of antidepressant drug therapy. *Psychiatr Dev.* 1987;**5**(2):151–71.

4. Wehr TA. A 'clock for all seasons' in the human brain. *Prog Brain Res.* 1996;**111**:321–42.

5. Moore RY, Silver R. Suprachiasmatic nucleus organization. *Chronobiol Int.* 1998;**15**(5):475–87.

6. Moore RY, Lenn NJ. A retinohypothalamic projection in the rat. *J Comp Neurol.* 1972;**146**(1):1–14.

7. Stratmann M, Schibler U. Properties, entrainment, and physiological functions of mammalian peripheral oscillators. *J Biol Rhythms.* 2006;**21**(6):494–506.

8. von Schantz M. Phenotypic effects of genetic variability in human clock genes on circadian and sleep parameters. *J Genet.* 2008;**87**(5):513–9.

9. Abe H, Honma S, Namihira M, *et al.* Clock gene expressions in the suprachiasmatic nucleus and other areas of the brain during rhythm splitting in CS mice. *Brain Res Mol Brain Res.* 2001;**87**(1):92–9.

10. Kondratov RV, Shamanna RK, Kondratova AA, Gorbacheva VY, Antoch MP. Dual role of the CLOCK/BMAL1 circadian complex in transcriptional regulation. *FASEB J.* 2006;**20**(3):530–2.

11. Yuan Q, Lin F, Zheng X, Sehgal A. Serotonin modulates circadian entrainment in *Drosophila*. *Neuron.* 2005;**47**(1):115–27.

12. McClung CA, Sidiropoulou K, Vitaterna M, *et al.* Regulation of dopaminergic transmission and cocaine reward by the Clock gene. *Proc Natl Acad Sci USA.* 2005;**102**(26):9377–81.

13. Spanagel R, Pendyala G, Abarca C, *et al.* The clock gene Per2 influences the glutamatergic system and modulates alcohol consumption. *Nat Med.* 2005;**11**(1):35–42.

14. Mansour HA, Wood J, Logue T, *et al.* Association study of eight circadian genes with bipolar I disorder, schizoaffective disorder and schizophrenia. *Genes Brain Behav.* 2006;**5**(2):150–7.

15. Mendlewicz J, Linkowski P, Kerkhofs M, *et al.* Diurnal hypersecretion of growth hormone in depression. *J Clin Endocrinol Metab.* 1985;**60**(3):505–12.

16. Linkowski P, Mendlewicz J, Leclercq R, *et al.* The 24-hour profile of adrenocorticotropin and cortisol in major depressive illness. *J Clin Endocrinol Metab.* 1985;**61**(3):429–38.

17. Wirz-Justice A. Diurnal variation of depressive symptoms. *Dialogues Clin Neurosci.* 2008;**10**(3):337–43.

18. Reinink E, Bouhuys N, Wirz-Justice A, van den Hoofdakker R. Prediction of the antidepressant response to total sleep deprivation by diurnal variation of mood. *Psychiatry Res.* 1990;**32**(2):113–24.

19. Wirz-Justice A, Benedetti F, Berger M, *et al.* Chronotherapeutics (light and wake therapy) in affective disorders. *Psychol Med.* 2005;**35**(7):939–44.

20. Benedetti F, Barbini B, Colombo C, Smeraldi E. Chronotherapeutics in a psychiatric ward. *Sleep Med Rev.* 2007;**11**(6):509–22.

21. Kafka MS, Wirz-Justice A, Naber D, Moore RY, Benedito MA. Circadian rhythms in rat brain neurotransmitter receptors. *Fed Proc.* 1983;**42**(11):2796–801.

22. Wesemann W, Weiner N. Circadian rhythm of serotonin binding in rat brain. *Prog Neurobiol.* 1990;**35**(6):405–28.

23. Shieh KR, Chu YS, Pan JT. Circadian change of dopaminergic neuron activity: effects of constant light and melatonin. *Neuroreport.* 1997;**8**(9–10):2283–7.

24. Castaneda TR, de Prado BM, Prieto D, Mora F. Circadian rhythms of dopamine, glutamate and GABA in the striatum and nucleus accumbens of the awake rat: modulation by light. *J Pineal Res.* 2004;**36**(3):177–85.

25. Manev H, Uz T. Clock genes: influencing and being influenced by psychoactive drugs. *Trends Pharmacol Sci.* 2006;**27**(4):186–9.

26. Rowe MK, Wiest C, Chuang DM. GSK-3 is a viable potential target for therapeutic intervention in bipolar disorder. *Neurosci Biobehav Rev.* 2007;**31**(6):920–31.

27. Klemfuss H. Rhythms and the pharmacology of lithium. *Pharmacology.* 1992;**56**:53–78.

28. Ogden CA, Rich ME, Schork NJ, *et al.* Candidate genes, pathways and mechanisms for bipolar (manic-depressive) and related disorders: an expanded convergent functional genomics approach. *Mol Psychiatry.* 2004;**9**(11):1007–29.

29. Partonen T, Treutlein J, Alpman A, *et al.* Three circadian clock genes Per2, Arntl, and Npas2 contribute to winter depression. *Ann Med.* 2007;**39**(3):229–38.

30. Nievergelt CM, Kripke DF, Barrett TB, *et al.* Suggestive evidence for association of the circadian genes PERIOD3 and ARNTL with bipolar disorder. *Am J Med Genet B Neuropsychiatr Genet.* 2006;**141B**(3):234–41.

31. Ebisawa T, Uchiyama M, Kajimura N, *et al.* Association of structural polymorphisms in the human period3 gene with delayed sleep phase syndrome. *EMBO Rep.* 2001;**2**(4):342–6.

32. Benedetti F, Dallaspezia S, Colombo C, *et al.* A length polymorphism in the circadian clock gene Per3 influences age at onset of bipolar disorder. *Neurosci Lett.* 2008;**445**(2):184–7.

33. Martinek S, Inonog S, Manoukian AS, Young MW. A role for the segment polarity gene shaggy/GSK-3 in the *Drosophila* circadian clock. *Cell.* 2001;**105**(6):769–79.

34. Badenhop RF, Moses MJ, Scimone A, *et al.* A genome screen of 13 bipolar affective disorder pedigrees

27

Section 1: Basic science

provides evidence for susceptibility loci on chromosome 3 as well as chromosomes 9, 13 and 19. Mol Psychiatry. 2002;7(8):851–9.

35. Benedetti F, Bernasconi A, Lorenzi C, et al. A single nucleotide polymorphism in glycogen synthase kinase 3-beta promoter gene influences onset of illness in patients affected by bipolar disorder. Neurosci Lett. 2004;355(1–2):37–40.

36. Benedetti F, Serretti A, Colombo C, et al. A glycogen synthase kinase 3-beta promoter gene single nucleotide polymorphism is associated with age at onset and response to total sleep deprivation in bipolar depression. Neurosci Lett. 2004;368(2):123–6.

37. Benedetti F, Serretti A, Pontiggia A, et al. Long-term response to lithium salts in bipolar illness is influenced by the glycogen synthase kinase 3-beta -50 T/C SNP. Neurosci Lett. 2005;376(1):51–5.

38. Beaulieu JM, Zhang X, Rodriguiz RM, et al. Role of GSK3 beta in behavioral abnormalities induced by serotonin deficiency. Proc Natl Acad Sci USA. 2008;105(4):1333–8.

39. Bailer U, Wiesegger G, Leisch F, et al. No association of clock gene T3111C polymorphism and affective disorders. Eur Neuropsychopharmacol. 2005;15(1):51–5.

40. Katzenberg D, Young T, Finn L, et al. A CLOCK polymorphism associated with human diurnal preference. Sleep. 1998;21(6):569–76.

41. Benedetti F, Dallaspezia S, Cigala Fulgosi M, et al. Actimetric evidence that CLOCK 3111 T/C SNP influences depressive insomnia and activity patterns in bipolar depression. Am J Med Genet B Neuropsychiatr Genet. 2007;144(5):631–5.

42. Benedetti F, Radaelli D, Bernasconi A, et al. Clock genes beyond the clock: CLOCK genotype biases neural correlates of moral valence decision in depressed patients. Genes Brain Behav. 2008;7:20–5.

43. Serretti A, Benedetti F, Mandelli L, et al. Genetic dissection of psychopathological symptoms: insomnia in mood disorders and CLOCK gene polymorphism. Am J Med Genet. 2003;121B(1):39–43.

44. Serretti A, Cusin C, Benedetti F, et al. Insomnia improvement during antidepressant treatment and CLOCK gene polymorphism. Am J Med Genet B Neuropsychiatr Genet. 2005;10:10.

45. Benedetti F, Serretti A, Colombo C, et al. Influence of CLOCK gene polymorphism on circadian mood fluctuation and illness recurrence in bipolar depression. Am J Med Genet. 2003;123B(1):23–6.

46. Greene JD, Sommerville RB, Nystrom LE, Darley JM, Cohen JD. An fMRI investigation of emotional engagement in moral judgment. Science. 2001;293(5537):2105–8.

47. Vogt BA. Pain and emotion interactions in subregions of the cingulate gyrus. Nat Rev Neurosci. 2005;6(7):533–44.

48. Benedetti F, Bernasconi A, Blasi V, et al. Neural and genetic correlates of antidepressant response to sleep deprivation: a functional magnetic resonance imaging study of moral valence decision in bipolar depression. Arch Gen Psychiatry. 2007;64(2):179–87.

49. Elliott R, Rubinsztein JS, Sahakian BJ, Dolan RJ. The neural basis of mood-congruent processing biases in depression. Arch Gen Psychiatry. 2002;59(7):597–604.

50. Roybal K, Theobold D, Graham A, et al. Mania-like behavior induced by disruption of CLOCK. Proc Natl Acad Sci USA. 2007;104(15):6406–11.

51. Benedetti F, Fresi F, Maccioni P, Smeraldi E. Behavioural sensitization to repeated sleep deprivation in a mice model of mania. Behav Brain Res. 2008;187(2):221–7.

52. Gessa GL, Pani L, Fadda P, Fratta W. Sleep deprivation in the rat: an animal model of mania. Eur Neuropsychopharmacol. 1995;5 Suppl:89–93.

53. Sprouse J. Pharmacological modulation of circadian rhythms: a new drug target in psychotherapeutics. Expert Opin Ther Targets. 2004;8(1):25–38.

54. Sprouse J, Braselton J, Reynolds L. Fluoxetine modulates the circadian biological clock via phase advances of suprachiasmatic nucleus neuronal firing. Biol Psychiatry. 2006;60(8):896–9.

55. Wirz-Justice A, Benedetti F, Terman M. Chronotherapeutics for Affective Disorders. A Clinician's Manual for Light and Wake Therapy. (Basel: Karger, 2009).

56. Deboer T, Vansteensel MJ, Detari L, Meijer JH. Sleep states alter activity of suprachiasmatic nucleus neurons. Nat Neurosci. 2003;6(10):1086–90.

57. Benedetti F, Barbini B, Fulgosi MC, et al. Combined total sleep deprivation and light therapy in the treatment of drug-resistant bipolar depression: acute response and long-term remission rates. J Clin Psychiatry. 2005;66(12):1535–40.

58. Benedetti F, Dallaspezia S, Fulgosi MC, et al. Phase advance is an actimetric correlate of antidepressant response to sleep deprivation and light therapy in bipolar depression. Chronobiol Int. 2007;24(5):921–37.

59. Bhattacharjee Y. Psychiatric research. Is internal timing key to mental health? Science. 2007;317(5844):1488–90.

60. Bunney JN, Potkin SG. Circadian abnormalities, molecular clock genes and chronobiological treatments in depression. Br Med Bull. 2008;86:23–32.

28

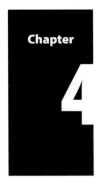

Neurochemistry and neurophysiology of sleep abnormalities associated with depression

Christopher Michael Sinton and Robert W. McCarley

Abstract

Major depressive disorder (MDD) is associated with well characterized sleep abnormalities. The differences in rapid eye movement (REM) sleep that are observed in the depressed patient can be related to an imbalance between monoaminergic and cholinergic systems, a difference that could therefore underlie the neurochemical basis of the disorder. The sleep disruption that is typically present in MDD has recently been identified as a possible causative factor for the cellular and synaptic changes in brain morphology that are seen in depression, so providing additional insight and potential new treatments. Bodyweight dysregulation also occurs in MDD in conjunction and correlated with the differences in sleep, implying fundamental changes in the control of energy balance. This has led to revised hypotheses about the etiology of depression to implicate two hypothalamic neuropeptides, orexin (i.e., hypocretin) and melanin-concentrating hormone (MCH). These neuropeptides are important for the regulation of metabolic status and also are now known to influence sleep, especially REM sleep. Although speculative, data from rodent sleep and behavioral studies, anatomy, molecular genetics, and initial clinical trials of an MCH receptor antagonist converge to link differences in MCH activity with depression.

Sleep abnormalities in depression

Mood disorders and disorders of sleep are seemingly inextricably linked; indeed it has been known since antiquity that depression is often accompanied by insomnia [1]. Not only is the overlap in the patient populations with these disorders considerable, since about 90% of patients with major depressive disorder show some sleep abnormality [2], but there is also evidence that sleep is most affected in the severest cases of depression [3]. This relationship between sleep and depression may eventually prove to be important for an understanding of the neuropathology of MDD. Here we focus on the neurochemistry of sleep and wakefulness to interpret the sleep abnormalities that accompany MDD in terms of possible causative neurochemical differences. Although the exact neuropathology in mood disorders remains unknown, the potential neurochemical imbalances in these patients as revealed by dysregulated sleep could provide insight into the pathophysiology of the disorder.

Abnormal sleep in depressed patients has been characterized over many years from polysomnographic studies in the sleep laboratory. These data are based primarily on recordings of the electroencephalogram (EEG), the electrooculogram (EOG), and the electromyogram (EMG). Summarized briefly, the EEG in the human shows, during wakefulness, a high-frequency, low-amplitude signal that is gradually replaced by lower frequencies and higher amplitudes as non-rapid eye movement (NREM) sleep progresses. As the depth of NREM sleep increases, the frequencies in the EEG signal become slower, and their amplitude progressively higher. NREM sleep can be subdivided into Stages 1 through 4, based on the degree of this slowing, especially in the 0.5–4.0 Hz range (i.e., the delta frequency range). Slow-wave sleep (SWS) is synonymous with Stages 3 and 4, when delta frequencies predominate. Periodically, NREM sleep is interrupted by periods of REM sleep when the EEG is almost indistinguishable from that recorded during wakefulness. Electroencephalogram signals are in fact so similar that reference must

Sleep and Mental Illness, eds. S. R. Pandi-Perumal and M. Kramer. Published by Cambridge University Press.
© Cambridge University Press 2010.

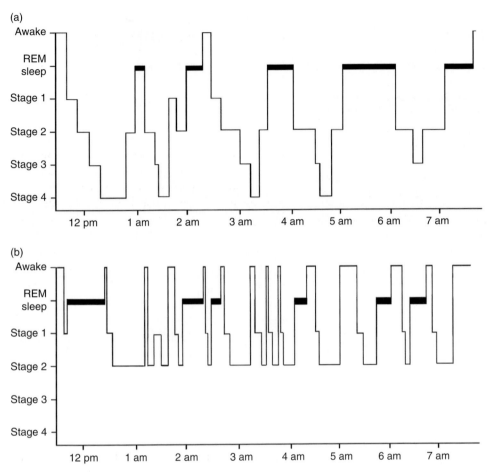

Figure 4.1 Typical all night hypnograms derived from the polygraphic recordings of (a) a healthy young adult, and (b) a depressed patient. In the normal subject, note the cyclical alternation between NREM and REM sleep, the preponderance of Stage 3 and 4 NREM sleep (i.e., SWS) earlier in the night and that of REM sleep towards morning. In contrast, the depressed patient exhibits a shortened first REM sleep latency (i.e., the time from sleep onset to the first period of REM sleep) and an increased duration of the first REM sleep episode. These REM sleep differences are combined with a notable loss of SWS, and decreased total sleep time and sleep efficiency. The latter are due both to fragmented sleep and early morning awakening.

be made to muscle activity (EMG) and eye movements (EOG) to enable REM sleep to be distinguished reliably from wakefulness. Both wakefulness and REM sleep are thus marked by an activated or aroused forebrain (for more detail see McCarley [4]) but can be differentiated by the muscle atonia and rapid eye movements that are observed during REM sleep. Over the course of a night, this cyclical change from NREM to REM sleep, which lasts about 90 minutes in the normal adult, is repeated several times. The depth of NREM sleep is greater during those cycles that occur early in the night, whereas the time spent in REM sleep is increased in the later cycles (Figure 4.1a).

The sleep abnormalities that accompany depression can most effectively be grouped into three categories, namely those that involve REM sleep, those that affect deep SWS, and those that affect the duration and overall continuity of sleep during the night (Figure 4.1b).

REM sleep abnormalities

The interval, or latency, between sleep onset and the beginning of the first REM sleep period is typically reduced in MDD. The average REM sleep latency in normal adults is 65–80 minutes, but is usually 40–50 minutes in depressed patients, and this is often combined with a prolonged duration for the first REM sleep period. Furthermore, some patients exhibit a greater number of rapid eye movements per unit time (i.e., an increased "REM density"), especially during the first REM sleep episode. The REM density and the REM sleep episode durations may also be increased in other early night bouts of REM sleep in addition to the first. Hence the depressed patient shows more REM sleep in the first half of the night when compared with normal controls. Several studies have suggested that these REM sleep abnormalities can persist beyond the stage of clinical recovery from the disorder [5, 6].

In summary, REM sleep abnormalities in MDD show that there is an increased propensity for this stage of sleep in these patients combined with a greater intensity of REM sleep. These differences could result either from an enhancement in the processes that generate REM sleep, or a reduced influence of the processes that normally inhibit the appearance of REM sleep after sleep onset. The fact that these REM sleep characteristics can frequently remain after clinical recovery suggests that they reflect the susceptibility to depression (i.e., a trait marker) rather than a state marker of the disorder.

Slow-wave sleep abnormalities

Most MDD patients also exhibit a marked reduction in the time spent in Stages 3 and 4 (SWS), or delta sleep. This is especially important during the first NREM sleep episode, or the period between sleep onset and the first REM sleep episode, which is a time when delta sleep is normally at a maximum (see Figure 4.1). Frequency analysis of the EEG also shows a reduced power in the delta bandwidth in these patients [7]. Conversely, there is an increase in the time spent in light (Stage 1) NREM sleep in depression.

Importantly, SWS abnormalities in depression divide patients into two groups. The first group comprises those patients who show the pattern of reduced SWS described above. These patients are also usually hypophagic and exhibit weight loss, and especially among those who are older, agitated, or psychotic, frequently complain of insomnia as a result of early morning awakening [8]. In contrast, there is a smaller group of about 10 to 15% of depressed patients, described as atypical depressives, who do not exhibit reduced SWS. In fact they sleep excessively, especially

those who are younger, lethargic, and bipolar, and they are also hyperphagic and exhibit weight gain. Another mood disorder, recurrent seasonal affective disorder, is frequently associated with hypersomnia [9].

Disturbances in the continuity of sleep

Sleep architecture is profoundly changed by the presence of depression and all stages of NREM sleep can be affected. In fact, the association of insomnia with MDD, which has long been recognized, has been extended to a prospective study in which patients with insomnia were found to be at a higher risk of developing depression at a one-year follow-up interval [10]. Insomnia, however, is neither as specific nor as sensitive an indicator of MDD as the REM sleep and SWS abnormalities [2]. The disturbances of sleep typically found in depressed patients include reductions in both total sleep time and sleep efficiency [3]. The causes include difficulty in falling asleep, early morning awakenings, and/or increased fragmentation of sleep resulting from nocturnal awakenings (Figure 4.1b).

Disturbances in sleep continuity and SWS as well as hypersomnia are primarily state markers for depression, i.e., they are not typically present when the disorder is in clinical remission.

Fatigue and sleepiness are frequently observed in depressed patients and fatigue can even be a prodromal symptom [11]. In addition to the hypersomnia associated with atypical depression, daytime sleepiness can result from the disturbed continuity of sleep. In fact, fatigue, especially severe, can be a symptom of the disorder. Following treatment that ameliorates depression, continuing complaints of fatigue and sleepiness can be particularly difficult to treat in these patients, and this has led to the use of adjunctive drug treatments (e.g., Fava and collaborators [12]).

Neurochemical changes associated with sleep and wakefulness

A brief synopsis of those aspects of the neurochemical mechanisms of sleep and wakefulness that are relevant to depression are reviewed here. The interested reader is referred to recent reviews for a more complete presentation of this information [13, 14].

Wakefulness

Wakefulness is supported by several, apparently redundant, excitatory neurotransmitter pathways: none of

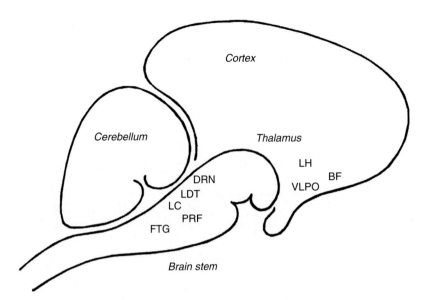

Figure 4.2 A schematic of a sagittal section of a mammalian brain to indicate the locations of the principal brain areas that are mentioned in the text. LH, lateral hypothalamus; BF, basal forebrain; DRN, dorsal raphe nucleus; FTG, gigantocellular tegmental field; LC, locus coeruleus; LDT, laterodorsal tegmentum; PRF, pontine reticular formation; VLPO, ventrolateral preoptic area.

these, which include acetylcholine (ACh) and the monoamines (e.g., norepinephrine, NE), is required for the expression of wakefulness, but all contribute [15]. These neurotransmitters send an excitatory innervation to forebrain centers in the thalamus and cortex to depolarize thalamic and cortical neurons and so induce cortical arousal on the EEG. Wakefulness is thus the result of arousing input from these neurotransmitter pathways at forebrain levels and, conversely, NREM sleep is the absence of such input.

Figure 4.2 displays a schematic of the location of brain centers important for sleep and wakefulness. Acetylcholine-containing cells in the brain stem are localized to the laterodorsal tegmentum and pedunculopontine tegmentum (LDT/PPT) region. These cholinergic neurons project to the thalamus, and they are active whenever the EEG is desynchronized. Conversely, they have a low discharge rate during NREM sleep [16]. A second important cholinergic ascending pathway originates in the substantia inominata and nucleus basalis of the Meynert of the basal forebrain (BF) and sends widespread projections directly to the cortex. There is also a BF cholinergic innervation of the thalamus, particularly the nucleus reticularis. Like LDT/PPT neurons, most BF neurons show an increased discharge rate when the EEG is desynchronized (see Jones [17] for a review) in either wakefulness or REM sleep.

The ascending monoaminergic projections include those that contain NE and serotonin (5-hydroxytryptamine, 5-HT), originating, respectively, in the locus coeruleus (LC) and the raphe nuclei (e.g., the dorsal raphe nucleus, DRN). These neurons also influence EEG activation and wakefulness [18], and project widely throughout the forebrain, including the thalamus and cortex, and exhibit highly significant state-related changes in discharge rates, being highest in wakefulness, decreasing during NREM sleep, and becoming virtually quiescent during REM sleep [19, 20]. This pattern of discharge is therefore an important distinction from that of the two major ascending cholinergic systems, which discharge in correlation with an activated EEG.

NREM sleep

Sleep begins when excitatory drive from the activating neurotransmitters to the forebrain is reduced. As sleep deepens, the state is increasingly characterized by a low-frequency, synchronized EEG and subsequently by the appearance of high-voltage, slow-wave delta activity. Confirmation of the role of the reduction in cholinergic and monoaminergic forebrain innervation in these EEG changes has been obtained from both in vitro and in vivo electrophysiological studies of thalamic and cortical cells [21]. Summarized briefly, thalamocortical cellular activity exhibits a rapid single spike discharge mode during wakefulness (i.e., when the cells are depolarized). Then, during drowsiness and NREM sleep, as the excitatory drive diminishes and depolarization is replaced by relative hyperpolarization, the activity of these cells becomes dominated by rhythmic synchronized oscillations that are in turn transmitted to become network oscillations in the cortex. As sleep progresses, the frequency of these oscillations continues to decline, and more cortical cells are recruited. This change in the discharge pattern in thalamic and cortical cells, which is the basis for the EEG observed in wakefulness and NREM sleep, can be replicated in the in vitro preparation by application or removal, respectively, of ACh or monoamines.

Data support the hypothesis that an increase in extracellular adenosine in the BF during wakefulness inhibits the group of BF wake–active neurons, including those that contain ACh, and so promotes sleepiness [22–24]. This increase in adenosine is an important mechanism of the homeostatic sleep drive, and may result from a decrease in high-energy adenosine triphosphate with a consequent increase in adenosine.

REM sleep

Following a period of NREM sleep, the normal progression is to REM sleep. As noted above, monoaminergic cells become quiescent during REM sleep and their discharge rate falls to zero, i.e., they can be described as "REM-off" cells. One inhibitory influence that reduces the discharge rate of the monoaminergic cells during sleep originates from a group of sleep-active neurons in the ventrolateral preoptic area (VLPO). These neurons, which contain the inhibitory neurotransmitters, γ-amino butyric acid (GABA) and/or galanin [25], first become active with the onset of NREM sleep. This process then continues into REM sleep when neighboring cells, comprising an area known as the extended VLPO [26], are also recruited. Cells in the extended VLPO are thus at least in part responsible for the enhanced inhibition of the brainstem monoaminergic nuclei during REM sleep. The VLPO is important for integrating a "sleepiness" signal and beginning the process of sleep and then of REM sleep, but there are other significant inhibitory GABAergic influences on the monoaminergic nuclei during REM sleep. These are known to be both local interneurons as well as pathways that originate from the pontine reticular formation (PRF) [27]. These

GABAergic influences are important for the mutual interaction between pontine cholinergic and mono-aminergic cell populations during REM sleep that is discussed below.

This quiescence in monoaminergic cell discharge rate is critical for the expression of REM sleep. As monoaminergic influence decreases, a group of brainstem LDT/PPT cholinergic neurons, which are not active during wakefulness, become disinhibited [28]. In fact, 5-HT specifically inhibits this group of REM-active LDT/PPT neurons but has no effect on neighboring LDT/PPT neurons that are active during both wakefulness and REM sleep [29]. The LDT/PPT cholinergic cells that are active only during REM sleep are described as "REM-on" cells. They project caudally to several populations of cells in the PRF to release the various pontine-generated REM sleep components, such as rapid eye movements and muscle atonia. Other LDT/PPT cholinergic cells act during REM sleep to promote forebrain arousal, as they do during wakefulness. The first evidence to implicate LDT/PPT cholinergic neurons in the executive control of REM sleep came from anatomical studies (see McCarley [4] for a review). Direct projections were found from the LDT/PPT to those areas of the PRF in which local injections of cholinomimetics had been shown to be most effective in producing an REM-like state. Furthermore, lesions and electrical stimulation of the LDT/PPT produced, respectively, a decrease and an increase in REM sleep. Direct in vivo measurements of ACh also demonstrated that pontine levels of this neurotransmitter were higher during REM sleep.

However, a recent anatomical study has extended the concept of populations of REM-off and REM-on cells [30]. This work was based on data showing that lesions of the cholinergic or monoaminergic cell populations per se are not sufficient to make major differences in the duration of REM sleep. This suggested that although these neurotransmitters play a role in the executive control, and also possibly in the function of REM sleep, other neurons must be primarily responsible for the onset and offset of the state. Lu and colleagues [30] thus identified more extensive regions of REM-off and REM-on cells that, when lesioned, had a significant impact on the time spent in REM sleep. Both the REM-off and REM-on regions contain populations of GABA-containing neurons that send projections to the other region. The two populations are thus in a mutually inhibitory arrangement that reinforces any change in discharge rate to ensure a rapid switch at the beginning and end of an episode of REM sleep. Described briefly, the REM-off region extends laterally from the dorsal raphe into the lateral pontine tegmentum, and the REM-on region, in the area of the subcoeruleus, lies ventral of the fourth ventricle and lateral to the LDT. They can thus be considered as extensions of the cholinergic and monoaminergic cell fields, more precisely defined but possibly inclusive of the PRF and local GABA influences in the REM-on area that had previously been identified [27]. These results are important to the present discussion because they demonstrate that REM sleep bout length is influenced by GABA-containing cells over a large area of the mesopontine tegmentum, a concept that is relevant below.

The reciprocal interaction model of REM sleep control

We have noted that the expression of REM sleep is potentially dependent on the mutually inverse discharge activities of groups of neurons, particularly those that contain ACh and the monoamines. This relationship was more formally described in the reciprocal interaction model, which is a mathematical model of REM sleep control proposed by McCarley and Hobson [31]. The idea for the model came from early electrophysiological data demonstrating that the change in the discharge rate of neurons over the sleep cycle in the LC area was the inverse of that of PRF neurons [32]. This led to a concept of mutually interacting and inhibiting populations of REM-on and REM-off neurons, and thus, in developing the model, McCarley and Hobson [31] adapted equations that had originally been derived for predator–prey interactions (Figure 4.3). Several aspects of the model, especially the mutually inhibitory influence of the two cell populations, were considered controversial for many years. Indeed, when first formulated, the neurochemical identity of the relevant PRF neurons was unknown and at that time they were considered equivalent to neurons in the gigantocellular tegmental field (FTG). The FTG field is now considered to largely comprise cells that are not specifically responsive to changes in the sleep cycle. Subsequently the REM-on cells of the model were identified as the subset of the mesopontine cholinergic neurons described above. Furthermore, the REM-off cells in the LC region could only be tentatively identified at

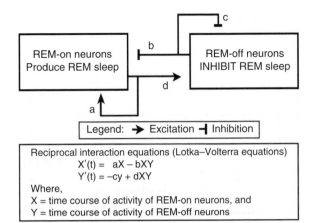

Figure 4.3 A schematic of the circuits that were proposed for the reciprocal interaction model of REM sleep control showing the two populations of neurons, one being REM-off and the other REM-on in a mutually inhibitory/excitatory relationship. The equations on which this model was based (the Lotka–Volterra equations) were first formulated to describe the population numbers in a predator–prey relationship.

that time as being equivalent to NE neurons and in fact it was several years after the model was first formulated before definitive neurochemical identification was possible.

The reciprocal interaction model has therefore been adapted as new results have become available to allow its refinement and improvement. This process began with the neurochemical identification of the relevant cholinergic and monoaminergic cell groups, and the interested reader is referred to a recent review of the history and the current formulation of the model [33]. Data have been accumulated over many years in support of the relevant mechanisms involved. Importantly, and throughout this development, the basic premise of the mutually inverse discharge rates of two neuronal populations has remained unchanged. As an example of supporting data, the inhibition of the REM-on cholinergic neurons by REM-off monoaminergic neurons has only been demonstrated relatively recently. The first studies that showed that 5-HT directly inhibits a subpopulation of LDT/PPT cholinergic neurons [34–36] were conducted in vitro and described the hyperpolarization (i.e., a decrease in discharge rate) of these LDT/PPT cells by 5-HT. This inhibition was found to be particularly reliable for LDT/PPT neurons that fire in bursts, and such burst firing had been shown to be highly correlated with lateral geniculate nucleus ponto–geniculo–occiptal (PGO) waves, another important REM sleep component. Other data indicated

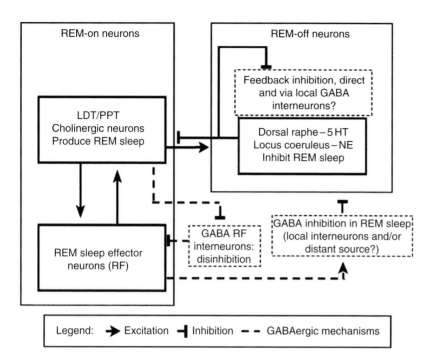

Figure 4.4 The reciprocal interaction model was refined and extended as the limit cycle model, shown in this simplified schematic of some of the anatomical and structural relationships between the REM-off and REM-on neuronal populations. The neurochemical identity of these neuronal populations was identified and the important influence of GABAergic inhibition was recognized. RF = reticular formation. For other abbreviations see text.

that the effect of NE on these LDT/PPT cholinergic neurons was also inhibitory [37]. Moreover, non-cholinergic, presumably GABAergic, interneurons are excited by NE [38]; GABAergic interneurons would act to inhibit cholinergic neurons so providing another mechanism of inhibition of cholinergic LDT/PPT neurons by NE. In fact, continuing in vivo studies have demonstrated that serotonergic and noradrenergic inhibitory control of the LDT/PPT REM sleep-generating region is sufficiently strong to influence the expression of REM sleep [39, 40].

A later important refinement of the model constrained the maximal discharge rate of the REM-off and REM-on neuronal populations and also included a parameter to reflect a circadian influence. These changes, termed the limit cycle model, significantly improved the model [41, 42]. Figure 4.4 is a simplified schematic of this model. Initially a descriptive tool that could demonstrate, for example, how mutually inhibiting neuronal populations might interact, the model became a much closer approximation to the underlying neurophysiology with potential predictive power. Finally, as noted above, recent neurophysiological data are likely to require eventual extension of the model to include other GABA-containing REM-off and REM-on cell fields [14].

Cholinergic–aminergic imbalance in MDD and associated sleep abnormalities

It is evident from the foregoing that a possible explanation for the REM sleep abnormalities observed in depression is a cholinergic–aminergic imbalance, i.e., that the monoaminergic inhibitory influence on the LDT/PPT cholinergic cells is weakened and/or that the cholinergic drive in the PRF is strengthened. Such differences would result in a greater propensity for REM sleep and increased intensity of REM sleep. Evidence has been established from several studies over many years that such an imbalance is likely in depression.

Rodent models, for example, have consistently suggested that differences in cholinergic and/or monoaminergic systems can induce behavioral effects that mimic the symptoms of depression. Thus, the Flinders sensitive line (FSL) of rats, which express an increased number of cholinergic muscarinic receptors, were found to show such behavioral differences as well as to exhibit shorter REM sleep latencies [43, 44], indicating that this marker of depression might also be caused by a cholinergic abnormality. However, FSL rats have increased total REM sleep time, which does not occur in depressed patients [45]. Recently, by using the tail suspension test, which has been validated as revealing antidepressant activity, selective breeding of mice that were more "helpless" in this test created another example of a rodent expressing depressive-like behavior [46]. These mice also show reduced REM sleep latency as well as a lighter and more fragmented sleep pattern, and also behave in a more "depressed" way in other tests such as the forced-swim test. Interestingly, these mice were found to have decreased serotoninergic neuronal activity.

Clinical data also support these preclinical results. For example, Gillin and collaborators found that many MDD patients had increased sensitivity to the induction of REM sleep following infusion of cholinergic agonists [47, 48], suggesting that they may have a primary cholinergic abnormality. In view of the equal importance of monoaminergic and cholinergic systems in the control of REM sleep, however, it is possible that a monoamine deficiency is primarily responsible for the enhanced effectiveness of cholinergic agonists in inducing REM sleep in depressed patients. Alternatively, different subgroups of the disorder, for example the atypical–typical groups, could involve various causative factors to differing degrees. Hence both ACh and/or monoamine abnormalities could be present in mood disorders. Considered overall, however, the evidence points to a more important monoaminergic role as the causative factor in depression in parallel with a similarly more important role in the control of REM sleep [49]. Thus lessened monoaminergic inhibition is more likely to lead to the REM sleep differences observed in MDD.

Monoaminergic abnormalities in depression

A longstanding monoamine theory of depression proposes that a deficiency in monoaminergic activity (NE and/or 5-HT) is responsible for the occurrence of some, if not all, types of depression [50, 51]. The strongest evidence for this thesis comes from the neurochemical action of the current generation of drugs that alleviate MDD. A wide range of drugs with varying mechanisms of action targeting the monoamines is now available to treat depression [52]. Importantly, a delay of about two weeks is needed for their clinical effectiveness to be apparent, and significant neurochemical effects of these compounds in preclinical models also appear gradually over a period that corresponds closely to this delay. For example, it has been known for many years that

almost all clinically effective tricyclic antidepressants (TCAs), including the atypical compounds such as iprindole, which does not inhibit the uptake of monoamines acutely, affect NE and 5-HT receptor binding after chronic administration [53–55]. Furthermore, the functional relevance of these binding data was demonstrated by early electrophysiological studies: chronic, but not acute, administration of TCAs, including the atypical compounds, increases the responsiveness of monoaminergic neurons to monoamines administered directly at the cell body level [56, 57].

Initial insight into the mechanism by which antidepressants acted at the neuronal level came from a study that demonstrated increased 5-HT transmission, but only after two weeks of drug treatment [58]. The compound tested, zimelidine, a selective serotonin reuptake inhibitor (SSRI), first reduced 5-HT transmission because of depolarization blockade but this effect gradually disappeared over the subsequent two weeks of treatment as 5-HT_{1A} autoreceptor desensitization occurred. Subsequent work showed that 5-HT_{1A} autoreceptor desensitization was also apparent in the action of many different types of antidepressant and putative antidepressant drugs. In each case, the increased 5-HT neurotransmission occurred after repeated treatment, though in some instances after only two or three days of treatment, and thus a shorter time course than the usual therapeutic response. Most of these compounds demonstrate affinity for 5-HT receptors and thus have direct effects on 5-HT neurons, making the mechanism of their action on 5-HT_{1A} autoreceptor desensitization and 5-HT neurotransmission understandable. But other antidepressants, most notably bupropion, which shows no significant binding affinity at any 5-HT receptor, also affected 5-HT neurotransmission accompanied by 5-HT_{1A} autoreceptor desensitization. Clearly, the primary excitatory influence from these compounds must be extra-serotoninergic.

Rodent behavioral studies had demonstrated that the effects of bupropion could be inhibited by prazosin, an adrenergic α_1 receptor antagonist [59]. Additionally, the increase in activity of 5-HT neurons after chronic bupropion administration could not be observed in NE-lesioned animals [60]. Since 5-HT neuronal activity can be modulated by NE release in the raphe via an effect at the adrenergic α_1 receptor [61], this led to the hypothesis that bupropion might be altering 5-HT neurotransmission through NE release. Interestingly, a two-week treatment of vagal nerve stimulation, which is used clinically as a treatment for epilepsy but which has also exhibited consistent mood elevating effects, was found to increase 5-HT neuronal activity in the rat [62]. This effect was not associated with 5-HT_{1A} autoreceptor desensitization, however, but occurred through adrenergic α_1 receptor activation. Recent data from an electrophysiological study of the effects of chronic bupropion have now shown that, in addition to 5-HT_{1A} autoreceptor desensitization and increased 5-HT neurotransmission which occurred within a few days of the onset of treatment and then remained for the two-week duration of the study, NE neuronal activity was also changed by the drug [63]. An initial decline in the discharge rate of NE cells gradually recovered over the two-week treatment period and this was accompanied by desensitization of the adrenergic α_2 receptor. However, the net effect of the recovery of NE neuronal activity was to increase 5-HT neurotransmission through NE release and adrenergic α_1 activation in the raphe [63]. Hence in the case of bupropion, and possibly for other antidepressants, a primary effect on NE activation is translated into increased 5-HT neurotransmission.

In summary, the varying mechanisms of action of antidepressant drugs indicate a greater complexity and variety of action than was previously considered. However, the commonality among them remains the increased neurotransmission of NE and/or 5-HT systems. This underlines the continuing importance of the monoamines in the effective treatment of mood disorders. Thus, despite limitations in a simple monoamine deficiency theory of depression, data still point convincingly to the involvement of monoamine systems, albeit at a more sophisticated level of understanding.

Antidepressant drugs and changes in REM sleep

The monoamines are also critical for the regulation of REM sleep and this indicates a possible connection between the mechanisms of REM sleep and the neuropathology of depression. In fact, one of the best predictors of the clinical effectiveness of amitriptyline, a TCA, in the treatment of depressed patients was found to be the prolongation of the short latency to the first REM sleep period [64]. This change to the REM sleep latency occurred as early as ten days prior to a clinical response. Essentially all clinically effective antidepressant treatments, including the TCAs and monoamine oxidase inhibitors (MAOIs), have a marked suppressant effect on REM sleep, and also induce a characteristic REM sleep rebound when they are discontinued [65, 66]. Further support for the link between the mechanisms of REM sleep and depression comes from a preclinical study of REM sleep deprivation [67]. Deprivation of REM sleep improves the symptoms of depression, and with about the same efficacy as TCAs though the effect does not outlast the recovery sleep [68]. Importantly, results from the study by Basheer and colleagues [67] in the rat showed that REM sleep deprivation increased the messenger RNA (mRNA) levels of tyrosine hydoxylase (TH) and the norepinephrine transporter (NET) in the LC. Tricyclic antidepressant treatment also increases TH and NET mRNA in the LC. REM sleep deprivation has also been shown to decrease rat cortical high-affinity binding sites for the antidepressant imipramine [69], with the likely mediating event being the deprivation-induced increased discharge rate of monoaminergic neurons. The commonality of mechanism in the alleviation of mood and REM sleep control systems thus supports the hypothesis that the REM sleep abnormalities in MDD are the result of monoaminergic disturbances.

Predictions from the reciprocal interaction model and REM sleep in depressives

The limit cycle form of the reciprocal interaction model has enabled predictions to be made about the changes in REM sleep that would result from altering the values of various parameters in the model [33, 42]. This work has provided additional insight into the factors that might cause the REM sleep differences that are observed in MDD. For example, the presence of a factor that replicates a circadian influence has provided a way to examine how variations in this and related parameters might affect the REM sleep of depressives. Thus a phase advance in the propensity for REM sleep was found to be insufficient to explain the observed differences in REM sleep in MDD. Importantly, however, the model has shown that a more rapid decline in the activity of the REM-off monoaminergic cell population results in a shorter latency, larger amplitude, and longer episode duration of the first bout of REM sleep. This result therefore replicates to a good approximation the differences in REM sleep that are observed in MDD patients: the larger amplitude of REM sleep produced by the model can be considered equivalent to a greater intensity of REM sleep (i.e., REM density). Furthermore, these changes to REM sleep occur independently of the circadian time of entry into the first REM sleep bout.

These results suggested that the REM sleep abnormalities in MDD patients might be realistically modeled by differences in the discharge activity of the monoaminergic cell population at sleep onset. This finding of a reduced monoaminergic influence is compatible with the neurochemical and neurophysiological differences in MDD patients described above, as well as the normalization of REM sleep abnormalities by antidepressants. Thus both a qualitative review of evidence of the relative importance of the monoaminergic and cholinergic mechanisms in depression and REM sleep [49] and the subsequent quantitative modeling [41, 42, 70] have pointed to the conclusion that the activity of monoaminergic neurons may be less at sleep onset in MDD patients than in normal people.

Summary

Several different lines of evidence converge to suggest that the REM sleep abnormalities that are associated with MDD are the result of an imbalance in the cholinergic–monoaminergic control system. Furthermore, a decreased monoaminergic influence at sleep onset is the most likely explanation for this imbalance. The commonality in the mechanisms of action of the antidepressant drugs is consistent with this viewpoint since they increase the effectiveness of the monoaminergic systems over a time course that is similar to the delay needed for their clinical efficacy.

Morphological and cellular changes associated with depression

Recent work has provided evidence of brain morphometric changes associated with both MDD and animal models of depression. These include changes in cellular and synaptic structure and in neurogenesis, especially in the hippocampus [71, 72]. Importantly, such changes may underlie the cognitive deficits associated with MDD, such as the impairment in attention, memory, and problem solving [73]. Although the mechanisms that result in these structural and morphometric changes in the brains of depressed patients are currently unknown, recent findings suggest that they could be mediated by the sleep disturbances that occur in depression. On the basis of this evidence, we propose that sleep disruption in MDD might be responsible for at least some of these effects. That is, that certain brain structural changes associated with depression are the result of the alterations in sleep observed in this disorder.

In fact, there appears to be a direct relationship between the degree of sleep abnormality and prognosis in depression. For example, abnormalities in the sleep EEG have been found to be associated with the severity of clinical symptoms based on the Hamilton scale [74]. Moreover, there is a correlation between the extent that delta activity is diminished during sleep in MDD and a greater recurrence of the disorder following termination of treatment [75]. This association between decreased delta power and MDD is likely to be particularly significant for future research into the disorder. The known neurobiology of SWS can potentially allow physiological and proteomic measures of the relationship between abnormalities in delta power and the variables altered in both MDD and animal models of depression to be explored.

Evidence from studies of adenosine

As noted above, studies have shown that increasing wakefulness leads to the increased accumulation of BF adenosine, which in turn progressively inhibits the wake-active neurons in this region. The result is greater sleepiness. Interestingly, over prolonged periods of sleep deprivation or restriction, this inhibition is further enhanced by an intracellular cascade of events activated by higher extracellular adenosine concentrations over longer periods [14]. The outcome is amplified transcription and translation of adenosine A1 receptors on wake-active neurons, so effectively "resetting the gain" of this homeostatic system, i.e., inhibition is enhanced for a given level of adenosine. Moreover, BF proteins associated with the cytoskeleton and synapse show quantitative and qualitative changes following sleep deprivation [76], pointing to sleep as a time of synaptic alteration.

Modeling the disrupted sleep of the depressed patient

Sleep interruption (SI) studies in rodents are based on the disruption and fragmentation of sleep so as to restrict delta sleep (i.e., SWS), increase wakefulness,

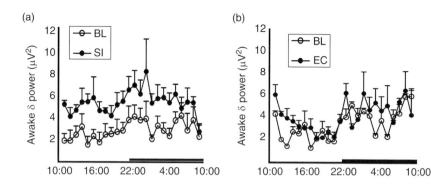

Figure 4.5 Delta power (i.e., the power in the EEG in the 1–4 Hz frequency band) during wakefulness is increased during sleep interruption (SI). Graphs represent the mean (± SEM, N = 5) delta power for each hour during the light and dark phases; the dark phase is marked by the horizontal bar on the time axis. (a) SI resulted in a significant increase in wakefulness delta power compared with the baseline (BL) recording. (b) In contrast, the exercise control (EC) rats exhibited no change in delta power during wakefulness. Data from which this figure is derived have been previously published [77].

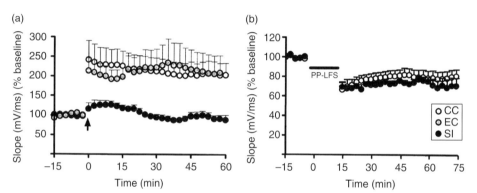

Figure 4.6 Long-term potentiation (LTP) is impaired in hippocampal slices taken from the brains of rats that had been subjected to 24 hours of sleep interruption (SI). Hippocampal synaptic plasticity was examined in rats after SI and compared with rats from the exercise control (EC) and cage control (CC) conditions. (a) Data are averaged and plotted in two-minute bins as mean (+SEM) for N = 6 (SI, EC) and N = 8 (CC) rats. Sleep interruption prevented the appearance of LTP that was observed in both the EC and CC groups. The arrow marks the time at which tetanic stimulation to induce LTP was applied. (b) In contrast, long-term depression (LTD) was unaffected by SI (N = 6) in this comparison with CC (N = 6) rats. Long-term depression was induced by five minutes of paired-pulse low-frequency stimulation (PP-LFS). Data from which this figure is derived have been previously published [77].

and disturb sleep continuity (Figure 4.5). This procedure thus mimics some of the features of sleep in depression without resorting to total sleep deprivation, which, like REM sleep deprivation, actually has antidepressant properties. Hippocampal slices taken from the brains of rats after 24 hours of SI demonstrate a profound depression in long-term potentiation (LTP) [77], an exogenously induced form of synaptic plasticity in this region, and considered a model of learning and memory [78] (see Figure 4.6). This result replicates similar findings reported after total sleep deprivation [79] and REM sleep deprivation [80]. Additionally, using the water maze, a spatial memory task that is dependent on hippocampal

function [81], SI was found to impair acquisition of spatial memory in comparison with control animals. Hippocampal synaptic plasticity has been shown to be sensitive to changes in stress, which can be measured by plasma corticosterone levels. However, plasma corticosterone after SI was elevated to the same extent as that in exercise control (EC) rats that did not show a reduction in LTP (Figure 4.6) [77]. Hence the increase in plasma corticosterone after SI was unlikely to be the cause of the diminished LTP in these animals. The mechanism of SI-induced changes in LTP and learning remains unknown, though increasing adenosine levels in the hippocampus is one possible mechanism. Importantly, with respect to SI as a model of brain morphometric changes linked to fragmented sleep, SI, like other animal models of depression, reduces neurogenesis in the hippocampal dentate gyrus [82]. Most of this effect is not due to increased corticosterone.

Summary

Evidence from a range of different studies indicates that sleep is a time of synaptic change and neuronal plasticity, processes that might themselves be linked to brain adaptation during sleep. Modeling the disrupted sleep of the depressed patient has revealed profound changes to these processes at the hippocampal level in the rat, together with associated behavioral deficits. This model is thus likely to provide a basis for studying potential brain morphometric changes that result from the interrupted sleep of the depressed patient, while avoiding the potential confounding antidepressant effects of either REM sleep or total sleep deprivation.

Depression, the regulation of bodyweight, and sleep

Depression is typically associated with abnormalities in bodyweight. As noted above, depressed patients can be divided into two principal clusters: one group exhibits weight loss that is associated with reduced SWS, but the second group of atypical depressives shows weight gain with increased sleep, including SWS. We have reviewed the evidence for an altered balance between central cholinergic and monoaminergic systems in the disorder (i.e., with relatively increased ACh activity and decreased NE/5-HT activity), and that this imbalance appears sufficient to explain the basis of the accompanying REM sleep abnormalities. Furthermore, increased cholinergic activity may result in decreased delta power during NREM sleep and thus reduced SWS. This would follow from the cholinergically mediated relatively greater depolarization of cortical and thalamic cells during NREM sleep if ACh activity is higher [21]. Although other symptoms associated with the disorder, such as reduced drive or motivation or increased fatigue, could be responsible for bodyweight differences, neurochemical alterations may also underlie this characteristic of MDD.

For example, 5-HT has consistently been linked over many years with differences in food intake and thus an influence on bodyweight [83]. Indeed,

fenfluramine, an SSRI, and sibutramine, a mixed 5-HT and NE reuptake inhibitor, were first recognized as potential anti-obesity agents during their clinical trials as antidepressants [84]. An important locus of this serotoninergic action on energy balance has been identified as being in the hypothalamus, primarily in the region of the paraventricular nuclei (PVN) and the ventromedial hypothalamic nuclei [85], but also in the arcuate nucleus [86]. The interaction between 5-HT and energy balance is complex, however, and the interested reader is referred to a recent review [86]. But summarized briefly, studies of the effect of 5-HT on feeding behavior demonstrate unequivocally that potentiating 5-HT suppresses food intake. Conversely, 5-HT antagonists and compounds that decrease the activity of 5-HT systems enhance food consumption and thus tend to increase bodyweight. However, as noted above, the evidence from the REM sleep abnormalities in depressed patients, and from the mood elevating properties of treatments that enhance 5-HT, suggest that depression is associated with decreased 5-HT activity. Thus any influence of 5-HT on the bodyweight abnormalities observed in MDD would more likely be apparent as a weight gain, assuming similar levels of energy expenditure. This is incompatible with the weight loss seen in most depressed patients. In summary, the bodyweight abnormalities that are evident in depressed patients are unlikely to be explicable in terms of 5-HT differences alone.

The first detailed study of the influence of NE on feeding behavior also identified the PVN as the primary locus of action of this neurotransmitter [87]. Unlike 5-HT, however, increasing NE stimulates food intake. In a series of studies over several years, Leibowitz and her colleagues demonstrated that this noradrenergic stimulatory effect was mediated through the α_2 receptor [88, 89]. They also confirmed that the actions of NE and 5-HT on food intake were primarily localized to the PVN, and in particular, that they could not be elicited from the lateral hypothalamus (LH), another area known to be important for energy balance [90]. Thus, based on the same reasoning applied to 5-HT above, the decreased NE activity associated with depression would result in decreased appetite, and, especially in combination with decreased sleep, could be sufficient to explain the loss of bodyweight in the majority of depressed patients.

Although it is therefore feasible that the loss in weight that accompanies MDD is directly related to an underlying decrease in NE activity, this

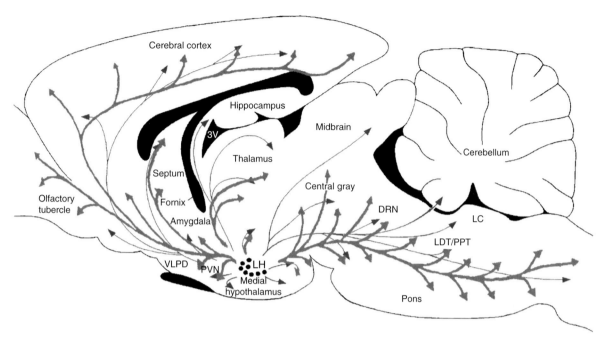

Figure 4.7 This schematic of a sagittal section from a rodent brain displays the overlap and concordance of the projections throughout the neuraxis of the orexin- (thin arrows) and MCH- (thick arrows) containing neurons. Cell bodies for both systems are located primarily in the lateral hypothalamus [130]. For abbreviations see text and the legend for Figure 4.2.

neurotransmitter imbalance appears insufficient to explain the weight gain observed in atypical depression. Furthermore, the monoamines principally affect feeding behavior and have less effect on other aspects of energy balance, in particular metabolic status. The latter is another critical component in the maintenance of bodyweight since it is coupled not only to food intake but also to energy expenditure, for example as activity. Knowledge of the mechanisms of energy balance was recently expanded with the discovery of two hypothalamic neuropeptides, orexin (i.e., hypocretin) and melanin-concentrating hormone (MCH), that are implicated in metabolic status and feeding behavior [91, 92]. Importantly, they also modulate sleep, in particular REM sleep [93, 94]. The neurons containing these neuropeptides project widely throughout the neuraxis (Figure 4.7). Interestingly, the cell bodies of the two systems are independent yet closely intermingled and localized around the perifornical hypothalamus and LH [95, 96]. Their projections also exhibit considerable overlap and innervate many of the areas that are known to be involved in the control of sleep and wakefulness, including the DRN, the LC, and the LPD/PPT region.

Orexin

The LH had been identified as critical for energy balance in early studies in which the area was lesioned to produce a hypophagic syndrome. Thus, when orexin was found uniquely localized to cell bodies in and around the LH, the neuropeptide was initially believed to be involved only in the mechanisms of feeding and metabolic status [92]. The subsequent discovery that the absence of the neuropeptide resulted in narcolepsy, a disabling sleep disorder, was unexpected [93]. The interested reader is referred to extensive reviews of the disorder and potential mechanisms by which the absence of orexin causes narcolepsy (e.g., [97–99]). Importantly, in defining these mechanisms, orexin was found to have excitatory effects in the LC and raphe nuclei as well as on ventral tegmental dopamine neurons, a likely component of reward and motivation circuitry [100, 101]. These results thus implicated orexin in the modulation of systems that control REM sleep and/or have been linked with a defining symptom of depression. In fact, narcolepsy is associated with a highly significant reduction in the latency to REM sleep, to the extent that direct transitions from wakefulness to

REM sleep occur [99]. Since a reduction in REM sleep latency is also an important characteristic of sleep in depression, decreased orexinergic cell activity was hypothesized as a potential factor in the pathogenesis of MDD [102]. Evidence in favor of this hypothesis was obtained. For example, increased orexin levels were noted in the cerebrospinal fluid (CSF) of rats following REM sleep deprivation, providing a potential mechanism by which REM sleep deprivation could enhance mood [103]. Furthermore, when compared with normal controls, the circadian variation of CSF orexin levels of depressed patients is damped, also potentially implicating orexin in mood regulation [102]. However, in this study the average 24-hour level of orexin in CSF was not affected in the patient population, indicating that reduced orexinergic cell activity was unlikely to be causative for the disorder, at least in the small group of patients tested. In another preclinical study, Wistar–Kyoto rats, considered a potential rodent model of depression because of their reduced REM sleep latency, were found to have fewer orexinergic immunoreactive cell bodies in the LH [104].

Tricyclic antidepressants, including imipramine and chlorimipramine, have been used to treat REM sleep abnormalities in narcolepsy for many years, and depression is frequently associated with narcolepsy [105]. Rye and colleagues, for example, reported that a narcoleptic patient with atypical depression was successfully treated with bupropion with the symptoms of both disorders being alleviated by the drug treatment [106]. However, as the authors noted, this study actually supports the differentiation of narcolepsy and depression because the positive effects of the bupropion treatment occurred rapidly without chronic administration. This indicated that the symptoms of depression were likely the result of narcolepsy rather than a separate nosological entity. Furthermore, chronic bupropion treatment did not alter mean CSF orexin levels in the study of damped orexin rhythm noted above, despite effective treatment of the depressive symptoms in these patients [102].

Taken together therefore, these findings provide little support for the hypothesis of a direct relationship between altered orexin functionality and the pathogenesis of MDD, even if many narcoleptics present with the symptoms of depression. In fact, rating of the depression associated with narcolepsy has demonstrated that only about 25% of these patients have mild clinical depression or MDD, making the association less conclusive [107]. Even the shortened REM sleep latency, which first led to the hypothesis of a mechanistic link between depression and narcolepsy, exhibits important differences when examined more closely [108]. For example, the distributions of REM latency are significantly different between the two populations. In narcolepsy there is a bimodal distribution, with REM sleep initiated either immediately following sleep onset or after at least 60 minutes. In contrast, in MDD, REM sleep occurs primarily between 1 and 60 minutes after sleep onset [108].

Another important symptom of narcolepsy, however, is daytime sleepiness, frequently associated with lethargy and fatigue [99]. This is similar to the fatigue and sleepiness seen in depressives and, even if the underlying causative factors are different, both disorders are responsive to wakefulness promoting agents, including psychostimulants and modafinil [11]. Modafinil, in particular, is effective in narcolepsy and is used clinically, although currently off-label, to treat the fatigue and sleepiness that accompanies depression, whether symptomatic of the disorder itself or as a side effect of the antidepressant therapy. For example, several studies have reported that modafinil is effective in alleviating fatigue and excessive sleepiness as an adjunctive therapy with SSRIs in depression [109–111]. Importantly, this extends to significantly improved mood with the combined therapy over that achieved with the SSRI alone, a result which might reflect reduced sleepiness but also could relate to the underlying neuropathology in depression. Unfortunately, despite intense research in recent years and the identification of possible mechanisms of action of modafinil, the relevance of this effect of the drug to the neuropathology of depression remains unknown. Hence the clinical findings with modafinil as an adjunctive treatment do not yet provide additional insight into depression, other than in a negative sense. For example, modafinil does not act through the orexin system [112]. Hence orexin is unlikely to be implicated in the neuropathology of depression as a result of the improvement in depressive symptoms seen with modafinil.

Melanin-concentrating hormone (MCH)

The neuropeptide MCH is expressed in neurons with cell bodies closely intermingled with those that exhibit orexin immunoreactivity in the LH [95]. Melanin-concentrating hormone and orexin are not colocalized

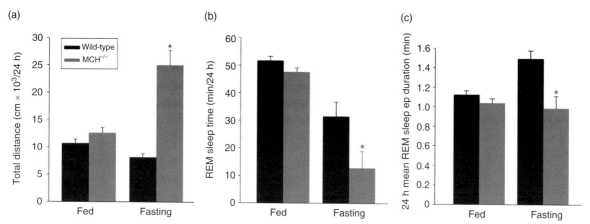

Figure 4.8 $MCH^{-/-}$ mice respond abnormally to fasting when compared with wild-type mice in terms of hyperactivity in an open field and reduction in REM sleep time. Bars represent cumulative totals (mean + SEM) over 24 hours of (a) distance travelled in the open field (cm); (b) total time spent in REM sleep (minutes); (c) mean REM sleep episode duration (minutes). Graphs (b) and (c) demonstrate that wild-type mice adapt to the fasting condition with a smaller reduction in REM sleep time, combined with a partially compensating increase in REM sleep mean bout duration. An asterisk denotes a significant difference between the genotypes. Data from which this figure is derived have been previously published [94].

within the same neurons, however, though their projections show remarkable concordance and overlap throughout the neuraxis (Figure 4.7). The likely importance of MCH in energy homeostasis was identified prior to the discovery of orexin when MCH gene expression was found to be upregulated in the *ob/ob* mouse, a leptin-deficient model that exhibits an obese phenotype [113]. Generation of the MCH knockout ($MCH^{-/-}$) mouse, which is hypophagic and lean, subsequently showed that MCH was important for energy expenditure as well as the initiation of feeding [114]. Interestingly, the $MCH^{-/-}$ mouse was considered behaviorally normal in other respects at the time of its initial characterization and it was only when these mice were tested under fasting conditions that a notable hyperactivity was revealed (Figure 4.8a) [94].

Intracerebroventricular injection of MCH enhances sleep [115], but a specific link between MCH and REM sleep was first indicated by the increased activity of MCH neurons during this state [116]. Subsequently, MCH-1 receptor antagonists were found to decrease sleep, including REM sleep [117], but paradoxically, a mouse with the gene for the MCH-1 receptor deleted expresses increased REM sleep [118]. MCH-1 is the only MCH receptor expressed in the mouse, so in principle the MCH-1 receptor knockout mouse should also have the same phenotype as the $MCH^{-/-}$ mouse. However, that is not the case and the apparent complexity of the

relationship between MCH and REM sleep was revealed by a recent study of the $MCH^{-/-}$ mouse [94]. These mice, when normally fed, expressed essentially the same REM sleep as wild-type mice, both in terms of the total time spent in the state and the distribution and duration of REM sleep bouts. But under conditions of fasting, REM sleep was profoundly reduced in the $MCH^{-/-}$ genotype, an effect that was significantly greater than that observed in wild-type mice both in terms of time spent in the state and bout duration (Figure 4.8b and 4.8c). In contrast, NREM sleep was similarly reduced in both genotypes during fasting. Clearly, $MCH^{-/-}$ mice responded abnormally to fasting: REM sleep was dysregulated and they become hyperactive. Furthermore, this did not reflect a general inability to deal with exogenous stress since these mice responded unexceptionally to sleep deprivation.

In summary, MCH may be implicated in the regulation of sleep, particularly REM sleep, and it also plays a role in energy balance. The combination of these two factors was recently demonstrated unexpectedly during clinical trials of a drug being developed as a potential anti-obesity treatment. In this trial of a novel MCH-1 antagonist (NGD-4715), the compound was administered to healthy, obese subjects under a restricted caloric diet. Under these conditions, half the subjects reported vivid dreams and sleep disturbances, which did not occur when subjects were placed on a high-calorie diet. In fact, the sleep reports from the subjects under caloric restriction are reminiscent of those that are described during REM sleep rebound, or increased need for REM sleep [119, 120]. In the current context we note, possibly coincidentally, that effective antidepressant drugs induce a rebound in REM sleep when they are discontinued.

It is intriguing that MCH has also been shown to affect mood and anxiety in typical rodent models, though these data are conflicting and remain controversial at this time. Anxiolytic effects, for example, have been observed under conditions of both increased and decreased MCH signaling [121, 122]. Furthermore, in another recent study, four different MCH-1 receptor antagonists were examined in the rat forced-swim and mouse tail suspension tests, both measures of learned helplessness and considered valid indicators of potential antidepressant activity [123]. No evidence of antidepressant efficacy was found. In contrast, when C57Bl/6 mice were exposed to chronic mild stress (CMS) for five weeks, MCH-1 receptor gene expression was upregulated in the hippocampus [124]. Chronic mild stress has been shown to induce anhedonia in rodents and mimic some of the behavioral and neurochemical correlates of a depressive-like state. Furthermore, chronic fluoxetine, administered after completion of the CMS paradigm, reversed both the upregulation of MCH-1 gene expression and the depressive-like behavior in these mice. Behavioral tests of anxiolytic activity in MCH-1 knockout mice were also conducted in this study and these mice exhibited reduced anxiety. Interestingly, however, when the MCH-1 knockout mice were tested in forced-swim and tail suspension tests only the female mice in this cohort showed antidepressant activity, and the male mice did not [124].

This is a remarkable finding, which the authors suggested may have relevance to the increased incidence of depression in women, who are twice as likely to develop MDD [125]. Roy and colleagues [124] also analyzed the pattern of results in detail and concluded that noradrenergic neurotransmission could be increased in the female MCH-1 knockout mice, though no explanation of any potential causative mechanism was offered. Another difference between male and female rodents in the expression of MCH has been reported, however, and this finding may be relevant here [126]. In the original description of MCH-containing cell bodies and projections in rat brain, a few cells with MCH immunostaining were noted in the PRF, an area that we have described as being important for REM sleep [95]. In the recent study, Rondini and colleagues [126] re-examined and confirmed this result but also found additional MCH-containing cell bodies in the caudal LDT, adjacent to the previously described PRF area, but only in female rats. These immunostained cells in the LDT were not observed in the males. Furthermore, these MCH-containing cells in the LDT of the females also stained for the GABA processing enzyme, glutamic acid decarboxylase [126]. Hence these neurons, which colocalize MCH and GABA, may be identical to those in this area of the pons that are implicated in the mutual interaction between cholinergic and monoaminergic cell populations during REM sleep. Alternatively this MCH-containing group of neurons could modulate REM sleep as part of an extended REM-on cell field [127].

Although it is premature to speculate on the possibility that MCH abnormalities might be involved in depression, it is conceivable that reduced MCH activity is associated with the disorder. Furthermore, increased MCH neurotransmission could underlie the pattern of symptoms seen in atypical depression. Certainly the convergent evidence from the effects of MCH on anxiety, mood, and sleep in rodents is potentially important. And it is relevant that the neuropeptide is apparently expressed in neurons in the PRF (and the LDT in female rats) that have been closely linked with the mechanisms of an underlying neurochemical imbalance in depression. However, the lack of consistency in the rodent behavioral studies remains a difficulty with this hypothesis. Background strain effects may be important, as well as sex differences for some of the studies. The relevance of metabolic status should also be emphasized. This is because of the large differences in behavior and sleep in $MCH^{-/-}$ mice once food is withdrawn (Figure 4.8), together with the results from the clinical trial of NGD-4715 under caloric restriction. Finally, an additional complicating factor must be noted. The prepro-MCH gene that is deleted in the $MCH^{-/-}$ mouse encodes not only the MCH sequence, but also two other sequences, neuropeptide EI (NEI) and NGE [128]. Neuropeptide EI is extensively colocalized with MCH, probably throughout the projection system, and is known to have behavioral effects, at least when locally administered in the hypothalamus of female rats [129]. There is little other published work on NEI, but some of the phenotypic differences in sleep and behavior between the $MCH^{-/-}$ mouse and the MCH-1 receptor knockout might be due to the lack of NEI in the former model.

Summary and conclusions

The sleep abnormalities associated with MDD have been well characterized and are observed sufficiently frequently that they can be used as a marker. In reviewing these abnormalities, we have noted that evidence has accrued over many years in support of the hypothesis that an imbalance between monoaminergic and cholinergic systems could underlie the neurochemical pathophysiology in the disorder. We have also considered research into MDD from the point of view that considers the sleep disruption associated with depression as a causative factor for the structural brain changes that are associated with the disorder. This approach may provide additional insight and potential new treatments.

Significant bodyweight dysregulation also occurs in MDD in conjunction and correlated with the differences in sleep, and these weight changes are not entirely explicable in terms of a monoaminergic–cholinergic imbalance. Despite the established link between the monoamines and feeding behavior, metabolic data suggest that a more fundamental dysregulation of energy balance may be associated with MDD. Two hypothalamic neuropeptides, orexin and MCH, are important for the regulation of metabolic status and also influence sleep, in particular REM sleep. Hypotheses have been proposed to link these neuropeptides with the etiology of depression, and it is possible, though unlikely, that orexin pathophysiology might cause mood disorder. In contrast, increasing evidence has recently become available to suggest that differences in MCH activity could change the balance between aminergic and cholinergic systems, alter REM sleep, and affect bodyweight regulation. Although speculative, data from rodent sleep and behavioral studies, anatomy, molecular genetics, and initial clinical trials of a MCH-1 receptor antagonist converge to link MCH with depression.

Future studies with this neuropeptide and other related neurochemical systems involved in bodyweight regulation could therefore be relevant for research into the mechanisms of depression. The study of sleep remains not only an essential way to understand the disorder but also potentially a critical step in the development of new therapies.

References

1. Gillin JC, Borbely AA. Sleep: a neurobiological window on affective disorders. *Trends Neurosci.* 1985;**8**:537–42.

2. Kupfer DJ. EEG sleep as biological markers in depression. In: Usdin E, Hanin I, eds. *Biological Markers in Psychiatry and Neurology.* (New York: Pergamon, 1982;387–96).

3. Kupfer DJ, Reynolds CF. Sleep and affective disorders. In: Paykel ES, ed. *Handbook of Affective Disorders,* 2nd edn. (New York: Guilford, 1992;311–23).

4. McCarley RW. Sleep neurophysiology: basic mechanisms underlying control of wakefulness and sleep. In: Chokroverty S, ed. *Sleep Disorders Medicine: Basic Science, Technical Considerations, and Clinical Aspects,* 2nd edn. (Woburn, MA: Butterworth-Heinemann, 1999;21–50).

5. Coble P, Foster FG, Kupfer DJ. Electroencephalographic sleep diagnosis of primary depression. *Arch Gen Psychiatry.* 1976;**33**:1124–7.

6. Foster FG, Kupfer DJ, Coble P, McPartland RJ. Rapid eye movement sleep density. An objective indicator in severe medical-depressive syndromes. *Arch Gen Psychiatry.* 1976;**33**:1119–23.

7. Borbely AA, Tobler I, Loepfe M, *et al.* All-night spectral analysis of the sleep EEG in untreated depressives and normal controls. *Psychiatry Res.* 1984;**12**:27–33.

8. Kvist J, Kirkegaard C. Effect of repeated sleep deprivation on clinical symptoms and the TRH test in endogenous depression. *Acta Psychiatr Scand.* 1980;**62**:494–502.

9. Dalgleish T, Rosen K, Marks M. Rhythm and blues: the theory and treatment of seasonal affective disorder. *Br J Clin Psychol.* 1996;**35** (Pt 2):163–82.

10. Ford DE, Kamerow DB. Epidemiologic study of sleep disturbances and psychiatric disorders. An opportunity for prevention? *JAMA.* 1989;**262**:1479–84.

11. Baldwin DS, Papakostas GI. Symptoms of fatigue and sleepiness in major depressive disorder. *J Clin Psychiatry.* 2006;**67** Suppl 6:9–15.

12. Fava M, Thase ME, DeBattista C, *et al.* Modafinil augmentation of selective serotonin reuptake inhibitor therapy in MDD partial responders with persistent fatigue and sleepiness. *Ann Clin Psychiatry.* 2007;**19**:153–9.

13. Sinton CM, McCarley RW. Neurophysiological mechanisms of sleep and wakefulness: a question of balance. *Semin Neurol.* 2004;**24**:211–23.

14. McCarley RW. Neurobiology of REM and NREM sleep. *Sleep Med.* 2007;**8**:302–30.

15. Jones BE. From waking to sleeping: neuronal and chemical substrates. *Trends Pharmacol Sci.* 2005;**26**:578–86.

16. el Mansari M, Sakai K, Jouvet M. Unitary characteristics of presumptive cholinergic tegmental neurons during the sleep-waking cycle in freely moving cats. *Exp Brain Res.* 1989;**76**:519–29.

17. Jones BE. Activity, modulation and role of basal forebrain cholinergic neurons innervating the cerebral cortex. *Prog Brain Res.* 2004;**145**:157–69.

18. McCormick DA. Cholinergic and noradrenergic modulation of thalamocortical processing. *Trends Neurosci.* 1989;**12**:215–21.

19. McGinty DJ, Harper RM. Dorsal raphe neurons: depression of firing during sleep in cats. *Brain Res.* 1976;**101**:569–75.

20. Aston-Jones G, Bloom FE. Activity of norepinephrine-containing locus coeruleus neurons in behaving rats anticipates fluctuations in the sleep-waking cycle. *J Neurosci.* 1981;**1**:876–86.

21. McCormick DA, Bal T. Sleep and arousal: thalamocortical mechanisms. *Annu Rev Neurosci.* 1997;**20**:185–215.

22. Strecker RE, Morairty S, Thakkar MM, *et al.* Adenosinergic modulation of basal forebrain and preoptic/anterior hypothalamic neuronal activity in the control of behavioral state. *Behav Brain Res.* 2000;**115**:183–204.

23. Porkka-Heiskanen T, Strecker RE, Thakkar M, *et al.* Adenosine: a mediator of the sleep-inducing effects of prolonged wakefulness. *Science.* 1997;**276**:1265–8.

24. Kalinchuk AV, McCarley RW, Stenberg D, Porkka-Heiskanen T, Basheer R. The role of cholinergic basal forebrain neurons in adenosine-mediated homeostatic control of sleep: lessons from 192 IgG-saporin lesions. *Neuroscience.* 2008;**157**:238–53.

25. Sherin JE, Elmquist JK, Torrealba F, Saper CB. Innervation of histaminergic tuberomammillary neurons by GABAergic and galaninergic neurons in the ventrolateral preoptic nucleus of the rat. *J Neurosci.* 1998;**18**:4705–21.

26. Lu J, Bjorkum AA, Xu M, *et al.* Selective activation of the extended ventrolateral preoptic nucleus during rapid eye movement sleep. *J Neurosci.* 2002;**22**:4568–76.

27. Gervasoni D, Peyron C, Rampon C, *et al.* Role and origin of the GABAergic innervation of dorsal raphe serotonergic neurons. *J Neurosci.* 2000;**20**:4217–25.

28. Steriade M, Datta S, Pare D, *et al.* Neuronal activities in brain-stem cholinergic nuclei related to tonic activation processes in thalamocortical systems. *J Neurosci.* 1990;**10**:2541–59.

29. Thakkar MM, Strecker RE, McCarley RW. Behavioral state control through differential serotonergic inhibition in the mesopontine cholinergic nuclei: a simultaneous unit recording and microdialysis study. *J Neurosci.* 1998;**18**:5490–7.

30. Lu J, Sherman D, Devor M, Saper CB. A putative flip-flop switch for control of REM sleep. *Nature.* 2006;**441**:589–94.

31. McCarley RW, Hobson JA. Neuronal excitability modulation over the sleep cycle: a structural and mathematical model. *Science.* 1975;**189**:58–60.

32. Hobson JA, McCarley RW, Wyzinski PW. Sleep cycle oscillation: reciprocal discharge by two brainstem neuronal groups. *Science.* 1975;**189**:55–8.

33. Steriade M, McCarley RW. *Brain Control of Wakefulness and Sleep.* (New York, NY: Kluwer Academic/Plenum, 2005).

34. Muhlethaler M, Khateb A, Serafin M. Effects of monoamines and opiates on pedunculopontine neurons. In: Mancia M, Marini G, eds. *The Diencephalon and Sleep.* (New York: Raven Press, 1990; 367–78).

35. Luebke JI, Greene RW, Semba K, *et al.* Serotonin hyperpolarizes cholinergic low-threshold burst neurons in the rat laterodorsal tegmental nucleus in vitro. *Proc Natl Acad Sci USA.* 1992;**89**:743–7.

36. Leonard CS, Llinas R. Serotonergic and cholinergic inhibition of mesopontine cholinergic neurons controlling REM sleep: an in vitro electrophysiological study. *Neuroscience.* 1994;**59**:309–30.

37. Williams JA, Reiner PB. Noradrenaline hyperpolarizes identified rat mesopontine cholinergic neurons in vitro. *J Neurosci.* 1993;**13**:3878–83.

38. Kohlmeier KA, Reiner PB. Noradrenaline excites non-cholinergic laterodorsal tegmental neurons via two distinct mechanisms. *Neuroscience.* 1999;**93**:619–30.

39. Portas CM, Thakkar M, Rainnie D, McCarley RW. Microdialysis perfusion of 8-hydroxy-2-(di-n-propylamino)tetralin (8-OH-DPAT) in the dorsal raphe nucleus decreases serotonin release and increases rapid eye movement sleep in the freely moving cat. *J Neurosci.* 1996;**16**:2820–8.

40. Horner RL, Sanford LD, Annis D, Pack AI, Morrison AR. Serotonin at the laterodorsal tegmental nucleus suppresses rapid-eye-movement sleep in freely behaving rats. *J Neurosci.* 1997;**17**:7541–52.

41. McCarley RW, Massaquoi SG. A limit cycle mathematical model of the REM sleep oscillator system. *Am J Physiol.* 1986;**251**:R1011–29.

42. McCarley RW, Massaquoi SG. Neurobiological structure of the revised limit cycle reciprocal interaction model of REM cycle control. *J Sleep Res.* 1992;**1**:132–7.

43. Overstreet DH. Selective breeding for increased cholinergic function: development of a new animal model of depression. *Biol Psychiatry.* 1986;**21**:49–58.

44. Overstreet DH, Friedman E, Mathe AA, Yadid G. The Flinders Sensitive Line rat: a selectively bred putative animal model of depression. *Neurosci Biobehav Rev.* 2005;**29**:739–59.

45. Shiromani PJ, Overstreet D, Levy D, Goodrich CA, Campbell SS, Gillin JC. Increased REM sleep in rats selectively bred for cholinergic hyperactivity. *Neuropsychopharmacology.* 1988;**1**:127–33.

46. El Yacoubi M, Bouali S, Popa D, *et al.* Behavioral, neurochemical, and electrophysiological characterization of a genetic mouse model of depression. *Proc Natl Acad Sci USA.* 2003;**100**:6227–32.

47. Gillin JC, Sitaram N, Mendelson WB. Acetylcholine, sleep, and depression. *Hum Neurobiol.* 1982;**1**:211–19.

48. Sitaram N, Nurnberger JI, Jr., Gershon ES, Gillin JC. Cholinergic regulation of mood and REM sleep: potential model and marker of vulnerability to affective disorder. *Am J Psychiatry.* 1982;**139**:571–6.

49. McCarley RW. REM sleep and depression: common neurobiological control mechanisms. *Am J Psychiatry.* 1982;**139**:565–70.

50. Schildkraut JJ, Kety SS. Biogenic amines and emotion. *Science.* 1967;**156**:21–37.

51. Maas JW. Biogenic amines and depression. Biochemical and pharmacological separation of two types of depression. *Arch Gen Psychiatry.* 1975;**32**:1357–61.

52. Slattery DA, Hudson AL, Nutt DJ. Invited review: the evolution of antidepressant mechanisms. *Fundam Clin Pharmacol.* 2004;**18**:1–21.

53. Gandolfi O, Barbaccia ML, Costa E. Comparison of iprindole, imipramine and mianserin action on brain serotonergic and beta adrenergic receptors. *J Pharmacol Exp Ther.* 1984;**229**:782–6.

54. Peroutka SJ, Snyder SH. Long-term antidepressant treatment decreases spiroperidol-labeled serotonin receptor binding. *Science.* 1980;**210**:88–90.

55. Wolfe BB, Harden TK, Sporn JR, Molinoff PB. Presynaptic modulation of beta adrenergic receptors in rat cerebral cortex after treatment with antidepressants. *J Pharmacol Exp Ther.* 1978;**207**:446–57.

56. de Montigny C, Aghajanian GK. Tricyclic antidepressants: long-term treatment increases responsivity of rat forebrain neurons to serotonin. *Science.* 1978;**202**:1303–6.

57. Menkes DB, Aghajanian GK, McCall RB. Chronic antidepressant treatment enhances alpha-adrenergic and serotonergic responses in the facial nucleus. *Life Sci.* 1980;**27**:45–55.

58. Blier P, De Montigny C. Electrophysiological investigations on the effect of repeated zimelidine administration on serotonergic neurotransmission in the rat. *J Neurosci.* 1983;**3**:1270–8.

59. Ferris RM, Beaman OJ. Bupropion: a new antidepressant drug, the mechanism of action of which is not associated with down-regulation of postsynaptic beta-adrenergic, serotonergic (5-HT2), alpha 2-adrenergic, imipramine and dopaminergic receptors in brain. *Neuropharmacology.* 1983;**22**:1257–67.

60. Dong J, Blier P. Modification of norepinephrine and serotonin, but not dopamine, neuron firing by sustained bupropion treatment. *Psychopharmacology (Berl).* 2001;**155**:52–7.

61. Svensson TH, Bunney BS, Aghajanian GK. Inhibition of both noradrenergic and serotonergic neurons in brain by the alpha-adrenergic agonist clonidine. *Brain Res.* 1975;**92**:291–306.

62. Dorr AE, Debonnel G. Effect of vagus nerve stimulation on serotonergic and noradrenergic transmission. *J Pharmacol Exp Ther.* 2006;**318**:890–8.

63. El Mansari M, Ghanbari R, Janssen S, Blier P. Sustained administration of bupropion alters the neuronal activity of serotonin, norepinephrine but not dopamine neurons in the rat brain. *Neuropharmacology.* 2008;**55**:1191–8.

64. Kupfer DJ, Spiker DG, Coble PA, Neil JF, Ulrich R, Shaw DH. Sleep and treatment prediction in endogenous depression. *Am J Psychiatry.* 1981;**138**:429–34.

65. Vogel G, Neill D, Hagler M, Kors D. A new animal model of endogenous depression: a summary of present findings. *Neurosci Biobehav Rev.* 1990;**14**:85–91.

66. Vogel GW, Buffenstein A, Minter K, Hennessey A. Drug effects on REM sleep and on endogenous depression. *Neurosci Biobehav Rev.* 1990;**14**:49–63.

67. Basheer R, Magner M, McCarley RW, Shiromani PJ. REM sleep deprivation increases the levels of tyrosine hydroxylase and norepinephrine transporter mRNA in the locus coeruleus. *Brain Res Mol Brain Res.* 1998;**57**:235–40.

68. Giedke H, Schwarzler F. Therapeutic use of sleep deprivation in depression. *Sleep Med Rev.* 2002;**6**:361–77.

69. Mogilnicka E, Arbilla S, Depoortere H, Langer SZ. Rapid-eye-movement sleep deprivation decreases the density of 3H-dihydroalprenolol and 3H-imipramine binding sites in the rat cerebral cortex. *Eur J Pharmacol.* 1980;**65**:289–92.

70. McCarley RW, Massaquoi SG. Further discussion of a model of the REM sleep oscillator. *Am J Physiol.* 1986;**251**:R1033–6.

71. Manji HK, Drevets WC, Charney DS. The cellular neurobiology of depression. *Nat Med.* 2001;**7**:541–7.

72. Duman RS. Synaptic plasticity and mood disorders. *Mol Psychiatry.* 2002;**7** Suppl 1:S29–34.

73. Chamberlain SR, Sahakian BJ. Cognition in mania and depression: psychological models and clinical implications. *Curr Psychiatry Rep.* 2004;**6**:451–8.

74. Perlis ML, Giles DE, Buysse DJ, Thase ME, Tu X, Kupfer DJ. Which depressive symptoms are related to which sleep electroencephalographic variables? *Biol Psychiatry.* 1997;**42**:904–13.

75. Germain A, Nofzinger EA, Kupfer DJ, Buysse DJ. Neurobiology of non-REM sleep in depression: further evidence for hypofrontality and thalamic dysregulation. *Am J Psychiatry.* 2004;**161**:1856–63.

76. Basheer R, Brown R, Ramesh V, Begum S, McCarley RW. Sleep deprivation-induced protein changes in basal forebrain: implications for synaptic plasticity. *J Neurosci Res.* 2005;**82**:650–8.

77. Tartar JL, Ward CP, McKenna JT, *et al.* Hippocampal synaptic plasticity and spatial learning are impaired in a rat model of sleep fragmentation. *Eur J Neurosci.* 2006;**23**:2739–48.

78. Shapiro ML, Eichenbaum H. Hippocampus as a memory map: synaptic plasticity and memory encoding by hippocampal neurons. *Hippocampus.* 1999;**9**:365–84.

79. Campbell IG, Guinan MJ, Horowitz JM. Sleep deprivation impairs long-term potentiation in rat hippocampal slices. *J Neurophysiol.* 2002;**88**:1073–6.

80. McDermott CM, LaHoste GJ, Chen C, *et al.* Sleep deprivation causes behavioral, synaptic, and membrane excitability alterations in hippocampal neurons. *J Neurosci.* 2003;**23**:9687–95.

81. Morris RG, Garrud P, Rawlins JN, O'Keefe J. Place navigation impaired in rats with hippocampal lesions. *Nature.* 1982;**297**:681–3.

82. Guzman-Marin R, Bashir T, Suntsova N, Szymusiak R, McGinty D. Hippocampal neurogenesis is reduced by sleep fragmentation in the adult rat. *Neuroscience.* 2007;**148**:325–33.

83. Leibowitz SF, Shor-Posner G. Brain serotonin and eating behavior. *Appetite.* 1986;**7** Suppl:1–14.

84. Adan RA, Vanderschuren LJ, Elf S. Anti-obesity drugs and neural circuits of feeding. *Trends Pharmacol Sci.* 2008;**29**:208–17.

85. Leibowitz SF, Alexander JT. Hypothalamic serotonin in control of eating behavior, meal size, and body weight. *Biol Psychiatry.* 1998;**44**:851–64.

86. Tecott LH. Serotonin and the orchestration of energy balance. *Cell Metab.* 2007;**6**:352–61.

87. Booth DA. Mechanism of action of norepinephrine in eliciting an eating response on injection into the rat hypothalamus. *J Pharmacol Exp Ther.* 1968;**160**:336–48.

88. Paez X, Leibowitz SF. Changes in extracellular PVN monoamines and macronutrient intake after idazoxan or fluoxetine injection. *Pharmacol Biochem Behav.* 1993;**46**:933–41.

89. Wellman PJ, Davies BT, Morien A, McMahon L. Modulation of feeding by hypothalamic paraventricular nucleus alpha 1- and alpha 2-adrenergic receptors. *Life Sci.* 1993;**53**:669–79.

90. Leibowitz SF. Pattern of drinking and feeding produced by hypothalamic norepinephrine injection in the satiated rat. *Physiol Behav.* 1975;**14**:731–42.

91. Tritos NA, Maratos-Flier E. Two important systems in energy homeostasis: melanocortins and melanin-concentrating hormone. *Neuropeptides.* 1999;**33**:339–49.

92. Sakurai T, Amemiya A, Ishii M, *et al.* Orexins and orexin receptors: a family of hypothalamic neuropeptides and G protein-coupled receptors that regulate feeding behavior. *Cell.* 1998;**92**:573–85.

93. Chemelli RM, Willie JT, Sinton CM, *et al.* Narcolepsy in orexin knockout mice: molecular genetics of sleep regulation. *Cell.* 1999;**98**:437–51.

94. Willie JT, Sinton CM, Maratos-Flier E, Yanagisawa M. Abnormal response of melanin-concentrating hormone deficient mice to fasting: hyperactivity and rapid eye movement sleep suppression. *Neuroscience.* 2008;**156**:819–29.

95. Bittencourt JC, Presse F, Arias C, *et al.* The melanin-concentrating hormone system of the rat brain: an immuno- and hybridization histochemical characterization. *J Comp Neurol.* 1992;**319**:218–45.

96. Peyron C, Tighe DK, van den Pol AN, *et al.* Neurons containing hypocretin (orexin) project to multiple neuronal systems. *J Neurosci.* 1998;**18**:9996–10015.

97. de Lecea L, Sutcliffe JG. The hypocretins and sleep. *FEBS J.* 2005;**272**:5675–88.

98. Kilduff TS, Peyron C. The hypocretin/orexin ligand-receptor system: implications for sleep and sleep disorders. *Trends Neurosci.* 2000;**23**:359–65.

99. Aldrich MS. Narcolepsy. *Neurology.* 1992;**42**:34–43.

100. Korotkova TM, Sergeeva OA, Eriksson KS, Haas HL, Brown RE. Excitation of ventral tegmental area dopaminergic and nondopaminergic neurons by orexins/hypocretins. *J Neurosci.* 2003;**23**:7–11.

101. Brown RE, Sergeeva OA, Eriksson KS, Haas HL. Convergent excitation of dorsal raphe serotonin

neurons by multiple arousal systems (orexin/hypocretin, histamine and noradrenaline). *J Neurosci.* 2002;**22**:8850–9.

102. Salomon RM, Ripley B, Kennedy JS, *et al.* Diurnal variation of cerebrospinal fluid hypocretin-1 (Orexin-A) levels in control and depressed subjects. *Biol Psychiatry.* 2003;**54**:96–104.

103. Pedrazzoli M, D'Almeida V, Martins PJ, *et al.* Increased hypocretin-1 levels in cerebrospinal fluid after REM sleep deprivation. *Brain Res.* 2004;**995**:1–6.

104. Allard JS, Tizabi Y, Shaffery JP, Trouth CO, Manaye K. Stereological analysis of the hypothalamic hypocretin/orexin neurons in an animal model of depression. *Neuropeptides.* 2004;**38**:311–15.

105. Reynolds CF 3rd, Christiansen CL, Taska LS, Coble PA, Kupfer DJ. Sleep in narcolepsy and depression. Does it all look alike? *J Nerv Ment Dis.* 1983;**171**:290–5.

106. Rye DB, Dihenia B, Bliwise DL. Reversal of atypical depression, sleepiness, and REM-sleep propensity in narcolepsy with bupropion. *Depress Anxiety.* 1998;**7**:92–5.

107. Adda C, Lefevre B, Reimao R. Narcolepsy and depression. *Arq Neuropsiquiatr.* 1997;**55**:423–6.

108. Pollmacher T, Mullington J, Lauer CJ. REM sleep disinhibition at sleep onset: a comparison between narcolepsy and depression. *Biol Psychiatry.* 1997;**42**:713–20.

109. Schwartz TL, Azhar N, Cole K, *et al.* An open-label study of adjunctive modafinil in patients with sedation related to serotonergic antidepressant therapy. *J Clin Psychiatry.* 2004;**65**:1223–7.

110. Thase ME, Fava M, DeBattista C, Arora S, Hughes RJ. Modafinil augmentation of SSRI therapy in patients with major depressive disorder and excessive sleepiness and fatigue: a 12-week, open-label, extension study. *CNS Spectr.* 2006;**11**:93–102.

111. Ninan PT, Hassman HA, Glass SJ, McManus FC. Adjunctive modafinil at initiation of treatment with a selective serotonin reuptake inhibitor enhances the degree and onset of therapeutic effects in patients with major depressive disorder and fatigue. *J Clin Psychiatry.* 2004;**65**:414–20.

112. Willie JT, Renthal W, Chemelli RM, *et al.* Modafinil more effectively induces wakefulness in orexin-null mice than in wild-type littermates. *Neuroscience.* 2005;**130**:983–95.

113. Zhang Y, Proenca R, Maffei M, *et al.* Positional cloning of the mouse obese gene and its human homologue. *Nature.* 1994;**372**:425–32.

114. Shimada M, Tritos NA, Lowell BB, Flier JS, Maratos-Flier E. Mice lacking melanin-concentrating hormone are hypophagic and lean. *Nature.* 1998;**396**:670–4.

115. Verret L, Goutagny R, Fort P, *et al.* A role of melanin-concentrating hormone producing neurons in the central regulation of paradoxical sleep. *BMC Neurosci.* 2003;**4**:19.

116. Modirrousta M, Mainville L, Jones BE. Orexin and MCH neurons express c-Fos differently after sleep deprivation vs. recovery and bear different adrenergic receptors. *Eur J Neurosci.* 2005;**21**:2807–16.

117. Ahnaou A, Drinkenburg WH, Bouwknecht JA, *et al.* Blocking melanin-concentrating hormone MCH1 receptor affects rat sleep-wake architecture. *Eur J Pharmacol.* 2008;**579**:177–88.

118. Adamantidis A, Salvert D, Goutagny R, *et al.* Sleep architecture of the melanin-concentrating hormone receptor 1-knockout mice. *Eur J Neurosci.* 2008;**27**:1793–800.

119. Cartwright RD, Monroe LJ. Relation of dreaming and REM sleep: the effects of REM deprivation under two conditions. *J Pers Soc Psychol.* 1968;**10**:69–74.

120. Schlosberg A, Benjamin M. Sleep patterns in three acute combat fatigue cases. *J Clin Psychiatry.* 1978;**39**:546–9.

121. Monzon ME, De Barioglio SR. Response to novelty after i.c.v. injection of melanin-concentrating hormone (MCH) in rats. *Physiol Behav.* 1999;**67**:813–17.

122. Borowsky B, Durkin MM, Ogozalek K, *et al.* Antidepressant, anxiolytic and anorectic effects of a melanin-concentrating hormone-1 receptor antagonist. *Nat Med.* 2002;**8**:825–30.

123. Basso AM, Bratcher NA, Gallagher KB, *et al.* Lack of efficacy of melanin-concentrating hormone-1 receptor antagonists in models of depression and anxiety. *Eur J Pharmacol.* 2006;**540**:115–20.

124. Roy M, David N, Cueva M, Giorgetti M. A study of the involvement of melanin-concentrating hormone receptor 1 (MCHR1) in murine models of depression. *Biol Psychiatry.* 2007;**61**:174–80.

125. Sloan DM, Kornstein SG. Gender differences in depression and response to antidepressant treatment. *Psychiatr Clin North Am.* 2003;**26**:581–94.

126. Rondini TA, Rodrigues Bde C, de Oliveira AP, Bittencourt JC, Elias CF. Melanin-concentrating hormone is expressed in the laterodorsal tegmental nucleus only in female rats. *Brain Res Bull.* 2007;**74**:21–8.

127. Brown RE, McKenna JT, Winston S, *et al.* Characterization of GABAergic neurons in rapid-eye-movement sleep controlling regions of the brainstem reticular formation in GAD67-green fluorescent protein knock-in mice. *Eur J Neurosci.* 2008;**27**:352–63.

128. Marsh DJ, Weingarth DT, Novi DE, *et al.* Melanin-concentrating hormone 1 receptor-deficient mice are lean, hyperactive, and hyperphagic and have altered metabolism. *Proc Natl Acad Sci USA.* 2002;**99**:3240–5.

129. Gonzalez MI, Baker BI, Hole DR, Wilson CA. Behavioral effects of neuropeptide E-I (NEI) in the female rat: interactions with alpha-MSH, MCH and dopamine. *Peptides.* 1998;**19**:1007–16.

130. Karteris E, Randeva HS, Grammatopoulos DK, Jaffe RB, Hillhouse EW. Expression and coupling characteristics of the CRH and orexin type 2 receptors in human fetal adrenals. *J Clin Endocrinol Metab.* 2001;**86**:4512–19.

Neurobiology of insomnia

Joëlle Adrien and Lucile Garma

Introduction

Insomnia is the most frequent of sleep disorders, but its physiopathology remains largely unknown. Recently, major breakthroughs have brought novel insights in the field of sleep research, at both the basic and clinical levels. Conducted notably by using molecular biology, cellular physiology, functional imagery, and cognitive approach, these studies allow proposal of new hypotheses addressing the neurobiology of insomnia.

Here, we will focus on deciphering the similarities and differences between the diverse types of insomnias, and in particular psychophysiological insomnia (or primary insomnia, PI) that affects, using stringent diagnostic criteria, about 1 to 3% of the general population, and insomnia associated with major depression (MDDI) that affects 6 to 10% with an almost two-fold increased incidence in women compared to men [1, 2, 3]. Each of these types is associated with clinical signs, biological traits, and physiopathological features that will be detailed. Some of these characteristics are common to both types of insomnia whereas others are specific of either one.

The neurobiological approach to insomnia relies on a model of sleep–wakefulness regulations that can be schematized as interactions between four main systems: those controlling wakefulness and sleep initiation that are organized as a sleep–wake "flip-flop" switch, and those regulating non-rapid eye movement sleep (NREM) and REM sleep that interact as another switch. Insomnia is symptomatic of an imbalance between these various partners.

Features common to primary insomnia and to insomnia associated with major depression

These features concern the mechanisms of transition from wakefulness to sleep rather than those of sleep processes themselves.

From wakefulness to sleep

Sleep–wakefulness regulations depend on two main systems that alternatively induce waking or sleep: the sleep–wake "switch" [4]. These systems are schematized in Figure 5.1. It should be noted that these regulations depend also on biological clocks, but these will not be described herein.

The main systems controlling wakefulness

These systems correspond to structures that are interconnected but whose hierarchical organization is still largely unknown. Schematically, they involve broadly distributed neurotransmitter systems:

Cholinergic systems in the pontine reticular formation and basal nuclei play a primary role in cortical activation, i.e., the low-amplitude fast frequencies of the EEG signal. Their influences are transmitted also through glutamatergic systems, the major network underlying cortical activation and behavioral arousal [5].

The noradrenergic system in the locus coeruleus is involved in cortical activation and behavioral arousal, essentially by global stimulation of vigilance.

Sleep and Mental Illness, eds. S. R. Pandi-Perumal and M. Kramer. Published by Cambridge University Press.
© Cambridge University Press 2010.

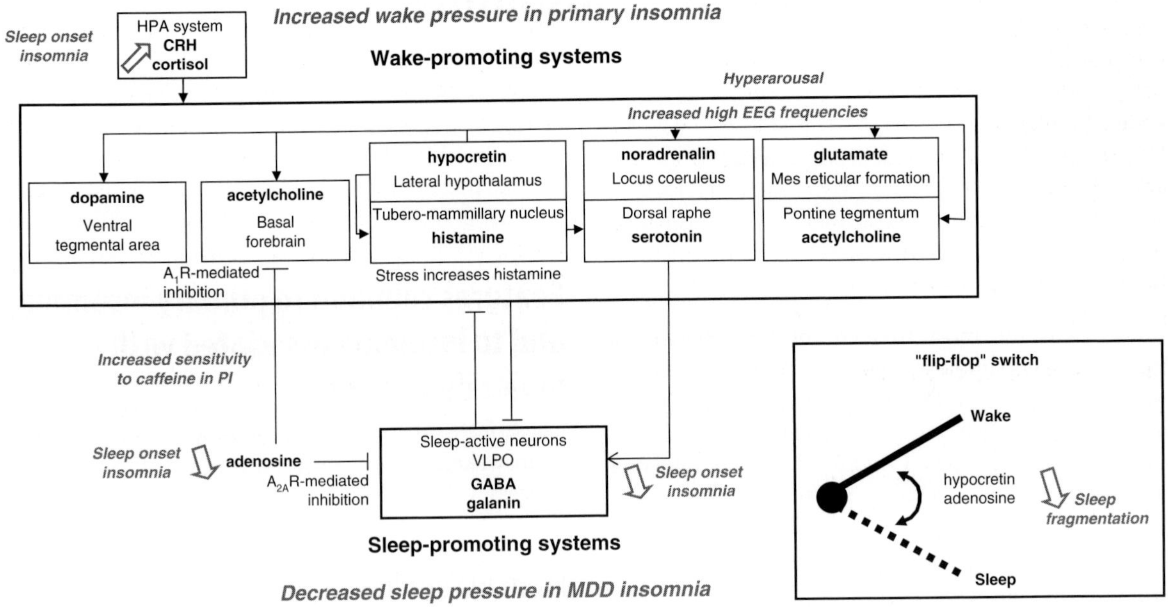

Figure 5.1 The waking (on top) and sleep-inducing (bottom) systems develop mutually inhibitory interactions. The alternative expression of wakefulness or sleep depends on a "flip-flop" switch (right) whose functioning mode reduces transitional states and state fragmentation. Hypocretin and adenosine participate in the latter processes. In insomnia, the switch tends to remain in the upward position due to hyperactivity of the waking systems (essentially in PI) or hypoactivity of the sleep-inducing systems (essentially in MDDI). Sleep misperception could be accounted for by the lack of contrast between waking and sleep, resulting from the reduced amplitude of the switch oscillation. Thin arrows represent excitation and bars represent inhibition between structures. Large arrows and text in italics summarize the dysfunctions that would account for the various symptoms of insomnia.

The dopaminergic system (substantia nigra and ventral tegmental area) is essential in cortical/behavioral wakefulness and cognitive functions [5].

The histaminergic system in the posterior hypothalamus sends afferents to all other waking systems, as well as to sleep-initiating structures [6]. It is involved mainly in the cognitive component of wakefulness [7].

The hypocretins (or orexins) are the most recently identified sleep-related peptides. They play a role in stimulating wakefulness, essentially its behavioral (motor) component [8], through activation of other waking systems. Hypocretins facilitate stabilization of behavioral states and are also involved in appetite and neuroendocrine controls [9, 10].

The stress system, notably the corticotropin releasing hormone (CRH), also participates significantly in facilitating wakefulness. In particular, CRH enhances vigilance by stimulating wakefulness structures in the brainstem (notably through cortisol acting at glucocorticoid receptors on noradrenergic and serotonergic neurons) and forebrain, as well as autonomic-related systems in the brainstem and spinal cord [11]. Conversely, sleep loss results in cortisol increase [12].

Two other systems are part of the wakefulness network but they behave differently from the former ones; schematically, their activity during wakefulness contributes to building up the sleep pressure:

The serotoninergic system, originating in the raphe nuclei, is involved in the processes of sleep initiation possibly through facilitation of peptidergic sleep mechanisms [13].

Adenosine accumulates during wakefulness, in relation to the energy demand. It secondarily induces sleepiness through inhibition of the waking systems, by notably inhibiting acetylcholine release in the basal forebrain through A_1 receptors [14]. Blockade of these adenosine receptors (by caffeine) prevents this inhibiting action [15] and thus increases alertness.

Systems promoting sleep

To date, the main system known to promote sleep is located in the anterior hypothalamus. It comprises the ventrolateral preoptic area (VLPO) and adjacent part of the basal forebrain. This "sleep inducing" system contains GABAergic [16] and galaninergic [17] inhibitory neurons that send projections to most arousal structures. Adenosine would facilitate the activation of these neurons [18] through A_{2A} adenosinergic receptors [19]. Serotonin also excites these neurons together with participating in increasing the sleep pressure [19].

The sleep–wake flip-flop switch

There is mutual inhibition between the VLPO and the major waking systems, which operates according to a "flip-flop" circuit [4]. This system generates two possible stable states (wakefulness or sleep), with minimization of intermediate states through modulation by hypocretins (wakefulness) and adenosine (sleep) that both stabilize behavioral states.

The transition to sleep depends on a homeostatic drive related to the sleep pressure that depends on the accumulation of sleep inducing/promoting factors [20] such as adenosine [19], vasoactive intestinal polypeptide [13], or cytokines [21]. Among these influences, the best known is that of adenosine at the level of VLPO and basal forebrain where it promotes the transitions from wakefulness to sleep [19].

This flip-flop switch represents the wake–sleep (day–night) contrast, a requirement for optimal functioning. Impairment of this sleep–wake switch by either hyperactivity of the arousal systems or hypoactivity of the sleep-promoting systems will induce insomnia.

Impairment of the sleep–wake switch
Clinical aspects

Both PI and MDDI share most of the classical complaints of insomnia, i.e., problems with falling asleep, waking up several times during the night, having difficulties going back to sleep, and feeling of insufficient and/or non-restorative sleep. In addition, the homeostatic regulation of sleep in insomniac patients is poorly efficient, with lack of recovery sleep after sleep loss that adds to the exhaustion feeling, and reinforces sleep-related anxiety [22].

Polysomnographic recordings indicate major sleep fragmentation, and frequent awakenings with notably in PI increased episodes of wakefulness after sleep onset (WASO) [23], and in MDDI early morning awakenings. These impairments are associated with sympathetic hyperactivity such as increased heart rate and elevated rectal temperature [24]. The HPA system is hyperactive, with an increase in adrenocorticotropic hormone (ACTH) and cortisol secretion notably during the evening and the first part of the night, a positive correlation between the cortisol level and time awake, and an exaggerated corticotropin-releasing factor (CRF) response to stress [25].

The EEG signal is impaired with either an increase of rapid EEG frequencies in the beta-1 frequency range (14–20 Hz) or a decrease of activity in the slow delta range (0.5–2.5 Hz) [2, 23, 24]. In parallel, whole-brain glucose metabolism is enhanced [26], notably during NREM sleep in the pontine tegmentum and thalamo-cortical networks in correlation with WASO [27].

Neurobiology

The neurobiological processes that underlie these alterations involve dysfunction of the sleep–wake switch with hyperactivity of the wakefulness networks or hypoactivity of the systems promoting sleep in PI and MDDI, respectively [28].

Hyperactivity of the wakefulness systems

This is observed in both PI and MDDI, but more pronounced in the former, thus preventing sleep onset even though sleep promoting systems are not necessarily altered.

Hyperarousal is expressed at somatic, metabolic, electroencephalographic, and cognitive levels. It is one of the main physiopathological substrates of PI and it persists all along the 24 hour-period. This hyperarousal around sleep onset, illustrated by the increased power of rapid EEG bands and reduced delta activity [29], could account for the difficulties in initiating sleep. In the same manner, hyperarousal during the whole night, illustrated by the decreased contrast between fast and slow EEG frequencies [23, 24], might account for WASO and the feeling of light, unrefreshing sleep, as well as for the sleep misperception that affects most insomniac patients.

Besides enhanced glucose metabolism in the brain, the mechanisms underlying such hyperarousal could involve the glutamatergic system [30], and the cholinergic network notably through adenosine: in fact, insomniacs exhibit hypersensitivity to caffeine [15], suggesting that their adenosine metabolism or

53

adenosinergic receptors would be upregulated. The HPA axis activation, illustrated by the increase of ACTH and cortisol release [31] and the enhancement of catecholamine metabolism [32], contributes to such increased tone of the wakefulness systems. In turn, the HPA axis stimulates histaminergic [33] and hypocretinergic [34] neurotransmissions, two of the major wake-promoting systems [5].

Hypoactivity of the sleep systems

In MDDI, the sleep–wake switch is altered mainly through a deficit in the sleep promoting systems. Comparatively to PI, MDDI is associated with a larger deficit in EEG synchronization [2] notably in the delta band [23], and decreased glucose metabolism in the basal ganglia and frontal cortex [35]. This could be accounted for by hypoactivity of the GABAergic system in the VLPO and basal forebrain, and by a deficit in adenosine processes [36]. In addition, a reduced serotonergic neurotransmission at VLPO level, together with the decrease of adenosine, could participate in the relative lack of sleep pressure. Indeed, a reduction of serotonergic neurotransmission is observed in depressed patients and in animal models of this pathology [37], and the inhibition of serotonin synthesis induces a depression relapse [38] associated with insomnia [39]. These adenosinergic and serotonergic impairments could underlie notably the difficulties in initiating sleep and the sleep fragmentation.

Thus, common mechanisms underlying PI and MDDI concern an alteration of the sleep–wake flip-flop switch, with enhanced wakefulness processes in PI and decreased sleep-promoting processes in MDDI.

Insomnia in major depression is associated with impairments of the sleep architecture

Insomnia is one of the main symptoms of major depressive episodes. Schematically, the mechanisms accounting for this disorder would concern essentially the systems generating NREM, notably slow-wave sleep (SWS), and REM sleep (Figure 5.2).

Neurobiology of NREM and REM sleep

The processes leading to alternation of NREM and REM sleep depend on a second flip-flop switch that involves structures regulating respectively each of these states [40].

NREM sleep mechanisms are still largely unknown. Schematically, slow EEG rhythms are generated in thalamo-cortical networks under conditions of GABAergic activation and cholinergic disinhibition [41]. GABAergic neurons of the basal forebrain play a key role in this process. They inhibit both locally the cholinergic, and distally the histaminergic and orexinergic neurons, all three systems known to be essential for maintaining cortical arousal [5]. These GABAergic neurons also project directly to cortical areas, and exhibit reduced activity during fast EEG frequencies and enhanced firing during delta slow oscillations [42]. Adenosine would facilitate these processes, notably the synchronized activity of deep SWS according to a homeostatic drive [14, 43].

REM sleep regulatory mechanisms, which have been revisited recently, depend on complex reciprocal interactions between various neuronal networks, and can be schematized as follows [14, 40].

Basic structures in the brainstem contain neurons responsible for the production of REM sleep. Schematically, they comprise mutually inhibitory REM-executive (REM-on) and REM-suppressive (REM-off) systems [14, 40, 44, 45].

REM-on systems are active during the whole REM phase, and are composed of essentially GABAergic (peri coeruleus, PC; dorsal paragigantocellular nucleus, DPGI), mixed GABAergic/glutamatergic (sub-laterodorsal nucleus, SLD), and glutamatergic (pontine reticular formation, PRF) structures. They are considered as the actual REM sleep generator areas. In parallel, cholinergic neurons in the pontine tegmentum (laterodorsal, LDT and pedunculopontine tegmentum, PPT) are also REM-on structures, but they modulate rather than generate the REM state [46].

REM-off systems are quiescent during the whole REM sleep phase. They comprise mainly GABAergic or mixed GABAergic/glycinergic neuronal groups (lateral pontine tegmentum, LPT; ventrolateral periacqueducal gray, vlPAG). Other systems such as the serotonergic (DRN) and noradrenergic (LC) neuronal groups act as a parallel modulatory REM-off system.

These REM-on and REM-off structures at the brainstem level function like a flip-flop system, with notably mutually inhibitory GABAergic areas [46]. In addition, the switch to a REM or NREM state is

NREM–REM Sleep

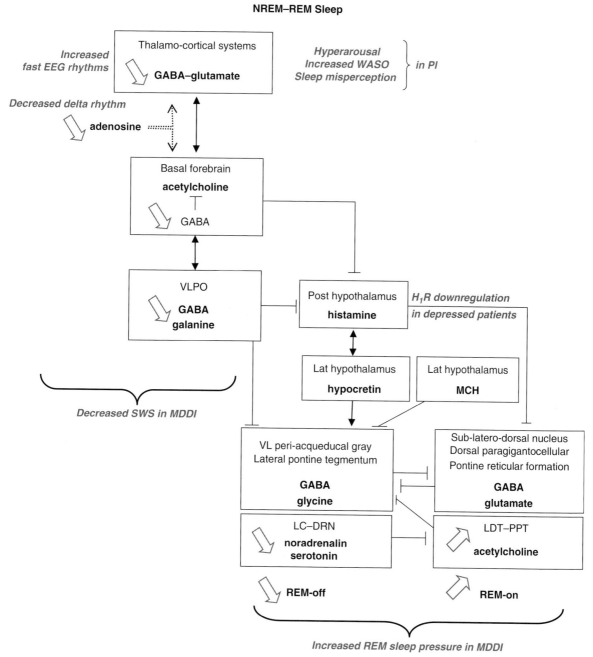

Figure 5.2 The networks involved in the regulation of NREM sleep (top left) are located in the VLPO and basal forebrain. These two systems exert a GABAergic and galaninergic tonic inhibitory drive on most of the waking structures, and notably on the histaminergic neurons in the posterior hypothalamus. Synchronized waves in the cortex are generated within GABAergic and glutamatergic thalamo-cortical systems (top) under the facilitatory influence of the basal forebrain through notably adenosine. The REM sleep state (bottom right) depends on interactions between REM-on/executive and REM-off/inhibiting systems, involving primarily GABAergic systems. The silencing of REM-off structures, notably under the influence of MCH neurons in the lateral hypothalamus and of GABA/galanine neurons in the VLPO, induces a disinhibition of REM-on systems, and thus the expression of REM sleep. In MDDI, the profound impairments of the sleep architecture can be accounted for by the same neurobiological deficits as those involved in the mood alteration. These are mainly: (1) Functional deficit of serotonergic/noradrenergic and enhancement of cholinergic systems, as well as decrease of the histaminergic tone. These imbalances facilitate REM-on mechanisms and thus increase the REM sleep "pressure". (2) Reduction of the adenosine- and GABA-related processes would account for the decrease of SWS and of EEG delta activity. Same symbols as in Figure 5.1.

influenced by structures localized more rostrally in the brain.

Modulatory structures in the hypothalamus are thought to regulate the alternate activation of REM-on or REM-off systems. It is the hypothalamic neurons expressing the melanin concentrating hormone that facilitate REM sleep through inhibition of REM-on structures [47]. Conversely, REM sleep is inhibited by the hypocretinergic system, in the posterolateral hypothalamus, through activation of REM-off structures [14], and by the histaminergic system, in the posterior hypothalamus, through inhibition of REM-on structures [7].

Differences between PI and MDDI are related to impairment of internal sleep organization

Clinical aspects

As we have seen above, in both types of insomnias patients suffer from frequent waking episodes during the night, but the early morning awakenings are most characteristic of MDDI, and even constitute a clinical marker of this pathology. Furthermore, in contrast to PI, MDDI is associated with deep alteration of the sleep architecture. In particular, SWS is almost absent at the beginning of the sleep period while REM sleep latency is reduced, and REM time is increased during the first part of the night together with enhancement in the density of rapid eye movements [48].

Regarding the EEG signal, MDDI is associated with an impairment of essentially delta activity: its power is decreased or delta waves are abnormally distributed across the sleep period, with a dramatic decline in the second part of the sleep period, and an inter-hemispheric asymmetry increased during all sleep states [23]. These alterations are more pronounced in women than in men, which is in favour of gender differences in the physiopathology of depression [49].

Neurobiology: slow-wave sleep in MDDI

The SWS deficit and reduced activity of the delta frequency range in depressed patients would be accounted for by at least the following alterations. The first one concerns the GABAergic/glutamatergic systems, one of the main actors of thalamo-cortical synchronization/desynchronization: GABA levels in the cortex are decreased while those of glutamate are enhanced [30]. This imbalance would underlie notably the lack of contrast between high- and low-frequency EEG rhythms during the whole night [23]. Second, a deficit in adenosine has been evidenced in depressed patients [36] that could also participate in the decrease of EEG delta activity [14, 50]. Finally, the serotonergic system is affected, with notably a hypersensitivity of $5-HT_2$ receptors [37] that would lead primarily to reducing the amounts of SWS [51]. In fact, antidepressants with antagonistic properties at $5-HT_2$ receptors are the most efficient to restore SWS [52].

Altogether, the neurobiological deficits leading to a decrease in NREM sleep and associated delta activity would account for the sleep fragmentation and the feeling of non-restorative sleep, while the abnormal distribution of EEG delta waves and their rapid decline in the second part of the night might underlie the early morning awakenings.

REM sleep in MDDI

Schematically, major depression is associated with a global increase in cholinergic [53] and decrease in serotonergic and noradrenergic [38] neurotransmissions. Indeed, the REM sleep susceptibility to cholinergic agents is enhanced in depressed patients [54, 55]. Conversely, the serotonergic tone is reduced, through altered sensitivity of $5-HT_2$ and $5-HT_{1A}$ receptors [56], as well as functional impairment of the serotonin transporter [57] notably in relation with estrogens [58].

Altogether, these alterations generate an imbalance between REM-on and REM-off systems that results in an enhanced REM sleep pressure illustrated by the reduced REM sleep latency and the increased density of rapid eye movements during the first REM periods [48].

Other dysfunctional systems might also account for these anomalies. Such is the case of hypocretin, whose levels and cirdadian oscillations are impaired in depressed patients [59]; of histamine with H1 receptors hyposensitivity [38]; or of melanin concentrating hormone since antagonists at type 1 receptors have an antidepressant action [60, 61]. All these deficits will tend to induce a disinhibition of REM-on systems and in turn a facilitation of REM sleep.

Conclusion

Recent studies allow better characterization of primary insomnia versus insomnia associated with major depression. In primary insomnia, the underlying processes address essentially the interactions between wake- and sleep-promoting systems, i.e., an imbalance in the sleep–wake flip-flop switch. Sleep is difficult to initiate, and cannot be stabilized due to continuous underlying hyperarousal. According to this view, sleep mechanisms are not primarily altered but sleep is impaired due to intruding waking processes inside the sleep period: PI would be primarily a disorder of hyperarousal.

In contrast in MDD insomnia, even though it shares with PI the sleep–wake balance alteration that induces common difficulties in initiating sleep and frequent awakenings, the main characteristic concerns the sleep organization itself. The mechanisms that underlie the impairments of NREM/SWS and even more of REM sleep are similar to those accounting for some symptoms of depression [37]. Insomnia is not a "cause" or a "consequence" of major depression, and contrary to common opinion, one is not "depressed because of poor sleep". The reverse even occurs in 60% of depressed patients whose mood is improved after one night of sleep deprivation [37]. Thus, both disorders would be the expression of common physiopathological mechanisms. In turn, the fact that insomnia is often the first sign of a major depression or of a depressive relapse [1, 3, 62, 63] should be viewed not as a causal factor but rather as the first manifestation of a neurobiological impairment that is observed on sleep regulation prior to being evidenced at the level of mood.

Finally, investigating the neurobiological substrates of each type and symptom of insomnia should help us to understand the alterations leading to the main characteristics of insomnia sufferers' complaints, including sleep misperception. Such analysis should bring some clues for improving treatment strategies addressing physiological and cognitive alterations associated with this highly prevalent sleep disorder.

References

1. Ohayon MM, Roth T. Place of chronic insomnia in the course of depressive and anxiety disorders. *J Psychiatr Res*. 2003;**37**:9–15.

2. Cortoos A, Verstraeten E, Cluydts R. Neurophysiological aspects of primary insomnia: implications for its treatment. *Sleep Med Rev*. 2006;**10**:255–66.

3. Buysse DJ, Angst J, Gamma A, *et al*. Prevalence, course, and comorbidity of insomnia and depression in young adults. *Sleep*. 2008;**31**:473–80.

4. Saper CB, Chou TC, Scammell TE. The sleep switch: hypothalamic control of sleep and wakefulness. *Trends Neurosci*. 2001;**24**:726–31.

5. Jones BE. From waking to sleeping: neuronal and chemical substrates. *Trends Pharmacol Sci*. 2005;**26**:578–86.

6. Lin JS. Brain structures and mechanisms involved in the control of cortical activation and wakefulness, with emphasis on the posterior hypothalamus and histaminergic neurons. *Sleep Med Rev*. 2000;**4**:471–503.

7. Parmentier R, Ohtsu H, Djebbara-Hannas Z, *et al*. Anatomical, physiological, and pharmacological characteristics of histidine decarboxylase knock-out mice: evidence for the role of brain histamine in behavioral and sleep-wake control. *J Neurosci*. 2002;**22**:7695–711.

8. Mileykovskiy BY, Kiyashchenko LI, Siegel JM. Behavioral correlates of activity in identified hypocretin/orexin neurons. *Neuron*. 2005;**46**:787–98.

9. Taheri S, Zeiter JM, Mignot E. The role of hypocretins (orexins) in sleep regulation and narcolepsy. *Ann Rev Neurosci*. 2002;**25**:283–313.

10. Sakurai T. Roles of orexin/hypocretin in regulation of sleep/wakefulness and energy homeostasis. *Sleep Med Rev*. 2005;**9**:231–41.

11. Chang FC, Opp MR. Corticotropin-releasing hormone (CRH) as a regulator of waking. *Neurosci Biobehav Rev*. 2001;**25**:445–53.

12. Steiger A. Sleep and the hypothalamo-pituitary-adrenocortical system. *Sleep Med Rev*. 2002;**6**:125–38.

13. Jouvet M. The regulation of paradoxical sleep by the hypothalamo-hypophysis. *Arch Ital Biol*. 1988;**126**:259–74.

14. McCarley RW. Neurobiology of REM and NREM sleep. *Sleep Med*. 2007;**8**:302–30.

15. Salin-Pascual RJ, Valencia-Flores M, Campos RM, Castano A, Shiromani PJ. Caffeine challenge in insomniac patients after total sleep deprivation. *Sleep Med*. 2006;**7**:141–5.

16. Gallopin T, Fort P, Eggermann E, *et al*. Identification of sleep-promoting neurons in vitro. *Nature*. 2000;**404**:992–5.

17. Szymusiak R, Gvilia I, McGinty D. Hypothalamic control of sleep. *Sleep Med*. 2007;**8**:291–301.

18. Morairty S, Rainnie D, McCarley R, Greene R. Disinhibition of ventrolateral preoptic area sleep-active neurons by adenosine: a new mechanism for sleep promotion. *Neuroscience*. 2004;**123**:451–7.

19. Gallopin T, Luppi PH, Cauli B, *et al.* The endogenous somnogen adenosine excites a subset of sleep-promoting neurons via A2A receptors in the ventrolateral preoptic nucleus. *Neuroscience.* 2005;**134**:1377–90.

20. Borbely A, Tobler I. Endogenous sleep-promoting substances and sleep regulation. *Physiol Rev.* 1989;**2**:605–70.

21. Krueger JM, Fang J, Hansen MK, Zhang J, Obál F Jr. Humoral regulation of sleep. *News Physiol Sci.* 1998;**13**:189–94.

22. Pigeon WR, Perlis ML. Sleep homeostasis in primary insomnia. *Sleep Med Rev.* 2006;**10**:247–54.

23. Perlis ML, Kehr EL, Smith MT, *et al.* Temporal and stagewise distribution of high frequency EEG activity in patients with primary and secondary insomnia and in good sleeper controls. *J Sleep Res.* 2001;**10**:93–104.

24. Basta M, Chrousos GP, Vela-Bueno A, Vgontzas AN. Chronic insomnia and stress system. *Sleep Med Clin.* 2007;**2**:279–91.

25. Vgontzas AN, Bixler EO, Lin HM, *et al.* Chronic insomnia is associated with nyctohemeral activation of the hypothalamic-pituitary-adrenal axis: clinical implications. *J Clin Endocrinol Metab.* 2001;**86**:3787–94.

26. Nofzinger EA, Buysse DJ, Germain A, *et al.* Functional neuroimaging evidence for hyperarousal in insomnia. *Am J Psychiatry.* 2004;**161**:2126–8.

27. Nofzinger EA, Nissen C, Germain A, *et al.* Regional cerebral metabolic correlates of WASO during NREM sleep in insomnia. *J Clin Sleep Med.* 2006;**2**:316–22.

28. Bastien CH, St-Jean G, Morin CM, Turcotte I, Carrier J. Chronic psychophysiological insomnia: hyperarousal and/or inhibition deficits? An ERPs investigation. *Sleep.* 2008;**31**:887–98.

29. Staner L, Cornette F, Maurice D, *et al.* Sleep microstructure around sleep onset differentiates major depressive insomnia from primary insomnia. *J Sleep Res.* 2003;**12**:319–30.

30. Sanacora G, Gueorguieva R, Epperson CN, *et al.* Subtype-specific alterations of gamma-aminobutyric acid and glutamate in patients with major depression. *Arch Gen Psychiatry.* 2004;**61**:705–13.

31. Roth T, Roehrs T, Pies R. Insomnia: pathophysiology and implications for treatment. *Sleep Med Rev.* 2007;**11**:71–9.

32. Berridge CW. Noradrenergic modulation of arousal. *Brain Res Rev.* 2008;**58**:1–17.

33. Yanai K, Tashiro M. The physiological and pathophysiological roles of neuronal histamine: an insight from human positron emission tomography studies. *Pharmacol Ther.* 2007;**113**:1–15.

34. Winsky-Sommerer R, Boutrel B, de Lecea L. Stress and arousal: the corticotrophin-releasing factor/hypocretin circuitry. *Mol Neurobiol.* 2005;**32**:285–94.

35. Drummond SP, Smith MT, Orff HJ, Chengazi V, Perlis ML. Functional imaging of the sleeping brain: review of findings and implications for the study of insomnia. *Sleep Med Rev.* 2004;**8**:227–42.

36. Hines LM, Tabakoff B. WHO/ISBRA study on state and trait markers of alcohol use and dependence investigators. Platelet adenylyl cyclase activity: a biological marker for major depression and recent drug use. *Biol Psychiatry.* 2005;**58**:955–62.

37. Adrien J. Neurobiological bases for the relation between sleep and depression. *Sleep Med Rev.* 2002;**6**:341–52.

38. Ruhé HG, Mason NS, Schene AH. Mood is indirectly related to serotonin, norepinephrine and dopamine levels in humans: a meta-analysis of monoamine depletion studies. *Mol Psychiatry.* 2007;**12**:331–59.

39. Riemann D, Feige B, Hornyak M, *et al.* The tryptophan depletion test: impact on sleep in primary insomnia: a pilot study. *Psychiatry Res.* 2002;**109**:129–35.

40. Lu J, Sherman D, Devor M, Saper CB. A putative flip-flop switch for control of REM sleep. *Nature.* 2006;**441**:589–94.

41. Steriade M. Brain electrical activity and sensory processing during waking and sleep states. In Kryger MH, Roth T, Dement WC, eds. *Principles and Practice of Sleep Medicine*, 4th edn. (Philadelphia: Elsevier, 2005;101–19).

42. Manns ID, Alonso A, Jones BE. Discharge profiles of juxtacellularly labeled and immunohistochemically identified GABAergic basal forebrain neurons recorded in association with the electroencephalogram in anesthetized rats. *J Neurosci.* 2000;**20**:9252–63.

43. Landolt HP. Sleep homeostasis: a role for adenosine in humans? *Biochem Pharmacol.* 2008;**75**:2070–9.

44. Pace-Schott EF, Hobson JA. The neurobiology of sleep: genetics, cellular physiology and subcortical networks. *Nature Neuroscience.* 2002;**3**:591–605.

45. Goutagny R, Luppi PH, Salvert D, *et al.* Role of the dorsal paragigantocellular reticular nucleus in paradoxical (rapid eye movement) sleep generation: a combined electrophysiological and anatomical study in the rat. *Neuroscience.* 2008;**152**:849–57.

46. Fuller PM, Saper CB, Lu J. The pontine REM switch: past and present. *J Physiol.* 2007;**584**:735–41.

47. Verret L, Goutagny R, Fort P, *et al.* A role of melanin-concentrating hormone producing neurons in the central regulation of paradoxical sleep. *BMC Neurosci.* 2003;**4**:19–25.

48. Peterson MJ, Benca RM. Sleep in mood disorders. *Psychiatr Clin North Am.* 2006;**29**:1009–32.

49. Armitage R, Hoffmann RF. Sleep EEG, depression and gender. *Sleep Med Rev.* 2001;**5**:237–46.

50. Adrien J. L'adénosine dans la régulation du sommeil. *Rev Neurol* (Paris). 2001;**157**:5S7–5S11.

51. Ursin R. Serotonin and sleep. *Sleep Med Rev.* 2002;**6**:55–67.

52. Thase ME. Antidepressant treatment of the depressed patient with insomnia. *J Clin Psychiatry.* 1999; **60** Suppl 17:28–31.

53. Shytle RD, Silver AA, Lukas RJ, *et al.* Nicotinic acetylcholine receptors as targets for antidepressants. *Mol Psychiatry.* 2002;**7**:525–35.

54. Perlis ML, Smith MT, Orff HJ, *et al.* The effects of an orally administered cholinergic agonist on REM sleep in major depression. *Biol Psychiatry.* 2002;**51**:457–62.

55. Riemann D. Insomnia and comorbid psychiatric disorders. *Sleep Med.* 2007;**8** Suppl 4:S15–20.

56. Drevets WC, Thase ME, Moses-Kolko EL, *et al.* Serotonin-1A receptor imaging in recurrent depression: replication and literature review. *Nucl Med Biol.* 2007;**34**:865–77.

57. Canli T, Lesch KP. Long story short: the serotonin transporter in emotion regulation and social cognition. *Nat Neurosci.* 2007;**10**:1103–9.

58. Bouali S, Evrard A, Chastanet M, *et al.* Sex hormone-dependent desensitization of 5-HT1A autoreceptors in knockout mice deficient in the 5-HT transporter. *Eur J Neurosci.* 2003;**18**:2203–12.

59. Salomon RM, Ripley B, Kennedy JS, *et al.* Diurnal variation of cerebrospinal fluid hypocretin-1 (orexin-A) levels in control and depressed subjects. *Biol Psychiatry.* 2003;**54**:96–104.

60. Chaki S, Yamaguchi J, Yamada H, *et al.* ATC0175: an orally active melanin-concentrating hormone receptor 1 antagonist for the potential treatment of depression and anxiety. *CNS Drug Rev.* 2005;**11**:341–52.

61. Basso AM, Bratcher NA, Gallagher KB, *et al.* Lack of efficacy of melanin-concentrating hormone-1 receptor antagonists in models of depression and anxiety. *Eur J Pharmacol.* 2006;**540**:115–20.

62. Chang PP, Ford DE, Mead LA, Cooper-Patrick L, Klag MJ. Insomnia in young men and subsequent depression. The John Hopkins precursors study. *Am J Epidemiol.* 1997;**146**:105–14.

63. Gillin JC. Are sleep disturbances risk factors for anxiety, depressive and addictive disorders? *Acta Psychiatr Scand Suppl.* 1998;**393**:39–43.

Chapter 6

Animal models of sleep and stress: implications for mental illness

Deborah Suchecki

Introduction

The influence of stress on sleep is beyond any doubt. However, there are more subtleties to this relation than previously thought. Therefore, the nature and the length of the stressor, and, most of all, the individual who faces the stressful challenge determine the outcome. Moreover, not only does stress alter the sleep pattern but also inadequate sleep influences the stress response, i.e., whether one is sleep-deprived or not determines the ability to respond to stress. This bidirectional association can, thus, represent a vicious circle with detrimental consequences to mental health.

In this chapter, I will describe the sleep changes obtained with animal models of psychopathologies and how they relate to the findings in humans. Moreover, I will discuss possible mechanisms of stress-induced sleep changes and even venture to propose a new function for sleep in the processing of emotional events.

Sleep pattern in stress-related psychopathologies: major depression, anxiety and post-traumatic stress disorder

The goal of this chapter is not to give details about the sleep pattern in these pathologies, for there are specific chapters that deal with this issue. However, it is important to give some information in order to understand how the animal models are useful to study the neurobiology of sleep disorders under these conditions. A common feature to these three pathologies is the presence of insomnia in some form, either represented by difficulty to initiate (anxiety)

or maintain sleep (post-traumatic stress disorder, PTSD), or due to early wakening (major depression). The fact that stress is a major triggering factor for insomnia reinforces the relationship between adverse life events and sleep alterations in mental disorders. Nonetheless, stress rarely causes, by itself, permanent sleep problems [1]. The changes in sleep pattern are usually transient, ending a short time after the resolution of the stressful event, even when the stressor is chronic, such as problems in the work environment [2], divorce [3], or loss of loved ones [4–6]. Interestingly, non-depressed elderly volunteers who were mourning for their lost spouse presented more REM density than non-bereaved control volunteers, but no other change in REM sleep. The bereaved group did not develop depression within a two-year follow-up period, indicating that maintenance of normal sleep after a major adverse life event may represent a protective mechanism for health [6].

Interestingly, an important feature of insomniacs is the fact that although they experience just as many minor life stressors as good sleepers, they interpret these events as more stressful and may, therefore, have greater predisposition to ruminate about the stressors and, consequently, to suffer a greater impact of these events, which would lead to longer lasting sleep disturbances [7]. Moreover, it has been shown in a group of primary insomnia (PI) patients that intrusive thoughts of stressful nature impact on sleep quality, producing more beta activity in the EEG and less delta power [8].

Sleep disturbances are hallmarks of depression and PTSD. These psychiatric pathologies are also triggered by stressful events, but individual vulnerability is again a predominant feature. In depression, delta sleep is impaired and latency to REM sleep is

Sleep and Mental Illness, eds. S. R. Pandi-Perumal and M. Kramer. Published by Cambridge University Press.
© Cambridge University Press 2010.

shortened, whereas the percentage of REM sleep is augmented [9, 10]. In a recent meta-analysis, it was reported that sleep disturbances in PTSD include decreased total sleep time due to shorter delta sleep, increased wake time after sleep onset with sleep disruptions due to nightmares and increased REM density [11, 12].

Animal models for the study of stress-induced sleep changes

The use of experimental models of human diseases is advantageous insofar as many of the mechanisms involved in the installation of the disease can be disclosed, not to mention the development of potential therapeutic agents and preventive actions. Nonetheless, there is special difficulty in modeling human psychopathologies because these involve higher cognitive functions that cannot yet be tested in animals. Still, these models are extremely useful to unveil the neurobiology and, in some cases, even conditions that may trigger or prevent the development of such pathologies.

From animal studies it becomes clear that sleep plays an adaptive role in coping with stress. As long as the stress response is within the protection range, i.e., healthy coping, a compensatory and more intense sleep pattern will ensue. That is to say, after the stressor, animals will sleep more (sleep rebound) and more "deeply" than they did before the event (baseline sleep).

In the next pages I will explore the impact of stress on sleep in healthy and pathological conditions and how different hormonal responses to stress can lead to protection or damage of the sleep pattern. Based on animal studies of genetic and behavioral differences of stress response we will propose models of sleep disorders in PTSD and depression and possible neurobiological mediators of these disorders.

Changes in sleep pattern induced by stressful events result from an integration of genetic, neuroendocrine, and neurophysiological mechanisms. Therefore, most of the studies involve one or a combination of the following strategies: (1) environmental influences, which evaluate the effects of stressors that may or not represent an ethologic situation (social defeat and footshock, respectively) and (2) genetic influences, which evaluate how the sleep of animals with different genetic backgrounds respond to stress.

Environmental influences

For almost three decades the influence of stress on the sleep of rodents has been evaluated. In these species, it is generally accepted that sleep is increased after an acute stressful event, and this increase is believed to function as a coping strategy and an adaptive response that help the animal to recover. However, sleep is not induced immediately after the stress event. There is a prolonged latency for sleep to occur, inasmuch as during stress exposure, both SWS and PS are inhibited, regardless of how long is the stressor [13]. Thereafter, sleep remains inhibited for at least two hours after the end of the stimulus [14, 15], when it begins to rise, reaching the highest levels during the dark phase of the cycle [14–18].

It is worth remembering that the hormonal stress response involves the locus coeruleus–adrenal medulla branch, resulting in the secretion of noradrenalin and adrenaline and the hypothalamic–pituitary–adrenal (HPA) axis, with its major hormones corticotropin-releasing factor (CRF), vasopressin, adrenocorticotropic hormone (ACTH) and glucocorticoids (cortisol or corticosterone). But other hormones are also essential for an appropriate stress response, including oxytocin, prolactin, and endorphins. Noradrenalin, adrenaline, and CRF are essentially pro-waking hormones, whereas prolactin and endorphins are pro-sleep hormones and glucocorticoids depend on optimal levels to induce paradoxical sleep (PS, Figure 6.1); either low or sustained high levels impair PS [13] in rats or REM in humans [19].

Interestingly, there appears to be an optimal time frame within which immobilization stress leads to sleep rebound, being neither too short nor too long, with optimal quality of sleep occurring with one hour of immobilization [13, 20, 21]. Nonetheless, the resulting sleep pattern observed after exposure to stress depends, in great part, on the nature of the stressor. Thus, acute cold stress has been shown to induce SWS, whereas acute footshock induces sustained waking during the subsequent six hours of recording in the daytime period [22] or a later rebound during the day, but not during the dark period [23, 24]. Other studies corroborate the waking-promoting effect of footshock using different paradigms. For instance, in mice, the association of tone with shock (conditioned fear), either in single or multiple training schedules, produces a reduction of SWS and PS. For mice submitted to the multiple training schedule sleep reduction is still evident on the day after

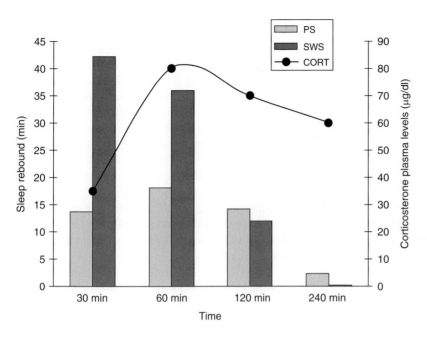

Figure 6.1 Schematic illustration of the inverted U-curve of corticosterone plasma levels, as a consequence of length of immobilization stress, and the expression of PS rebound. Note that SWS is progressively inhibited by increasing levels of the hormone. The illustration is a modification of some findings reported by Marinesco and coworkers [13].

training. Presentation of the tone to this same group up to 27 days after the training elicits reduction of PS, indicating that the reminder of the adverse situation is, by itself, able to elicit waking [25]. These results suggest that context fear conditioning procedure could be used as a model of PTSD, since these patients exhibit increased psychologic and physiologic discomfort when they are reminded of the traumatic event. With this idea in mind Pawlyk and coworkers [26] studied the sleep pattern of rats submitted to situational reminders of a series of five shocks. When sleeping in the same context where shock was delivered, rats exhibit longer latencies to sleep and to PS and reduced percentage of PS; however, when sleeping in a neutral context they display SWS and PS rebound, being thus able to distinguish between neutral and aversive contexts, confirming the occurrence of aversive conditioning. However, there are some issues to keep in mind. First, these studies tend to record the sleep of animals for short periods after footshock, which may not be sufficient to detect the rebound period. Second, and most important, PTSD is not manifested immediately or shortly after the trauma, but some months after. Moreover, PTSD patients seldom need to sleep in the traumatic context. Ideally, one should expose the animals to the traumatic context and assess the impact on sleep in a different cage and, preferably, some weeks after the event.

In human beings the most powerful stressors are those that involve a social context, such as job strains, professional hierarchy, family problems, and interpersonal relationships. In rodents, one example of a social stressor is the social defeat paradigm, accomplished by the resident–intruder paradigm. This method is based on the establishment of a territory by a male and its defense against unfamiliar male intruders. The experimental male (the "intruder") is introduced into the home cage of an aggressive male (the "resident"), the former being attacked and forced to submit by the latter [27]. Social defeat by a male conspecific induces not only strong neuroendocrine responses in plasma catecholamines and corticosterone, but also acute responses in heart rate, blood pressure, body temperature, prolactin, and testosterone [27]. Studies of social defeat-induced sleep rebound show increased slow-wave activity (SWA) but not time spent in SWS, reflecting augmented intensity, but not quantity of sleep. Moreover, SWA is believed to take place in order to restore internal balance after a traumatic event [28, 29].

It is quite interesting that these responses are also modulated by the genetic background and previous stress history of the animals. The gene–environment diathesis hypothesis has permeated numerous studies on the impact of stress on behavior, both in humans and in animal models. According to this hypothesis, the resulting resilience or vulnerability to stress-induced

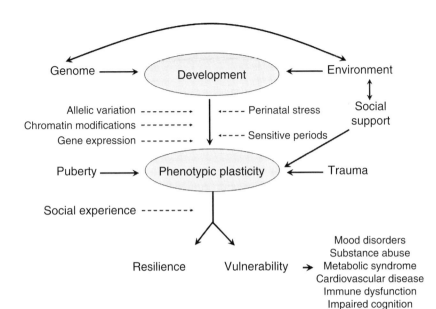

Figure 6.2 Schematic illustration of the genetic–environmental diathesis influence on the build up of resilience or vulnerability to stress-related disorders. The illustration is based on a paper by Plotsky and colleagues [30] and on an oral presentation by Paul Plotsky at the XXXVI ISPNE Annual Meeting September 24 to 27, 2005, Montreal, Quebec, Canada.

disorders are the consequence of an interplay between the genetic background and the environmental influences during specific time-windows, including infancy and adolescence. Adversity during these periods may result in augmented vulnerability, whereas social support throughout life may lead to resilience [30]. A schematic representation of this proposition is presented in Figure 6.2.

With the idea that adversity during infancy might constitute a risk factor for psychopathologic behavior-type in rats, we performed a series of experiments employing the long maternal separation (LMS). Numerous studies have shown that three to six hours of daily maternal separation – LMS – results in increased novelty-induced fear [31] and propensity to consume alcohol [32], two well known features of anxiety-like behavior. Moreover, these animals present hyper-responsiveness of the hypothalamic–pituitary–adrenal (HPA) axis to stress [33]. Given the waking-promoting effect of CRF [34] and corticosterone [23], we hypothesized that LMS could result in a phenotype of vulnerability for stress-induced insomnia. The rationale for the use of the LMS model was based on the fact that anxious individuals are at greater risk to develop chronic insomnia after a stressful situation [7, 35, 36].

We initiated this series of studies by challenging Wistar rats submitted to brief maternal separation (BMS – 15 minutes of separation from the mother during the first two weeks of life, which presumably results in a hypo-responsive HPA axis) with a one-hour restraint stress and assessed their sleep pattern before and after the challenge. We reasoned that early-handled rats would display more sleep rebound than control rats, but to our surprise, they showed the same amount of sleep rebound as control non-manipulated rats, i.e., increased time spent in SWS and in PS [16]. We then proceeded to test LMS rats, expecting that they would exhibit changes compatible with anxiety- and depressive-like behaviors and, consequently, less sleep rebound. But again, to our surprise we found that male rats displayed more paradoxical sleep in the light period of the baseline sleep than control and BMS rats, and a sleep rebound in the dark period of the light–dark cycle similar to the other groups. In addition, all groups exhibited a similar corticosterone response to the challenge.

Female rats, in turn, exhibited a significant PS rebound in the dark period after one hour of cold stress; however, the sleep rebound was greater in LMS rats. Moreover, both manipulated groups (BMS and LMS) exhibited a smaller secretion of corticosterone, although this did not reach statistical significance [15]. Therefore, although we reported on gender differences for stress-induced sleep rebound we were unable to establish a model of vulnerability to insomnia induced by stress.

Another paradigm that has produced stress hyper-responsiveness is prenatal stress. The most effective period to expose pregnant rats to the stressor so as the offspring becomes hyper-responsive is the third – and last – week of pregnancy. The offspring of mothers exposed to gestational stress present hormonal and behavioral changes that are compatible with depression-type behavior [37], including altered sleep regulation, with shorter latency to PS, more PS time, and more awakenings [38].

Genetic influences

The genetic background is a major variable for determination of behavioral expression. Therefore, the same stimulus may lead to different outcomes, depending on how animals react to it. Animal models that attempt to represent human individual differences employ two main strategies: (1) selection of high and low responders to a given stimulus in genetically heterogeneous outbred strains; (2) comparison of inbred strains, which are genetically identical within strain but vary genetically and phenotypically across strains.

In regard to the first strategy, selection of Wistar rats, which intensely explore the open arms of the elevated plus maze (thus considered low anxiety-related behavior or LAB rats), or intensely avoid it (thus considered high anxiety-related behavior or HAB rats), has provided neuroendocrine and behavioral phenotypes that reflect different coping strategies and fearful behaviors to novel situations [39, 40]. High anxiety-related behavior rats display less baseline pre-PS and greater stress-induced sleep impairment, reflected by augmented wakefulness, and reduced SWS and pre-PS, than LAB animals. Interestingly, blockade of CRF-R1 receptors results in more SWS in HAB animals [41], confirming, by means of a different approach, that hyperactivity of the CRF system in "anxious" rats is most likely involved with stress-induced wakefulness.

Using locomotor activity as the behavioral endpoint for selection, Bouyer and colleagues [42] reported on the sleep pattern of high (HR – high novelty-induced locomotor activity) and low responders (LR – low novelty-induced locomotor activity) exposed to immobilization stress. Initially, there was a positive correlation between novelty-induced locomotor activity and corticosterone plasma levels. Peak corticosterone levels were similar between low and high responders, but the latter exhibited an impaired negative feedback, leading to sustained levels of the hormone. Compared to LR, the amount of wakefulness is greater in HR, at the expense of SWS, whereas PS is similar between both phenotypes. In response to acute immobilization, both LR and HR increase their time spent in PS; however, for LR there is a reduction in the time spent in SWS, whereas for HR the reduction takes place in the time spent in wakefulness, which means that stress-induced sleep rebound was evident only in HR.

The second approach consists of comparing different strains that basically differ in their behavioral and neuroendocrine responsiveness to stress. For instance, Lewis (LEW) rats, which are deficient in CRF production, exhibit less wakefulness and more SWS than Fisher 344 (F344) and Sprague–Dawley (Sp-D) rats [43, 44]. Lewis and F344 strains are derived from Sp-D rats and when compared to Sp-D or to outbred Wistar strains, F344 rats show adrenocortical and prolactin hyper-responsiveness to footshock stress and display more anxiety-related behavior in the open field and elevated plus maze. In their home cages, F344 and Wistar rats are more active during the dark period and baseline sleep indicates that these two strains also sleep less than LEW and Sp-D rats. The shorter time of sleep is due to reduction of both SWS and PS, but interestingly, the proportion of PS in regard to total sleep time is similar for all strains [45]. In response to a conditioning fear paradigm, performed in two days, LEW rats exhibit the largest sleep loss during the daytime period and the least recovery during the night-time period, compared to F344 and Wistar rats. Curiously, F344 and LEW exhibit similar levels of freezing behavior, which are higher than those exhibited by Wistar rats, indicating that the reaction to an aversive stimulus may not predict the sleep alteration [46].

In mice strains that differ in reactivity to noxious stimuli such as footshock and contextual fear conditioning a clear and persistent loss of SWS and PS is observed in the more "anxious" BALB/cJ mice, whereas the less "anxious" C57BL/6J mice only show a loss of PS within the hour that follows shock presentation [47, 48]. A similar pattern of sleep reactivity is also seen in response to non-noxious manipulations, such as exposure to an open field [49] or restraint stress [50]: C57BL/6J mice display the characteristic rebound, whereas the BALB/cJ strain displays sleep impairment.

Finally, the use of the Wistar–Kyoto rat, a genetic model of depression, has shed some light on the regulation of sleep in this disorder. These rats present the typical changes in sleep architecture found in depressive patients [51]. Treatment with antidepressants, however, was shown to not reduce PS in Wistar–Kyoto as much as in Wistar rats, suggesting that they may be less sensitive to this class of drugs [52]. Nonetheless, we recently performed a study with Wistar–Kyoto rats using citalopram and showed that not only was PS reduced after the first administration of the drug but also that prolonged treatment resulted in a normalization of the PS in response to a learning paradigm that involves footshock. Therefore, we believe that 21 days of citalopram treatment is able to normalize PS to the levels shown by Wistar rats (unpublished data). A recent study also demonstrated that PS deprivation, an effective, although transient, treatment for depression, increases the expression of orexin in both Wistar–Kyoto and Wistar rats, indicating that contrary to the author's hypothesis, orexin may not be the mediator of PS deprivation-induced antidepressant effect [53].

Mechanisms and mediators of stress-induced sleep changes

Being a global phenomenon, it is only natural to believe that stress alters numerous neurotransmitter and hormonal systems in and out of the central nervous system. The major hormones that participate in the stress response are those of the HPA axis, the locus coeruleus–adrenal medulla system, and hypophysial hormones such as prolactin. A close relationship between these hormones and sleep has already been determined, especially in human beings who exhibit a monophasic pattern of sleep. Major pulses of growth hormone secretion occur during delta sleep, when the lowest levels of HPA and adrenaline activity are observed. Therefore, a negative relationship between cortisol, adrenaline, and delta sleep has been established [54].

Of particular interest is stress-induced prolactin (PRL) secretion and its relationship with PS. It has been well established in human beings that the rise in prolactin levels is observed after sleep onset and that maximal values occur in the early morning hours [55]. The PS-promoting effects of PRL have been demonstrated in cats, rats, and rabbits, although they seem to be time-dependent inasmuch as PS is induced only when PRL is administered in the light period, whereas PRL injection during the dark period inhibits PS [56]. More recently, intracerebroventricular (icv) administration of low doses of PRL-releasing peptide was shown to increase PRL levels and to induce PS [57]. Moreover, intact rats exposed to ether stress exhibit increased levels of PRL and of PS, but animals previously hypophysectomised do not, suggesting that PRL is involved in the augmented PS [58]. We have recently shown that animals sleep deprived for 96 hours and submitted to footshock during the deprivation period exhibit a very pronounced PS rebound afterwards and very high prolactin plasma levels, suggesting that endogenous prolactin is also related to the occurrence of PS [24]. Therefore, prolactin may represent the mediating mechanism of stress-induced sleep rebound and animals that failed to secrete sufficient amounts of this hormone after stress exposure may be at higher risk of developing behavioral alterations that may resemble the human psychopathology.

References

1. Hall M, Thayer JF, Germain A, *et al.* Psychological stress is associated with heightened physiological arousal during NREM sleep in primary insomnia. *Behav Sleep Med.* 2007;**5**:178–93.

2. Akerstedt T, Knutsson A, Westerholm P, *et al.* Sleep disturbances, work stress and work hours: a cross-sectional study. *J Psychosom Res.* 2002;**53**:741–8.

3. Cartwright RD, Wood E. Adjustment disorders of sleep: the sleep effects of a major stressful event and its resolution. *Psychiatry Res.* 1991;**39**:199–209.

4. Hall M, Buysse DJ, Dew MA, *et al.* Intrusive thoughts and avoidance behaviors are associated with sleep disturbances in bereavement-related depression. *Depress Anxiety.* 1997;**6**:106–12.

5. Hardison HG, Neimeyer RA, Lichstein KL. Insomnia and complicated grief symptoms in bereaved college students. *Behav Sleep Med.* 2005;**3**:99–111.

6. Reynolds CF 3rd, Hoch CC, Buysse DJ, *et al.* Sleep after spousal bereavement: a study of recovery from stress. *Biol Psychiatry.* 1993;**34**:791–7.

7. Morin CM, Rodrigue S, Ivers H. Role of stress, arousal, and coping skills in primary insomnia. *Psychosom Med.* 2003;**65**:259–67.

8. Hall M, Buysse DJ, Nowell PD, *et al.* Symptoms of stress and depression as correlates of sleep in primary insomnia. *Psychosom Med.* 2000;**62**:227–30.

9. Holsboer-Trachsler E, Seifritz E. Sleep in depression and sleep deprivation: a brief conceptual review. *World J Biol Psychiatry.* 2000;**1**:180–6.

10. Riemann D, Berger M, Voderholzer U. Sleep and depression: results from psychobiological studies: an overview. *Biol Psychol.* 2001;**57**:67–103.

11. Kobayashi I, Boarts JM, Delahanty DL. Polysomnographically measured sleep abnormalities in PTSD: a meta-analytic review. *Psychophysiology.* 2007;**44**:660–9.

12. Raboni MR, Tufik S, Suchecki D. Treatment of PTSD by eye movement desensitization reprocessing (EMDR) improves sleep quality, quality of life, and perception of stress. *Ann N Y Acad Sci.* 2006;**1071**:508–13.

13. Marinesco S, Bonnet C, Cespuglio R. Influence of stress duration on the sleep rebound induced by immobilization in the rat: a possible role for corticosterone. *Neuroscience.* 1999;**92**:921–33.

14. Tiba PA, Tufik S, Suchecki D. Effects of maternal separation on baseline sleep and cold stress-induced sleep rebound in adult Wistar rats. *Sleep.* 2004;**27**: 1146–53.

15. Tiba PA, Tufik S, Suchecki D. Long lasting alteration in REM sleep of female rats submitted to long maternal separation. *Physiol Behav.* 2008;**93**:444–52.

16. Tiba PA, Palma BD, Tufik S, Suchecki D. Effects of early handling on basal and stress-induced sleep parameters in rats. *Brain Res.* 2003; **975**:158–66.

17. Koehl M, Bouyer JJ, Darnaudery M, Le Moal M, Mayo W. The effect of restraint stress on paradoxical sleep is influenced by the circadian cycle. *Brain Res.* 2002;**937**:45–50.

18. Dewasmes G, Loos N, Delanaud S, Dewasmes D, Ramadan W. Pattern of rapid-eye movement sleep episode occurrence after an immobilization stress in the rat. *Neurosci Lett.* 2004;**355**:17–20.

19. Garcia-Borreguero D, Wehr TA, Larrosa O, *et al.* Glucocorticoid replacement is permissive for rapid eye movement sleep and sleep consolidation in patients with adrenal insufficiency. *J Clin Endocrinol Metab.* 2000;**85**:4201–6.

20. Rampin C, Cespuglio R, Chastrette N, Jouvet M. Immobilisation stress induces a paradoxical sleep rebound in rat. *Neurosci Lett.* 1991;**126**:113–18.

21. Cespuglio R, Marinesco S, Baubet V, Bonnet C, el Kafi B. Evidence for a sleep-promoting influence of stress. *Adv Neuroimmunol.* 1995;**5**:145–54.

22. Palma BD, Suchecki D, Tufik S. Differential effects of acute cold and footshock on the sleep of rats. *Brain Res.* 2000;**861**:97–104.

23. Vazquez-Palacios G, Velazquez-Moctezuma J. Effect of electric foot shocks, immobilization, and corticosterone administration on the sleep–wake pattern in the rat. *Physiol Behav.* 2000;**71**:23–8.

24. Machado RB, Tufik S, Suchecki D. Chronic stress during paradoxical sleep deprivation increases paradoxical sleep rebound: association with prolactin plasma levels and brain serotonin content. *Psychoneuroendocrinology.* 2008;**33**:1211–24.

25. Sanford LD, Fang J, Tang X. Sleep after differing amounts of conditioned fear training in BALB/cJ mice. *Behav Brain Res.* 2003;**147**:193–202.

26. Pawlyk AC, Jha SK, Brennan FX, Morrison AR, Ross RJ. A rodent model of sleep disturbances in posttraumatic stress disorder: the role of context after fear conditioning. *Biol Psychiatry.* 2005;**57**:268–77.

27. Koolhaas JM, De Boer SF, De Rutter AJ, Meerlo P, Sgoifo A. Social stress in rats and mice. *Acta Physiol Scand Suppl.* 1997;**640**:69–72.

28. Meerlo P, de Bruin EA, Strijkstra AM, Daan S. A social conflict increases EEG slow-wave activity during subsequent sleep. *Physiol Behav.* 2001;**73**:331–5.

29. Meerlo P, Pragt BJ, Daan S. Social stress induces high intensity sleep in rats. *Neurosci Lett.* 1997;**225**:41–4.

30. Plotsky PM, Owens MJ, Nemeroff CB. Psychoneuroendocrinology of depression. Hypothalamic–pituitary–adrenal axis. *Psychiatr Clin North Am.* 1998;**21**:293–307.

31. Caldji C, Francis D, Sharma S, Plotsky PM, Meaney MJ. The effects of early rearing environment on the development of GABAA and central benzodiazepine receptor levels and novelty-induced fearfulness in the rat. *Neuropsychopharmacology.* 2000;**22**:219–29.

32. Huot RL, Thrivikraman KV, Meaney MJ, Plotsky PM. Development of adult ethanol preference and anxiety as a consequence of neonatal maternal separation in Long Evans rats and reversal with antidepressant treatment. *Psychopharmacology (Berl).* 2001;**158**:366–73.

33. Plotsky PM, Meaney MJ. Early, postnatal experience alters hypothalamic corticotropin-releasing factor (CRF) mRNA, median eminence CRF content and stress-induced release in adult rats. *Brain Res Mol Brain Res.* 1993;**18**:195–200.

34. Chang FC, Opp MR. Corticotropin-releasing hormone (CRH) as a regulator of waking. *Neurosci Biobehav Rev.* 2001;**25**:445–53.

35. Waters WF, Adams SG Jr., Binks P, Varnado P. Attention, stress and negative emotion in persistent sleep-onset and sleep-maintenance insomnia. *Sleep.* 1993;**16**:128–36.

36. Larsson MR, Backstrom M, Johanson A. The interaction between baseline trait anxiety and trauma

exposure as predictor of post-trauma symptoms of anxiety and insomnia. *Scand J Psychol.* 2008;**49**:447–50.

37. Weinstock M. The long-term behavioural consequences of prenatal stress. *Neurosci Biobehav Rev.* 2008;**32**:1073–86.

38. Dugovic C, Maccari S, Weibel L, Turek FW, Van Reeth O. High corticosterone levels in prenatally stressed rats predict persistent paradoxical sleep alterations. *J Neurosci.* 1999;**19**:8656–64.

39. Liebsch G, Montkowski A, Holsboer F, Landgraf R. Behavioural profiles of two Wistar rat lines selectively bred for high or low anxiety-related behaviour. *Behav Brain Res.* 1998;**94**:301–10.

40. Neumann ID, Wigger A, Liebsch G, Holsboer F, Landgraf R. Increased basal activity of the hypothalamo–pituitary–adrenal axis during pregnancy in rats bred for high anxiety-related behaviour. *Psychoneuroendocrinology.* 1998;**23**:449–63.

41. Lancel M, Muller-Preuss P, Wigger A, Landgraf R, Holsboer F. The CRH1 receptor antagonist R121919 attenuates stress-elicited sleep disturbances in rats, particularly in those with high innate anxiety. *J Psychiatr Res.* 2002;**36**:197–208.

42. Bouyer JJ, Vallee M, Deminiere JM, Le Moal M, Mayo W. Reaction of sleep–wakefulness cycle to stress is related to differences in hypothalamo–pituitary–adrenal axis reactivity in rat. *Brain Res.* 1998;**804**:114–24.

43. Opp MR, Imeri L. Rat strains that differ in corticotropin-releasing hormone production exhibit different sleep–wake responses to interleukin 1. *Neuroendocrinology.* 2001;**73**:272–84.

44. Opp MR. Rat strain differences suggest a role for corticotropin-releasing hormone in modulating sleep. *Physiol Behav.* 1997;**63**:67–74.

45. Tang X, Liu X, Yang L, Sanford LD. Rat strain differences in sleep after acute mild stressors and short-term sleep loss. *Behav Brain Res.* 2005;**160**:60–71.

46. Tang X, Yang L, Sanford LD. Rat strain differences in freezing and sleep alterations associated with contextual fear. *Sleep.* 2005;**28**:1235–44.

47. Sanford LD, Tang X, Ross RJ, Morrison AR. Influence of shock training and explicit fear-conditioned cues on sleep architecture in mice: strain comparison. *Behav Genet.* 2003;**33**:43–58.

48. Sanford LD, Yang L, Tang X. Influence of contextual fear on sleep in mice: a strain comparison. *Sleep.* 2003;**26**:527–40.

49. Tang X, Xiao J, Liu X, Sanford LD. Strain differences in the influence of open field exposure on sleep in mice. *Behav Brain Res.* 2004;**154**:137–47.

50. Meerlo P, Easton A, Bergmann BM, Turek FW. Restraint increases prolactin and REM sleep in C57BL/6J mice but not in BALB/cJ mice. *Am J Physiol Regul Integr Comp Physiol.* 2001;**281**:R846–54.

51. Dugovic C, Solberg LC, Redei E, Van Reeth O, Turek FW. Sleep in the Wistar-Kyoto rat, a putative genetic animal model for depression. *Neuroreport.* 2000;**11**:627–31.

52. Ivarsson M, Paterson LM, Hutson PH. Antidepressants and REM sleep in Wistar-Kyoto and Sprague-Dawley rats. *Eur J Pharmacol.* 2005;**522**:63–71.

53. Allard JS, Tizabi Y, Shaffery JP, Manaye K. Effects of rapid eye movement sleep deprivation on hypocretin neurons in the hypothalamus of a rat model of depression. *Neuropeptides.* 2007;**41**:329–37.

54. Born J, Fehm HL. The neuroendocrine recovery function of sleep. *Noise Health.* 2000;**2**:25–38.

55. Roky R, Obal F, Jr., Valatx JL, *et al.* Prolactin and rapid eye movement sleep regulation. *Sleep.* 1995;**18**:536–42.

56. Roky R, Valatx JL, Jouvet M. Effect of prolactin on the sleep–wake cycle in the rat. *Neurosci Lett.* 1993;**156**:117–20.

57. Zhang SQ, Inoue S, Kimura M. Sleep-promoting activity of prolactin-releasing peptide (PrRP) in the rat. *Neuroreport.* 2001;**12**:3173–6.

58. Bodosi B, Obal F, Jr., Gardi J, *et al.* An ether stressor increases REM sleep in rats: possible role of prolactin. *Am J Physiol Regul Integr Comp Physiol.* 2000;**279**:R1590–8.

Insomnia and brain orexin alterations in depressive illness

Pingfu Feng and Kumaraswamy Budur

Summary

Chronic insomnia is characterized by long-lasting behavioral and physiologic hyperarousal, elevated orexinergic and hypothalamic–pituitary–adrenal (HPA) systems, and is causatively associated with chronic stress. The overfunctioning wake-promoting background mainly contributed by the orexinergic system is hypothesized in the following review mostly based on preclinical evidence. Elevated brain orexin(s) could result from genetic issues, chronic stress, or insufficient aminergic suppression such as the reduction of dopamine (DA) and serotonin (5-hydroxytryptamine, 5-HT), which could be associated with reduced social/physical activity, chronic disease, or surgery since the production of these neurotransmitters is dependent on social and physical activity.

General review of insomnia

Insomnia is defined as difficulty initiating sleep, maintaining sleep, early awakening, or non-restorative sleep despite adequate opportunity and is accompanied by one or more of the following: fatigue or daytime sleepiness; attention, concentration, or memory impairment; poor social, occupational or academic performance; mood disturbance or irritability; reduction in motivation, energy or initiative; errors/accidents at work or while driving; tension; headaches; gastrointestinal distress; and worries about sleep [1]. It is estimated that about 10 to 20% of the population suffers from chronic insomnia [2, 3]. Primary insomnia accounts for about 25% of patients with chronic insomnia [4]. Insomnia is associated with significant impairment in social and occupational functioning and the direct costs on society are huge [5].

Patients with chronic primary insomnia are characterized by a state of hyperarousal. An overwhelming amount of evidence supports the concept of hyperarousal in insomnia patients. Insomnia patients, despite lack of sleep at night and complaints of fatigue during the day, are not sleepier during the day compared with controls with normal nocturnal sleep. On the contrary, insomniacs are more alert than normal sleepers. On multiple sleep latency tests (MSLT), insomniacs either have a normal or prolonged sleep latency compared with control subjects [4, 6]. This is suggestive of insomnia being a 24-hour hyperarousal disorder, rather than just nocturnal sleep loss. Sympathetic nervous system hyperarousal in patients with chronic insomnia is evidenced by various objective findings including a higher basal metabolic rate [7] and elevated catecholamine levels [8].

The findings on neuroimaging studies are also consistent with hyperarousal in insomnia. Patients with insomnia show elevated global cerebral metabolism during sleep compared with normal sleepers. Shifting from wakefulness to sleep states is associated with a smaller decline in metabolic rates in the areas that promote wakefulness in insomniacs compared with normal sleepers. It is suggested that elevated brain metabolism can explain the subjective symptoms of disturbed sleep in insomniacs and the inability of the arousal system to decrease its activity, while shifting from wakefulness to sleep states, may account for the difficulty in sleep initiation [9, 10].

Various EEG findings again support the hypothesis of hyperarousal in insomnia. During wakefulness, and at the sleep onset period, insomniacs have an elevated relative beta power and lower delta power [11, 12]. During rapid eye movement (REM) sleep, alpha and beta powers are increased, while theta and delta powers are lower [13].

It is hypothesized that elevated corticotropin-releasing hormone (CRH) activity, causing hyperarousal, is responsible for the pathogenesis of primary insomnia [14]. This is based on the fact that both animal and human studies reveal an overactive HPA axis in insomniacs. Primary insomnia patients have elevated levels of urinary cortisol that correlate with the duration of wakefulness at night [8]. Richardson and Roth concluded that CRH hyperactivity, because of either a genetic diathesis or stress, results in an exaggerated CRH response to stress. Any further re-exposure to stress leads to an amplification of the abnormal stress response; this sequence leads to significant difficulties with sleeping in the face of stressful situations and an exaggerated and prolonged sleep disturbance following stress, and eventually chronic primary insomnia [14]. Chronic insomnia is associated with increased adrenocorticotropic hormone (ACTH) levels [15]. Furthermore, patients with insomnia have significantly higher plasma cortisol levels in the evening and night and a reduced duration of the quiescent period of circadian cortisol secretion compared with controls. This is thought to be secondary to the diminished negative feedback of cortisol on CRH [16, 17]. Middle-aged adults are more sensitive to the arousal effects of cortisol compared to young adults and this might explain increasing age as a risk factor for insomnia. In a study to examine the effects of exogenous administration of CRH on arousal and wakefulness, it was noted that only middle-aged men, and not young men, had increased wakefulness and this was more pronounced during the first half of the night. Also, only middle-aged men, and not young men, had decreases in slow-wave sleep in response to CRH [18]. A study to examine the effects of doxepin, a tricyclic antidepressant, on nocturnal sleep and plasma cortisol levels in patients with primary insomnia showed that doxepin improved sleep and reduced mean cortisol levels, suggesting that beneficial effects of the medication are at least partially mediated by the normalization of the HPA axis [19].

The vast objective evidence including findings on sleep measures, neuroimaging, EEG, and cortisol findings supports the notion of chronic insomnia as a state of hyperarousal rather than just sleep loss. This hyperarousal feature is likely a regulatory offset resulting from a wake/sleep imbalanced regulatory background (WIRB) integrated with multiple wake/sleep regulatory systems. The WIRB has either an elevated wake promoting or a reduced sleep promoting regulation or a combination. Obviously, the WIRB in chronic insomnia is not likely a single neuronal or humoral alteration; instead, multiple neuronal and humoral regulatory systems may be involved.

Wake/sleep regulation by neurotransmitters

Although it is not quite clear how each basic neuronal regulatory system participates in the WIRB, understanding these wake/sleep regulatory systems is quite critical.

Wake- and arousal-promoting regulation

The concept for the function of aminergic neurons in sleep/wake regulation has been changed dramatically in the last decade. These neurons including serotonergic (5-HT), noradrenergic (NA), dopaminergic (DA), and histaminergic (HA) neurons are now recognized as strong wake-promoting neurons.

5-HT neurons are located in the raphé nucleus and project widely to the entire central nervous system (CNS) and act via the release of 5-HT. 5-HT dorsal raphé nucleus (DRN) neurons fire at their highest rate during wakefulness, at a lower rate during non-REM sleep, and completely cease to fire during REM sleep [20–23]. Extracellular level of 5-HT in the DRN [24], medial medullary reticular formation [25], laterodorsal and pedunculopontine tegmentum (LDT/PPT) [26], hippocampus [27], and frontal cortex [24] exhibited a similar pattern, i.e., highest in waking, lower in slow-wave sleep and lowest in REM sleep. 5-HT activates the cortex through the activation of $5-HT_{2a}$ receptors on thalamocortical neuronal terminals and thereby increases glutamate release, which in turn activates cortical neurons as demonstrated by an increase of c-Fos expression [28]. Systemic administration of a $5-HT_{2a}$ receptor agonist, DOI, significantly decreases neocortical high-voltage spindle activity, and this effect may be blocked by different $5-HT_2$ receptor antagonists [29]. 5-HT neurons are widely involved in the regulation of sleep/wake states, mood, and behavioral and basic physiologic activities. Deficiency in 5-HT neurons has been accepted as being the cause of the depression in a large portion of the insomniac population.

Norepinephrine (NE) is one of the main brain monoamines synthesized and released by NA neurons located in the locus coeruleus (LC) [30]. The LC

NE neurons give rise to local axon projections to forebrain structures within the dorsal noradrenergic bundle and innervate the thalamus, hippocampus, and cortex and also projections to motor neurons [31]. Similar to 5-HT, spontaneous discharge of NE-containing neurons is the highest during waking, lower during slow-wave sleep, and virtually absent during REM sleep. The discharge anticipated sleepwalking stages as well as phasic cortical activity, such as spindles, during slow-wave sleep [21, 32, 33]. At the end of the REM sleep period and a few seconds prior to behavioral arousal, the discharges are resumed [32]. Norepinephrine neurons innervate the cortex, with the highest density of cortical innervation being in layers III and IV [34]. The tonic release of NE in the cortex is increased with vigilance level [35]. The pontine [36] and prefrontal [37] release of NE is highest during waking and is strongly decreased during REM sleep. When there is a novel stimulation or event, a phasic mode of discharge quickly occurs [38]. Infusion of $\alpha2$ adrenergic receptor agonist clonidine into LC suppressed NA neurons firing and decreased waking and increased sleep without affecting REM sleep [39]. Norepinephrine excites $\alpha1$ receptors in the forebrain to promote cortical activation and excites $\alpha2$ receptors in the brainstem to inhibit REM sleep [40, 41].

Histamine has been suggested as a "waking substance" due to the sedative "side effects" of antihistamines that triggered early work [42]. The HA nucleus is located between the mamillary bodies and the chiasma opticum at the tuber cinereum [43]. Similar to most aminergic neurons, HA neurons fire the most when awake, slower during NREM sleep, and the least in REM sleep [44]. Extracellular HA levels in the preoptic/anterior hypothalamus were the most during wakefulness, lower during NREM sleep, and the least during REM sleep [45]. This level also exhibits a marked circadian rhythmicity in accordance with the firing of HA neurons during waking [46]. All HA receptors, H_{1R}–H_{4R}, have excitatory actions on enteric neurons and are found in the whole intestine and enteric nervous system in humans [47]. More severe autoimmune diseases and neuroinflammation are observed in mice lacking H_{3R} [48]. In the brain, HA excites cholinergic neurons [49], 5-HT neurons in the DRN [50], and DA neurons in the striatum [51], and NA neurons in the locus coeruleus [52]. Microinjection of HA or 2-thiazolylethylamine (an H_{1R} agonist) caused a long-lasting suppression

of cortical slow activity and an increase in quiet wakefulness [49]. Histamine maintains wakefulness through direct projections of the tuberomammillary nucleus (TMN) to the thalamus and the cortex, and indirectly through activation of other ascending arousal systems, mainly cholinergic and aminergic nuclei [52].

Dopamine-containing cell bodies were previously thought to be almost exclusively confined to the substantia nigra pars compacta, ventral tegmental area, and tuberoinfundibular system. Numerous cell bodies that stained for tyrosine hydroxylase in the dorsal and median raphe nuclei area were also found. A dopamine neuron has very different electrophysiologic features in the firing rate and pattern from all other aminergic neurons. Dopamine neurons in the substantia nigra recorded in freely moving cats displayed the highest discharge rate during active waking, which was greater than the discharge rate during quiet waking. The firing activity has no correlation with phasic electromyography (EMG) changes, and there is no significant change when an animal progresses from quiet waking through NREM sleep and REM sleep. Interestingly, the firing rate has also no correlation with either sleep spindles or PGO waves. However, this stability can be dramatically altered under special circumstances, such as during and following orienting responses [53–55]. These brought an initial concept that dopamine is not critically involved in the sleep/wake regulation. However, a big differences in terminal DA release between states was observed, i.e., the release of DA in postsynaptic target regions decreased significantly during sleep and increased about 50% during movement [55]. Lesions of DA cell groups in the ventral tegmentum that project to the forebrain produce marked reduction in behavioral arousal [56]. Dopamine-specific reuptake blockers promote wakefulness in normal and sleep-disordered narcoleptic animals [57]. In mice, deletion of the DA transporter (DAT) gene reduces NREM sleep time and increases wakefulness independently from locomotor effects. DAT knockout mice are also unresponsive to the normally robust wake-promoting action of modafinil, methamphetamine, and the selective DAT blocker GBR12909 but are hypersensitive to the wake-promoting effects of caffeine [58].

Cholinergic neurons are one of the major components in the ascending reticular formation system [59] and were found to be critical in maintaining cortical wakefulness in brain transaction studies in the 1940s by Moruzzi and Magoun. They found that cholinergic basal forebrain neurons lie in the path of the major ascending fiber system from the brainstem reticular activating system and thus serve as the ventral extra-thalamic relay to the cerebral cortex [60, 61]. Cortical activation evoked by stimulation of the reticular formation has been shown to depend upon two pathways, one through the thalamus and the other through the basal forebrain [62]. The neurons that provide the major cholinergic innervation to the cerebral cortex are located in the nucleus basalis of Meynert [63–65]. Through activation of the basal forebrain relay, cholinergic nucleus basalis neurons project to cerebral cortex and release acetylcholine (ACh) from their terminals. Cholinergic cells are modulated in turn by afferents ascending from the pontomesencephalic tegmentum [66]. Lesions of the basal forebrain cholinergic cells are associated with a decrease in cortical ACh release and a parallel decrease in cortical activation [67–69]. Reciprocally, electrical or chemical stimulation of the cholinergic basalis neurons in anesthetized or brainstem-transected animals leads to a parallel increase in cortical ACh release and cortical activation [70, 71].

Sleep-promoting neuronal and humoral regulation

Two basic sleep states, REM sleep and NREM sleep, are identified in human and most warm-blooded animals. Non-REM sleep generally occurs from a decreasing wake level such as drowsiness and is displayed as progressively increased amplitude and decreased frequency of cortical EEG and decreased amplitude of EMG. When the amplitude of the EEG becomes very high and the frequency decreases to 4 Hz or below, it is also called slow-wave sleep (SWS). Rapid eye movement sleep features are low amplitude and high frequency of EEG and low amplitude EMG. This stage is also called paradoxical sleep and active sleep in the neonatal period. One feature of REM sleep is that the EEG is dominated by a frequency band 4–7 Hz, called theta rhythm, which can be best recorded in the hippocampus area or the cortex above the hippocampus. Rapid eye movement sleep is so named because rapid eye movements occur during this stage in the human and the cat. Although it is rarely recorded in rodents, the name REM sleep remains widely used.

GABAergic neurons are one of the major inhibitory neuronal systems in the nervous system. GABAergic neurons in the median preoptic nucleus (MnPN) ventrolateral preoptic (VLPO) area play a major role in the initiation, and neurons in the VLPO play a major role in the maintenance of slow-wave NREM sleep [59, 72, 73]. Blocking $GABA_A$ receptors in this area increases quiet wakefulness but significantly reduces deep NREM and REM sleep [74]. Common hypnotic drugs and anesthetics enhance GABA-mediated neurotransmission acting at $GABA_A$ receptors [75–77]. Activation of $GABA_B$ receptors, which are G-protein-coupled receptors linked to PKC channels, enhances cortical slow-wave activity and sleep, and simultaneously diminishes peripheral muscle tone [73, 78]. The VLPO GABA neurons are inhibited by NE, 5-HT, and ACh, which are all transmitters that promote wakefulness [79]. GABA neurons from VLPO and pontine ventral periaqueductal gray including the DRN itself innervate DRN neurons. GABA is reduced in the plasma and cerebrospinal fluid (CSF) of depressives [80, 81]. The reduction of GABA is seen more in severely depressed patients [82]. Interestingly, GABA activation by diazepam enhances immobility [83, 84] and either $GABA_B$ –/– mice or those given a selective $GABA_B$ receptor antagonist had decreased immobility in the forced-swim test [85]. The number of Fos-immunoreactive neurons in the VLPO is positively correlated with total sleep time recorded during the 60 minutes prior to sacrifice [59].

Adenosine is also a ubiquitous neuromodulator that increases sleep, particularly high-amplitude NREM sleep, and suppresses wakefulness. Many of these effects are mediated by adenosine A1 receptors and are thought to be functioning in the basal forebrain [86–88]. The neuronal activity of wakefulness-active neurons in the magnocellular basal forebrain, with the highest discharge activity during wakefulness, showed marked reduction in activity just before and during the entry to NREM sleep. The adenosine concentrations in the basal forebrain are increased following prolonged wakefulness. This suggests that the reduction of wake-related discharges is due to an increase in the extracellular concentration of adenosine during wakefulness. Adenosine acts via the A_1 receptor to reduce the activity of wakefulness-promoting neurons [89]. Microdialysis perfusion of A_1 receptor antisense in the basal forebrain significantly reduces NREM sleep with an increase in wakefulness. After six hours of sleep deprivation, the antisense-treated animals spend significantly less time in NREM sleep, and show an even greater post-deprivation reduction in delta power (60–75%) and a concomitant increase in wakefulness [90]. Adenosine perfusion into the basal forebrain increases the relative power in the delta frequency band, whereas higher frequency bands (theta, alpha, beta, and gamma) show a decrease [91]. There is a significant diurnal variation in enzyme activities in the cortex and the basal forebrain brain areas. Adenosine kinase and both nucleotidases show their lowest activity in the middle of the rest phase, suggesting the level of adenosine metabolism is related to activity and may be associated with the lower level of energy metabolism during sleep compared to wakefulness [92].

Cholinergic LDT/PPT neurons are responsible for the generation of REM sleep. These neurons project to cholinoceptive medial pontine reticular formation neurons to provide ACh, which activates muscarinic cholinergic receptor m2/m4 to contribute to cholinergic REM sleep generation [66, 93, 94, 95, 96]. LDT/PPT neurons fire tonically during wakefulness and increase firing before and throughout REM sleep [97, 98]. Microinjection of a cholinergic agonist, carbachol, into the pontine reticular formation of chronically instrumented intact or acutely decerebrated rats and cats has been used extensively to study REM sleep mechanisms [99, 100]. Activation of the cholinergic cell compartment of the PPT by GABA also initiates REM sleep in the rat [101]. The effects of carbachol on REM sleep can be reduced by the muscarinic receptor antagonist atropine [100, 102] and scopolamine [103].

Orexin regulation of wake/sleep states

Orexins were originally studied as part of the hypothalamic network for energy homeostasis and were found to promote wakefulness and suppress sleep via orexin type 1 and type 2 receptors (OX1R and OX2R) [104, 105]. Orexins, including orexin A and orexin B, are isolated from the hypothalamus [106, 107] and are synthesized in neurons of the perifornical region and the lateral hypothalamus. Fibers of these neurons innervate most brain regions including the brainstem and basal forebrain, cortex, and spinal cord [108, 109]. Orexin-immunopositive neurons are characterized by biphasic broad spikes and are waking-active neurons. These neurons exhibit tonic discharge highly specific to wakefulness. All orexin waking-active neurons exhibit slow tonic discharges during wakefulness and cease firing shortly after the onset of EEG synchronization, the EEG sign of sleep. They remain virtually silent during NREM sleep, but display transient discharges during REM sleep. During the transition from sleep to wakefulness, orexin neurons fire in clusters prior to the onset of EEG activation, the EEG sign of wakefulness, and respond with a short latency to an arousing sound stimulus given during sleep [110]. Local application of orexin A in the basal forebrain [111] or the LDT/PPT [112] increases wakefulness dramatically. Intracerebroventricular administration of orexin A promotes both quiet wake and active wake, but orexin B promotes active wake only in normal adult rats. Orexin A promotes quiet wake only if administered into the medial preoptic area, medial septal area, and substantia innominata [104]. Brain injection of orexin A in the hypothalamic paraventricular nucleus, rostral lateral hypothalamic area, and substantia nigra pars compacta significantly increased time spent vertical and ambulating [113]. c-Fos expression in orexin neurons correlates positively with the amount of wakefulness and negatively with the amounts of NREM and REM sleep [114]. The majority of orexinergic neurons express c-Fos during active waking [114]. In rat brain slices of centromedial nuclei and rhomboid nuclei in the thalamus, orexin depolarizes and excites all neurons tested through a direct postsynaptic action.

Orexin excites almost all wake-promoting neurons including cholinergic, DA, NA [115], and 5-HT neurons [50, 116]. In rat brain slices, orexins have a strong and direct excitatory effect on the cholinergic neurons of the contiguous basal forebrain. This effect of orexins' action depends upon OX2R. OX2R, which is lacking in narcoleptic dogs [117], has a strong and direct excitatory effect on the cholinergic neurons of the contiguous basal forebrain [111]. These results suggest that the orexins excite cholinergic neurons that release acetylcholine in the cerebral cortex and thereby contribute to the cortical activation associated with wakefulness [115].

Orexins excite 5-HT neurons directly via a tetrodotoxin-insensitive, Na^+/K^+ non-selective cation current [50, 116]. Orexin A and orexin B induce dose-dependent inward currents in most 5-HT neurons. At higher concentrations, orexins also increase spontaneous postsynaptic currents in 5-HT neurons. These effects can be mostly blocked by the $GABA_A$

receptor antagonist bicuculline. In rat brain slices of the centromedial nuclei and rhomboid nuclei in the thalamus, orexin depolarizes and excites all neurons tested through a direct postsynaptic action [115]. Further study indicated that the effect of orexins on 5-HT activation is different. Orexin A increases 5-HT in the dorsal raphe nucleus, but not in the median raphe nucleus. However, orexin B elicited a small but significant effect in both the dorsal raphe nucleus and the median raphe nucleus [118]. Orexins may have regionally selective effects on 5-HT release in the CNS, implying a unique interaction between orexins and 5-HT in the regulation of activities including sleep–wakefulness. Immunolabeling showed that orexin fibers project to 5-HT neurons in the dorsal raphe nucleus.

Orexins administered in the ventral tegmental area yielded a marked increase in the rewarding effect place preference test, and the release of dopamine and calcium in the nucleus accumbens. This orexin-induced DA and calcium release can be inhibited by selective PKC inhibitor [119–122]. In summary, orexins excite or promote all aminergic neurons, which are all involved in the pathology of depression. In feedback, orexins are inhibited by 5-HT [123], DA, and NA neurons [124]. This closed circuit of regulation of wake/sleep states may also provide a homeostatic regulation for the need of wake-regulating substrates and for the sleep/wake cycle as well.

Orexins induce wakefulness by means of the TMN HA neurons via H_{1R}. Perfusion of orexin A into the TMN through a microdialysis probe promptly increased wakefulness with a reduction in REM and NREM sleep. Microdialysis studies showed that application of orexins into the TMN increased histamine release from both the medial preoptic area and the frontal cortex in a dose-dependent manner [125–128]. Morphologically and electrophysiologically identified HA neurons are depolarized and excited by the orexins through a direct postsynaptic action. The effect of orexins is likely mediated by OX2R [128, 129].

Orexins respond to stress and HPA activation

Stress induces the response of orexins. A tremendous amount of data has shown that stress exerts complex effects on the brain and periphery, dependent on the temporal profile and intensity of the stressor. Cold stress but not immobilization stress increased

the expression of orexin mRNA in the LHA in older but not younger rats. Interestingly intracerebroventricular injection of orexin induced dose-dependent increase of corticosterone levels [130] and plasma ACTH, corticosterone and c-Fos mRNA in the paraventricular nucleus (PVN) of the rat [131]. Orexin A is increased after short-term forced swimming and is decreased after long-term immobilization [132]. The involvement of glucocorticoids in stress processes as well as in bodyweight regulation is well known. Lateral hypothalamic prepro-orexin mRNA expression is decreased after adrenalectomy. Peripheral glucocorticoid treatment with dexamethasone restores its expression to normal levels indicating that orexin expression in the lateral hypothalamus is modulated by the glucocorticoids status [133]. Noxious stimuli significantly induced Fos protein in orexin neurons [134]. This evidence indicates that orexins constitute one of the neuronal systems that respond to stress.

Classically, the stress response is mediated by the HPA system. In an acute stress stimulation, neurons in the hypothalamic paraventricular nucleus synthesize and release CRH, which starts the response of HPA axis to stress. The CRH neurons induce ACTH release from the pituitary, which subsequently causes cortisol release from the adrenal cortex. Corticotropin-releasing hormone neurons project not only to the median eminence but also into brain areas where they regulate, for example, adrenal innervation of the autonomic system and affect mood [135, 136]. Simultaneously, an increase of CRH in the brain also increases wakefulness [137] and suppression of CRH by intracerebroventricular administration of antisense CRH DNA oligodeoxynucleotides reduces CRH mRNA and wakefulness [138]. In animal studies, chronic stress by footshock and immobilization by restraining or forced swimming induces enhanced wake regulation as indicated by either an increase of wakefulness or decrease of total sleep [139, 140].

Corticotropin-releasing hormone suppresses sleep and increases wakefulness through an elevation of orexin [141] but not necessarily by ACTH and cortisol [142, 143]. New data indicate that the CRF peptidergic system directly innervates orexin-expressing neurons. Corticotropin-releasing hormone activates orexinergic neurons, which in turn alter vigilance, while both ACTH [144] and cortisol [145] do not increase wakefulness [142, 143]. Application of CRF to hypothalamic slices containing identified orexin neurons depolarizes membrane potential and increases firing rate in a subpopulation of orexinergic cells. Corticotropin-releasing factor induced depolarization is tetrodotoxin insensitive and is blocked by the peptidergic CRH_{R1} antagonist astressin. In CRH_{R1} knockout mice, activation of orexin neurons in response to acute stress is severely impaired. This evidence indicates that after stressor stimuli, CRH-stimulated release of orexin contributes to the activation and maintenance of arousal associated with the stress response [141]. Orexins inhibit pain transmission. In prepro-orexin (precursor of orexin A and B) knockout mice, baseline pain thresholds are not different between the knockout and wild-type mice. However, knockout mice present a greater degree of hyperalgesia induced by peripheral inflammation and less stress-induced analgesia than wild-type mice [146]. OX1R immunoreactivity is dramatically increased and peaked in the hippocampus and cortex two days after ischemia stress induced by transient common carotid artery occlusion [147]. In addition, administration of alpha-helical CRH or CRH antagonist blocks the orexin-induced grooming and face-washing behaviors in rats. These findings indicated that wake or vigilance regulation is an important feature of a stress response and that orexinergic systems are a critical mediator in stress-induced wake increase or insomnia.

Elevated orexin content is implicated in human and animal models of insomnia

The aforementioned discussion implied that an elevated orexinergic system may exist and play a critical role in the WIRB in chronic insomniacs. Poor and disturbed sleep or insomnia is a major symptom in major depressive disorders (MDD) [148–151]. Studies in the past 30 years have consistently demonstrated that MDD is characterized by poor sleep maintenance, reduced slow-wave NREM sleep, disturbances of sleep continuity, reduced REM latency, and an increase in REM density [152, 153]. Some patients with depression have abnormal central arousal (either hypo- or hyper-) and orexins could be one of the key wake-promoting neural components influencing sleep [154]. For the limited resource of human studies, orexinergic measurements are only carried out in peripheral samples including blood and CSF. Cerobrospinal fluid orexin A levels are

slightly increased in depressed patients. But, the diurnal variations of orexin A levels are dampened. In the same study, treatment with sertraline (a selective serotonin reuptake inhibitor) for five weeks resulted in a slight decrease in orexin A levels, but a similar effect is not noted after treatment with bupropion, another potent antidepressant medication. This might be due to the 5-HT effect on orexin tone [155]. Orexin levels correlate with specific psychiatric symptoms. A significant negative correlation is noted between orexin levels and the symptoms of lassitude (difficulty in initiating activities), slowness of movements, and rating of global illness [156]. Suicide ideation is one of the features of depression and suicide is one of the important causes of mortality in patients with depression [157, 158]. Interestingly, suicidal patients with depression have significantly lower CSF orexin-A levels compared to suicidal patients with dysthymia or adjustment disorder [159]. This indicates that the suicidal patients with depression have a dysfunction of the hypothalamic region involving neuropeptides that regulate arousal and vigilance.

We have recently modeled chronic insomnia in the rat by a treatment of chronic neonatal stress, i.e., maternal deprivation (MD). A large body of data has shown that neonatal MD leads to long-lasting alterations of stress at behavioral, physiologic, and molecular levels including elevated activation of the HPA axis, a marker for chronic stress [160]. Behaviorally, the MD rat is more sensitive to stressful stimulation and has increased anxiety [161, 162]. Molecularly, the MD rat has increased plasma ACTH and corticosterone at baseline and in response to stressful stimulation [160], hyper-expression of CRH mRNA from the hypothalamus [163], and elevated brain CRH levels [164]. We found that an adult rat neonatally treated with ten days of MD showed features of chronic insomnia including decreased total sleep and increased total wake time during the subjective night [165]. In this chronic model of insomnia, hypothalamic CRH and orexin A levels are highly increased but hippocampal orexin B is decreased [165]. Similar results are also found in a rat model of depression induced by neonatal administration of clomipramine. The rat model of depression has shown increases in both hypothalamic orexin A and orexin B [166].

These facts imply that both CRH and orexin alterations play a critical role in the neurobiological regulation of hyperarousal in insomnia and that rehabilitation of neuronal and hormonal elevation may be the key for symptomatic recovery of insomnia.

These findings indicate that this model of chronic stress is likely a model of chronic insomnia and that orexins may play a critical role in the features of hyperarousal seen in the clinical syndrome.

Our hypothesis for insomnia

Hyperarousal is one of the most common features of insomnia [167] and one of the stronger predictors of chronic insomnia [168]. Hyperarousal is important to the clinical presentation of primary insomnia [14, 169, 170]. Symptomatic and phenotype changes of hyperarousal indicate an over-functioned wake promotion in the WIRB, which involves multiple aminergic neuronal systems, cholinergic neuronal systems, and orexinergic neuronal systems [171, 172]. The discovery of orexinergic neurons and their role in wake promotion shed light on the better understanding of insomnia in neuronal regulation. A working concept for the pathology of insomnia is that the orexinergic system plays a key role in chronic or primary insomnia due to its effect in responding to stress, in facilitating wake-promoting aminergic and cholinergic neurons, and in promoting wakefulness. The amazing fact is that all aminergic neurons have a negative feedback effect on the orexinergic neurons, that is, orexinergic neurons are inhibited by 5-HT [123], DA, and NA neurons [124]. This closed circuit of wake/sleep regulation may provide a homeostatic regulation for the need of wake-regulating substrates and for the sleep/wake cycle as well. We hypothesize that stress-associated chronic insomnia mainly results from increased brain orexin levels, which could be induced by various types of factors including being genetically coded with higher level of orexinergic activity and chronic stress invoked elevation of orexins. Disinhibition from wake-promoting aminergic neurons, especially DA and 5-HT, could also be a cause for elevation of orexins and/or CRH because the activity-dependent release features during movement [55, 173–175] (Figure 7.1). In addition, the supportive evidence includes (1) that epidemiologic data have shown that reduced social activity is a risk factor in depression [176]; (2) that the reduction of social/physical activity is often seen in chronic disease and post surgery, etc.; and (3) antidepressants reduce orexin levels [155, 177]. Certainly, an orexinergic pathway may

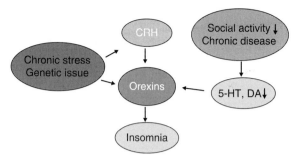

Figure 7.1 A tentative hypothesis of chronic insomnia. This hypothesis indicated that insomnia could result from elevated brain orexins, which can be induced by (1) genetic issue, (2) stress induced elevation of HPA, and (3) the reduction of 5-HT and DA, which might result from reduced social activity, exercise, chronic disease, surgery, etc.

not be shared by all causes of insomnia such as narcolepsy, which has insomnia with undetectable orexin levels [178, 179].

References

1. AASM. *International Classification of Sleep Disorders (ICSD)*, 2nd edn. *Diagnostic and Coding Manual.* (Westchester, IL: The American Academy of Sleep Medicine, 2005).

2. Ancoli-Israel S, Cooke JR. Prevalence and comorbidity of insomnia and effect on functioning in elderly populations. *J Am Geriatr Soc.* 2005;**53**: S264–71.

3. NSF. *Sleep in America Poll 2005.* (National Sleep Foundation, 2005).

4. Stepanski E, Zorick F, Roehrs T, Young D, Roth T. Daytime alertness in patients with chronic insomnia compared with asymptomatic control subjects. *Sleep.* 1988;**11**:54–60.

5. Walsh JK, Engelhardt CL. The direct economic costs of insomnia in the United States for 1995. *Sleep.* 1999; **22** Suppl (2):S386–93.

6. Bonnet MH, Arand DL. Activity, arousal, and the MSLT in patients with insomnia. *Sleep.* 2000;**23**:205–12.

7. Bonnet MH, Arand DL. 24-hour metabolic rate in insomniacs and matched normal sleepers. *Sleep.* 1995;**18**:581–8.

8. Vgontzas AN, Tsigos C, Bixler EO, *et al.* Chronic insomnia and activity of the stress system: a preliminary study. *J Psychosom Res.* 1998;**45**:21–31.

9. Nofzinger E, Nowell P, Buysee D. Towards a neurobiology of sleep disturbance in primary insomnia and depression: a comparison of subjective, visually scored and measures. *Sleep.* 1999;**22**:S99.

10. Nofzinger EA, Buysse DJ, Germain A, *et al*. Functional neuroimaging evidence for hyperarousal in insomnia. *Am J Psychiatry*. 2004;**161**:2126–8.

11. Lamarche CH, Ogilvie RD. Electrophysiological changes during the sleep onset period of psychophysiological insomniacs, psychiatric insomniacs, and normal sleepers. *Sleep*. 1997;**20**:724–33.

12. Staner L, Cornette F, Maurice D, *et al*. Sleep microstructure around sleep onset differentiates major depressive insomnia from primary insomnia. *J Sleep Res*. 2003;**12**:319–30.

13. Merica H, Blois R, Gaillard JM. Spectral characteristics of sleep EEG in chronic insomnia. *Eur J Neurosci*. 1998;**10**:1826–34.

14. Richardson GS, Roth T. Future directions in the management of insomnia. *J Clin Psychiatry*. 2001; **62** Suppl 10:39–45.

15. Vgontzas AN, Bixler EO, Lin HM, *et al*. Chronic insomnia is associated with nyctohemeral activation of the hypothalamic-pituitary-adrenal axis: clinical implications. *J Clin Endocrinol Metab*. 2001; **86**:3787–94.

16. Rodenbeck A, Hajak G. Neuroendocrine dysregulation in primary insomnia. *Rev Neurol* (*Paris*). 2001; **157**:S57–61.

17. Young EA, Haskett RF, Grunhaus L, *et al*. Increased evening activation of the hypothalamic-pituitary-adrenal axis in depressed patients. *Arch Gen Psychiatry*. 1994;**51**:701–7.

18. Vgontzas AN, Bixler EO, Wittman AM, *et al*. Middle-aged men show higher sensitivity of sleep to the arousing effects of corticotropin-releasing hormone than young men: clinical implications. *J Clin Endocrinol Metab*. 2001;**86**:1489–95.

19. Rodenbeck A, Cohrs S, Jordan W, *et al*. The sleep-improving effects of doxepin are paralleled by a normalized plasma cortisol secretion in primary insomnia. A placebo-controlled, double-blind, randomized, cross-over study followed by an open treatment over 3 weeks. *Psychopharmacology* (*Berl*). 2003;**170**:423–8.

20. Aston-Jones G, Akaoka H, Charlety P, Chouvet G. Serotonin selectively attenuates glutamate-evoked activation of noradrenergic locus coeruleus neurons. *J Neurosci*. 1991;**11**:760–9.

21. Hobson JA, McCarley RW, Wyzinski PW. Sleep cycle oscillation: reciprocal discharge by two brainstem neuronal groups. *Science*. 1975;**189**:55–8.

22. McGinty DJ, Harper RM. Dorsal raphe neurons: depression of firing during sleep in cats. *Brain Res*. 1976;**101**:569–75.

23. Trulson ME, Jacobs BL. Raphe unit activity in freely moving cats: correlation with level of behavioral arousal. *Brain Res*. 1979;**163**:135–50.

24. Portas CM, Bjorvatn B, Fagerland S, *et al*. On-line detection of extracellular levels of serotonin in dorsal raphe nucleus and frontal cortex over the sleep/wake cycle in the freely moving rat. *Neuroscience*. 1998;**83**:807–14.

25. Blanco-Centurion CA, Salin-Pascual RJ. Extracellular serotonin levels in the medullary reticular formation during normal sleep and after REM sleep deprivation. *Brain Res*. 2001;**923**:128–36.

26. Strecker RE, Thakkar MM, Porkka-Heiskanen T, *et al*. Behavioral state-related changes of extracellular serotonin concentration in the pedunculopontine tegmental nucleus: a microdialysis study in freely moving animals. *Sleep Res Online*. 1999;**2**:21–7.

27. Park SP, Lopez-Rodriguez F, Wilson CL, *et al*. In vivo microdialysis measures of extracellular serotonin in the rat hippocampus during sleep-wakefulness. *Brain Res*. 1999;**833**:291–6.

28. Scruggs JL, Patel S, Bubser M, Deutch AY. DOI-induced activation of the cortex: dependence on 5-HT2A heteroceptors on thalamocortical glutamatergic neurons. *J Neurosci*. 2000;**20**:8846–52.

29. Jakala P, Sirvio J, Koivisto E, *et al*. Modulation of rat neocortical high-voltage spindle activity by 5-HT1/5-HT2 receptor subtype specific drugs. *Eur J Pharmacol*. 1995;**282**:39–55.

30. Dahlstrom A, Fuxe K. Localization of monoamines in the lower brain stem. *Experientia*. 1964;**20**:398–9.

31. Fenik V, Marchenko V, Janssen P, Davies RO, Kubin L. A5 cells are silenced when REM sleep-like signs are elicited by pontine carbachol. *J Appl Physiol*. 2002;**93**:1448–56.

32. Aston-Jones G, Bloom FE. Activity of norepinephrine-containing locus coeruleus neurons in behaving rats anticipates fluctuations in the sleep-waking cycle. *J Neurosci*. 1981;**1**:876–86.

33. Rasmussen K, Morilak DA, Jacobs BL. Single unit activity of locus coeruleus neurons in the freely moving cat. I. During naturalistic behaviors and in response to simple and complex stimuli. *Brain Res*. 1986;**371**:324–34.

34. Berridge CW, Waterhouse BD. The locus coeruleus-noradrenergic system: modulation of behavioral state and state-dependent cognitive processes. *Brain Res Brain Res Rev*. 2003;**42**:33–84.

35. Aston-Jones G. Brain structures and receptors involved in alertness. *Sleep Med*. 2005;**6** Suppl 1:S3–7.

36. Shouse MN, Staba RJ, Saquib SF, Farber PR. Monoamines and sleep: microdialysis findings in pons and amygdala. *Brain Res*. 2000;**860**:181–9.

37. Lena I, Parrot S, Deschaux O, *et al.* Variations in extracellular levels of dopamine, noradrenaline, glutamate, and aspartate across the sleep–wake cycle in the medial prefrontal cortex and nucleus accumbens of freely moving rats. *J Neurosci Res.* 2005;**81**:891–9.

38. Bouret S, Sara SJ. Network reset: a simplified overarching theory of locus coeruleus noradrenaline function. *Trends Neurosci.* 2005;**28**:574–82.

39. Sakai K, Crochet S. Role of the locus coeruleus in the control of paradoxical sleep generation in the cat. *Arch Ital Biol.* 2004;**142**:421–7.

40. Gottesmann C. Noradrenaline involvement in basic and higher integrated REM sleep processes. *Prog Neurobiol.* 2008;**85**:237–72.

41. Jones BE. Paradoxical REM sleep promoting and permitting neuronal networks. *Arch Ital Biol.* 2004;**142**:379–96.

42. Monnier M, Fallert M, Battacharya IC. The waking action of histamine. *Experientia.* 1967;**23**:21–2.

43. Ericson H, Watanabe T, Kohler C. Morphological analysis of the tuberomammillary nucleus in the rat brain: delineation of subgroups with antibody against L-histidine decarboxylase as a marker. *J Comp Neurol.* 1987;**263**:1–24.

44. Lin JS. Brain structures and mechanisms involved in the control of cortical activation and wakefulness, with emphasis on the posterior hypothalamus and histaminergic neurons. *Sleep Med Rev.* 2000;**4**:471–503.

45. Strecker RE, Nalwalk J, Dauphin LJ, *et al.* Extracellular histamine levels in the feline preoptic/anterior hypothalamic area during natural sleep-wakefulness and prolonged wakefulness: an in vivo microdialysis study. *Neuroscience.* 2002;**113**:663–70.

46. Mochizuki T, Yamatodani A, Okakura K, *et al.* Circadian rhythm of histamine release from the hypothalamus of freely moving rats. *Physiol Behav.* 1992;**51**:391–4.

47. Breunig E, Michel K, Zeller F, *et al.* Histamine excites neurones in the human submucous plexus through activation of H1, H2, H3 and H4 receptors. *J Physiol.* 2007;**583**:731–42.

48. Teuscher C, Subramanian M, Noubade R, *et al.* Central histamine H3 receptor signaling negatively regulates susceptibility to autoimmune inflammatory disease of the CNS. *Proc Natl Acad Sci USA.* 2007;**104**:10146–51.

49. Lin JS, Hou Y, Sakai K, Jouvet M. Histaminergic descending inputs to the mesopontine tegmentum and their role in the control of cortical activation and wakefulness in the cat. *J Neurosci.* 1996;**16**:1523–37.

50. Brown RE, Sergeeva OA, Eriksson KS, Haas HL. Convergent excitation of dorsal raphe serotonin neurons by multiple arousal systems (orexin/hypocretin, histamine and noradrenaline). *J Neurosci.* 2002;**22**:8850–9.

51. Schlicker E, Malinowska B, Kathmann M, Gothert M. Modulation of neurotransmitter release via histamine H3 heteroreceptors. *Fundam Clin Pharmacol.* 1994;**8**:128–37.

52. Haas HL, Sergeeva OA, Selbach O. Histamine in the nervous system. *Physiol Rev.* 2008;**88**:1183–241.

53. Steinfels GF, Heym J, Strecker RE, Jacobs BL. Behavioral correlates of dopaminergic unit activity in freely moving cats. *Brain Res.* 1983;**258**:217–28.

54. Steriade M, McCarley RW. *Brainstem Control of Wakefulness and Sleep.* (New York: Plenum Press, 1990).

55. Trulson ME. Simultaneous recording of substantia nigra neurons and voltammetric release of dopamine in the caudate of behaving cats. *Brain Res Bull.* 1985;**15**:221–3.

56. Crochet S, Sakai K. Dopaminergic modulation of behavioral states in mesopontine tegmentum: a reverse microdialysis study in freely moving cats. *Sleep.* 2003;**26**:801–6.

57. Nishino S, Mignot E. Pharmacological aspects of human and canine narcolepsy. *Prog Neurobiol.* 1997;**52**:27–78.

58. Wisor JP, Nishino S, Sora I, *et al.* Dopaminergic role in stimulant-induced wakefulness. *J Neurosci.* 2001;**21**:1787–94.

59. Szymusiak R, McGinty D. Hypothalamic regulation of sleep and arousal. *Ann N Y Acad Sci.* 2008;**1129**:275–86.

60. Moruzzi G, Magoun H. Brain stem reticular formation and activation of the EEG. *Electroenceph Clin Neurophysiol.* 1949;**1**:455.

61. Starzl TE, Taylor CW, Magoun HW. Ascending conduction in reticular activating system, with special reference to the diencephalon. *J. Neurophysiol.* 1951;**14**:461–477.

62. Hagan JJ, Leslie RA, Patel S, *et al.* Orexin A activates locus coeruleus cell firing and increases arousal in the rat. *Proc Natl Acad Sci USA.* 1999;**96**:10911–16.

63. Lehmann J, Nagy JI, Atmadia S, Fibiger HC. The nucleus basalis magnocellularis: the origin of a cholinergic projection to the neocortex of the rat. *Neuroscience.* 1980;**5**:1161–74.

64. Rye DB, Wainer BH, Mesulam MM, Mufson EJ, Saper CB. Cortical projections arising from the basal forebrain: a study of cholinergic and non-cholinergic components employing combined retrograde tracing and immunohistochemical localization of choline acetyltransferase. *Neuroscience.* 1984;**13**:627–43.

65. Shute CC, Lewis PR. The ascending cholinergic reticular system: neocortical, olfactory and subcortical projections. *Brain.* 1967;**90**:497–520.

66. Saper CB, Chou TC, Scammell TE. The sleep switch: hypothalamic control of sleep and wakefulness. *Trends Neurosci.* 2001;**24**:726–31.

67. Buzsaki G, Bickford RG, Ponomareff G, *et al.* Nucleus basalis and thalamic control of neocortical activity in the freely moving rat. *J Neurosci.* 1988;**8**:4007–26.

68. Lo Conte G, Casamenti F, Bigl V, Milaneschi E, Pepeu G. Effect of magnocellular forebrain nuclei lesions on acetylcholine output from the cerebral cortex, electrocorticogram and behaviour. *Arch Ital Biol.* 1982;**120**:176–88.

69. Stewart DJ, MacFabe DF, Vanderwolf CH. Cholinergic activation of the electrocorticogram: role of the substantia innominata and effects of atropine and quinuclidinyl benzilate. *Brain Res.* 1984;**322**:219–32.

70. Casamenti F, Deffenu G, Abbamondi AL, Pepeu G. Changes in cortical acetylcholine output induced by modulation of the nucleus basalis. *Brain Res Bull.* 1986;**16**:689–95.

71. Rasmusson DD, Clow K, Szerb JC. Modification of neocortical acetylcholine release and electroencephalogram desynchronization due to brainstem stimulation by drugs applied to the basal forebrain. *Neuroscience.* 1994;**60**:665–77.

72. Gvilia I, Turner A, McGinty D, Szymusiak R. Preoptic area neurons and the homeostatic regulation of rapid eye movement sleep. *J Neurosci.* 2006;**26**:3037–44.

73. Jones BE. From waking to sleeping: neuronal and chemical substrates. *Trends Pharmacol Sci.* 2005;**26**:578–86.

74. Ali M, Jha SK, Kaur S, Mallick BN. Role of GABA-A receptor in the preoptic area in the regulation of sleep-wakefulness and rapid eye movement sleep. *Neurosci Res.* 1999;**33**:245–50.

75. Gottesmann C. GABA mechanisms and sleep. *Neuroscience.* 2002;**111**:231–9.

76. Lancel M. Role of GABA-A receptors in the regulation of sleep: initial sleep responses to peripherally administered modulators and agonists. *Sleep.* 1999;**22**:33–42.

77. Rudolph U, Antkowiak B. Molecular and neuronal substrates for general anaesthetics. *Nat Rev Neurosci.* 2004;**5**:709–20.

78. Williams SR, Turner JP, Crunelli V. Gamma-hydroxybutyrate promotes oscillatory activity of rat and cat thalamocortical neurons by a tonic GABAB, receptor-mediated hyperpolarization. *Neuroscience* 1995;**66**:133–41.

79. Guidotti A. Role of DBI in brain and its posttranslational processing products in normal and abnormal behavior. *Neuropharmacology.* 1991;**30**:1425–33.

80. Lloyd KG, Morselli PL, Bartholini G. GABA and affective disorders. *Med Biol.* 1987;**65**:159–65.

81. Petty F, Kramer GL, Fulton M, Moeller FG, Rush AJ. Low plasma GABA is a trait-like marker for bipolar illness. *Neuropsychopharmacology.* 1993;**9**:125–32.

82. Roy A, Dejong J, Ferraro T. CSF GABA in depressed patients and normal controls. *Psychol Med.* 1991;**21**:613–8.

83. Nagatani T, Sugihara T, Kodaira R. The effect of diazepam and of agents which change GABAergic functions in immobility in mice. *Eur J Pharmacol.* 1984;**97**:271–5.

84. Nakagawa Y, Ishima T, Ishibashi Y, Yoshii T, Takashima T. Involvement of GABA(B) receptor systems in action of antidepressants: baclofen but not bicuculline attenuates the effects of antidepressants on the forced swim test in rats. *Brain Res.* 1996;**709**:215–20.

85. Mombereau C, Kaupmann K, Froestl W, *et al.* Genetic and pharmacological evidence of a role for GABA (B) receptors in the modulation of anxiety- and antidepressant-like behavior. *Neuropsychopharmacology.* 2004;**29**:1050–62.

86. Porkka-Heiskanen T, Strecker RE, McCarley RW. Brain site-specificity of extracellular adenosine concentration changes during sleep deprivation and spontaneous sleep: an in vivo microdialysis study. *Neuroscience.* 2000;**99**:507–17.

87. Strecker RE, Morairty S, Thakkar MM, *et al.* Adenosinergic modulation of basal forebrain and preoptic/anterior hypothalamic neuronal activity in the control of behavioral state. *Behav Brain Res.* 2000;**115**:183–204.

88. Szymusiak R, Alam N, McGinty D. Discharge patterns of neurons in cholinergic regions of the basal forebrain during waking and sleep. *Behav Brain Res.* 2000;**115**:171–82.

89. Thakkar MM, Delgiacco RA, Strecker RE, McCarley RW. Adenosinergic inhibition of basal forebrain wakefulness-active neurons: a simultaneous unit recording and microdialysis study in freely behaving cats. *Neuroscience.* 2003;**122**:1107–13.

90. Thakkar MM, Winston S, McCarley RW. A1 receptor and adenosinergic homeostatic regulation of sleep-wakefulness: effects of antisense to the A1 receptor in the cholinergic basal forebrain. *J Neurosci.* 2003;**23**:4278–87.

91. Portas CM, Thakkar M, Rainnie DG, Greene RW, McCarley RW. Role of adenosine in behavioral state modulation: a microdialysis study in the freely moving cat. *Neuroscience.* 1997;**79**:225–35.

92. Alanko L, Heiskanen S, Stenberg D, Porkka-Heiskanen T. Adenosine kinase and 5′-nucleotidase activity after prolonged wakefulness in the cortex and the basal forebrain of rat. *Neurochem Int.* 2003;**42**:449–54.

93. Jones SV, Barker JL, Goodman MB, Brann MR. Inositol trisphosphate mediates cloned muscarinic receptor-activated conductances in transfected mouse fibroblast A9 L cells. *J Physiol.* 1990;**421**:499–519.

94. Mitani A, Ito K, Hallanger AE, *et al.* Cholinergic projections from the laterodorsal and pedunculopontine tegmental nuclei to the pontine gigantocellular tegmental field in the cat. *Brain Res.* 1988;**451**:397–402.

95. Semba K, Reiner PB, Fibiger HC. Single cholinergic mesopontine tegmental neurons project to both the pontine reticular formation and the thalamus in the rat. *Neuroscience.* 1990;**38**:643–54.

96. Shiromani PJ, Armstrong DM, Berkowitz A, Jeste DV, Gillin JC. Distribution of choline acetyltransferase immunoreactive somata in the feline brainstem: implications for REM sleep generation. *Sleep.* 1988;**11**:1–16.

97. el Mansari M, Sakai K, Jouvet M. Unitary characteristics of presumptive cholinergic tegmental neurons during the sleep-waking cycle in freely moving cats. *Exp Brain Res.* 1989;**76**:519–29.

98. Kayama Y, Ohta M, Jodo E. Firing of 'possibly' cholinergic neurons in the rat laterodorsal tegmental nucleus during sleep and wakefulness. *Brain Res.* 1992;**569**:210–20.

99. Horner RL, Kubin L. Pontine carbachol elicits multiple rapid eye movement sleep-like neural events in urethane-anaesthetized rats. *Neuroscience.* 1999;**93**:215–26.

100. Marks GA, Birabil CG. Enhancement of rapid eye movement sleep in the rat by cholinergic and adenosinergic agonists infused into the pontine reticular formation. *Neuroscience.* 1998;**86**:29–37.

101. Datta S. Evidence that REM sleep is controlled by the activation of brain stem pedunculopontine tegmental kainate receptor. *J Neurophysiol.* 2002;**87**:1790–8.

102. Baghdoyan HA, Lydic R, Fleegal MA. M2 muscarinic autoreceptors modulate acetylcholine release in the medial pontine reticular formation. *J Pharmacol Exp Ther.* 1998;**286**:1446–52.

103. Poland RE, McCracken JT, Lutchmansingh P, *et al.* Differential response of rapid eye movement sleep to cholinergic blockade by scopolamine in currently depressed, remitted, and normal control subjects. *Biol Psychiatry.* 1997;**41**:929–38.

104. Espana RA, Baldo BA, Kelley AE, Berridge CW. Wake-promoting and sleep-suppressing actions of hypocretin (orexin): basal forebrain sites of action. *Neuroscience.* 2001;**106**:699–715.

105. Trivedi P, Yu H, MacNeil DJ, *et al.* Distribution of orexin receptor mRNA in the rat brain. *FEBS Lett.* 1998;**438**:71–5.

106. de Lecea L, Kilduff TS, Peyron C, *et al.* The hypocretins: hypothalamus-specific peptides with neuroexcitatory activity. *Proc Natl Acad Sci USA.* 1998;**95**:322–7.

107. Sakurai T, Amemiya A, Ishii M, *et al.* Orexins and orexin receptors: a family of hypothalamic neuropeptides and G protein-coupled receptors that regulate feeding behavior. *Cell.* 1998;**92**:1 page following 696.

108. Peyron C, Tighe DK, van den Pol AN, *et al.* Neurons containing hypocretin (orexin) project to multiple neuronal systems. *J Neurosci.* 1998;**18**:9996–10015.

109. Zhang JH, Sampogna S, Morales FR, Chase MH. Orexin (hypocretin)-like immunoreactivity in the cat hypothalamus: a light and electron microscopic study. *Sleep.* 2001;**24**:67–76.

110. Takahashi K, Lin JS, Sakai K. Neuronal activity of orexin and non-orexin waking-active neurons during wake-sleep states in the mouse. *Neuroscience.* 2008;**153**:860–70.

111. Thakkar MM, Ramesh V, Strecker RE, McCarley RW. Microdialysis perfusion of orexin-A in the basal forebrain increases wakefulness in freely behaving rats. *Arch Ital Biol.* 2001;**139**:313–28.

112. Xi MC, Morales FR, Chase MH. Effects on sleep and wakefulness of the injection of hypocretin-1 (orexin-A) into the laterodorsal tegmental nucleus of the cat. *Brain Res.* 2001;**901**:259–64.

113. Kotz CM, Wang C, Teske JA, *et al.* Orexin-A mediation of time spent moving in rats: Neural mechanisms. *Neuroscience.* 2006;**142**(1):29–36.

114. Estabrooke IV, McCarthy MT, Ko E, *et al.* Fos expression in orexin neurons varies with behavioral state. *J Neurosci.* 2001;**21**:1656–62.

115. Eggermann E, Serafin M, Bayer L, *et al.* Orexins/hypocretins excite basal forebrain cholinergic neurones. *Neuroscience.* 2001;**108**:177–81.

116. Liu RJ, van den Pol AN, Aghajanian GK. Hypocretins (orexins) regulate serotonin neurons in the dorsal raphe nucleus by excitatory direct and inhibitory indirect actions. *J Neurosci.* 2002;**22**:9453–64.

117. Lin L, Faraco J, Li R, *et al*. The sleep disorder canine narcolepsy is caused by a mutation in the hypocretin (orexin) receptor 2 gene. *Cell.* 1999;**98**:365–76.

118. Tao R, Ma Z, McKenna JT, *et al*. Differential effect of orexins (hypocretins) on serotonin release in the dorsal and median raphe nuclei of freely behaving rats. *Neuroscience.* 2006;**141**:1101–5.

119. Muroya S, Funahashi H, Yamanaka A, *et al*. Orexins (hypocretins) directly interact with neuropeptide Y, POMC and glucose-responsive neurons to regulate Ca^{2+} signaling in a reciprocal manner to leptin: orexigenic neuronal pathways in the mediobasal hypothalamus. *Eur J Neurosci.* 2004;**19**:1524–34.

120. Muroya S, Uramura K, Sakurai T, Takigawa M, Yada T. Lowering glucose concentrations increases cytosolic Ca^{2+} in orexin neurons of the rat lateral hypothalamus. *Neurosci Lett.* 2001;**309**:165–8.

121. Narita M, Nagumo Y, Miyatake M, *et al*. Implication of protein kinase C in the orexin-induced elevation of extracellular dopamine levels and its rewarding effect. *Eur J Neurosci.* 2007;**25**:1537–45.

122. Uramura K, Funahashi H, Muroya S, *et al*. Orexin-a activates phospholipase C- and protein kinase C-mediated Ca^{2+} signaling in dopamine neurons of the ventral tegmental area. *Neuroreport.* 2001;**12**:1885–9.

123. Muraki Y, Yamanaka A, Tsujino N, *et al*. Serotonergic regulation of the orexin/hypocretin neurons through the 5-HT1A receptor. *J Neurosci.* 2004;**24**:7159–66.

124. Li Y, van den Pol AN. Direct and indirect inhibition by catecholamines of hypocretin/orexin neurons. *J Neurosci.* 2005;**25**:173–83.

125. Hong ZY, Huang ZL, Qu WM, Eguchi N. Orexin A promotes histamine, but not norepinephrine or serotonin, release in frontal cortex of mice. *Acta Pharmacol Sin.* 2005;**26**:155–9.

126. Huang ZL, Qu WM, Li WD, *et al*. Arousal effect of orexin A depends on activation of the histaminergic system. *Proc Natl Acad Sci USA.* 2001;**98**:9965–70.

127. Ishizuka T, Yamamoto Y, Yamatodani A. The effect of orexin-A and -B on the histamine release in the anterior hypothalamus in rats. *Neurosci Lett.* 2002;**323**:93–6.

128. Yamanaka A, Tsujino N, Funahashi H, *et al*. Orexins activate histaminergic neurons via the orexin 2 receptor. *Biochem Biophys Res Commun.* 2002;**290**:1237–45.

129. Eriksson KS, Sergeeva O, Brown RE, Haas HL. Orexin/hypocretin excites the histaminergic neurons of the tuberomammillary nucleus. *J Neurosci.* 2001;**21**:9273–9.

130. Ida T, Nakahara K, Murakami T, *et al*. Possible involvement of orexin in the stress reaction in rats. *Biochem Biophys Res Commun.* 2000;**270**:318–23.

131. Kuru M, Ueta Y, Serino R, *et al*. Centrally administered orexin/hypocretin activates HPA axis in rats. *Neuroreport* 2000;**11**:1977–80.

132. Martins PJ, D'Almeida V, Pedrazzoli M, *et al*. Increased hypocretin-1 (orexin-A) levels in cerebrospinal fluid of rats after short-term forced activity. *Regul Pept.* 2004;**117**:155–8.

133. Stricker-Krongrad A, Beck B. Modulation of hypothalamic hypocretin/orexin mRNA expression by glucocorticoids. *Biochem Biophys Res Commun.* 2002;**296**:129–33.

134. Zhu L, Onaka T, Sakurai T, Yada T. Activation of orexin neurones after noxious but not conditioned fear stimuli in rats. *Neuroreport.* 2002;**13**:1351–3.

135. Linthorst AC, Reul JM. Stress and the brain: solving the puzzle using microdialysis. *Pharmacol Biochem Behav.* 2008;**90**:163–73.

136. McEwen BS. Central effects of stress hormones in health and disease: Understanding the protective and damaging effects of stress and stress mediators. *Eur J Pharmacol.* 2008;**583**:174–85.

137. Opp MR. Corticotropin-releasing hormone involvement in stressor-induced alterations in sleep and in the regulation of waking. *Adv Neuroimmunol.* 1995;**5**:127–43.

138. Chang FC, Opp MR. A corticotropin-releasing hormone antisense oligodeoxynucleotide reduces spontaneous waking in the rat. *Regul Pept.* 2004;**117**:43–52.

139. Papale LA, Andersen ML, Antunes IB, Alvarenga TA, Tufik S. Sleep pattern in rats under different stress modalities. *Brain Res.* 2005;**1060**:47–54.

140. Rabat A, Bouyer JJ, Aran JM, Le Moal M, Mayo W. Chronic exposure to an environmental noise permanently disturbs sleep in rats: inter-individual vulnerability. *Brain Res.* 2005;**1059**:72–82.

141. Winsky-Sommerer R, Yamanaka A, Diano S, *et al*. Interaction between the corticotropin-releasing factor system and hypocretins (orexins): a novel circuit mediating stress response. *J Neurosci.* 2004;**24**:11439–48.

142. Bohlhalter S, Murck H, Holsboer F, Steiger A. Cortisol enhances non-REM sleep and growth hormone secretion in elderly subjects. *Neurobiol Aging.* 1997;**18**:423–9.

143. Friess E, V Bardeleben U, Wiedemann K, Lauer CJ, Holsboer F. Effects of pulsatile cortisol infusion on sleep-EEG and nocturnal growth hormone release in healthy men. *J Sleep Res.* 1994;**3**:73–9.

144. Wetzel W, Wagner T, Vogel D, Demuth HU, Balschun D. Effects of the CLIP fragment ACTH

20–24 on the duration of REM sleep episodes. *Neuropeptides.* 1997;**31**:41–5.

145. Young AH, Sharpley AL, Campling GM, Hockney RA, Cowen PJ. Effects of hydrocortisone on brain 5-HT function and sleep. *J Affect Disord.* 1994;**32**:139–46.

146. Watanabe S, Kuwaki T, Yanagisawa M, Fukuda Y, Shimoyama M. Persistent pain and stress activate pain-inhibitory orexin pathways. *Neuroreport.* 2005;**16**:5–8.

147. Nakamachi T, Endo S, Ohtaki H, *et al.* Orexin-1 receptor expression after global ischemia in mice. *Regul Pept.* 2005;**126**:49–54.

148. Fava M. Daytime sleepiness and insomnia as correlates of depression. *J Clin Psychiatry.* 2004, **65** Suppl 16:27–32.

149. Kessler RC, McGonagle KA, Zhao S, *et al.* Lifetime and 12-month prevalence of DSM-III-R psychiatric disorders in the United States. Results from the National Comorbidity Survey. *Arch Gen Psychiatry.* 1994;**51**:8–19.

150. Kessler RC, Merikangass KR. The National Comorbidity Survey Replication (NCS-R): background and aims. *Int J Methods Psychiatr Res.* 2004;**13**:60–8.

151. Murray JL, Lopez ADL. *The Global Burden of Disease: A Comprehensive Assessment of Mortality and Disability from Diseases, Injuries, and Risk Factors in 1990 and Projected to 2020.* (Cambridge, MA: Harvard University Press, 1996).

152. Benca RM, Obermeyer WH, Thisted RA, Gillin JC. Sleep and psychiatric disorders. A meta-analysis. *Arch Gen Psychiatry.* 1992;**49**:651–68; discussion 669–70.

153. Riemann D, Voderholzer U, Berger M. Sleep and sleep–wake manipulations in bipolar depression. *Neuropsychobiology.* 2002;**45** Suppl 1:7–12.

154. Nofzinger EA, Price JC, Meltzer CC, *et al.* Towards a neurobiology of dysfunctional arousal in depression: the relationship between beta EEG power and regional cerebral glucose metabolism during NREM sleep. *Psychiatry Res.* 2000;**98**:71–91.

155. Salomon RM, Ripley B, Kennedy JS, *et al.* Diurnal variation of cerebrospinal fluid hypocretin-1 (Orexin-A) levels in control and depressed subjects. *Biol Psychiatry.* 2003;**54**:96–104.

156. Brundin L, Petersen A, Bjorkqvist M, Traskman-Bendz L. Orexin and psychiatric symptoms in suicide attempters. *J Affect Disord.* 2007;**100**:259–63.

157. Goodwin FK, Jamison KR. Suicide. In: *Manic-Depressive Illness.* (New York: Oxford University Press, 1990).

158. Guze SB, Robins E. Suicide and primary affective disorders. *Br J Psychiatry.* 1970;**117**:437–8.

159. Brundin L, Bjorkqvist M, Petersen A, Traskman-Bendz L. Reduced orexin levels in the cerebrospinal fluid of suicidal patients with major depressive disorder. *Eur Neuropsychopharmacol.* 2007;**17**:573–9.

160. Plotsky PM, Meaney MJ. Early, postnatal experience alters hypothalamic corticotropin-releasing factor (CRF) mRNA, median eminence CRF content and stress-induced release in adult rats. *Brain Res Mol Brain Res.* 1993;**18**:195–200.

161. Boccia ML, Pedersen CA. Brief vs. long maternal separations in infancy: contrasting relationships with adult maternal behavior and lactation levels of aggression and anxiety. *Psychoneuroendocrinology.* 2001;**26**:657–72.

162. Wigger A, Neumann ID. Periodic maternal deprivation induces gender-dependent alterations in behavioral and neuroendocrine responses to emotional stress in adult rats. *Physiol Behav.* 1999;**66**:293–302.

163. Ladd CO, Owens MJ, Nemeroff CB. Persistent changes in corticotropin-releasing factor neuronal systems induced by maternal deprivation. *Endocrinology.* 1996;**137**:1212–18.

164. Plotsky PM, Thrivikraman KV, Nemeroff CB, *et al.* Long-term consequences of neonatal rearing on central corticotropin-releasing factor systems in adult male rat offspring. *Neuropsychopharmacology.* 2005;**30**:2192–204.

165. Feng P, Vurbic D, Wu Z, Strohl KP. Brain orexins and wake regulation in rats exposed to maternal deprivation. *Brain Res.* 2007;**1154C**:163–72.

166. Feng P, Vurbic D, Wu Z, Hu Y, Strohl K. Changes in brain orexin levels in a rat model of depression induced by neonatal administration of clomipramine. *J Psychopharmacol.* 2008;**22**:784–91.

167. Bonnet MH, Arand DL. Hyperarousal and insomnia. *Sleep Med Rev.* 1997;**1**:97–108.

168. Griffiths MF, Peerson A. Risk factors for chronic insomnia following hospitalization. *J Adv Nurs.* 2005;**49**:245–53.

169. Billiard M, Bentley A. Is insomnia best categorized as a symptom or a disease? *Sleep Med.* 2004;**5** Suppl 1: S35–40.

170. Drake C, Richardson G, Roehrs T, Scofield H, Roth T. Vulnerability to stress-related sleep disturbance and hyperarousal. *Sleep.* 2004;**27**:285–91.

171. Espana RA, Scammell TE. Sleep neurobiology for the clinician. *Sleep.* 2004;**27**:811–20.

172. Zee P. Physiology of sleep and wake. In: Richardson G, ed., *Update on the Science, Diagnosis and Management of Insomnia.* (London: The Royal Society of Medicine Press Limited, 2006; 3–20).

173. Heidbreder CA, Weiss IC, Domeney AM, *et al.* Behavioral, neurochemical and endocrinological characterization of the early social isolation syndrome. *Neuroscience.* 2000;**100**:749–68.

174. Matthews K, Dalley JW, Matthews C, Tsai TH, Robbins TW. Periodic maternal separation of neonatal rats produces region- and gender-specific effects on biogenic amine content in postmortem adult brain. *Synapse.* 2001;**40**:1–10.

175. Trulson ME. Simultaneous recording of dorsal raphe unit activity and serotonin release in the striatum using voltammetry in awake, behaving cats. *Life Sci.* 1985;**37**:2199–204.

176. Morgan K. Daytime activity and risk factors for late-life insomnia. *J Sleep Res.* 2003;**12**:231–8.

177. Feng P, Hu Y, Li D, *et al.* The effect of clomipramine on wake/sleep and orexinergic expression in rats. *J Psychopharmacol.* 2009;**23**(5):559–66.

178. Gerashchenko D, Blanco-Centurion CA, Miller JD, Shiromani PJ. Insomnia following hypocretin2-saporin lesions of the substantia nigra. *Neuroscience.* 2006;**137**:29–36.

179. Mignot E, Lammers GJ, Ripley B, *et al.* The role of cerebrospinal fluid hypocretin measurement in the diagnosis of narcolepsy and other hypersomnias. *Arch Neurol.* 2002;**59**:1553–62.

Pathophysiology of changes in sleep EEG and hormone secretion

Axel Steiger and Mayumi Kimura

Introduction

Impaired sleep is a key symptom in patients with depression [1]. Accordingly characteristic sleep-EEG changes occur in depression. Furthermore the activity of several endocrine systems shows aberrances in affective disorders. In normal subjects and in depressed patients as well sleep is associated with characteristic patterns of secretion of various hormones. Therefore the simultaneous analysis of sleep EEG and, by blood sampling during sleep, of nocturnal hormone secretion is used to discover sleep–endocrine changes in depressed patients. It is now well established that there is a bidirectional interaction between the electrophysiological (sleep EEG) and sleep–endocrine (nocturnal hormone secretion) components of sleep. Certain hormones, particularly neuropeptides, have been identified in clinical and preclinical studies as common regulators of sleep EEG and sleep-related hormone secretion. This chapter aims to present the state of the art in the pathophysiology of sleep–endocrine changes in affective disorders.

Sleep–endocrine changes in patients with depression

In young normal human subjects during the first half of the night the major amounts of slow-wave sleep (SWS), slow-wave activity (SWA), and the growth hormone (GH) peak are found; whereas the secretion of the hypothalamo–pituitary–adrenocortical (HPA) hormones, cortisol and corticotropin (ACTH), is low. In contrast, during the second half of the night cortisol and ACTH levels increase until awakening and rapid eye movement sleep (REMS) preponderates, whereas the amounts of SWS and GH are low [2, 3].

(Figure 8.1). Prominent changes of these patterns in affective disorders are disinhibition of REMS, elevated ACTH and cortisol levels, and decreases of SWS and GH.

In detail characteristic sleep-EEG changes in depression include disturbed sleep continuity (prolonged sleep latency, increased intermittent wakefulness, early morning awakenings), changes of non-REMS (NREMS) (decreases of stage 2 and SWS, in younger patients the major portions of SWS and SWA are shifted from the first to the second sleep cycle) and REMS disinhibition (shortened REMS latency, prolonged first REMS period and enhanced REMS density, a measure for the amount of rapid eye movement during REMS) [4] (Figure 8.1). Most sleep–endocrine studies in depressed patients showed elevated cortisol and ACTH secretion during the night or throughout 24 hours when compared to normal control subjects [5]. A positive correlation was found between age and cortisol levels [6]. Blunted GH secretion was found in several studies [7, 8].

Interestingly during normal aging changes of sleep–endocrine activities similar to those in patients with depression occur. Already during the third decade of lifespan distinct decreases of SWS, SWA, and GH release start. Correspondingly in elderly subjects the amount of SWS is low or SWS is even absent. Furthermore sleep continuity is altered as sleep efficiency and sleep period time decrease and nocturnal awakenings increase. In senescence REMS time and REMS latency decrease. Elevated and unchanged cortisol has also been reported in the elderly. In most studies the amplitude of the cortisol rhythm is reduced. In elderly patients with depression due to a synergistic effect of depression and aging sleep–endocrine changes are most distinct (Figure 8.1).

Sleep and Mental Illness, eds. S. R. Pandi-Perumal and M. Kramer. Published by Cambridge University Press.
© Cambridge University Press 2010.

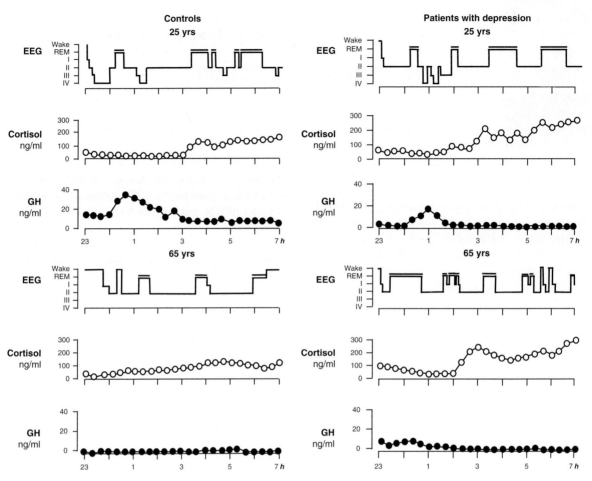

Figure 8.1 Hypnograms (sleep EEG) and nocturnal secretion patterns of cortisol and growth hormone (GH) in young and elderly control subjects and patients with depression. REM-rapid eye movement sleep; I–IV mean stages of non-rapid eye movement sleep.
Steiger, A. Neuroendocrinology of sleep disorders. In: Textbook of Biological Psychiatry *(D'haenen, H., den Boer, J. A., Westenberg, H., Willner, P., eds.), pp. 1229–1246. John Wiley & Sons, Ltd, London, 2002. Copyright (2002), with kind permission from Wiley.*

Two studies compared sleep–endocrine activity longitudinally between acute depression and recovery. One study reported decreases of cortisol and ACTH levels throughout 24 hours and normalized REMS after remission [5]. Since some of the patients received antidepressants that suppress REMS at the retest it is difficult to disentangle effects of remission and of drugs. A decrease of cortisol was confirmed by intra-individual comparison of male drug-free patients [7]. In this study testosterone levels increased after recovery [9], whereas prolactin levels remained unchanged and did not differ from those of younger normal subjects [10]. The blunted GH levels did not differ between acute depression and recovery. Sleep EEG even further deteriorated as stage 4 sleep decreased and the number of awakenings increased after recovery [7]. Both studies [5, 7] confirm that HPA hypersecretion is a robust symptom of acute depression. Similarly challenge tests of the HPA system and CRH cerebrospinal fluid levels normalize in depressed patients after recovery [11]. The persistence of most sleep-EEG changes [12] and of blunted GH secretion [8] in remitted patients has been replicated over three years. These findings indicate that HPA activity normalizes independently from sleep architecture. Hence hypercortisolism in depression is not a consequence of shallow sleep. Blunted testosterone levels may, however, be the consequence of HPA overactivity. The persistence of sleep EEG and GH changes in remitted patients may represent a biological scar due to the metabolic aberrances during the acute episode of depression. Alternatively these changes may represent a trait in depressed patients. As long as no intra-individual comparison is available between the premorbid and depressed state in patients, this issue remains unclear.

Interestingly in young male patients who survived severe brain injury, sleep EEG and nocturnal hormone secretion were similar to those of remitted depressed patients. The amounts of stage 2 sleep and GH levels of these patients were lower than in healthy volunteers several months after the injury, whereas cortisol levels did not differ between groups [13]. In the survivors of brain injury either elevated HPA activity due to stress during intensive care or treatment with glucocorticoids in a subgroup may have contributed to the changes of sleep and GH.

Elevated HPA hormones were observed in patients with primary insomnia [14]. These findings point to similarities in the pathophysiology of depression and of primary insomnia. This is of interest in the light of an elevated risk for depression in patients with persisting insomnia [15].

Besides impaired sleep, loss of appetite and weight are other frequent symptoms of depression. Therefore the secretion of ghrelin and leptin in depressed patients is of interest. A reciprocal interaction between the orexigenic ghrelin and the anorexigenic leptin is thought to play a key role in the regulation of the energy balance [16]. Nocturnal leptin levels were significantly higher in drug-free patients with depression than in controls [17]. Higher leptin concentrations in women than in men were found in patients and healthy subjects as described before. Leptin levels were correlated with body mass index in the controls but not in the patients. This finding suggests a change of leptin secretion in depression. An increase in leptin during the night was found neither in the male controls nor in the patients, whereas others [18] had reported an increase between 00:00 and 04:00 hours in normal male subjects. In the group of younger healthy women leptin increased during this interval and was greater by trend than in age-matched depressed patients. This finding suggests that the nocturnal leptin peak is blunted in young female patients with depression. As expected cortisol was elevated in the patients. Since glucocorticoids are able to prevent the decrease of leptin after fasting, it appears likely that hypercortisolism in depressed patients counteracts the decrease of leptin secretion due to a decreased

food intake and weight loss. On the other hand elevated leptin levels may further stimulate CRH secretion in depressed patients similar to preclinical findings [19] and may contribute to HPA overdrive. In contrast to leptin, ghrelin levels in drug-free patients with depression did not differ from those in normal controls [20].

Nocturnal thyroid stimulating hormone (TSH) levels were blunted and ACTH levels were enhanced in drug-free male depressed patients compared to normal controls. ACTH was negatively correlated to TSH during the first half of the night. This observation points to a common regulation of the hypothalamic–pituitary–thyroid and the HPA systems in depression [21].

The role of neuropeptides and steroids in sleep–endocrine changes in depression

Already the sleep–endocrine pattern in normal controls points to a reciprocal interaction between the hypothalamo–pituitary–somatotrophic (HPS) and the HPA systems with GH and cortisol, respectively, as their peripheral endpoints. This view is further supported by the similar changes of sleep–endocrine activity during depression and normal aging.

The HPA system

The HPA system mediates the reaction to acute physical and psychological stress. It is essential for individual survival. The stress reaction starts with the release of CRH from the parvocellular portion of the paraventricular nucleus of the hypothalamus resulting in the secretion of ACTH from the anterior pituitary and finally in the secretion of cortisol (in humans) or corticosterone (in rats) from the adrenocortex. Various cofactors contribute to this cascade [11].

After intracerebroventricular (icv) administration of CRH, SWS decreased in rats [22], rabbits [23], and mice [24]. Even after sleep deprivation lasting 72 hours, icv CRH decreased SWS but increased sleep latency and REMS in rats [25]. The synthesis and secretion of CRH is reduced in the Lewis rat, which has a hypothalamic gene defect in comparison to other rat strains. Wakefulness was decreased and SWS was increased in Lewis rats compared to intact strains [26]. After the CRH antagonist α-helical CRH and astressin wakefulness decreased in a

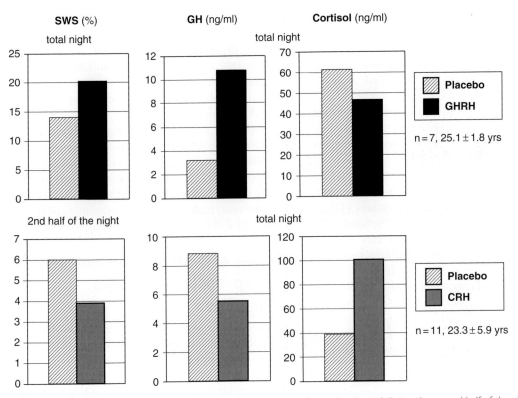

Figure 8.2 Sleep–endocrine variables (slow-wave sleep [SWS] during the total night and during the second half of the night, respectively, growth hormone [GH] and cortisol) after placebo and GH-releasing hormone (GHRH) (upper part) and after placebo and corticotropin-releasing hormone (CRH) (bottom) in young normal male control subjects. GHRH and CRH exert opposite effects on these variables.

dose-dependent manner after administration before the dark period [27]. These findings suggest that CRH participates in the regulation of physiological waking periods. In another study, however, α-helical CRH was effective only in stressed rats, which showed enhanced REMS. Rapid eye movement sleep decreased to values of the non-stressed condition after α-helical CRH [28]. Furthermore α-helical CRH diminished selectively the REMS rebounds after sleep deprivation in rats. The authors suggest that stress acting via CRH is the major factor that induces this rebound [29].

In homozygous CRH-overexpressing mice REMS is elevated compared to the wild type [30]. The REMS rebound after sleep deprivation is enhanced even in the heterozygous mice. When the CRH-1 receptor antagonist DMP 696 was administered orally one hour before the end of six-hour sleep deprivation, the levels of increased REMS during recovery sleep in hetero- and homozygous mice did not differ from those in control and wild-type mice. These findings show that CRH-1-receptor antagonism normalizes

sleep changed due to stress or CRH. Similar findings were observed when another CRH-1-receptor antagonist, NBI 30775, was tested in stressed rats with selective low (LAB) or high (HAB) anxiety-related behavior [31]. Whereas in these rats sleep patterns did not differ distinctly during baseline related to their anxiety, the stress-induced sleep attenuation in the HAB rats was normalized after the treatment to the level of LAB rats, which showed weaker stress responses.

Similarly to the findings in laboratory animals [22, 23], SWS and REMS decreased after pulsatile intravenous (iv) administration of CRH (23:00 to 03:00 hours) in young normal male human subjects. Furthermore the GH peak was blunted and cortisol was elevated during the first half of the night [32] (Figure 8.2). Also, in young normal female subjects CRH impaired sleep [33]. After hourly iv injections of a lower dose of CRH (08:00 to 18:00 hours) sleep remained unchanged during the following night, whereas melatonin was blunted [34]. Both after a single iv injection of CRH during the first SWS period and during wakefulness EEG activity in the sigma frequency range increased

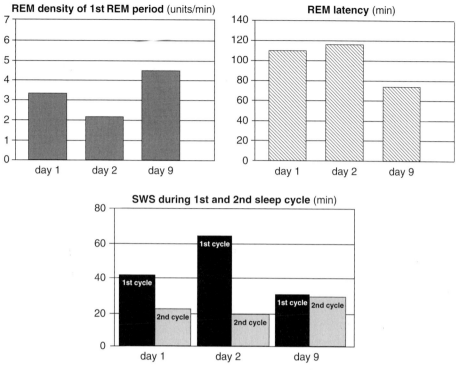

Figure 8.3 Sleep-EEG variables during high dose corticosteroid treatment in patients with multiple sclerosis. REM density during the first REM period (upper part left) decreased significantly after acute treatment (day 2) compared to baseline, but increased after prolonged treatment compared to day 2. REM latency (upper part right) decreased at day 9 compared to baseline. Slow-wave sleep (SWS) duration (bottom) during the first two sleep cycles was modulated by treatment. SWS markedly declined from the first to the second sleep cycle at baseline. After prolonged treatment (day 9) this decline was abolished due to similar time spent in SWS in the first two sleep cycles. *Reprinted from* Psychoneuroendocrinology, 28, I. A. Antonijevic and A. Steiger, Depression-like changes of the sleep-EEG during high dose corticosteroid treatment in patients with multiple sclerosis, 780–795, Copyright (2003), with kind permission from Elsevier.

during the first three sleep cycles in young normal controls [35]. The vulnerability of the sleep EEG to CRH appears to increase during aging. This view derives from the comparison of the effects of a single CRH injection given ten minutes after sleep onset in young and middle-aged normal males. Whereas in the young subjects sleep remained unchanged, SWS decreased and wakefulness increased in the middle-aged subjects [36].

After infusions of ACTH, REMS decreased and cortisol and GH increased in normal subjects [37]. The ACTH (4–9) analogue ebiratide induced sleep-EEG changes corresponding to a general central nervous system (CNS) activation. Rapid eye movement sleep, GH, and cortisol remained unchanged in this study [38].

After cortisol administration SWS, SWA, and GH increased and REMS decreased in young [39] and elderly [40] normal subjects. Since CRH [32] and cortisol influenced SWS and GH [39, 40], it appears

unlikely that changes of peripheral cortisol levels mediate these changes. Probably feedback inhibition of endogenous CRH induces these effects. CRH [32], ACTH [37], and cortisol [39, 40] all diminished REMS, whereas ebiratide [38] did not share these effects. Hence it appears likely that REMS suppression is mediated by cortisol after each of these hormones. Similarly after metyrapone, an inhibitor of cortisol synthesis, REMS remained unchanged, whereas SWS and cortisol decreased in normal subjects [41]. In this study ACTH was distinctly elevated. This finding suggests that endogenous CRH was increased.

The effects of acute and long-lasting glucocorticoid administration on sleep are different. After nine days of treatment of patients with multiple sclerosis with the glucocorticoid receptor agonist methylprednisolone, REMS latency decreased, REMS density increased, and major portions of SWS and SWA shifted from the first to the second sleep cycle (Figure 8.3).

These effects resemble sleep-EEG changes in depressed patients [42].

In patients with depression, nocturnal cortisol administration prompted changes resembling those in normal controls [39, 40]. Growth hormone, NREMS, and SWS increased [43].

In a clinical trial the CRH-1-receptor antagonist NBI 30775 exerted antidepressive effects. In a subgroup of these patients sleep EEG was recorded before treatment, after one and after four weeks of active treatment. Compared with baseline, SWS increased after one week and after four weeks. The number of awakenings and REMS density decreased by trend during the same period. Separate evaluations of these effects in panels of two dose ranges showed no significant change at the lower dose, whereas in the higher dose range REMS density decreased and SWS increased between baseline and the fourth week (Figure 8.4). These data suggest that CRH-1-receptor antagonism induces normalization of sleep-EEG changes in depressed patients. It appears that CRH overdrive contributes to shallow sleep and REMS disinhibition in depression and CRH-1-receptor antagonism appears to help to counteract these changes, as supported also by the results from the conditional CRH-overexpressing mice.

The HPS system

Described as above, all components of the HPA system are involved in sleep regulation. Similarly, the HPS hormones are reported to play some roles in the sleep-regulatory mechanism. In general, growth-hormone-releasing hormone (GHRH) and ghrelin stimulate GH release, whereas somatostatin shows the opposite effect.

Growth-hormone-releasing hormone is an important endogenous sleep-promoting substance. Hypothalamic GHRH mRNA expression shows a circadian rhythm. In the rat the highest levels are found when sleep propensity is highest in these night-active animals at the beginning of the light periods [44]. In the giant transgenic mice plasma GH is permanently elevated. During the light period NREMS is slightly increased and REMS is almost doubled in these animals compared to normal mice. After sleep deprivation the giant mice sleep more than controls [45]. In dwarf rats the central GHRHergic transmission is impaired and hypothalamic GHRH contents are reduced. These animals show less NREMS and REMS than normal

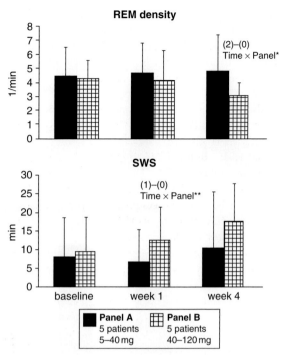

Figure 8.4 REM density (1/min, upper part) and slow-wave sleep (SWS) during the second half of the night (min, bottom) of three examinations (baseline, first week, end of treatment) compared for panel A and panel B during treatment with the CRH-1-receptor antagonist R121919. Panel B showed a significant reduced REM density at week 4 (end of the treatment period and a significant increase of SWS (second half of the night) between baseline and week 1. *Reprinted from* Journal of Psychiatric Research, *38, K. Held, H. Künzel, M. Ising, D. A. Schmid, A. Zobel, H. Murck, F. Holsboer and A. Steiger, Treatment with the CRH1-receptor-antagonist R121919 Improves sleep-EEG in patients with depression, 129–136, Copyright (2004), with kind permission from Elsevier.*

rats [46]. Similarly in dwarf homozygous mice with non-functional GHRH receptors the amounts of NREMS and REMS are lower than in normal mice. Growth-hormone-releasing hormone, ghrelin, and the somatostatin analogue octreotide had no effect on sleep EEG in the dwarf mice. Obviously the actions of these substances on sleep EEG require intact GHRH receptor signaling [47].

After icv GHRH, SWS increased in rats and rabbits [22, 48]. The same effect was found after injection of GHRH into the ventrolateral preoptic area in rats and after systemic administration to rats. Vice versa NREMS decreased after GHRH antagonists. The sleep-promoting effect of sleep deprivation is antagonized by GHRH antibodies and by microinjections of the GHRH antagonist into the area preoptica.

These findings suggest that GHRH promotes NREMS. The amount of NREMS is high when GHRH activity is high, whereas inhibition of GHRH is linked with reduced NREMS. Growth-hormone-releasing hormone appears to be involved in the sleep promotion after sleep deprivation [49].

Also, in humans, GHRH promotes sleep. After repetitive iv GHRH (22:00 to 01:00 hours) SWS and GH increased and cortisol was blunted in young normal male subjects [50] (Figure 8.2). The sleep-promoting effect of GHRH in young men was confirmed after iv and intranasal administration [51]. However, when GHRH was given in the early morning hours while endogenous HPA activity is high, no major changes of sleep EEG were found. Growth hormone increased, but ACTH and cortisol remained unchanged. Only a weak sleep-promoting effect of GHRH was found in a sample of elderly healthy controls. The first NREMS period was prolonged and the number of awakenings decreased [51]. Similarly intranasal GHRH exerted only a weak sleep-promoting effect in elderly normal subjects [52]. A sexual dimorphism of the effects of GHRH was found in a large sample of patients with depression and normal controls of both genders of a wide age range. In male patients and controls sleep was improved and HPA hormones were reduced, whereas in normal and depressed women NREMS decreased and wakefulness and HPA hormones increased [6].

Ghrelin was identified in the stomach and hypothalamus of humans and rats as an endogenous ligand of the GH secretagogue (GHS) receptor. Besides promoting GH release, ghrelin stimulates HPA hormones and prolactin. Furthermore it has a key role in energy balance by increasing food intake and weight gain [16]. Already prior to the discovery of ghrelin synthetic GHSs were known. After GHRP-6, stage 2 sleep increased [53]. In contrast after hexarelin, SWS and SWA decreased. It is thought that the change of the GHRH/CRH ratio in favor of CRH prompted this effect [54]. After oral administration of the GHS MK-677 for one week a distinct sleep-promoting effect occurred in young male subjects [55].

In mice, systemic administration of ghrelin promoted NREMS [47]. A sleep-promoting effect of ghrelin is supported by the observation of decreases of NREMS and REMS in ghrelin knockout mice [56]. In contrast, wakefulness was increased during the first two hours after icv and intrahypothalamic ghrelin in rats [57]. A sleep-promoting effect of ghrelin is further supported by studies in normal human subjects. Similar to the effects of GHRH, pulsatile iv injections of ghrelin increased SWS and GH in young male subjects. The effects on HPA hormones differed between GHRH, which blunted cortisol in young men [50] and ghrelin, which increased ACTH and cortisol, particularly during the first few hours of the night [58]. Also in elderly men NREMS was elevated after ghrelin. In young and elderly women, however, sleep EEG remained unchanged after ghrelin [59].

The somatostatin analogue, octreotide, decreased NREMS in rats after systemic and icv administration [60]. Similarly SWS decreased during the total night and intermittent wakefulness increased during the second half of the night after subcutaneous administration of octreotide in young normal men. Octreotide is more potent than exogenous somatostatin. This explains the lack of effects of iv somatostatin in young normal subjects, whereas it impaired sleep in normal elderly women and men [51]. These data suggest a reciprocal interaction of GHRH and somatostatin in sleep regulation similar to their opposite action on GH release. The same dose of somatostatin that had no effect in young men impaired sleep in elderly subjects probably due to a decline of endogenous GHRH.

Galanin

The peptide galanin is widely located in the mammalian brain. A cluster of galaninergic and GABAergic neurons was found in the ventrolateral preoptic area, which stimulates NREMS [61]. This observation is in line with the finding that iv administration of galanin (22:00 to 01:00 hours) increased SWA and EEG activity in the theta range, whereas hormone secretion remained unchanged [62]. In patients with depression who were medicated with the antidepressant trimipramine, galanin was injected hourly between 09:00 and 12:00 hours. The Hamilton Depression Rating Scale was determined before and after the last injection. The improvement in this rating was significantly greater after galanin compared to placebo. During the following night REMS latency increased. These data suggest an acute antidepressive effect of galanin, which may resemble that of therapeutic sleep deprivation [63].

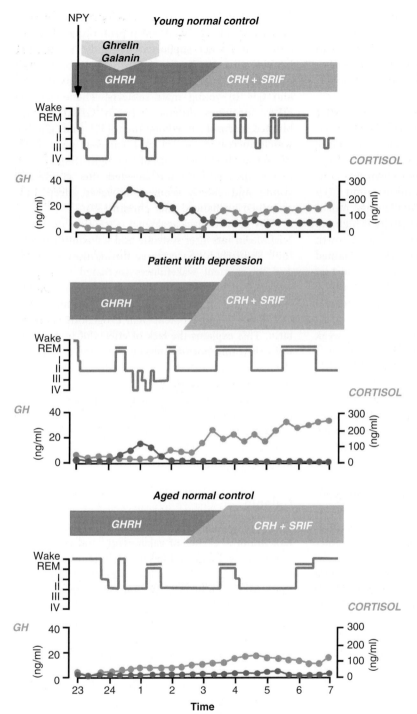

Figure 8.5 Model of peptidergic sleep-endocrine regulation. CRH, corticotropin-releasing hormone; GHRH, growth hormone-releasing hormone; NPY, neuropeptide Y; SRIF, somatostatin. Characteristic hypnograms and patterns of cortisol and GH secretion are shown in a young and in an elderly normal subject and in a depressed patient. It is thought that GHRH is released during the first half of the night, whereas CRH preponderates during the second half of the night. GHRH stimulates GH and SWS around sleep onset, whereas CRH is related to cortisol release and REMS in the morning hours. NPY is a signal for sleep onset. Besides GHRH, galanin and ghrelin promote sleep, whereas somatostatin impairs sleep. During depression (CRH overactivity) and during normal aging, similar changes of sleep–endocrine activity are found. Changes in the GHRH/CRH balance in favor of CRH appear to play a key role in these aberrances. *Nervenarzt (1995), 66: 15–27, Schlafendokrinologie, Axel Steiger, (Fig.2), Copyright Springer-Verlag 1995, with kind permission of Springer Science and Business Media.*

Neuropeptide Y (NPY)

Besides GHRH, neuropeptide Y (NPY) appears to be a physiological antagonist to CRH. Opposite effects of both peptides were found in animal models of anxiety. Intracerebroventricular NPY prompted benzodiazepine-like effects in the sleep EEG of rats [64]. The increase of sleep latency after CRH was antagonized in a dose-dependent fashion by NPY in rats [65].

In contrast an awake-promoting effect of NPY was reported [66]. Repetitive iv NPY decreased sleep latency, the duration of the first REMS period, and HPA hormones but increased stage 2 sleep and sleep period time [67]. In depressed patients of both genders and a wide age range, and in age and sex-matched controls, NPY prompted shortened sleep latency whereas HPA hormones and other sleep-EEG variables remained unchanged [68]. It appears that the effect of NPY on the timing of sleep onset is robust since it was found in young normal male controls, in normal controls of both sexes with a higher age, in patients with depression, and in the animal model as well.

Conclusions

The data reported in this chapter suggest a key role of hormones in the pathophysiology of sleep–endocrine changes during depression.

Figure 8.5 shows a model of peptidergic sleep regulation. The neuropeptides GHRH and CRH are common regulators of sleep EEG and sleep-associated hormone secretion. During the first few hours of the night GHRH is active and stimulates GH and, at least in males, it promotes sleep and inhibits ACTH and cortisol. In contrast CRH enhances vigilance and impairs NREMS. Whereas acute CRH administration decreases REMS in male subjects, several data, particularly sleep recordings in conditional CRH-overexpressing mice, suggest that CRH promotes REMS. Furthermore CRH decreases GH and stimulates HPA hormones. Changes in the GHRH/CRH ratio in favour of CRH result in shallow sleep, REMS disinhibition, elevated cortisol and blunted GH secretion during depression, and in a similar vein during normal aging. In depression elevated CRH activity is well documented, whereas during aging the activity of GHRH declines. Somatostatin as another sleep-impairing peptide is more effective, when the influence of GHRH is reduced in the elderly. Interestingly in women GHRH exerts CRH-like effects as it impairs sleep and increases HPA hormones. This gender difference may contribute to the higher risk of depression in women in comparison to male subjects. After acute administration of cortisol, SWS and GH increased in young and elderly normal human subjects and in patients with depression, probably due to feedback inhibition of endogenous CRH. Prolonged administration of the glucocorticoid receptor agonist methylprednisolone in patients with multiple sclerosis, however, induced sleep-EEG changes similar to those that are characteristic for patients with depression. This finding suggests that synergism of elevated CRH and of its peripheral effect, elevated glucocorticoid concentrations, contribute to the sleep-EEG changes in depression. In the mouse model and in depressed patients CRH-1-receptor antagonists were shown to be capable of counteracting the effects of CRH. Neuropeptide Y appears to be an endogenous antagonist of CRH, particularly in the timing of sleep onset. Besides GHRH, galanin and ghrelin were shown to promote NREMS in male subjects. Whereas ghrelin shared the sleep- and GH-promoting effects of GHRH in male subjects, it exerted opposite effects on HPA hormones, which are blunted after GHRH and are increased after ghrelin. We suggest that ghrelin may act as an interphase between the HPA and HPS systems. In patients with depression galanin showed acute antidepressive effects. The HPA system and galanin are targets for the development of novel principles in the therapy of affective disorders.

Acknowledgments

The studies from the first author's laboratory were supported by grants from the Deutsche Forschungsgemeinschaft (Ste 486/1–2, 5–1, 5–2, 5–3 and 5–4).

References

1. Holsboer-Trachsler E, Seifritz E. Sleep in depression and sleep deprivation: a brief conceptual review. *World J Biol Psychiatry*. 2000;**1**:180–6.

2. Weitzman ED. Circadian rhythms and episodic hormone secretion in man. *Annu Rev Med*. 1976;**27**:225–43.

3. Steiger A. Neuroendocrinology of sleep. In: Lajtha A, Blaustein J, eds. *Handbook of Neurochemistry and Molecular Neurobiology*, 3rd edn. (New York: Springer Science and Business Media, 2007; pp. 895–937).

4. Armitage R. Sleep and circadian rhythms in mood disorders. *Acta Psychiatr Scand*. 2007;**115** (Suppl. 433):104–15.

5. Linkowski P, Mendlewicz J, Kerkhofs M, *et al.* 24-hour profiles of adrenocorticotropin, cortisol, and growth hormone in major depressive illness: effect of antidepressant treatment. *J Clin Endocrinol Metab*. 1987;**65**:141–52.

6. Antonijevic IA, Murck H, Frieboes RM, Steiger A. Sexually dimorphic effects of GHRH on sleep-endocrine activity in patients with depression and normal

controls – part II: hormone secretion. *Sleep Res Online.* 2000;**3**:15–21.

7. Steiger A, von Bardeleben U, Herth T, Holsboer F. Sleep EEG and nocturnal secretion of cortisol and growth hormone in male patients with endogenous depression before treatment and after recovery. *J Affect Disord.* 1989;**16**:189–95.

8. Jarrett DB, Miewald JM, Kupfer DJ. Recurrent depression is associated with a persistent reduction in sleep-related growth hormone secretion. *Arch Gen Psychiatry.* 1990;**47**:113–18.

9. Steiger A, von Bardeleben U, Wiedemann K, Holsboer F. Sleep EEG and nocturnal secretion of testosterone and cortisol in patients with major endogenous depression during acute phase and after remission. *J Psychiatr Res.* 1991;**25**:169–77.

10. Steiger A, Holsboer F. Nocturnal secretion of prolactin and cortisol and the sleep EEG in patients with major endogenous depression during an acute episode and after full remission. *Psychiatry Res.* 1997;**72**:81–8.

11. Holsboer F. The rationale for corticotropin-releasing hormone receptor (CRH-R) antagonists to treat depression and anxiety. *J Psychiatr Res.* 1999;**33**:181–214.

12. Kupfer DJ, Ehlers CL, Frank E, *et al.* Electroencephalographic sleep studies in depressed patients during long-term recovery. *Psychiatry Res.* 1993;**49**:121–38.

13. Frieboes RM, Müller U, Murck H, *et al.* Nocturnal hormone secretion and the sleep EEG in patients several months after traumatic brain injury. *J Neuropsychiatry Clin Neurosci.* 1999;**11**:354–60.

14. Vgontzas AN, Bixler EO, Lin HM, *et al.* Chronic insomnia is associated with nyctohemeral activation of the hypothalamic-pituitary-adrenal axis: Clinical implications. *J Clin Endocrinol Metab.* 2001;**86**:3787–94.

15. Vollrath M, Wicki W, Angst J. The Zurich Study. VIII. Insomnia: Association with depression, anxiety, somatic syndromes, and course of insomnia. *Eur Arch Psychiatry Neurol Sci.* 1989;**239**:113–24.

16. Nogueiras R, Tschöp MH, Zigman JM. Central nervous system regulation of energy metabolism: ghrelin versus leptin. *Ann N Y Acad Sci.* 2008;**1126**:14–19.

17. Antonijevic IA, Murck H, Frieboes RM, *et al.* Elevated nocturnal profiles of serum leptin in patients with depression. *J Psychiatr Res.* 1998;**32**:403–10.

18. Licinio J, Mantzoros C, Negrao AB, *et al.* Human leptin levels are pulsatile and inversely related to pituitary-adrenal function. *Nat Med.* 1997;**3**:575–9.

19. Raber J, Chen S, Mucke L, Feng L. Corticotropin-releasing factor and adrenocorticotrophic hormone as potential central mediators of OB effects. *J Biol Chem.* 1997;**272**:15057–60.

20. Kluge M, Schüssler P, Kleyer S, and Steiger A. Nocturnal ghrelin secretion in major depression. *Eur Neuropsychopharmacol.* 2007;**17** (Suppl 4):S333.

21. Peteranderl C, Antonijevic IA, Steiger A, *et al.* Nocturnal secretion of TSH and ACTH in male patients with depression and healthy controls. *J Psychiatr Res.* 2002;**36**(3):189–96.

22. Ehlers CL, Reed TK, Henriksen SJ. Effects of corticotropin-releasing factor and growth hormone-releasing factor on sleep and activity in rats. *Neuroendocrinology.* 1986;**42**:467–74.

23. Opp M, Obál F Jr., Krueger JM. Corticotropin-releasing factor attenuates interleukin 1-induced sleep and fever in rabbits. *Am J Physiol Regul Integr Comp Physiol.* 1989;**257**:R528–R535.

24. Romanowski C, Fenzl F, Flachskamm C, Deussing JM, Kimura F. CRH-R1 is involved in effects of CRH on NREM, but not REM, sleep suppression. *Sleep Biol Rhythms.* 2007;**5** (Suppl. 1):A53.

25. Marrosu F, Gessa GL, Giagheddu M, Fratta W. Corticotropin-releasing factor (CRF) increases paradoxical sleep (PS) rebound in PS-deprived rats. *Brain Res.* 1990;**515**:315–18.

26. Opp MR. Rat strain differences suggest a role for corticotropin-releasing hormone in modulating sleep. *Physiol Behav.* 1997;**63**:67–74.

27. Chang FC, Opp MR. Blockade of corticotropin-releasing hormone receptors reduces spontaneous waking in the rat. *Am J Physiol Regul Integr Comp Physiol.* 1998;**275**:R793–R802.

28. Gonzalez MMC, Valatx JL. Effect of intracerebroventricular administration of alpha-helical CRH (9–41) on the sleep/waking cycle in rats under normal conditions or after subjection to an acute stressful stimulus. *J Sleep Res.* 1997;**6**:164–70.

29. Gonzalez MMC, Valatx JL. Involvement of stress in the sleep rebound mechanism induced by sleep deprivation in the rat: use of alpha-helical CRH (9–41). *Behav Pharmacol.* 1998;**9**:655–62.

30. Kimura M, Müller-Preuss P, Wiesner E, *et al.* REM sleep enhancement in CNS-specific CRH-overexpressing mice. *Neurosci Res.* 2007; **58** (Suppl. 1):S32.

31. Lancel M, Müller-Preuss P, Wigger A, Landgraf R, Holsboer F. The CRH1 receptor antagonist R121919 attenuates stress-elicited sleep disturbances in rats, particularly in those with high innate anxiety. *J Psychiatr Res.* 2002;**36**:197–208.

32. Holsboer F, von Bardeleben U, Steiger A. Effects of intravenous corticotropin-releasing hormone upon

sleep-related growth hormone surge and sleep EEG in man. *Neuroendocrinology.* 1988;**48**:32–8.

33. Schüssler P, Kluge M, Dresler M, Yassouridis A, Steiger A. Effects of intravenous corticotropin-releasing hormone upon sleep EEG in young healthy women. *J Sleep Res.* 2008;**17** (Suppl. 1): P382.

34. Kellner M, Yassouridis A, Manz B, *et al.* Corticotropin-releasing hormone inhibits melatonin secretion in healthy volunteers: a potential link to low-melatonin syndrome in depression? *Neuroendocrinology.* 1997;**16**:339–45.

35. Antonijevic IA, Murck H, Frieboes RM, Holsboer F, Steiger A. Hyporesponsiveness of the pituitary to CRH during slow wave sleep is not mimicked by systemic GHRH. *Neuroendocrinology.* 1999;**69**:88–96.

36. Vgontzas AN, Bixler EO, Wittman AM, *et al.* Middle-aged men show higher sensitivity of sleep to the arousing effects of corticotropin-releasing hormone than young men: clinical implications. *J Clin Endocrinol Metab.* 2001;**86**:1489–95.

37. Born J, Späth-Schwalbe E, Schwakenhofer H, Kern W, Fehm HL. Influences of corticotropin-releasing hormone, adrenocorticotropin, and cortisol on sleep in normal man. *J Clin Endocrinol Metab.* 1989;**68**:904–11.

38. Steiger A, Guldner J, Knisatschek H, *et al.* Effects of an ACTH/MSH(4–9) analog (HOE 427) on the sleep EEG and nocturnal hormonal secretion in humans. *Peptides.* 1991;**12**:1007–10.

39. Friess E, Tagaya H, Grethe C, Trachsel L, Holsboer F. Acute cortisol administration promotes sleep intensity in man. *Neuropsychopharmacology.* 2004;**29**:598–604.

40. Bohlhalter S, Murck H, Holsboer F, Steiger A. Cortisol enhances non-REM sleep and growth hormone secretion in elderly subjects. *Neurobiol Aging.* 1997;**18**:423–9.

41. Jahn H, Kiefer F, Schick M, *et al.* Sleep-endocrine effects of the 11-β–hydroxasteroid dehydrogenase inhibitor metyrapone. *Sleep.* 2003;**26**:823–9.

42. Antonijevic IA, Steiger A. Depression-like changes of the sleep-EEG during high dose corticosteroid treatment in patients with multiple sclerosis. *Psychoneuroendocrinology.* 2003;**28**:780–95.

43. Schmid DA, Brunner H, Lauer CJ, *et al.* Acute cortisol administration increases sleep depth and growth hormone release in patients with a major depression. *J Psychiatr Res.* 2008;**42**(12):991–9.

44. Bredow S, Taishi P, Obál F Jr., Guha-Thakurta N, Krueger JM. Hypothalamic growth hormone-releasing hormone mRNA varies across the day in rat. *NeuroReport.* 1996;**7**:2501–5.

45. Hajdu I, Obál F Jr., Fang J, Krueger JM, Rollo CD. Sleep of transgenic mice producing excess rat growth hormone. *Am J Physiol Regul Integr Comp Physiol.* 2002;**282**:R70–R76.

46. Obál F Jr., Fang J, Taishi P, *et al.* Deficiency of growth hormone-releasing hormone signaling is associated with sleep alterations in the dwarf rat. *J Neurosci.* 2001;**21**:2912–18.

47. Obál F Jr, Alt J, Taishi P, Gardi J, Krueger JM. Sleep in mice with non-functional growth hormone-releasing hormone receptors. *Am J Physiol Regul Integr Comp Physiol.* 2003;**284**:R131–R139.

48. Obál F Jr., Alföldi P, Cady AB, *et al.* Growth hormone-releasing factor enhances sleep in rats and rabbits. *Am J Physiol Regul Integr Comp Physiol.* 1988;**255**:R310–R316.

49. Obál F Jr., Krueger JM. GHRH and sleep. *Sleep Medicine Rev.* 2004;**8**:367–77.

50. Steiger A, Guldner J, Hemmeter U, *et al.* Effects of growth hormone-releasing hormone and somatostatin on sleep EEG and nocturnal hormone secretion in male controls. *Neuroendocrinology.* 1992;**56**:566–73.

51. Steiger A. Neurochemical regulation of sleep. *J Psychiatr Res.* 2007;**41**:537–52.

52. Perras B, Pannenborg H, Marshall L, *et al.* Beneficial treatment of age-related sleep disturbances with prolonged intranasal vasopressin. *J Clin Psychopharmacol.* 1999;**19**:28–36.

53. Frieboes RM, Murck H, Maier P, *et al.* Growth hormone-releasing peptide-6 stimulates sleep, growth hormone, ACTH and cortisol release in normal man. *Neuroendocrinology.* 1995;**61**:584–9.

54. Frieboes RM, Antonijevic IA, Held K, *et al.* Hexarelin decreases slow-wave sleep and stimulates the sleep-related secretion of GH, ACTH, cortisol and prolactin during sleep in healthy volunteers. *Psychoneuroendocrinology.* 2004;**29**:851–60.

55. Copinschi G, Leproult R, Van Onderbergen A, *et al.* Prolonged oral treatment with MK-677, a novel growth hormone secretagogue, improves sleep quality in man. *Neuroendocrinology.* 1997;**66**:278–86.

56. Szentirmai E, Kapás L, Sun Y, Smith RG, Krueger JM. Spontaneous sleep and homeostatic sleep regulation in ghrelin knockout mice. *Am J Physiol Regul Integr Comp Physiol.* 2007;**293**:R510–R517.

57. Szentirmai E, Kapás L, Krueger JM. Ghrelin microinjection into forebrain sites induces wakefulness and feeding in rats. *Am J Physiol Regul Integr Comp Physiol.* 2007;**292**:R575–R585.

58. Weikel JC, Wichniak A, Ising M, *et al.* Ghrelin promotes slow-wave sleep in humans. *Am J Physiol Endocrinol Metab.* 2003;**284**:E407–E415.

59. Kluge M, Schüssler P, Zuber V, Yassouridis A, Steiger A. Ghrelin administered in the early morning

increases secretion of cortisol and growth hormone without affecting sleep. *Psychoneuroendocrinology.* 2007;**32**:287–92.

60. Beranek L, Hajdu I, Gardi J, *et al.* Central administration of the somatostatin analog octreotide induces captopril-insensitive sleep responses. *Am J Physiol Regul Integr Comp Physiol.* 1999;**277**: R1297–R1304.

61. Saper CB, Chou TC, Scammell TE. The sleep switch: hypothalamic control of sleep and wakefulness. *Trends Neurosci.* 2001;**24**:726–31.

62. Murck H, Antonijevic IA, Frieboes RM, *et al.* Galanin has REM-sleep deprivation-like effects on the sleep EEG in healthy young men. *J Psychiatr Res.* 1997;**33**:225–32.

63. Murck H, Held K, Ziegenbein M, *et al.* Intravenous administration of the neuropeptide galanin has fast antidepressant efficacy and affects the sleep EEG. *Psychoneuroendocrinology.* 2004;**29**:1205–11.

64. Ehlers CL, Somes C, Lopez A, Kirby D, Rivier JE. Electrophysiological actions of neuropeptide Y and its analogs: new measures for anxiolytic therapy? *Neuropsychopharmacology.* 1997;**17**:34–43.

65. Ehlers CL, Somes C, Seifritz E, Rivier JE. CRF/NPY interactions: a potential role in sleep dysregulation in depression and anxiety. *Depress Anxiety.* 1997;**6**:1–9.

66. Szentirmai E, Krueger JM. Neuropeptide Y promotes wakefulness in rats. *J Sleep Res.* 2006;**15** (Suppl. 1):59.

67. Antonijevic IA, Murck H, Bohlhalter S, *et al.* NPY promotes sleep and inhibits ACTH and cortisol release in young men. *Neuropharmacology.* 2000;**39**:1474–81.

68. Held K, Murck H, Antonijevic IA, *et al.* Neuropeptide Y (NPY) does not differentially affect sleep-endocrine regulation in depressed patients and controls. *Pharmacopsychiatry.* 1999;**32**:184.

Eating and sleep disorders: shared mechanisms?

Naomi L. Rogers and Bradley G. Whitwell

Eating and sleeping share a number of common elements. Regulation of both appetite and sleep–wake behaviors has been shown to involve both the hypothalamus and the paraventricular nucleus. Additionally, a number of neuroendocrine variables involved in the modulation of appetite and caloric intake are shared with (e.g., orexin) or are strongly influenced by the sleep–wake system (e.g., leptin, ghrelin, cortisol).

Glucose control

Maintaining optimal levels of glucose throughout the body is an essential homeostatic process. Circulating glucose levels fluctuate across the 24-hour day, depending on the activities engaged in at different times. Elevated glucose levels over an extended period can produce changes in the vasculature. Indeed, a compromised vascular system is a comorbid feature of diabetes, where glucose levels can be elevated for prolonged periods of time. Additionally, blindness, heart disease, kidney malfunction, and nerve damage may all result from a chronic exposure to high circulating glucose. Chronically low levels of glucose are also associated with negative effects, including impaired neurocognitive functioning and tissue development, and, in extreme cases, coma.

Circulating glucose levels are maintained via numerous, complex feedback loops. Throughout a 24-hour period, glucose levels are controlled via maintaining a balance between skeletal muscle and liver glucose uptake (signaled by insulin levels) and glucose production (signaled by glucagons). The control of caloric intake is maintained by the lateral ventromedial nucleus of the hypothalamus. The control of appetite and caloric intake is influenced by signals from both the central nervous system (CNS) and peripherary. Central nervous system signals involved in this control include the neuropeptidergic, monoaminergic, and endocannabinoid systems. Peripheral signals relating to satiety and adiposity are relayed via a number of neuroendocrine factors, including the hormones leptin and ghrelin. Cortisol, another important hormone involved in metabolism and glucose control, increases glucose production and release from the liver, and inhibits the uptake of glucose into peripheral tissues.

The secretion of cortisol is influenced by both the circadian timing system and the sleep–wake state. The 24-hour circadian variation in cortisol levels has been found to be related to the daily fluctuations in metabolism and fuel homeostasis. In addition to the circadian influence, sleep onset inhibits cortisol release, and the timing of the morning peak in cortisol is tightly linked with the timing of sleep offset (Rogers *et al.*, submitted).

Glucose control during sleep

During sleep, the body is commonly in a state of glucose intolerance. Increased levels of circulating glucose and insulin have been reported to range between 20 and 30% [1, 2]. Sleep itself, it has been proposed, may be at least partly responsible for the decrease in glucose uptake experienced during this time. It is likely that the CNS requirement for glucose is reduced during sleep, particularly during slow-wave sleep (SWS), during which time growth hormone also surges [3], owing to the reduction in muscle tone that occurs during sleep [4]. In the latter part of the nocturnal sleep period, glucose levels tend to normalize. This phenomenon may be due to the increased amounts of REM sleep that typically occur during the late nocturnal sleep period [1], the increasing levels of cortisol occurring throughout the second half of the

Sleep and Mental Illness, eds. S. R. Pandi-Perumal and M. Kramer. Published by Cambridge University Press.
© Cambridge University Press 2010.

sleep period, or in the preparation for waking, increasing activity, and metabolic requirements.

Sleep duration, appetite, and metabolism

Evidence from a number of studies is building, demonstrating a relationship between sleep duration and changes in metabolism, weight gain, obesity, and type-2 diabetes [5].

A small number of epidemiologic studies also suggest a link between sleep duration and increased incidence of type-2 diabetes, although the evidence is not conclusive. In a study of 70,000 females in the Nurses Heart Health Study, Ayas and colleagues found that both chronic short sleep durations (≤ 5 hours per night) and chronic long sleep durations (≥ 9 hours per night) were associated with an increased incidence of type-2 diabetes [6]. Similar relationships were also reported in male subjects in the Massachusetts Male Ageing Study [7] and in the Sleep Heart Health Study [8]. Other studies have reported significant effects of shortened sleep durations (≤ 5 hours per night) only in males [9], or no significant relationships between sleep durations (either short or long) and the incidence of diabetes [10].

A small number of controlled, in-laboratory studies have examined the relationship between sleep duration and various factors involved in metabolic control. Studies in which subjects have been exposed to either total sleep deprivation or a number of nights of sleep restriction have produced a decrease in glucose tolerance and increase in insulin sensitivity [11, 12].

In one study, 11 healthy male subjects were studied under conditions of both sleep restriction (four hours time in bed for six nights) and sleep extension (12 hours time in bed for six nights) [12]. Using intravenous glucose tolerance tests (IGTT) the authors demonstrated that following the sleep restriction condition, there was a significant reduction in glucose tolerance, resulting in subjects being described as being in a pre-diabetic state. In a subsequent study, the same research group compared the effects of more acute sleep restriction (two nights of four hours time in bed for sleep) with acute sleep extension (two nights of ten hours time in bed for sleep) in 12 healthy males [13]. Similar to their earlier study, sleep restriction was associated with a reduction in glucose tolerance, and glucose levels indicative of a pre-diabetic state.

Decreased levels of leptin (an appetite saiety hormone) and ghrelin (an appetite inducing hormone), as well as elevations in cortisol [14] have been associated with sleep restriction. The increased preference for high carbohydrate-containing foods and increased overall appetite [13] has also been associated.

Changes in eating, metabolism, and sleep in mood disorders

In the majority of serious psychiatric disorders, e.g., schizophrenia, bipolar disorder, depression, an associated disruption to the sleep–wake and circadian systems occurs. Additionally, many individuals with these disorders experience a disruption to their metabolic systems and appetite, with a resultant increase in weight gain and increased incidence of obesity. It has been posited that the increased occurrence of weight gain and increased incidence of obesity in these patient populations may be due to the medications administered for management of their disorder. However, it is now recognized that changes in appetite, weight gain, and obesity are present in these patients independent of their medications.

In patients with untreated first episode schizophrenia, there have been reports of increased central adiposity and elevated cortisol levels compared with control subjects [15]. Additionally, schizophrenia has been described as an independent risk factor for the development of diabetes. Approximately 15 to 18% of patients with schizophrenia have developed type-2 diabetes, and the prevalence of impaired glucose tolerance may be as high as 30% depending on age.

Many antipsychotic medications used in the treatment of schizophrenia increase the risk of obesity, and as a consequence may accelerate the development of metabolic syndrome. It has been proposed that the increase in weight gain and incidence of obesity may be driven by a disturbance to the hypothalamic systems that control energy balance [16, 17]. For example, pharmacological agents with antihistaminergic, antiadrenergic (α-1), and antiserotinergic (5-HT2a, 5-HT6) effects increase weight gain via actions on the metabolic regulatory pathways. We can therefore hypothesize that disturbances to the circadian and sleep–wake systems commonly reported in psychosis may disrupt the feedback mechanisms involved in energy regulation and metabolism, mimicking the pharmacological processes of the antipsychotic medications. Further studies are required to determine the nature of this relationship.

Eating and sleeping disorders
Night eating syndrome

Night eating syndrome (NES) was first described in 1955 and is characterized by morning anorexia, evening hyperphagia, sleep onset insomnia, and awakenings occurring at least once per night on at least three nights per week where food is consumed [18]. Although the majority of patients tend to be overweight or obese (BMI ≥25 or 30, respectively), some patients are considered to be in a normal weight range [19, 20]. Evidence suggesting a genetic component to NES exists, with relatives of patients more likely to have also experienced NES [21]. When patients with NES wake from sleep to eat, they do so consciously, and eat 'normal' foods. These characteristics are important in distinguishing NES from sleep related eating disorder (SRED), which will be discussed later.

There is strong evidence that NES is a circadian-based disorder [22, 23]. In patients with NES, it appears that as in healthy subjects the central circadian pacemaker, located in the suprachiasmatic nucleus (SCN) of the hypothalamus [24], maintains normal 24-hour timing in most of the physiological and behavioral systems under its control e.g., sleep–wake behavior. However, in NES patients there appears to be internal desynchrony with peripheral oscillators regulating caloric intake and appetite [22, 23, 25]. This internal circadian misalignment is similar to that induced in animal models where the circadian timing of caloric intake is desynchronized from other, centrally controlled, circadian rhythms [26].

Although there is no observable difference between NES patients and healthy subjects in their total caloric intake per 24 hours, the NES patients' timing of the daily caloric intake is markedly different. Patients with NES have significantly delayed eating rhythms, and tend to consume around 35% of their daily caloric intake after the evening meal, during their nocturnal sleep period [22].

There have been a number of studies examining the sleep characteristics of NES patients, relative to control subjects. When sleep behavior was assessed using at-home actigraphy across seven days [22] or in-laboratory polysomnography (PSG) assessed over three consecutive nights [23], no differences in the timing of sleep onset or sleep termination were reported between NES patients and obese controls.

In this same in-laboratory PSG study, reductions in the amount of stage 2 sleep, stage 3 sleep, total sleep time, and sleep quality were found in the NES patients compared to the control subjects. Interestingly, there were no differences in the total number of awakenings across the nocturnal sleep period between the two groups. During these awakenings, 93.3% of NES patients consumed food on all three nights, and in contrast, 92.9% of the control subjects did not eat during any awakenings. In two other PSG studies of patients with NES, there were a number of patients identified who did not experience evening hyperphagia and did not report hunger during their nocturnal awakenings where they ate [27, 28].

Changes in a number of neuroendocrine variables have been reported in NES, although it is unclear whether these changes are a cause or effect. Within a group of obese NES patients studied in a sleep laboratory, with a comparison group of obese control subjects, phase delays in the timing of the leptin (1.0 hour) and insulin (2.8 hours) rhythms were identified, while the timing of ghrelin secretion was phase advanced (5.2 hours) [25]. The circadian rhythm of circulating glucose levels was around 180° out of phase, i.e., either approximately 12-hour phase advanced or 12-hour phase delayed. In addition, the timing of the pineal hormone melatonin was also delayed, with a trend for cortisol to also be delayed. The amplitude of the circadian rhythms of ghrelin, insulin, and cortisol were reduced and TSH increased in NES patients relative to controls.

A relationship between NES and psychiatric disorders and mood disturbance has been proposed. Early reports indicated that psychosocial stressors were often temporally related to elevations in night eating symptoms [18]. In later studies, obese patients with NES attending either a clinic or studied in the laboratory reported higher depression scores and lower self-esteem scores compared to obese patients without NES [23, 29]. In one study that assessed mood in patients with NES and controls throughout a 24-hour day, it was reported that mood scores were lower in NES patients, with a decline in mood scores observed after 16:00 hours. Interestingly, the temporal profile of the decreasing mood scores differs from that typically seen in patients with depression, where mood tends to be lower earlier in the circadian cycle and higher in the late afternoon [30].

Night eating syndrome has also been reported to be comorbid with psychiatric disorders. Patients attending two outpatient clinics (n = 399) were assessed for the presence of NES. Of these, just over 12% were found to meet the criteria for NES [31]. Comparing patients from these clinics without NES, a higher proportion of those diagnosed with NES were found to also have a substance-abuse problem and to be obese.

Sleep related eating disorder

Distinct from NES, but sharing some common features, is sleep related eating disorder (SRED). The exact history of SRED, including a clear definition and the underlying nature of the disorder, has been somewhat unclear; however, SRED is now considered to be a parasomnia [32]. Similar to NES, patients with SRED engage in nocturnal eating and morning anorexia. Sleep related eating disorder patients are often also obese, and psychiatric disorders are commonly comorbid. However, in contrast to NES, other characteristics of SRED include: involuntary consumption of food; consuming strange combinations of food, uncooked foods or inedible substances; dangerous food preparation; not being easily awakened; and a lack of awareness of nocturnal eating activities (although this last feature varies both between and within patients) [33, 34].

In patients with SRED, consumption of calorie-rich food during nocturnal eating episodes is common, with patients typically preferring high carbohydrate and high fat content foods. Some patients also report binge eating. It is not unusual for the types of food consumed during these night-time episodes to differ from what the individual normally consumes during the daytime [34, 35]. Patients have reported eating frozen foods, raw meat, and cat food, as well consuming items such as coffee grounds, eggshells, cigarette butts, and cleaning products [33, 36]. The consumption of these substances places patients at a potential risk for poisoning, choking, and burns from hot liquids or foods. Many patients also report receiving injuries, such as cuts, due to unsafe food preparation.

It has been reported that approximately half of patients with SRED arouse from bed to eat at least once every night, with many of these patients reporting multiple eating episodes across the night [36, 37]. However, the incidence of multiple eating episodes per night may be higher than indicated in this early study. In one study, around 70% of participants (25 of 35) reported eating more than once each night, with an additional 22% of participants reporting rising and eating more than five times per night [35].

One characteristic of SRED is the lack of awareness associated with the night-time eating episodes. Patients with SRED exhibit difficulties in arousal during an episode, similar to that of sleep walking. This lack of awareness during episodes, however, is not universal nor agreed upon. One recent study reported that SRED patients were fully aware of their actions during their nocturnal eating episodes [35], while earlier studies have found partial awareness [33] or complete lack of awareness [36].

The presence of SRED is also often comorbid with other sleep disorders, such as restless legs syndrome (RLS), sleep apnea, and other parasomnias [36, 38]. Periodic limb movements during sleep (PLMS) are common, as is chewing or rhythmic masticatory muscle activity (RMMA) [33, 35].

Sleep related eating disorder has also been reported to be comorbid with psychiatric disorders. Patients with SRED have a higher incidence rate of depressed mood [35, 39]. Additionally, the onset of nocturnal eating and SRED is often associated with substance abuse or relationship problems [33, 36].

In an early report, nearly half of SRED patients studied were diagnosed with an Axis 1 disorder (DSM-IV) [36], with many of these patients displaying increased anxiety, particularly related to their night-time eating episodes, and fears of choking or starting a fire during food preparation. In a later study, just over half of patients were found to have experienced past abuse, and displayed some characteristics similar to those observed in patients with post-traumatic stress disorder (PTSD) [33].

Sleep related eating disorder has also been found to be associated with a number of CNS acting medications, including sedative hypnotics; newer hypnotic agents such as zolpidem; tricyclic antidepressants; mood stabilizers such as lithium; risperidone and anticholinergic compounds [32].

Summary

From the above discussions, it can be seen that the systems and processes that control caloric intake and sleep–wake behavior overlap in a number of respects, including the neurobiology, neuroendocrine signals, and pathologies. Further research is required in order to fully understand the nature of the relationship between these two systems. Understanding the relationship between caloric intake and sleep–wake behaviors potentially would improve the available treatment options for NES and SRED. Interventions to reduce the growing epidemic of obesity and metabolic disorders, such as type-2 diabetes, which is occurring in parallel with increasing numbers of individuals experiencing chronic sleep restriction, may also target both systems.

References

1. Scheen AJ, Byrne MM, Plat L, Leproult R, Van Cauter E. Relationships between sleep quality and glucose regulation in normal humans. *Am J Physiol.* 1996;**271**(2 Pt 1):E261–70.

2. Van Cauter E, Désir D, Decoster C, Féry F, Balasse EO. Nocturnal decrease in glucose tolerance during constant glucose infusion. *J Clin Endocrinol Metab.* 1989;**69**(3):604–11.

3. Sassin JF, Parker DC, Johnson LC, *et al.* Effects of slow wave sleep deprivation on human growth hormone release in sleep: preliminary study. *Life Sci.* 1969;**8**(1):1299–307.

4. Boyle PJ, Scott JC, Krentz AJ, *et al.* Diminished brain glucose metabolism is a significant determinant for falling rates of systemic glucose utilization during sleep in normal humans. *J Clin Invest.* 1994;**93**(2):529–35.

5. Trenell MI, Marshall NS, Rogers NL. Sleep and metabolic control: waking to a problem? *Clin Exper Pharmacol Physiol.* 2007;**34**(1):1–9.

6. Ayas NT, White DP, Manson JE, *et al.* A prospective study of sleep duration and coronary heart disease in women. *Arch Intern Med.* 2003;**163**(2):205–9.

7. Yaggi HK, Araujo AB, McKinlay JB. Sleep duration as a risk factor for the development of type-2 diabetes. *Diabetes Care.* 2006;**29**:657–61.

8. Gottlieb DJ, Punjabi NM, Newman AB, *et al.* Association of sleep time with diabetes mellitus and impaired glucose tolerance. *Arch Intern Med.* 2005;**165**(8):863–7.

9. Mallon L, Broman JE, Hetta J. High incidence of diabetes in men with sleep complaints or short sleep duration: a 12-year follow-up study of a middle-aged population. *Diabetes Care.* 2005;**28**:2762–7.

10. Björkelund C, Bondyr-Carlsson D, Lapidus L, *et al.* Sleep disturbances in midlife unrelated to 32-year diabetes incidence: the prospective population study of women in Gothenburg. *Diabetes Care.* 2005;**28**(11):2739–44.

11. VanHelder T, Symons JD, Radomski MW. Effects of sleep deprivation and exercise on glucose tolerance. *Aviat Space Environ Med.* 1993;**6**:487–92.

12. Spiegel K, Leproult R, Van Cauter E. Impact of sleep debt on metabolic and endocrine function. *Lancet.* 1999;**354**(9188):1435–9.

13. Spiegel K, Tasali E, Penev P, Van Cauter E. Sleep curtailment in healthy young men is associated with decreased leptin levels, elevated ghrelin levels, and increased hunger and appetite. *Ann Intern Med.* 2004;**141**(11):846–50.

14. Leproult R, Copinschi G, Buxton O, Van Cauter E. Sleep loss results in an elevation of cortisol levels the next evening. *Sleep.* 1997;**20**(10):865–70.

15. Thakore JH. Metabolic disturbance in first-episode schizophrenia. *B J Psychiatry Suppl.* 2004;**47**:S76–S9.

16. Kroeze WK, Hufeisen SJ, Popadak BA, *et al.* H1-histamine receptor affinity predicts short-term weight gain for typical and atypical antipsychotic drugs. *Neuropsychopharm.* 2003;**28**(3):519–26.

17. Kim SF, Huang AS, Snowman AM, Teuscher C, Snyder SH. Antipsychotic drug-induced weight gain mediated by histamine H1 receptor-linked activation of hypothalamic AMP-kinase. *Proc Natl Acad Sci USA.* 2007;**104**(9):3456–9.

18. Stunkard AJ, Grace WJ, Wolff HG. The night-eating syndrome: a pattern of food intake among certain obese patients. *Int J Med.* 1955;**19**:78–86.

19. de Zwaan M, Roerig DB, Crosby RD, Karaz S, Mitchell JE. Nighttime eating: a descriptive study. *Int J Eat Disord.* 2006;**39**(3):224–32.

20. Lundgren JD, Allison KC, O'Reardon JP, Stunkard AJ. A descriptive study of non-obese persons with night eating syndrome and a weight-matched comparison group. *Eating Behaviors.* 2008;**9**(3):343–51.

21. Lundgren JD, Allison KC, Stunkard AJ. Familial aggregation in the night eating syndrome. *Int J Eat Disord.* 2006;**39**(6):516–18.

22. O'Reardon JP, Ringel BL, Dinges DF, *et al.* Actigraphic and sleep diary assessment of rest-activity cycles in night eating syndrome. *Obes Res.* 2004;**12**(11):1789–96.

23. Rogers NL, Dinges DF, Allison KC, *et al.* Assessment of sleep in women with night eating syndrome. *Sleep.* 2006;**29**(6):814–19.

24. Moore RY. Organization and function of a central nervous system circadian oscillator: the suprachiasmatic hypothalamic nucleus. *Federation Proceedings.* 1983;**42**:2783–9.

25. Goel N, Stunkard AJ, Rogers NL, *et al.* Circadian rhythm profiles in women with night eating syndrome. *J Biol Rhythms.* 2009;**24**(1):85–94.

26. Damiola F, Le Minh N, Preitner N, *et al.* Restricted feeding uncouples circadian oscillators in peripheral tissues from the central pacemaker in the suprachiasmatic nucleus. *Genes Dev.* 2000; **14**(23):2950–61.

27. Spaggiari MC, Granella F, Parrino L, *et al.* Nocturnal eating syndrome in adults. *Sleep.* 1994;**17**:339–44.

28. Manni R, Ratti MT, Tartara A. Nocturnal eating: prevalence and features in 120 insomniac referrals. *Sleep.* 1997;**20**:734–8.

29. Gluck ME, Geliebter A, Satov T. Night eating syndrome is associated with depression, low self-esteem, reduced daytime hunger, and less weight loss in obese outpatients. *Obes Res.* 2001;**9**(4):264–7.

30. Birketvedt GS, Florholmen J, Sundsfjord J, *et al.* Behavioral and neuroendocrine characteristics of the night-eating syndrome. *J Am Med Assoc.* 1999; **282**(7):657–63.

31. Lundgren JD, Allison KC, Crow S, *et al.* Prevalence of the night eating syndrome in a psychiatric population. *Am J Psychiatry.* 2006;**161**(1):156–8.

32. Howell MJ, Schenck CH, Crow SJ. A review of nighttime eating disorders. *Sleep Med Rev.* 2009; **13**(1):23–34.

33. Schenck CH, Mahowald MW. Review of nocturnal sleep-related eating disorders. *Int J Eat Disord.* 1994;**15**(4):343–56.

34. Winkelman JW. Clinical and polysomnographic features of sleep-related eating disorder. *J Clin Psychiatry.* 1998;**59**:14–9.

35. Vetrugno R, Manconi M, Ferini-Strambi L, *et al.* Nocturnal eating: sleep-related eating disorder or night eating syndrome? A videopolysomnographic study. *Sleep.* 2006;**29**(7):949–54.

36. Winkelman JW. Clinical and polysomnographic features of sleep-related eating disorder. *J Clin Psychiatry.* 1998;**59**(1):14–19.

37. Schenck CH, Hurwitz TD, Bundlie SR, Mahowald MW. Sleep-related eating disorders: polysomnographic correlates of a heterogeneous syndrome distinct from daytime eating disorders. *Sleep.* 1991;**14**(5):419–31.

38. Striegel-Moore RH, Dohm FA, Hook JM, *et al.* Night eating syndrome in young adult women: prevalence and correlates. *Int J Eat Disord.* 2005;**37**(3):200–6.

39. Winkelman JW, Herzog DB, Fava M. The prevalence of sleep-related eating disorder in psychiatric and non-psychiatric populations. *Psychol Med.* 1999;**29**(6):1461–6.

Sleep–endocrine relationships in depressed women across the reproductive cycle

Charles J. Meliska, Luis Fernando Martínez, and Barbara L. Parry

Introduction

In their review of sleep and mood disorders, Peterson and Benca identified the most common subjective sleep complaints as initial, middle, and terminal insomnia, decreased amount of sleep, reduced restorative sleep, and disturbing dreams [1]. Common objective deficits, as measured by polysomnography (PSG) or wrist actigraphy, include delayed sleep onset, increased wake after sleep onset, increased early morning wake time, decreased total sleep time, decreased slow-wave sleep, and rapid eye movement (REM) sleep abnormalities, including reduced REM sleep latency and increased REM sleep percentage.

Parry and colleagues reviewed studies of sleep and depression in women across the reproductive cycle [2, 3]. The present chapter highlights recent studies of sleep–endocrine relationships in depressed women, focusing on studies that employ objective measures of sleep and biological rhythms (melatonin, cortisol, thyroid stimulating hormone [TSH], prolactin, temperature), and that document reproductive endocrine status. We also review studies of putative treatment interventions with light and wake therapy/sleep deprivation on mood and biological rhythms. Studies of estradiol, progesterone, follicle-stimulating hormone (FSH), and luteinizing hormone (LH) are presented primarily in relation to menopause. We address recent studies documenting the importance of age, body mass index (BMI), and obstructive sleep apnea (OSA) in sleep and circadian rhythm disruption in the section on menopause, the epoch during which, along with hot flashes, these problems become particularly salient.

Menstrual cycle studies

For menstrual cycle studies, measurements generally are made during menses (1 to 5 days after the onset of

bleeding); the follicular phase (1 to 14 days after menses onset, before ovulation, when FSH is secreted from the pituitary and the ovarian follicle is developing and secreting increasing estrogen); at ovulation (during the LH surge, 12 to 14 days after menses in a 28-day cycle); in the luteal phase (14 to 28 days after menses onset, after ovulation when the corpus luteum secretes progesterone); and in the premenstrual, late luteal phase (7 to 10 days before menses onset, when estradiol and progesterone levels are declining). See Figure 10.1.

Subjective sleep measures in healthy cycling women

At menarche, healthy girls start reporting poorer sleep quality before and during menstruation. Many studies of sleep and the menstrual cycle report poorer sleep quality, insomnia, and in some cases, hypersomnia, premenstrually. Delayed sleep onset and decreased luteal vs. follicular phase sleep efficiency and quality, as well as increased subjective daytime sleepiness, all unrelated to severity of other premenstrual symptoms, have been observed [2]. Baker and Driver refined earlier work by screening from study women with symptoms of premenstrual syndrome (PMS), including abdominal bloating or cramps, breast tenderness, headache, fatigue, stress, anxiety, joint or muscle pain, and identifying ovulation objectively by urine LH detection. These women reported poorer subjective sleep quality from three days before to four days after menstruation onset. Self-reported total sleep time, sleep onset latency, number and duration of awakenings, and morning vigilance did not differ significantly across menstrual cycle phases; sleep efficiency decreased slightly, premenstrually. Thus, while these healthy women perceived their sleep

Sleep and Mental Illness, eds. S. R. Pandi-Perumal and M. Kramer. Published by Cambridge University Press.

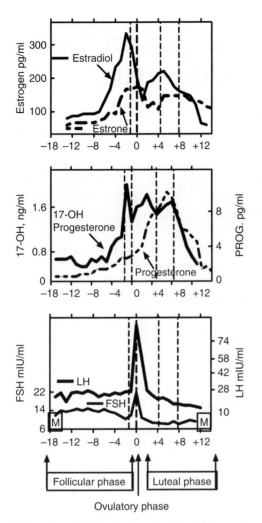

Figure 10.1 Variation in estrogens (estradiol, the major secretory product of the ovaries; estrone, the dominant plasma estrogen after menopause; and estriol, the metabolite of estradiol and estrone), progesterone, and gonadotropin (FSH, LH) levels during the menstrual cycle, as related to the LH peak (Day 0, lower panel). Days of menstrual bleeding are indicated by M. (Redrawn with permission from Yen SS, and Jaffe RB. *Reproductive Endocrinology: Physiology, Pathophysiology, and Clinical Management.* 2nd edition. Philadelphia: Saunders; 1986: p. 203.)

quality to be worse premenstrually and during menses, sleep continuity was not diminished [4].

Objective sleep measures in healthy cycling women

Although subjective reports of menstruation-related sleep disturbances are widespread, carefully controlled

studies using objective measures across the menstrual cycle provide a somewhat different picture. Driver *et al.* studied sleep electroencephalogram (EEG) changes in women who lacked PMS symptoms; ovulation and menstrual cycle stage were confirmed by body temperature, urinary LH, and midluteal plasma estrogen and progesterone levels. They found no significant variation across the menstrual cycle in *either* objective or subjective ratings of total sleep time, sleep efficiency, sleep latency, REM sleep latency, or slow-wave sleep, suggesting sleep disruption may be minimal when premenstrual dysphoria is absent [5].

Sleep in women with menstrual-cycle related mood symptoms

Women experiencing PMS or premenstrual dysphoric disorder (PMDD), a severe form of PMS characterized by depressed mood, report more subjective late luteal phase sleep disturbance, including hypersomnia and daytime sleepiness, than women without symptoms [2]. Based on objective measures, Parry *et al.* found women with premenstrual depression had more stage 2 (percentage) and less REM sleep (minutes and percentage) than healthy controls, irrespective of menstrual phase. Stage 3 sleep minutes decreased and intermittent awakenings increased during the late luteal phase in both symptomatic and asymptomatic women [6].

Menstruation-related sleep disturbances have not been confirmed in all carefully controlled studies employing objective measures [2]. In a rigorous study of polysomnographic changes in 18- to 40-year-old women, Baker *et al.* compared asymptomatic control subjects with women experiencing PMS/PMDD. Although those with severe PMS subjectively reported significantly poorer sleep quality during the late luteal phase, few significant differences in sleep variables were found in PSG measures related either to diagnostic category or menstrual phase. Only one variable, wake after sleep onset, was greater during the late luteal than in the follicular phase in both normal control (NC) subjects and women with PMS/PMDD. Women with premenstrual symptoms had a significantly longer latency to REM sleep onset than control women [7], in contrast to earlier work showing a shorter latency to REM onset in depressed vs. non-depressed subjects [2].

Biological rhythm studies

Melatonin

Melatonin circadian rhythms are relatively unaffected by normal menstrual cycle fluctuations in healthy women [2]. However, Shibui et al. found the 24-hour area under the curve (AUC) of serum melatonin was significantly decreased in the luteal compared with the follicular menstrual cycle phase, suggesting a decrease in the pacemaker amplitude regulating the melatonin rhythm [8]. Parry et al. found mood was related to melatonin chronobiology, such that melatonin onset time was delayed, duration was compressed, and AUC, amplitude and mean melatonin levels were decreased in PMDD, but not NC subjects during the luteal phase [9].

Temperature rhythms

Early studies reported decreased, increased, or no change in core body temperature (T_c) in association with menstrual cycle changes [2]. Wright and Badia observed higher core body temperatures in the luteal than in the follicular phase [10]. Baker et al. found higher mean in-bed temperatures in women with primary dysmenorrhea (but without menstrual-associated mood disturbances) compared with women with normal cycles. Higher body temperatures during luteal and menstrual phases were associated with reduced REM sleep [11]. In contrast, in a well controlled prospective study of women with PMDD vs. NC subjects, Parry et al. found that 24-hour T_c amplitude was significantly decreased in the luteal compared with the follicular menstrual cycle phase [12].

Reviewing earlier work, Baker and Driver reported body temperature reaches its nadir shortly after lights out and recovers to normal after lights on, independently of contraceptive use, and is higher during the luteal than in the follicular phase. In-bed temperatures were significantly higher in dysmenorrheic women than in controls [13].

Cortisol, TSH, and prolactin rhythms

Prolactin: Parry et al. found prolactin peak and amplitude were higher, and acrophase earlier in late luteal phase dysphoric disorder (LLPDD) patients than in NC subjects [2]. Comparing asymptomatic with dysmenorrheic women, Baker et al. found higher prolactin levels during the luteal and menstrual phases in dysmenorrheic women, in association with higher body temperatures and reduced REM sleep [11].

Cortisol: While reduced cortisol amplitude has been reported in the luteal compared with the follicular menstrual cycle phase, altered timing, but not quantitative, measures of cortisol secretion have been found in PMDD vs. NC subjects, with luteal phase cortisol acrophase occurring about one hour earlier in NC, but not PMDD subjects [2].

Thyroid stimulating hormone: In healthy women, amplitude of the TSH rhythm has been observed to be significantly decreased in the luteal compared with the follicular phase. As well, TSH rhythms have been found to occur earlier in PMDD compared with NC subjects [2].

Challenge studies: effects of wake therapy on mood, sleep, and biological rhythms

Parry and colleagues reported that wake therapy relieved depressive symptoms in women with PMDD. Both PMDD and NC groups showed longer REM latencies and less REM sleep (minutes and percentage) during the luteal compared with the follicular phase. Sleep quality improved during recovery nights in PMDD, but not in NC, subjects. Increases in REM sleep measures were associated with clinical improvement in responders to wake therapy. PMDD subjects, however, did not show sleep architecture changes similar to those of patients with major depressive disorders [2].

Effects of wake therapy on biological rhythms

Parry et al. evaluated whether the therapeutic benefit of wake therapy is mediated by altering sleep phase with melatonin secretion. They measured nocturnal plasma melatonin every 30 minutes in PMDD vs. NC women during late luteal interventions with early wake therapy (EWT) (sleep 03:00 to 07:00 hours; control condition) versus late wake therapy (LWT) (sleep 21:00 to 01:00 hours; active condition). Before treatment, melatonin offset was delayed and duration increased in the symptomatic luteal vs. asymptomatic follicular phase in both NC and PMDD subjects. LWT, but not EWT, advanced offset and decreased duration vs. the late luteal baseline, although mood improved equally after LWT and EWT. Later baseline luteal phase morning melatonin offset was associated with more depressed mood in PMDD patients; longer follicular phase melatonin duration predicted greater mood improvement following LWT. That

LWT, but not EWT, advanced melatonin offset and shortened duration while they were equally effective in improving mood suggests that decreasing morning melatonin secretion is not necessary for the therapeutic effects of wake therapy in PMDD [14].

The effect of sleep deprivation on cortisol timing measures also differed for PMDD versus NC subjects: during late partial sleep deprivation (when subjects' sleep was earlier), the cortisol acrophase was almost two hours earlier in PMDD subjects [2].

Effects of light therapy on biological rhythms

Because light suppresses melatonin secretion, controlled light exposure has been studied as a therapy for disorders in which melatonin dysregulation may play a role. Lam et al. conducted a carefully controlled test of dim vs. bright light exposure in women with LLPDD. During the luteal phase of each treatment cycle, patients received 30 minutes of either bright (10,000 lx) evening white light or dim (500 lx) red light (placebo condition). Results showed bright evening light vs. placebo reduced symptoms in women with LLPDD [15]. Morning bright light also is reported to shorten menstrual cycle length in women with abnormally long cycles, in whom dysphoric symptoms are more common [16], and to relieve symptoms of PMS, LLPDD, and/or PMDD [17].

Temperature: Parry et al. reported that T_c amplitude increased after recovery nights of sleep from wake therapy [12].

Prolactin: Danilenko and Samoilova found morning bright light (4,300 lx) during the follicular phase increased concentrations of prolactin and other hypophyseal hormones in women with long menstrual cycles (in whom dysphoria is more common) [16].

Pregnancy

Characteristic changes in estradiol, estriol, prolactin, and cortisol during pregnancy are illustrated in Figure 10.2.

Sleep studies in healthy pregnant women

Healthy pregnant women often report sleep disturbances that typically increase in frequency and intensity as pregnancy progresses [2]. In a large (N = 300) cross-sectional study Lopes et al. confirmed self-reported insomnia, excessive daytime sleepiness, and awakenings after sleep onset increased significantly from the first to the second, and from the second to the third trimesters of pregnancy [18].

Prospective PSG studies of sleep during pregnancy are rare, and the results inconsistent. Some studies report more awakenings and reduced deep sleep (stages 3 and 4) before delivery [2]. The stage of pregnancy when recordings are made is critical. In a cross-sectional study, Hertz et al. found increased stage 1 (lighter) sleep and greater wake after sleep onset, with decreased sleep efficiency and REM sleep in third-trimester women compared with age-matched, non-pregnant controls [19]. In contrast, Driver et al. found no reduction in stage 4 or REM sleep, and on the contrary, found increased slow-wave sleep (stages 3 and 4) at 27 to 39 weeks than at 8 to 16 weeks of pregnancy [20]. These findings support a restorative theory of sleep and are consistent with the effects of changing cortisol and progesterone levels on sleep. Lee et al. using home ambulatory monitoring from 11 to 36 weeks of gestation found total sleep time increased, but restorative sleep decreased significantly by 11 to 12 weeks gestation [21].

Using actigraphy and sleep diaries to study sleep in nulliparous and multiparous women, Signal et al. found parity influenced sleep quality. Nulliparas generally had lower sleep efficiency, spent more time in bed and had greater wake after sleep onset than multiparas during the second trimester [22].

Sleep studies in pregnant women with mood disorders

Sleep disturbance during pregnancy and postpartum is frequent, irrespective of a diagnosis of depression. Few prospective studies document sleep changes in relation to mood during pregnancy; even fewer rely on objective sleep measures. As noted, reduced subjective sleep quality, particularly during late pregnancy, as well as shorter (or longer) REM sleep during pregnancy may precede postpartum mood disorders [2]. Coble et al. recorded sleep EEGs in childbearing women with and without histories of mood disorder. Those with mood disorder histories had greater sleep disorder and REM latency reduction, evident from early pregnancy into the eighth postpartum month [23].

In a large prospective study, Field et al. studied 83 depressed and 170 non-depressed pregnant women during the second trimester, basing diagnosis on a Structured Clinical Interview for DSM-IV (SCID), and sleep assessment with a questionnaire. Consistent with earlier work, self-reports showed more sleep

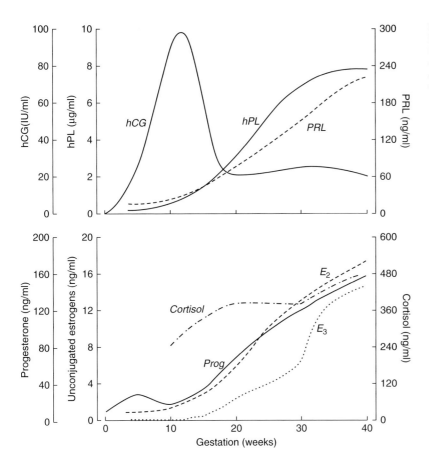

Figure 10.2 Serum concentrations of human chorionic gonadotropin (hCG), human placental lactogen (hPL), prolactin (PRL), progesterone (Prog), unconjugated estradiol (E_2) and estriol (E_3), and cortisol during pregnancy. (Redrawn with permission from Liu J, Rebar RW, Yen SS. Neuroendocrine control of the postpartum period. *Clin Perinatol.* 1983; 10(3):723–736.)

disturbance in depressed than non-depressed women during the second and third trimesters [24]. In contrast, in another large study (N = 273) in which depression was evaluated using the Beck Depression Inventory (BDI), and sleep was assessed at 15 to 23, 23 to 31, and 31 to 39 weeks of gestation using the Pittsburg Sleep Quality Index (PSQI), Skouteris *et al.* found sleep quality and depressive symptoms remained relatively stable across pregnancy; however, poor sleep quality early in pregnancy predicted higher BDI scores later in pregnancy. Depressive symptoms early in pregnancy were unrelated to sleep quality later [25].

Longitudinal studies of sleep and depression during pregnancy and postpartum

Numerous studies document a continuity of mood symptoms from pregnancy to postpartum. Wolfson *et al.* studied 38 primiparous women during the third trimester and again at 2 to 4 weeks, 12 to 16 weeks, and 12 to 15 months postpartum, using a sleep–wake diary and a self-rating depression scale. Mothers developing depressive symptoms 2 to 4 weeks postpartum reported greater total sleep time, later rise times, and more time napping at the end of pregnancy than non-depressed women [26]. Goyal *et al.* studied 124 primiparous women longitudinally, from their last prenatal month to three months postpartum, evaluating sleep with a self-report measure, and depression with the Center for Epidemiological Studies Depression Scale (CES-D). Three months postpartum, self-reported sleep onset latency, early awakenings, sleep disturbances, and sleep maintenance problems were significantly greater in women whose CES-D scores exceeded 16 than those with lower scores. Sleep disturbance in the fourth month of pregnancy was associated with depression symptoms three months after delivery. The authors concluded that initial insomnia during

105

pregnancy may be a strong predictor of postpartum depression [27].

Biological rhythms during pregnancy
Biological rhythms in healthy pregnant women

Melatonin: Serum melatonin levels increase progressively during pregnancy, becoming significantly higher during the third than during the first and second trimesters. While nocturnal melatonin amplitude and duration were higher in late pregnancy, there was no clear phase-shift [2, 28]. Parry *et al.* also found a positive association between melatonin quantity and week of gestation in 15 NC women – a relationship notably absent in a group of 10 women with major depressive disorder (MDD) [29].

Cortisol: Like melatonin, cortisol increases significantly during pregnancy in healthy women, while maintaining its characteristic diurnal pattern [2].

Thyroid stimulating hormone: Diurnal variation in TSH is reported to be maintained during pregnancy, with maximal values around midnight, as in nonpregnant women [2].

Prolactin: Prolactin secretion is reported to be episodic during pregnancy; while prolacting concentration is elevated during pregnancy, no relation to sleep quality has been noted [2]. Measuring at 20-minute intervals for 24 hours at 12, 20, and 32 weeks gestation, Boyar *et al.* found increased mean prolactin levels due to increased secretion per secretory episode during nocturnal sleep [30].

Biological rhythms in pregnant women with mood disorders

Melatonin: Extending earlier work, Parry *et al.* assayed nocturnal plasma melatonin from 18:00 to 11:00 hours in 15 NC and 10 depressed pregnant women. Melatonin was significantly lower in depressed relative to NC women, from 02:00 to 11:00 hours. Notably, melatonin AUC increased significantly across weeks of pregnancy in NC, but not in depressed, women. Women with personal or family histories of depression also had earlier melatonin synthesis and baseline offsets than women without histories, regardless of current diagnosis [29].

Cortisol: Based on single samples collected at unspecified times, Field *et al.* found elevated cortisol in depressed vs. non-depressed women during the second trimester. Cortisol level was also positively correlated with third trimester sleep disturbances

[31]. Jolley *et al.* recruited healthy pregnant women during late pregnancy, following up with ratings of depression 6 and 12 weeks postpartum. They sampled blood at approximately ten-minute intervals, for one hour, from 9 women with MDD and 13 non-depressed women, after 20 minutes of exercise. No significant differences between groups in adrenocorticotropic hormone (ACTH) or cortisol levels were found. However, while ACTH and cortisol were significantly related in healthy mothers, they were dissociated at both 6 and 12 weeks postpartum in depressed mothers, such that depressed mothers had higher ACTH and lower cortisol levels than non-depressed mothers [32]. Shea *et al.* compared the salivary cortisol rise upon awakening in NC and depressed women who were 25 to 36 weeks pregnant. Depressed women did not differ significantly from NC, but a history of childhood maltreatment was associated with lower baseline cortisol in normal and depressed groups, combined [33]. In a large sample of pregnant women (730 non-depressed, 70 probably depressed), Rich-Edwards *et al.* found elevated mid-pregnancy placental corticotropin-releasing hormone (CRH) levels were associated with prenatal depression symptoms [34]. It has been proposed that increased nocturnal CRH may be responsible for the increased awakenings associated with hypothalamic–pituitary–adrenal (HPA) axis hyperactivity [35].

Thyroid stimulating hormone: Parry *et al.* found a non-significant trend toward lower mean TSH levels in depressed compared with NC pregnant women [36].

Prolactin: Parry *et al.* found higher prolactin levels in women with MDD than NC women after controlling for weeks pregnant and BMI in the analyses [36].

Postpartum

Postpartum changes in estradiol, progesterone, FSH, LH, and prolactin are illustrated in Figure 10.3.

Sleep in healthy postpartum women
Subjective studies

Early studies in healthy women suggested sleep is disturbed, subjectively, during the early postpartum period, relative to sleep during pregnancy [2]. Recently, Signal *et al.* studied non-depressed nulliparous and multiparous women using actigraphy and sleep diaries

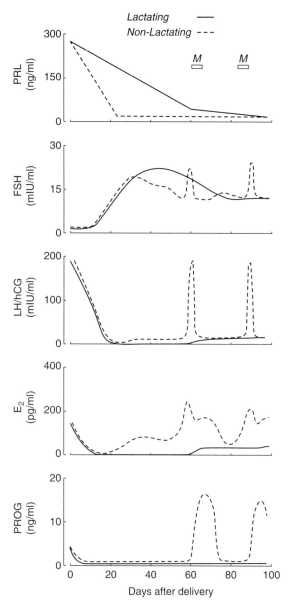

Figure 10.3 Serum concentrations of prolactin (PRL), follicle stimulating hormone (FSH), luteinizing hormone (LH), human chorionic gonadotropin (hCG), estradiol (E₂), and progesterone (PROG) in lactating and non-lactating women in the puerperium. The M bars refer to non-lactating women's menstrual periods. (Redrawn with permission from Liu J, Rebar RW, Yen SS. Neuroendocrine control of the postpartum period. *Clin Perinatol*. 1983;**10**(3):723–736.)

across seven nights, longitudinally, at four time periods: during the second trimester of pregnancy; one week before delivery; one week postpartum; and six weeks postpartum. Results confirmed the greatest

sleep changes occurred in the first postpartum week, with women averaging about 90 minutes less sleep than during pregnancy, and three times more sleep episodes in 24 hours. That 70% of women napped regularly during the day suggests nocturnal sleep loss may be compensated for with daytime naps [22].

Objective studies

Controlled PSG studies in healthy women show sleep efficiency increases and wake after sleep onset decreases relative to pregnant levels by 3 to 5 months postpartum; most (but not all) studies suggest REM sleep decreases after delivery [2]. Notably, women who breast-fed their babies had increased slow-wave sleep and less light non-REM sleep than age-matched control subjects, or women who bottle-fed infants [37]. However, some early studies using objective measures reported deterioration in total sleep time and sleep efficiency, and increased wake after sleep onset compared with late pregnancy [2].

Infant care issues may affect study results. Using PSG measures, Lee *et al.* found awake time increased and total sleep time and efficiency decreased by 3 to 4 weeks postpartum, relative to before delivery, in multiparas and first-time mothers. By three months postpartum, sleep characteristics improved; however, sleep efficiency remained significantly below baseline pre-pregnancy values. Initial sleep disturbances, which were greatest in primiparas, improved between the first and third postpartum months [21].

Breast-feeding

Parity and breast-feeding may affect mothers' sleep quality. Using sleep diaries, Thomas and Burr compared the sleep of 38 postpartum with 20 non-pregnant, nulliparous women, none of whom was depressed, 4 to 10 weeks after childbirth. Thirty of the mothers breast-fed their babies, exclusively, one fed only formula, and seven fed both breast and infant formula. The women reported more postpartum sleep disruption, ascribed primarily to infant care; their mean reported total sleep time was 7.2 hours per night, compared to a mean of 7.7 hours per night in nulliparous controls [38].

Studies using objective measures have produced different results. For example, Nishihara *et al.* compared EEG power spectra of breast-feeding mothers, 9 to 13 weeks postpartum, with those of non-pregnant women. Power spectra in the delta and theta frequency ranges during non-REM sleep were significantly higher for breast-feeding mothers than for non-pregnant women. The power spectra of mothers who experienced interrupted sleep due to child care did not differ significantly from those whose sleep was uninterrupted [39].

Groër found more positive mood and positive life events, and perceptions of lower stress in breast-feeding mothers compared with mothers who fed their infants formula, even though both groups reported comparable stressful life events [40]. While this suggests breast-feeding might protect against negative moods and stress, an alternative explanation is that depressed postpartum mothers may be less likely to breast-feed offspring than women with more positive moods, as Parry et al. [29] reported. Thus, sleep deficits could reflect greater clinical depression in non-breast-feeding mothers.

Doan et al. conducted a study at 3 months post-partum in 133 mothers challenging the notion that infant care disrupts postpartum sleep. Type of infant feeding (breast milk or formula) was determined from parent diaries. Using objective (actigraphy) as well as subjective (diary) measures, mothers who breast-fed infants in the evening and at night actually slept 40 to 45 minutes more, on average, than those who bottle fed. Self-reports also showed less sleep disturbance in mothers who exclusively breast-fed, than those who formula fed offspring. The authors concluded that supplementing breast-feeding with formula feeding did not improve mothers' sleep quality [41].

Sleep studies in women with postpartum mood disorders

In a large epidemiologic study (N = 43,093), Vesga-Lopez et al. confirmed depression risk increases postpartum, relative to the prepartum period [42]. Goyal et al. used questionnaires to characterize depressive symptoms and sleep in 124 primiparous women, from their last month of pregnancy through three months post-partum. Women who reported depression and sleep disturbances during the month before delivery also reported more depressive symptoms during the third month postpartum. The authors suggested that for new mothers, complaints of delayed sleep onset during pregnancy may be the most relevant marker for risk of postpartum depression [27].

Biological rhythms postpartum

Biological rhythms in healthy postpartum women: role of parity and breast-feeding

Melatonin: In the Thomas and Burr study, baseline levels of 6-sulfatoxymelatonin (a urinary melatonin metabolite) were significantly higher in postpartum than in the non-pregnant nulliparous controls, and melatonin secretion onset was significantly earlier in postpartum than in non-pregnant nulliparous women. However, the maximum, mean, and percentage rise in 6-sulfatoxymelatonin were lower in postpartum, relative to control subjects. The authors speculate that light exposure or sleep loss during night-time child care could reduce melatonin levels postpartum. Nevertheless, studies do not uniformly confirm reduced sleep in postpartum mothers due to childcare or breast-feeding [38].

Prolactin: Serum prolactin remains elevated in non-lactating mothers for 2 to 4 weeks postpartum, with a persistent diurnal pattern of secretion, and a subsequent decline across postpartum weeks [2].

Cortisol: Tu et al. found an interaction between breast-feeding, parity, and mood. Among multiparous mothers, cortisol was lower in breast-feeding mothers than in those who bottle fed, both at awakening and at 16:00 hours. Notably, no effect of infant feeding choice on cortisol was observed in primiparous mothers [43]. In fact, extensive work suggests lactation reduces stress responsiveness by dampening the HPA axis circadian rhythm [44]. For example, Altemus et al. compared lactating and non-lactating women, 7 to 18 weeks postpartum, after 20 minutes of treadmill exercise [45]. The last five minutes of exercise was set to elicit 90% of the maximal oxygen uptake. Plasma ACTH, cortisol, and glucose responses to exercise were significantly smaller in lactating women, as were basal norepinephrine levels, suggesting that lactation restrains stress-responsive hormonal systems.

Contrary to expectation, Groër found serum cortisol in breast- and formula-feeding mothers was associated with reduced stress and anxiety levels compared with controls; breast-feeding mothers reported lower perceived stress than controls, more positive life events, and less depression and anger than formula-feeders [40]. Groër et al. also found positive correlations between serum cortisol and sleepiness in breast-feeding mothers, 4 to 6 weeks postpartum [46].

Biological rhythms in women with postpartum mood disorders

Melatonin: Groër *et al.* studied mood in relation to melatonin and other neurohormones in 119 new mothers. Higher melatonin in mothers' milk, 4 to 6 weeks postpartum, was associated with lower milk prolactin ($r = -0.56$, $p = .01$). Sleepier, more fatigued mothers had higher melatonin levels in their morning milk. In general, stress, fatigue, and negative mood were associated with lower prolactin and higher melatonin levels in milk samples [46].

Parry *et al.* assessed plasma melatonin in postpartum NC and women diagnosed with MDD, every half hour from 18:00 to 11:00 hours. Depressed mothers displayed significantly higher nocturnal melatonin amplitudes across time intervals than NC women, and absolute AUC, melatonin synthesis AUC, and peak concentration were higher in postpartum DP vs. NC. Notably, in contrast to pregnant women with MDD (whose morning plasma melatonin concentrations were lower, compared with NC women), plasma melatonin levels were elevated in depressed postpartum subjects. Melatonin onset, offset, and duration were not significantly different in NC vs. depressed groups. The authors interpret these findings as evidence that regulation of the melatonin generating system is disturbed in postpartum depression [29].

Thyroid stimulating hormone: Parry *et al.* sampled TSH overnight at 30-minute intervals and found no statistically significant differences in depressed vs. NC women postpartum [36].

Prolactin: While some early work showed plasma prolactin was lower than normal in depressed women [2], Parry *et al.* reported mean prolactin amplitude was elevated in breast-feeding and non-breast-feeding MDD patients compared with NC women [36]. Asher *et al.* measured morning plasma prolactin just prior to and 3 days after delivery in 25 healthy women [47]. Postpartum prolactin was negatively correlated with Hamilton Anxiety Scale score: elevated prolactin was associated with reduced anxiety in lactating mothers. More recently, Groër *et al.* also found inverse correlations between serum prolactin and Profile of Mood States depression and fatigue scores in 119 new mothers, 4 to 6 weeks postpartum [46].

Effects of wake therapy on mood, sleep, and biological rhythms in depressed postpartum women

Parry and colleagues found beneficial effects, particularly of LWT, in postpartum depression. Hamilton Depression (Ham-D) scores were reduced after recovery sleep from LWT (sleep 21:00 to 01:00 hours), but not after EWT (sleep 03:00 to 07:00 hours) or dim red light. After the LWT intervention, 7 of 7 depressed women met criteria for response (greater than 40% decrease in symptoms) [2].

Menopause studies

The defining hormonal changes of menopause include a profound decrease in serum estradiol and estrone concentrations in conjunction with marked elevations of the gonadotropins, LH and FSH, due to diminished inhibitory feedback from estradiol. Reductions in androstenedione, dehydroepinadrosterone, and progesterone also occur [48].

Studies of sleep disturbance based on subjective measures

With few exceptions, women report sleep problems, including early, middle, and late insomnia, during and after the menopausal transition [49, 50]. In a study of 60- to 85-year-old women not complaining of sleep difficulties, Danker-Hopfe *et al.* found 34.5% endorsed PSQI items indicative of disturbed sleep (PSQI > 5), which were maintained at follow-up 16 months later [51]. Souza *et al.* obtained similar results regarding sleep habits of 271 pre-, peri-, and postmenopausal Brazilian women; 29% reported poor sleep quality, with perimenopausal women (aged 45 years to 1 year after menopause), and those having surgical menopause reporting worse sleep quality than premenopausal women. Menopausal status and self-perceived health status were the only statistically significant variables associated with sleep quality [52].

While implicated in sleep disturbances, menopausal status itself may not be a good predictor of disturbed sleep. Using standardized questionnaires, Chung and Tang examined factors associated with subjective sleep disturbance in 305 middle-aged (45 to 55 years) Chinese women. Cross-sectional analysis showed peri- and postmenopausal women were twice as likely to report poor sleep compared with premenopausal women, with sleep difficulty being one of the five most commonly reported climacteric symptoms. However, the association of menopausal status and sleep difficulty became non-significant when the investigators controlled for climacteric symptoms and recent stress. Risk of reporting disturbed sleep was four- to six-fold higher in women with prominent somatic complaints, psychological symptoms, and perceived stress [49].

Studies of sleep disturbance based on objective measures

Studies using objective measures show a less definitive relationship between menopause and sleep disturbances than subjective studies. Using PSG measures in 21 premenopausal (aged 45 to 51 years), 29 postmenopausal (aged 59 to 71 years), and 11 young (aged 20 to 26 years) women, Kalleinen et al. found that while total sleep time was similar in premenopausal (c. 405 minutes) and postmenopausal (c. 385 minutes) women, total sleep time was significantly longer in younger women (c. 448 minutes). Sleep efficiency was greater in younger women; pre- and postmenopausal women also had less slow-wave sleep and a higher frequency and duration of wake after sleep onset than younger women. The authors interpreted these differences as due primarily to the physiology of aging, rather than to menopausal changes, since sleep in premenopausal and postmenopausal women was actually quite similar [53].

Jean-Louis et al. provided further support for the effects of aging on objective sleep. They examined PSG home-recordings in postmenopausal women (aged 56 to 77 years). On average, women slept 439 minutes in 24 hours. Notably, 10% of accumulated sleep time occurred out of bed (i.e., naps), with greater age associated with more afternoon–evening sleep. Thus, more than younger women, older women may distribute total sleep time throughout the day [54].

Studies comparing objective vs. subjective sleep measures

As with the other reproductive epochs, whether objective sleep measurements confirm subjective reports in menopause is a source of continuing debate. In general, while some objective sleep measures confirm subjective reports, many studies reveal a large subjective–objective 'disconnect,' and substantially lower frequencies and intensities of sleep problems measured objectively [3].

Regestein et al. found low correlations between self-report and actigraphy sleep measures in 88 healthy, postmenopausal women, concluding that self-reported sleep disturbances may reflect subjective distress and reduced cognitive function, rather than actual sleep disturbance [55]. In a large epidemiologic study of objective and subjective measures in 589 pre-, peri-, and postmenopausal women, Young et al. found objective sleep quality was actually better during and after menopause, with postmenopausal women having more deep sleep and longer total sleep time than premenopausal women. The objective results conflicted with the women's subjective reports, as peri- and postmenopausal women expressed less satisfaction with their sleep than premenopausal women, particularly with initiating sleep. Women experiencing hot flashes reported more subjective sleep problems than women who did not [56].

Park et al. compared subjective with actigraphic sleep measures in 384 postmenopausal women (mean age: 67.9 years). Although actigraphic and self-reported sleep latencies were correlated, short self-reported sleep latencies tended to underestimate, whereas long self-reported sleep latencies overestimated actigraphy measures. Hypertension and anti-hypertensive drug use was positively correlated with sleep latency and measures of insomnia, mood, and hot flashes. Activity and light exposure were negatively related to global assessment of functioning [57].

In a study of 150 older men and women not complaining of sleep disturbances, Vitiello et al. found 33% of the women and 16% of the men endorsed substantial sleep disturbances (PSQI > 5). Correlations between PSG and subjective measures differed by gender; men with higher PSQI scores had longer PSG sleep latencies, less total sleep time, and lower sleep efficiencies than men with lower PSQI scores. This relationship was weaker in women, and absent in those taking estrogen replacement, despite the fact that women reported sleep disturbances more frequently than men. The authors suggested that objective measures of sleep quality may be appropriate for older men, but not women, as women and men may use different criteria to evaluate sleep quality [58].

Mechanisms of sleep disturbance

Several studies identify putative etiologies of sleep disturbances in menopausal women, including age, OSA, elevated blood pressure, psychological distress, mood, hormone levels, vasomotor symptoms (hot flashes), BMI, waist-to-hip ratio, and alterations in circadian phase (see review [3]).

Hot flashes and sleep

An association between hot flashes and self-reported sleep disturbance has been widely noted. In a large (N = 12,603) epidemiological study including Caucasian, African American, Asian, and Hispanic women, Kravitz et al. observed that menopausal status, rather than older age, per se, was significantly associated with sleep problems. However, they also identified vasomotor symptoms, arthritis, psychological, self-perceived health, and educational factors as associated with sleep difficulties [59]. Nevertheless, several contemporary studies raise questions about the relationship between hot flashes and sleep disturbances [3].

For example, after carefully screening 50 pre- and postmenopausal, 46- to 51-year-old women, Freedman and Roehrs excluded 19 (38%) from study due to drug use, sleep apnea, periodic limb movements, body mass index >30, hypertension, and the occurrence of hot flashes in asymptomatic women. Of those retained (11 cycling, 12 symptomatic, 11 asymptomatic for hot flashes), the groups did not differ significantly in PSG measures of total sleep time, awakenings after sleep onset, or other sleep measures. No evidence that hot flashes caused sleep disturbance was found. The authors suggested that studies attributing sleep disturbances to hot flashes may be confounded by inclusion of subjects whose sleep disorders arise from factors like drug use and sleep apnea [60].

In a recent follow-up study of 102 women reporting sleep disturbance, apnea, restless legs, or both occurred in 53% of subjects. Poor subjective sleep was linked to anxiety and hot flashes. Thus, reducing hot flashes may improve perceived sleep quality, but may not lessen underlying primary sleep disorders (apnea, restless legs syndrome) [61]. Similarly, Freeman et al. studied a cohort of over 400, 35- to 47-year-old women, longitudinally; all were premenopausal at the start. In the nearly 300 women who completed the study, hot flashes, pain, and depressed mood increased significantly over a nine-year period; however, poor sleep, vaginal dryness, and decreased libido were not associated with differences in menopausal stages [62].

Breathing disorders and anthropometric measures

Among the risks associated with menopause, sleep disordered breathing – including apnea (suspension of external breathing) and hypopnea (overly shallow breathing or abnormally low respiratory rate) – are common. In a cross-sectional study, Young et al. studied 589 pre-, peri-, and postmenopausal women, confirming menopausal status from menstrual history, gynecologic surgery, hormone replacement therapy, FSH levels, and vasomotor symptoms. Using PSG, they recorded frequency of apnea and hypopnea events per hour of sleep. Adjusted odds ratios for apnea and hypopnea events increased from peri- to postmenopause, supporting the conclusion that sleep-disordered breathing is a consequence of the menopausal transition, independent of confounding factors [63]. In that connection, Resta et al. studied sleep apnea in relation to obesity in 133 women with BMI of 30 or greater. Using PSG, they found disturbed respiration in 44% of their sample, which was predicted most strongly by neck circumference, BMI, and age. Obstructive sleep apnea was prevalent in 67% of postmenopausal vs. 31% of premenopausal women [64].

Dansey et al. confirmed the importance of anthropometric measures like height, weight, and neck circumference in menopausal sleep disorders. However, when controlling for BMI and neck circumference, the authors continued to observe more disturbed sleep in post- compared to premenopausal women, suggesting there may be functional, rather than anatomic, differences in the upper airway between the two groups [65].

Owens and Matthews' study of 521 middle-aged women showed that weight-related factors like elevated systolic and diastolic blood pressure and greater hip-to-waist ratios are associated with postmenopausal sleep difficulties. Furthermore, while there was no association between impaired sleep and menopausal status, per se, transition into menopause seems to impair sleep quality in women not taking hormone replacement, confirming the importance of hormonal fluctuations during this transitional period [66].

Estrogen and progesterone

An impressive body of evidence shows an association between sleep disturbed breathing and reduced levels of sex hormones during menopause [67]. However, the physiological basis of these ubiquitous sleep disturbances is undetermined. While the precise role played by altered endocrine function in menopausal insomnia is unclear, a few prospective, placebo-controlled studies exist. In one very large study, postmenopausal women (N = 1,043) who received conjugated equine estrogen plus medroxyprogesterone daily for one year reported significantly fewer sleep problems than controls who received placebo (N = 1,087). Whether improvements resulted from hormone replacement, per se, or were an indirect result of reductions in hot flashes or improved sexual functioning is unclear. Notably, hormone replacement did not significantly alter subjective baseline depression or anxiety [68].

Kravitz et al. studied hormone levels in relation to sleep disturbances in 630 pre- and perimenopausal women (aged 43 to 53 years). Perimenopausal women were 29% more likely than premenopausal women to report sleep difficulties, with the highest percentage of women reporting greater sleep disturbances in the beginning and end of menstrual cycles. Contrary to the literature, pregnanediol glucuronide level (a urinary progesterone metabolite) was actually associated with reduced sleep quality in perimenopausal women. The same was observed with FSH in premenopausal subjects [69].

While a potential mechanism of action for estrogen and progesterone is their effects on reducing sleep disordered breathing, D'Ambrosio's study of sleep in 12 healthy young women (aged 18 to 34 years) who underwent pharmacologically induced menopause conflicts with this position. Polysomnography sleep architecture and respiration were normal at baseline. As expected, after hormone suppression with leuprolide acetate (lupron), subjects ceased menstruating and plasma concentrations of 17 beta-estradiol and progesterone decreased to menopausal levels. While this "reversible oophorectomy" induced climacteric vasomotor symptoms (hot flashes and sweating), sleep latencies and architecture remained unchanged. Subjective reports of increased snoring were unconfirmed by PSG [70].

Mood and biological rhythms

Luteinizing hormone and follicle-stimulating hormone: With few exceptions, many studies show sleep and mood alterations such as depression or anxiety are associated with menopause [3]. Antonijevic et al.

compared sleep EEG in 16 female patients mostly with first episode MDD (7 pre- and 9 postmenopausal) with 19 controls (10 pre- and 9 postmenopausal) after growth-hormone-releasing hormone administration. Postmenopausal women displayed sleep alterations similar to those associated with depression, e.g., reduced sleep continuity and slow-wave sleep, and increased REM density. An inverse correlation between FSH and the decline in slow-wave sleep and sleep continuity was noted in depressed patients, suggesting a role of menopause in sleep–endocrine alterations associated with MDD [71].

Freeman et al. followed a cohort of premenopausal women longitudinally, for eight years. Depression risk increased 2.5 times in the menopause transition compared to the premenopausal period, after adjusting for smoking, BMI, PMS, hot flashes, poor sleep, employment, and marital status. Thus, menopause-related changes in the hormonal milieu of estradiol, LH, and FSH are strongly associated with new onset of depression [72].

In a longitudinal study of 41 women progressing into menopause, Woods et al. found links between specific endocrine levels and specific menopause symptoms. For example, serum FSH level was significantly and positively related to hot flash severity, vaginal dryness, forgetfulness, and sleep disruption. As might be expected (since estrone and FSH concentrations are inversely related), estrone level was negatively related to hot flash severity; however, estrone was unrelated to vaginal dryness. Decrease in estrone was correlated with decrease in sexual desire. Testosterone level was negatively correlated with vaginal dryness and with difficulty concentrating. Correlations among menopause symptoms showed hot flash severity was associated with sleep disruption and forgetfulness. Notably, hot flash severity and vaginal dryness were uncorrelated with depressed mood, despite the fact that depressed mood was correlated with sleep disruption, difficulty concentrating, and decreased sexual desire. Sleep disturbance severity and depressed mood were not significantly correlated with estrone, FSH, or testosterone. Frequency of night-time awakenings was correlated with decreased sexual desire and vaginal dryness, as well as hot flashes. Forgetfulness was associated with hot flashes and difficulty concentrating, whereas difficulty concentrating was associated with depressed mood and early awakening [73].

Murphy and Campbell studied ten women who were at least five years past menopause. Confirming previous work, they established that higher core body temperature prior to and during sleep was significantly correlated with higher LH levels and poorer sleep efficiency. Lower estradiol and higher LH levels were significantly correlated with poor sleep quality. However, as the observed effects of LH on sleep were more robust compared to those of estradiol, the authors suggested altering LH levels may be a potential alternative to traditional estrogen-based HRT for sleep disturbance [74].

Melatonin: Parry *et al.* measured plasma melatonin every 30 minutes in dim (<30 lx) light or dark from 18:00 to 10:00 hours in depressed and nondepressed, peri- and postmenopausal women. They found depressed patients had significantly delayed melatonin offset times, and elevated morning melatonin secretion compared with normal controls. Years past menopause predicted melatonin secretion duration; melatonin duration, body mass index, years past menopause, serum FSH level, and sleep end time were significant predictors of Ham-D and BDI depression ratings [75].

Studies of 6-sulfatoxymelatonin revealed a positive correlation between subjectively reported sleep latency and melatonin acrophase and offset time in postmenopausal women [57]. Furthermore, researching nap patterns in 436 postmenopausal women, Yoon *et al.* noted a significant inverse correlation between duration of evening naps (common in this population) and wake time; a 32-minute advance in 6-sulfatoxymelatonin onset time suggested a possible advance in circadian rhythms after menopause. No significant sleep differences between depressed women and controls were observed [76].

Cortisol: Few prospective studies have investigated relationships among menopause, cortisol, and sleep, and fewer still have established reliable relationships among them.

Prinz *et al.* studied 42 healthy women (mean age: 69 years), 20 of whom were on estrogen replacement therapy (ERT), at baseline and under mild stress (24 hours indwelling venous catheter). Groups were essentially the same in polysomnographic sleep variables at baseline. The catheter stress elevated urinary free cortisol and impaired sleep in both untreated women and women on ERT. Cortisol was inversely correlated with sleep efficiency, stages 2–4 sleep, REM minutes, and rise time. Women on ERT, however, experienced less stress-related sleep disruption than untreated women [77].

Woods *et al.* followed 169 women through the menopause transition and found cortisol levels increased with age, but there was no clear link to menopausal transition stages. Women with increased cortisol later in menopause had more severe vasomotor symptoms than those with smaller changes, but did not differ significantly in age, BMI, levels of FSH or estrone, health practices, exercise, mood, sleep, cognition, or stress levels [78].

A recent, placebo-controlled double-blind study compared 24-hour profiles of growth hormone (GH), prolactin, and cortisol (sampled every 20 minutes) in pre- and postmenopausal women, before and after 6 months of estrogen–progestin treatment (EPT). Results showed that while GH and PRL concentrations were lower in postmenopausal than premenopausal women, these differences disappeared after EPT. Cortisol levels did not differ between groups and were unaffected by EPT [79].

HRT treatment effects on sleep in menopause

Reviewing existing literature, Parry *et al.* concluded that unmedicated depressed women do not differ consistently or substantially from healthy menopausal women in cortisol, TSH, or prolactin. Estrogen treatment may affect these hormones differently, increasing prolactin but decreasing TSH in depressed women, without affecting levels of these hormones in healthy women [3].

Parry *et al.* examined HRT effects on objective and subjective sleep in depressed and healthy menopausal women. Subjectively, depressed patients reported more frequent and longer awakenings at baseline than healthy women, which persisted after eight weeks of estradiol treatment. Depressed women had less polysomnographic sleep efficiency, stage 3, and delta sleep than healthy women. Wake after sleep onset decreased in both groups after estradiol treatment, and sleep efficiency increased in healthy women along with reduced stage 1 minutes and percentage. In women with MDD, estradiol plus antidepressant (fluoxetine 10 to 40 mg) treatment increased REM density [80].

In contrast, one large study challenged the efficacy of HRT for menopausal symptoms. Maartens *et al.* studied menopausal complaints and depressive symptoms in 5,896 women (aged 47 to 54 years) and found that women on HRT showed the highest levels of menopausal symptoms. Women using oral contraceptives showed lower vasomotor symptoms than women on or off HRT. The authors noted that women presenting with symptoms other than vasomotor complaints during menopause might suffer from underlying depression, for which HRT has not been shown to be effective [81]. As part of the Women's Health Initiative Study, Wallace-Guy *et al.* found that in 154 postmenopausal women (mean age: 66.7 years), the total light exposure over 24 hours was negatively correlated with sleep latency, wake within sleep, and depressed mood (assessed by questionnaire) [82]. Additionally, short-wavelength light suppressed melatonin more in older/postmenopausal women than in younger/premenopausal women, perhaps due to age-related changes in density of the lens of the eye [83]. Thus, increased light exposure over 24 hours, particularly in the blue–green spectrum, may improve sleep quality and mood.

Conclusions

Well controlled, adequately powered, methodologically rigorous prospective studies of sleep in relation to other biological rhythms during the menstrual cycle, pregnancy, postpartum, and the postmenopausal period in healthy vs. depressed women are few in number and often present conflicting evidence.

Neuroendocrine studies suggests melatonin circadian rhythms are stable and resistant to menstrual cycle hormonal influences in healthy subjects, while changing across the menstrual cycle in women with PMDD [9]. Thus, sleep in relation to melatonin (sleep–melatonin phase angles) may be more important to understanding menstrual-related symptoms than either melatonin or sleep alone. Robust baseline differences were not observed between PMDD and NC in biological rhythms like core body temperature, cortisol, TSH, and prolactin.

Most studies of the circadian rhythms of cortisol, TSH, and prolactin suggest diurnal rhythms are maintained during pregnancy, with more changes observed in amplitude than in phase. Additionally, based on one small study, pregnant depressed women had lower mean melatonin amplitude (peak and AUC), and lower mean evening cortisol levels than healthy pregnant women.

In postpartum women, sleep appears to be disrupted immediately after delivery, but gradually returns to baseline levels after the infant's sleep and melatonin rhythms establish diurnal patterns. Depression and sleep disruption during pregnancy are reliable precursors of these symptoms, postpartum. Rather than disrupting sleep, breast-feeding may actually be associated with improved sleep in non-depressed mothers. However, it remains unclear whether improved sleep in breast-feeding mothers reflects breast-feeding, per se, or the self-selection of mothers whose low levels of anxiety and depression make breast-feeding – and sleep – easier for them than for women with mood disorders. Studies of circadian rhythmicity show melatonin, cortisol, and prolactin levels are associated with anxiety and depression in postpartum women. However, as in pregnancy, the causal relation between these disorders and sleep difficulties remains unclear. Critically timed wake therapy may benefit some depressed women during pregnancy and postpartum, but the effect on neuroendocrine rhythms in relation to sleep is unknown.

Earlier studies suggested that peri- and postmenopausal women experience more disturbed sleep and decreased sleep quality than cycling women, which was attributed, in part, to increased vasomotor symptoms. However, recent work shows little evidence to that effect, and suggests factors like age, BMI, hip-to-waist ratio, and depressed mood may play a greater role in disrupting sleep continuity and quality; however, data remain unclear as to their precise relation to menopausal status.

It must be noted that reliable objective evidence of sleep changes across reproductive epochs has not been consistently found. Rigorous studies using objective sleep measurements fail to confirm subjective sleep deficits widely reported by women during the luteal menstrual phase, pregnancy, postpartum, and peri- and postmenopausal periods. Comparisons of sleep disturbance studies suggest subjective reports often overestimate the magnitude of objective sleep difficulties. Similarly, although women typically report greater sleep disruption than men, they often display better sleep quality than men in studies where sleep is measured objectively [84]. Additionally, some night-time sleep losses may be compensated for with daytime naps.

Mood disorder symptoms present during the various reproductive stages may increase the perception of sleep difficulties without substantially affecting objectively measured sleep parameters. Clinicians should be aware that objective sleep difficulties may be relatively small or totally absent in most healthy women. And while some researchers identify sleep disturbance as a causal factor in depression, the bulk of the evidence suggests, rather, that depression contributes to sleep disturbance. However, sleep disturbance may antedate onset of depressive symptoms, particularly postpartum, and subjective reports of sleep disturbance may represent an important marker of depressed mood.

Acknowledgments

This work was supported in part by NIH grants 1 R01 MH63462–01A2, 1 R01 MH070788–01A2, and 1 R01 MH080159–01A1.

References

1. Peterson MJ, Benca RM. Sleep in mood disorders. *Psychiatr Clin North Am.* 2006;**29**(4):1009–32; abstract ix.

2. Parry BL, Martinez LF, Maurer EL, *et al.* Sleep rhythms and women's mood. Part I: Menstrual cycle, pregnancy and postpartum. *Sleep Med Rev.* 2006;**10**(2):129–44.

3. Parry BL, Martinez LF, Maurer EL, *et al.* Sleep, rhythms and women's mood. Part II: Menopause. *Sleep Med Rev.* 2006;**10**(3):197–208.

4. Baker FC, Driver HS. Self-reported sleep across the menstrual cycle in young, healthy women. *J Psychosom Res.* 2004;**56**(2):239–43.

5. Driver HS, Dijk DJ, Werth E, Biedermann K, Borbely AA. Sleep and the sleep electroencephalogram across the menstrual cycle in young healthy women. *J Clin Endocrinol Metab.* 1996;**81**(2):728–35.

6. Parry BL, Mendelson WB, Duncan WC, Sack DA, Wehr TA. Longitudinal sleep EEG, temperature, and activity measurements across the menstrual cycle in patients with premenstrual depression and in age-matched controls. *Psychiatry Res.* 1989;**30**(3):285–303.

7. Baker FC, Kahan TL, Trinder J, Colrain IM. Sleep quality and the sleep electroencephalogram in women with severe premenstrual syndrome. *Sleep.* 2007;**30**(10):1283–91.

8. Shibui K, Uchiyama M, Okawa M, *et al.* Diurnal fluctuation of sleep propensity and hormonal secretion across the menstrual cycle. *Biol Psychiatry.* 2000;**48**(11):1062–8.

9. Parry BL, Berga SL, Mostofi N, Klauber MR, Resnick A. Plasma melatonin circadian rhythms during the menstrual cycle and after light therapy in premenstrual dysphoric disorder and normal control subjects. *J Biol Rhythms.* 1997;**12**(1):47–64.

10. Wright KP, Badia P. Effects of menstrual cycle phase and oral contraceptives on alertness, cognitive performance, and circadian rhythms during sleep deprivation. *Behav Brain Res.* 1999;**103**(2):185–94.

11. Baker FC, Driver HS, Rogers GG, Paiker J, Mitchell D. High nocturnal body temperatures and disturbed sleep in women with primary dysmenorrhea. *Am J Physiol.* 1999;**277**(6 Pt 1):E1013–21.

12. Parry BL, LeVeau B, Mostofi N, *et al.* Temperature circadian rhythms during the menstrual cycle and sleep deprivation in premenstrual dysphoric disorder and normal comparison subjects. *J Biol Rhythms.* 1997;**12**(1):34–46.

13. Baker FC, Driver HS. Circadian rhythms, sleep, and the menstrual cycle. *Sleep Med.* 2007;**8**(6):613–22.

14. Parry BL, Meliska CJ, Martinez LF, *et al.* Late, but not early, wake therapy reduces morning plasma melatonin: relationship to mood in premenstrual dysphoric disorder. *Psychiatry Res.* 2008;**161**(1):76–86.

15. Lam RW, Carter D, Misri S, *et al.* A controlled study of light therapy in women with late luteal phase dysphoric disorder. *Psychiatry Res.* 1999;**86**(3):185–92.

16. Danilenko KV, Samoilova EA. Stimulatory effect of morning bright light on reproductive hormones and ovulation: results of a controlled crossover trial. *PLoS Clin Trials.* 2007;**2**(2):e7.

17. Barron ML. Light exposure, melatonin secretion, and menstrual cycle parameters: an integrative review. *Biol Res Nurs.* 2007;**9**(1):49–69.

18. Lopes EA, Carvalho LB, Seguro PB, *et al.* Sleep disorders in pregnancy. *Arq Neuropsiquiatr.* 2004;**62**(2A):217–21.

19. Hertz G, Fast A, Feinsilver SH, *et al.* Sleep in normal late pregnancy. *Sleep.* 1992;**15**(3):246–51.

20. Driver HS, Shapiro CM. A longitudinal study of sleep stages in young women during pregnancy and postpartum. *Sleep.* 1992;**15**(5):449–53.

21. Lee KA, Zaffke ME, McEnany G. Parity and sleep patterns during and after pregnancy. *Obstet Gynecol.* 2000;**95**(1):14–18.

22. Signal TL, Gander PH, Sangalli MR, *et al.* Sleep duration and quality in healthy nulliparous and multiparous women across pregnancy and post-partum. *Aust N Z J Obstet Gynaecol.* 2007;**47**(1):16–22.

23. Coble PA, Reynolds CF, 3rd, Kupfer DJ, *et al.* Childbearing in women with and without a history of affective disorder. II. Electroencephalographic sleep. *Compr Psychiatry.* 1994;**35**(3):215–24.

24. Field T, Diego M, Hernandez-Reif M, *et al.* Sleep disturbances in depressed pregnant women and their newborns. *Infant Behav Dev.* 2007;**30**(1):127–33.

25. Skouteris H, Germano C, Wertheim EH, Paxton SJ, Milgrom J. Sleep quality and depression during pregnancy: a prospective study. *J Sleep Res.* 2008; **17**(2):217–20.

26. Wolfson AR, Crowley SJ, Anwer U, Bassett JL. Changes in sleep patterns and depressive symptoms in first-time mothers: last trimester to 1-year postpartum. *Behav Sleep Med.* 2003;**1**(1):54–67.

27. Goyal D, Gay CL, Lee KA. Patterns of sleep disruption and depressive symptoms in new mothers. *J Perinat Neonatal Nurs.* 2007;**21**(2):123–9.

28. Kivela A. Serum melatonin during human pregnancy. *Acta Endocrinol (Copenh).* 1991;**124**(3):233–7.

29. Parry BL, Meliska CJ, Sorenson DL, *et al.* Plasma melatonin circadian rhythm disturbances during pregnancy and postpartum in depressed women and women with personal or family histories of depression. *Am J Psychiatry.* 2008;**165**(12):1551–8.

30. Boyar RM, Finkelstein JW, Kapen S, Hellman L. Twenty-four hour prolactin (PRL) secretory patterns during pregnancy. *J Clin Endocrinol Metab.* 1975; **40**(6):1117–20.

31. Field T, Diego M, Hernandez-Reif M, *et al.* Chronic prenatal depression and neonatal outcome. *Int J Neurosci.* 2008;**118**(1):95–103.

32. Jolley SN, Elmore S, Barnard KE, Carr DB. Dysregulation of the hypothalamic–pituitary–adrenal axis in postpartum depression. *Biol Res Nurs.* 2007; **8**(3):210–22.

33. Shea AK, Streiner DL, Fleming A, *et al.* The effect of depression, anxiety and early life trauma on the cortisol awakening response during pregnancy: preliminary results. *Psychoneuroendocrinology.* 2007;**32**(8–10):1013–20.

34. Rich-Edwards JW, Mohllajee AP, Kleinman K, *et al.* Elevated midpregnancy corticotropin-releasing hormone is associated with prenatal, but not postpartum, maternal depression. *J Clin Endocrinol Metab.* 2008;**93**(5):1946–51.

35. Buckley TM, Schatzberg AF. On the interactions of the hypothalamic–pituitary–adrenal (HPA) axis and sleep: normal HPA axis activity and circadian rhythm, exemplary sleep disorders. *J Clin Endocrinol Metab.* 2005;**90**(5):3106–14.

36. Parry BL, Meliska CJ, Martinez LF, *et al.* Neuroendocrine abnormalities in women with depression linked to the reproductive cycle. In: Sibley D, Hanin I, Kuhar M, Skolnick P, eds. *The Handbook of Contemporary Neuropharmacology.* (New York: John Wiley and Sons, 2007; pp. 843–57).

37. Blyton DM, Sullivan CE, Edwards N. Lactation is associated with an increase in slow-wave sleep in women. *J Sleep Res.* 2002;**11**(4):297–303.

38. Thomas KA, Burr RL. Melatonin level and pattern in postpartum versus nonpregnant nulliparous women. *J Obstet Gynecol Neonatal Nurs.* 2006;**35**(5):608–15.

39. Nishihara K, Horiuchi S, Eto H, Uchida S, Honda M. Delta and theta power spectra of night sleep EEG are higher in breast-feeding mothers than in non-pregnant women. *Neurosci Lett.* 2004;**368**(2):216–20.

40. Groer MW. Differences between exclusive breastfeeders, formula-feeders, and controls: a study of stress, mood, and endocrine variables. *Biol Res Nurs.* 2005;**7**(2):106–17.

41. Doan T, Gardiner A, Gay CL, Lee KA. Breast-feeding increases sleep duration of new parents. *J Perinat Neonatal Nurs.* 2007;**21**(3):200–6.

42. Vesga-Lopez O, Blanco C, Keyes K, *et al.* Psychiatric disorders in pregnant and postpartum women in the United States. *Arch Gen Psychiatry.* 2008;**65**(7):805–15.

43. Tu MT, Lupien SJ, Walker CD. Diurnal salivary cortisol levels in postpartum mothers as a function of infant feeding choice and parity. *Psychoneuroendocrinology.* 2006;**31**(7):812–24.

44. Brunton PJ, Russell JA, Douglas AJ. Adaptive responses of the maternal hypothalamic–pituitary–adrenal axis during pregnancy and lactation. *J Neuroendocrinol.* 2008; **20**(6):764–76.

45. Altemus M, Deuster PA, Galliven E, Carter CS, Gold PW. Suppression of hypothalmic-pituitary-adrenal axis responses to stress in lactating women. *J Clin Endocrinol Metab.* 1995;**80**(10):2954–9.

46. Groer M, Davis M, Casey K, *et al.* Neuroendocrine and immune relationships in postpartum fatigue. *MCN Am J Matern Child Nurs.* 2005;**30**(2):133–8.

47. Asher I, Kaplan B, Modai I, *et al.* Mood and hormonal changes during late pregnancy and puerperium. *Clin Exp Obstet Gynecol.* 1995;**22**(4):321–5.

48. Yen SS, Jaffe RB, Barbieri RL. *Reproductive Endocrinology: Physiology, Pathophysiology, and Clinical Management,* 4th edn. (Philadelphia: Saunders, 1999).

49. Chung KF, Tang MK. Subjective sleep disturbance and its correlates in middle-aged Hong Kong Chinese women. *Maturitas.* 2006;**53**(4):396–404.

50. Kalleinen N, Polo O, Himanen SL, Joutsen A, Polo-Kantola P. The effect of estrogen plus progestin treatment on sleep: a randomized, placebo-controlled, double-blind trial in premenopausal and late postmenopausal women. *Climacteric.* 2008;**11**(3):233–43.

51. Danker-Hopfe H, Hornung O, Regen F, *et al.* Subjective sleep quality in noncomplaining elderly subjects: results of a follow-up study. *Anthropol Anz.* 2006;**64**(4):369–76.

52. Souza CL, Aldrighi JM, Lorenzi Filho G. [Quality of sleep of climacteric women in Sao Paulo: some significant aspects.] *Rev Assoc Med Bras.* 2005; **51**(3):170–6.

53. Kalleinen N, Polo-Kantola P, Himanen SL, *et al.* Sleep and the menopause – do postmenopausal women experience worse sleep than premenopausal women? *Menopause Int.* 2008;**14**(3):97–104.

54. Jean-Louis G, Kripke DF, Assmus JD, Langer RD. Sleep–wake patterns among postmenopausal women: a 24-hour unattended polysomnographic study. *J Gerontol A Biol Sci Med Sci.* 2000;**55**(3): M120–3.

55. Regestein QR, Friebely J, Shifren JL, *et al.* Self-reported sleep in postmenopausal women. *Menopause.* 2004; **11**(2):198–207.

56. Young T, Rabago D, Zgierska A, Austin D, Laurel F. Objective and subjective sleep quality in premenopausal, perimenopausal, and postmenopausal women in the Wisconsin Sleep Cohort Study. *Sleep.* 2003; **26**(6):667–72.

57. Park DH, Kripke DF, Louis GJ, *et al.* Self-reported sleep latency in postmenopausal women. *J Korean Med Sci.* 2007;**22**(6):1007–14.

58. Vitiello MV, Larsen LH, Moe KE. Age-related sleep change: Gender and estrogen effects on the subjective-objective sleep quality relationships of healthy, noncomplaining older men and women. *J Psychosom Res.* 2004;**56**(5):503–10.

59. Kravitz HM, Ganz PA, Bromberger J, *et al.* Sleep difficulty in women at midlife: a community survey of sleep and the menopausal transition. *Menopause.* 2003;**10**(1):19–28.

60. Freedman RR, Roehrs TA. Lack of sleep disturbance from menopausal hot flashes. *Fertil Steril.* 2004; **82**(1):138–44.

61. Freedman RR, Roehrs TA. Sleep disturbance in menopause. *Menopause.* 2007;**14**(5):826–9.

62. Freeman EW, Sammel MD, Lin H, *et al.* Symptoms associated with menopausal transition and reproductive hormones in midlife women. *Obstet Gynecol.* 2007;**110**(2 Pt 1):230–40.

63. Young T, Finn L, Austin D, Peterson A. Menopausal status and sleep-disordered breathing in the Wisconsin Sleep Cohort Study. *Am J Respir Crit Care Med.* 2003;**167**(9):1181–5.

64. Resta O, Bonfitto P, Sabato R, De Pergola G, Barbaro MP. Prevalence of obstructive sleep apnoea in a sample of obese women: effect of menopause. *Diabetes Nutr Metab.* 2004;**17**(5):296–303.

65. Dancey DR, Hanly PJ, Soong C, Lee B, Hoffstein V. Impact of menopause on the prevalence and severity of sleep apnea. *Chest.* 2001;**120**(1):151–5.

66. Owens JF, Matthews KA. Sleep disturbance in healthy middle-aged women. *Maturitas.* 1998;**30**(1):41–50.

67. Netzer NC, Eliasson AH, Strohl KP. Women with sleep apnea have lower levels of sex hormones. *Sleep Breath.* 2003;**7**(1):25–9.

68. Welton AJ, Vickers MR, Kim J, *et al.* Health related quality of life after combined hormone replacement therapy: randomised controlled trial. *BMJ.* 2008; **337**:a1190.

69. Kravitz HM, Janssen I, Santoro N, *et al.* Relationship of day-to-day reproductive hormone levels to sleep in midlife women. *Arch Intern Med.* 2005;**165**(20):2370–6.

70. D'Ambrosio C, Stachenfeld NS, Pisani M, Mohsenin V. Sleep, breathing, and menopause: the effect of fluctuating estrogen and progesterone on sleep and breathing in women. *Gend Med.* 2005;**2**(4):238–45.

71. Antonijevic IA, Murck H, Frieboes RM, Uhr M, Steiger A. On the role of menopause for sleep-endocrine alterations associated with major depression. *Psychoneuroendocrinology.* 2003;**28**(3):401–18.

72. Freeman EW, Sammel MD, Lin H, Nelson DB. Associations of hormones and menopausal status with depressed mood in women with no history of depression. *Arch Gen Psychiatry.* 2006;**63**(4):375–82.

73. Woods NF, Smith-Dijulio K, Percival DB, *et al.* Symptoms during the menopausal transition and early postmenopause and their relation to endocrine levels over time: observations from the Seattle Midlife Women's Health Study. *J Womens Health (Larchmt).* 2007;**16**(5):667–77.

74. Murphy PJ, Campbell SS. Sex hormones, sleep, and core body temperature in older postmenopausal women. *Sleep.* 2007;**30**(12):1788–94.

75. Parry BL, Meliska CJ, Sorenson DL, *et al.* Increased melatonin and delayed offset in menopausal depression: role of years past menopause, follicle-stimulating hormone, sleep end time, and body mass index. *J Clin Endocrinol Metab.* 2008;**93**(1):54–60.

76. Yoon IY, Kripke DF, Elliott JA, Langer RD. Naps and circadian rhythms in postmenopausal women. *J Gerontol A Biol Sci Med Sci.* 2004;**59**(8):844–8.

77. Prinz P, Bailey S, Moe K, Wilkinson C, Scanlan J. Urinary free cortisol and sleep under baseline and stressed conditions in healthy senior women: effects of estrogen replacement therapy. *J Sleep Res.* 2001; **10**(1):19–26.

78. Woods NF, Carr MC, Tao EY, Taylor HJ, Mitchell ES. Increased urinary cortisol levels during the menopause transition. *Menopause.* 2006;13(2):212–21.

79. Kalleinen N, Polo-Kantola P, Irjala K, *et al.* 24-hour serum levels of growth hormone, prolactin, and cortisol in pre- and postmenopausal women: the effect of combined estrogen and progestin treatment. *J Clin Endocrinol Metab.* 2008; 93(5):1655–61.

80. Parry BL, Meliska CJ, Martinez LF, *et al.* Menopause: neuroendocrine changes and hormone replacement therapy. *J Am Med Womens Assoc.* 2004;59(2):135–45.

81. Maartens LW, Leusink GL, Knottnerus JA, Pop VJ. Hormonal substitution during menopause: what are we treating? *Maturitas.* 2000;34(2):113–18.

82. Wallace-Guy GM, Kripke DF, Jean-Louis G, *et al.* Evening light exposure: implications for sleep and depression. *J Am Geriatr Soc.* 2002;50(4):738–9.

83. Herljevic M, Middleton B, Thapan K, Skene DJ. Light-induced melatonin suppression: age-related reduction in response to short wavelength light. *Exp Gerontol.* 2005;40(3):237–42.

84. Lin TL, Ng SC, Chen YC, Hu SW, Chen GD. What affects the occurrence of nocturia more: menopause or age? *Maturitas.* 2005;50(2):71–7.

Melatonin and mental illness

Gregory M. Brown, Daniel P. Cardinali, and S. R. Pandi-Perumal

Abstract

There have been major advances in knowledge of the role of melatonin in body function and especially in mental illness. Originally isolated as a skin-lightening factor from the pineal gland, it is now known that at physiologic levels it has a key role in the regulation of circadian rhythms. At supraphysiologic levels it has been shown to have neuroprotective as well as cardioprotective effects. In this chapter the authors describe the regulation of melatonin and its relationship to circadian rhythm regulation. They then describe the interaction of melatonin with circadian rhythms and the sleep–wake cycle in major depressive disorder, bipolar depression, and seasonal affective disorder (SAD). An antidepressant has been introduced that represents a new class of antidepressant in that it also acts as an agonist at melatonin receptors and improves several sleep parameters. In seasonal affective disorder bright-light therapy has been shown to be an effective treatment: a treatment that is based on correcting a circadian rhythm misalignment as defined by examining the melatonin rhythm. Sleep–wake alterations in Alzheimer's disease are accompanied by major alterations in melatonin levels and in melatonin receptors in several brain regions. These findings raise the possibility that the melatonin decrease may be important not only for the rhythm disruption but might also have a role in the neurodegeneration itself. In autism spectrum disorders a decrease in melatonin levels along with the final enzyme in the melatonin synthetic pathway has been reported. Susceptibility to schizophrenia may be conferred by a polymorphism in the promoter region for the low affinity melatonin binding site QR2. Thus melatonin alterations are found in several mental disorders and appear to have a key role in those disorders.

Introduction

Melatonin, the hormone synthesized and secreted by the pineal gland, is secreted during darkness in all mammals. Production of melatonin is controlled by the master clock located in the suprachiasmatic nucleus (SCN) and is a messenger from the body clock that acts at both central and peripheral sites conveying the signal of darkness to the organism. In humans melatonin administration has two major effects on the sleep–wake cycle: it influences the timing of body rhythms and it produces drowsiness. Melatonin's effect on the timing of rhythms is due to feedback effects on the SCN while effects on sleepiness may be due to actions at other central sites.

Disruption in body rhythms together with sleep abnormalities has long been known to be a feature of various mental disorders. In major depressive disorder, bipolar depressive disorder, and seasonal affective disorder sleep symptoms are a prominent part of the diagnostic criteria. In Alzheimer's disease rhythm disorders may be prominent including "sundowning" – a symptom which features increased confusion toward the end of the day and into the night.

Several studies have addressed the possible causal links between melatonin abnormalities and rhythm disruption in mental illness. An early theory held that melatonin levels were decreased in depression and was followed by an alternative theory that the melatonin/cortisol ratio was decreased [1].

Subsequently theories have emphasized desynchronization of the melatonin and other rhythms. For example in SAD there is a well established therapeutic response to light therapy given in the morning. This treatment is based on the concept that there is a phase delay in body rhythms that is related to a delay in melatonin onset as revealed when melatonin is sampled under conditions of dim light. This treatment effect is the single best documented example of a physical treatment for a mental illness.

In this review the authors highlight factors regulating the melatonin system, including its relationship with circadian system regulation and then discuss what is known of melatonin systems in depression, Alzheimer's disease, anorexia nervosa, autism, and schizophrenia.

Regulation of melatonin

Under normal circumstances circulating melatonin comes entirely from the pineal gland [2] so that it functions as the hormone signal of that gland and as such is the primary hormonal signal of the circadian system. Pineal melatonin synthesis is regulated by the SCN, the site of the master pacemaker; although during light the clock signal is over-ridden downstream from the clock by a visual pathway through which light signals suppress melatonin synthesis. In mammals circulating melatonin shows a circadian rhythm with high levels during night time, falling precipitately during light so that there are virtually undetectable levels during daytime [3].

The SCN comprises a small group of hypothalamic nerve cells that coordinates timing of the sleep–wake cycle as well as circadian rhythms in other parts of the brain and peripheral tissues [4]. It consists of a set of individual oscillators that are coupled to form a pacemaker [5]. Anatomically the SCN comprises two major subdivisions, a core and a shell, although it is actually more complex than shown in simple line drawings. The photoperiod is the predominant influence on melatonin synthesis, acting by entrainment of the circadian rhythm generating system in the SCN of the hypothalamus via the retino-hypothalamic tract (RHT) and the geniculo-hypothalamic tract (GHT), which act on a population of non-rhythmic cells in the core that are responsive to light [5]. In contrast the shell largely receives input from non-visual hypothalamic, brainstem, and medial forebrain regions. However, there is overlap in cell populations and functions between these anatomical regions [5]. In the absence of periodic environmental synchronizers the circadian pacemaker is free running with a period very near to 24 hours.

The SCN influences neuronal firing in the sub-paraventricular zone (SVZ), which in turn acts via a multisynaptic pathway including the medial forebrain

bundle, reticular formation and intermediolateral cell column, the superior cervical ganglion, and postganglionic sympathetic fibers to stimulate synthesis of melatonin in the pineal gland.

Noradrenalin released from the sympathetic fibers in the pineal acts via a dual receptor adrenergic mechanism. It activates adenylyl cyclase via β_1-adrenergic receptors and protein kinase C activity via α_{1B}-adrenergic receptors thus potentiating β_1-adrenergic receptor activation of adenylyl cyclase [6]. This cross-talk causes a rapid, large increase in cyclic 3′,5′-adenosine monophosphate (cAMP), which leads to phosphorylation of the enzyme arylalkylamine N-acetyltransferase (AANAT; EC 2.3.1.87). Arylalkylamine N-acetyltransferase, which converts serotonin to N-acetylserotonin, has a pivotal role in the timing of melatonin synthesis and has been labeled the "the Timenzyme" [7]. It increases very rapidly with a doubling time of about 15 minutes in response to darkness onset and in response to light it shows an even more rapid half-life of degradation of 3.5 minutes. Since melatonin itself has a half-life in the circulation of about 30 minutes in humans, its levels change promptly in response to circadian signals and light [8].

The enzyme acetylserotonin methyltransferase (ASMT; EC 2.1.1.4), also known as hydroxyindole O-methyltransferase (HIOMT), catalyzes melatonin production from N-acetylserotonin and seems to be responsible for the amplitude of the nocturnal peak of melatonin in humans. In the Siberian hamster the amplitude of the nocturnal peak is related to ASMT activity rather than to AANAT [9] and in the rat N-acetylserotonin is present in vast excess during the night indicating that AA-NAT is not rate limiting for melatonin production [10].

Melatonin and the regulation of circadian rhythms

One of the most prominent effects of melatonin is the regulation of body rhythms. In humans melatonin can synchronize the sleep–wake cycle [11]. Moreover blind people with desynchronized sleep–wake cycles can be successfully treated with melatonin [12] as can sighted individuals with a desynchronized rhythm [13]. These effects raised the question of the brain target for synchronizing actions of melatonin.

Binding sites for melatonin initially identified in a wide variety of central and peripheral tissues using

^{3}H-melatonin and later 2-I^{125}-iodomelatonin were followed by the successful molecular cloning of the first high affinity melatonin receptor (MT$_1$) by Reppert and coworkers using a cDNA library constructed from a dermal cell line of melanophores, the first tissue in which melatonin's action had been demonstrated [14]. This initial finding led to the discovery of additional G$_i$-protein coupled melatonin receptors in humans. A second receptor (MT$_2$) is 60% identical in amino acid sequence to the MT$_1$ receptor [15] and a third receptor, now called GPR50, shares 45% of the amino acid sequence with MT$_1$ and MT$_2$ and is unusual in that it lacks N-linked glycosylation sites, has a C-terminal that is over 300 amino acids long, and does not bind melatonin [16].

A fourth 2-I^{125}-iodomelatonin binding site was identified in mammals (*MT$_3$*, initially called ML-2) [17]. Unlike the membrane receptors that have picomolar affinity it is a lower affinity nanomolar binding site with fast kinetics of association/dissociation [18]. This binding site has now been purified and characterized as quinone reductase type 2 (QR2 or NQO2) [19].

The MT$_1$ receptor acutely inhibits firing in SCN slices, and principally MT$_2$, but also MT$_1$, may contribute to phase shifting in these slices [20]. MT$_1$ and MT$_2$ also differentially regulate GABA$_A$ receptor function in SCN [21]. These findings point to the SCN as the target for the phase shifting actions of melatonin.

It is now established that many G protein-coupled receptors (GPCR), including the MT$_1$ and MT$_2$ receptors, exist in living cells as dimers. The relative propensity of the MT$_1$ homodimer and MT$_1$/MT$_2$ heterodimer formation are similar whereas that of the MT$_2$ homodimer is three- to four-fold lower [22]. Although the GPR50 receptor lacks the ability to bind melatonin it abolishes high affinity binding of the MT$_1$ receptor through heterodimerization [23]. Thus the GPR50 receptor can influence melatonin function by altering its binding to the MT$_1$ receptor.

Mapping of the MT$_1$ and MT$_2$ receptors in the brain and periphery using immunocytochemistry is ongoing. MT$_1$ and MT$_2$ receptors are present in the SCN [24, 25]. The MT$_1$ receptor is extremely widely distributed in the hypothalamus; of particular note it is colocalized with corticotropin in the paraventricular nucleus (PVN) and with oxytocin and vasopressin in the PVN and supraoptic nucleus [25]. MT$_1$ and MT$_2$ receptors have been identified in the hippocampus [26, 27], and in the occipital cortex [28], while MT$_1$ receptors and MT$_1$ and MT$_2$ RNA have been shown in the dopaminergic system [29, 30]. Effects produced by alterations in melatonin patterns or levels may be secondary to responses in any of these or in other regions yet to be characterized.

Major depressive disorder

Major depressive disorder (MDD), bipolar disorder, and seasonal affective disorder (SAD) are characterized by major disruptions in sleep architecture [31]. Moreover, sleep abnormalities with insomnia or hypersomnia form part of the diagnostic criteria for these conditions [32]. Because of the sleep abnormalities, changes in melatonin regulation have been of considerable interest to investigators.

An early study by Wetterberg and colleagues proposed a "low melatonin syndrome" or a low melatonin/cortisol ratio in MDD [1]. Although several studies replicated this finding of a low melatonin level, many others have found no difference or in fact found an increase, possibly because of subcategories of illness [33]. This discrepancy could also be related to the extremely high individual variance in melatonin levels, a variance that could obscure differences related to MDD [3]. Several studies have reported a phase advance of the melatonin rhythm in patients with MDD studied under dim light conditions (DLMO), while the offset may be delayed and the duration of secretion prolonged [33].

The tricyclic antidepressants and selective serotonin reuptake inhibitors most often used in treatment of MDD treat the depression but may fail to relieve the sleep abnormalities or may even cause worsening [31]. Moreover continuing treatment with the antidepressants desipramine, clomipramine, and fluoxetine has been shown to affect the distribution of melatonin receptor mRNAs in the brain. They decreased the amount of MT$_2$ receptor mRNA in hippocampal regions that decreased MT$_1$ receptor mRNA in the striatum [30]. The authors propose that prolonged treatment with classical antidepressant drugs alters the brain ratio of MT$_1$/MT$_2$ receptors to enable endogenous melatonin to potentiate antidepressant action [34].

Agomelatine, a naphthalenic compound chemically designated as N-[2-(7-methoxynaphth-1-yl) ethyl]acetamide, has been reported to be effective as an antidepressant not only in animal models of depression, but also in patients with MDD. Agomelatine has a novel mechanism of action, acting simultaneously as a melatonin MT_1 and MT_2 receptor agonist and as a 5-HT2C antagonist [35, 36]. This unique dual mechanism of action is undoubtedly the reason for both its antidepressant efficacy and its capacity to alleviate sleep–wakefulness rhythm disorders.

In a multicenter, multinational placebo-controlled study involving 711 patients from different European countries, agomelatine at doses of 25 mg/day was found both to improve depressive symptoms and to have a side-effects profile close to placebo [37]. Treatment with agomelatine was shown to produce subjective improvement and improvement of NREM sleep instability in 15 patients with major depressive disorder [38]. Moreover agomelatine demonstrated an absence of rebound effects in more complex cases of depression [39]. A double-blind, parallel-group study of 238 patients randomized to 25 mg/day agomelatine (with dose adjustment at two weeks to 50 mg/day in patients with insufficient improvement) showed a clinical improvement with agomelatine together with tolerability identical to placebo [40]. In a double-blind, placebo-controlled study of 25 mg and 50 mg agomelatine daily in 212 patients with major depressive disorder results supported the prescription of agomelatine 25 mg as the usual therapeutic dose, but suggested that increasing the dose to 50 mg could be beneficial for some patients without reducing tolerability [41]. In a double-blind comparison of venlafaxine and agomelatine it was reported that the drugs were equally effective but that agomelatine produced fewer problems with sexual functioning and a lower discontinuation rate [42].

The three major placebo-controlled studies of agomelatine were individually insufficient to demonstrate efficacy of agomelatine as an antidepressant [37, 40, 41]. Nonetheless, pooled data from these studies was sufficient to establish that agomelatine is an effective treatment for major depression [43]. Taken together there is evidence not only that agomelatine is an effective treatment for major depression but that it has very good tolerability and that unlike the majority of antidepressants it improves many aspects of sleep.

Bipolar depression

Because of its role in synchronizing rhythms and its effects on the sleep–wake cycle, melatonin is of particular interest in bipolar disorder. Nocturnal melatonin levels have been reported as decreased in several studies [33] and it has been proposed that low melatonin is a trait rather than a state marker for bipolar disorder [44]. A phase advance of melatonin secretion has been reported in manic patients [33, 45]. Thomson and coworkers reported a sex-specific association between bipolar affective disorder in women in south-eastern Scotland and a polymorphism in GPR50 [46]. However, no association was found in patients in a northern Swedish population [47]. Because bipolar disorder is complex and may have different genetic factors contributing to vulnerability it is possible that different risk factors are involved in northern Sweden, alternatively there may be a relationship with another functional polymorphism in or close to the GPR50 gene.

A preliminary adjunctive open-label study of the antidepressant efficacy of agomelatine in patients with bipolar I disorder experiencing a major depressive episode while on valpromide or lithium indicates effectiveness of combined therapy [48]. Thus, as for MDD, agomelatine appears to be an effective antidepressant medication in bipolar disorder. However, a double-blind study will be required to confirm the results.

Postmenopausal depression

It has been reported that in postmenopausal depression there is an increase in nocturnal melatonin that is phase delayed into the morning hours [49]. Based on preliminary evidence the author postulates that the increased and extended secretion of melatonin is secondary to low light exposure in these patients. Furthermore the changes in melatonin may be contributory to the depression.

Seasonal affective disorder

Seasonal affective disorder, according to the *Diagnostic and Statistical Manual of Mental Disorders* [32], is a subtype of major depressive or bipolar disorder characterized by recurrent affective episodes at the same time of the year. Most frequently the depressive episodes begin in fall or winter. Full remissions also occur at a characteristic time of year [32]. Symptoms of winter SAD including weight gain, increased sleep, loss of interest in sex, and decreased activity can also occur in animals that show photoperiod related changes. Because of the well established role of melatonin in animal seasonality it is reasonable to assume that melatonin might have a similar role in the winter form of SAD. Photoperiodic reproductive, body, and behavioral changes in photosensitive mammals are known to be mediated by changes in the circadian rhythm of pineal melatonin secretion [50]. The association of winter SAD with reduced day length and the ameliorative effect of bright light therapy on the disorder suggest that either photoperiodic time measurement or an altered circadian phase, or both, may play a role in the etiology of the disease as it does in photosensitive animals.

Several studies have failed to find any alteration in nocturnal melatonin levels in patients with SAD [51–53]. On the other hand there is evidence for an alteration of the phase of melatonin and other circadian rhythms in SAD. Both patients with winter depression and normal subjects can show a prolonged nocturnal melatonin rise when there are increased hours of darkness, although a study by Wehr and coworkers showed a longer nocturnal rise in SAD patients than in healthy volunteers [54]. Some but not all studies have suggested a delay in DLMO onset in SAD [55]. The majority of patients with winter depression respond better to early morning light treatment than to evening treatment [56, 57]. Lewy and coworkers have proposed that some patients with SAD are phase advanced and others phase delayed and that phase typing will lead to optimization of treatment [58]. Thus to produce a phase delay light treatment should be given in the evening and low-dose melatonin in the morning, while to cause a phase advance low-dose melatonin should be given in the evening and light treatment in the morning [59]. Further studies should help clarify this issue.

Antidepressant treatment has been used in treatment of patients with SAD when light therapy is ineffective or for logistic reasons. Thirty-seven acutely depressed patients with SAD in an open-label study with agomelatine (25 mg/day in the evening) over 14 weeks showed a significant improvement with good tolerability and an improvement both in sleep disturbance and in daytime sleepiness [60]. This study suggests that similarly to non-seasonal MDD, seasonal depression may be safely treated with agomelatine although double-blind studies are required.

Aging and Alzheimer's disease (AD)

With aging there is a fragmented sleep–wake pattern [61], which is even more pronounced in AD [62, 63].

The sleep complaints of aging are often comorbid with medical and psychiatric illness, associated with the medications used to treat those illnesses, or the result of circadian rhythm changes or other sleep disorders [64]. Demented patients frequently suffer from "sundowning", which is defined as "an exacerbation of symptoms indicating increased arousal or impairment in late afternoon, evening or at night, among elderly demented individuals" and is considered to be a chronobiological disturbance [65]. Thus in aging and especially in AD there is considerable evidence of a chronobiologic basis of sleep and behavior disorder.

The majority of studies of melatonin levels have shown a decrease with aging, a decrease that may well be instrumental in causing chronobiologic and hence sleep disruption [66]. Moreover, this decrease is greater in AD [67–69]. The pineal gland becomes calcified with age and as measured by computed tomography both the amount of calcification and the volume of uncalcified tissue have been reported to be decreased in patients with AD [70]. Thus the ability of the gland to secrete melatonin is decreased.

Studies of clock gene oscillation in autopsied pineal glands have shown that this rhythm is disrupted in AD, probably due to functional disconnection from the master clock, which is itself disrupted [71]. There are major changes in the rhythm of vasopressin expression in the SCN in later life [72], and there is a three times lower expression in AD patients [73]. Thus the regulation of the pineal gland is disrupted.

Studies of melatonin membrane receptor expression in aging and AD have also revealed changes. Immunohistochemical staining of the MT_1 receptor in the hippocampus is reported as increased in AD [26] while that of the MT_2 receptor is decreased [27]. MT_1 expression is decreased in the SCN in aging and even more so in AD [74]. More recently it was reported that pineal and cortical melatonin receptors MT_1 and MT_2 are decreased in AD [28].

It has been postulated that with degeneration of the SCN during aging and AD, the strength of the zeitgebers may be reduced, and the input of neural pathways involved in entrainment (synchronization) of the central clock may become dysfunctional or less sensitive during aging and even more so in AD [75]. In examining this concept studies have been done of the two main zeitgebers for the circadian system: light and melatonin.

A large multicenter trial showed only a trend to improvement in the circadian rhythm disturbance of AD when treatment was done using melatonin [76]. Because MT1 receptor expression in the SCN is decreased and the SCN is the primary target for circadian rhythm synchronization it is certainly possible that melatonin will be ineffective, alternatively a higher dose of melatonin may be required for effectiveness or a more potent melatonin agonist may be necessary [75]. Ramelteon is a novel agent that is a potent MT_1/MT_2 agonist documented as soporific agent with no abuse potential that synchronizes circadian rhythms [77–79]. No studies on ramelteon in AD have as yet been reported.

On the other hand, recently it has been reported that early morning light therapy improves the sleep–wake rhythm and daytime cognition and that evening melatonin increases nocturnal sleep time in patients with AD [80]. In yet other studies the combination of light therapy and melatonin was also effective in treating the rest–activity rhythm in AD [81, 82].

In addition to its synchronizing effects on circadian rhythms it is known that higher doses of melatonin have potent antioxidant effects. It has been postulated that these effects may be of use in diseases such as AD. Moreover, recent studies with the enzyme QR2 suggest that inhibition of QR2 may lead to "protective" effects and also that over-expression of this enzyme may have deleterious effects. There is an inhibitory effect of melatonin on QR2 observed in vitro, which may explain the protective effects reported for melatonin in different animal models, such as cardiac or renal ischemia effects that have been attributed to the controversial antioxidant properties of the hormone [83]. These effects of melatonin occur at concentrations that are similar to those reported for the antioxidant and/or protective effect of melatonin. The possibility that the protective effect of melatonin might involve QR2 is supported by a recent publication on the interaction between resveratrol and QR2. Resveratrol a phyto-polyphenol isolated from grapes, which is present in significant amounts in red wine, is claimed to have neuroprotective, cardioprotective, and anti-aging properties. There is evidence that resveratrol interacts with QR2 to produce an antioxidant effect [84, 85]. The development of specific ligands for QR2 may well lead to new anti-aging therapeutic agents.

For both melatonin and resveratrol there is evidence that they both prevent damage to mitochondria [86]

whether through an antioxidative action or by another route. Agents targeting mitochondria are under active development as they show promise as treatment for neurodegenerative diseases such as AD [87]. They are also under active exploration for diseases of aging such as type 2 diabetes [88].

Thus for AD there are at least two different actions of melatonin that are potentially useful, synchronization of the sleep–wake cycle and a neuroprotective effect. These actions are operative via different mechanisms.

Anorexia nervosa

In anorexia nervosa, nocturnal melatonin levels have been reported as elevated in several but not all studies [89]. Decreased caloric intake in anorexia nervosa has been established as the cause of several different endocrine changes. This may also be the case for the elevation of melatonin as underfeeding of rats has been shown to be associated with increased nocturnal melatonin [90].

Autism

A low melatonin level has been reported by three separate groups in patients with autism spectrum disorders (ASD) and these patients frequently show disruptions in sleep–wake cycles. A recent study has reported that ASD is associated with genetic polymorphisms of the ASMT gene, the gene that encodes the final enzyme of the melatonin synthetic pathway. Analyses of blood platelets and/or cultured cells revealed a highly significant decrease in ASMT activity and melatonin in both patients and their unaffected parents as compared to control subjects. These results indicate that a primary deficit in ASMT activity and its associated low melatonin level in ASD is a risk factor for ASD and support ASMT as a susceptibility gene for ASD [91]. These findings raise the question whether the lack of adequate melatonin at a crucial stage in development may cause a defect in human cognition and behavior.

Schizophrenia

Schizophrenia and Parkinson's disease have been reported to be associated with polymorphisms of QR2; a polymorphism that consists of an insertion/deletion of 29 base-pair nucleotides in the promoter region of the gene [92, 93]. This polymorphism may cause overexpression of this gene causing increased QR2 activity and may make individuals more susceptible to schizophrenia and Parkinsonism [83]. Polymorphisms of this gene together with decreased levels of QR2 mRNA are reported in patients with clozapine-associated agranulocytosis [94].

Conclusions

Several psychiatric disorders are associated with sleep and/or rhythm disorders raising the question of the relationship of melatonin to the disorder. In particular the strong association of MDD and other depressive disorders with sleep disorder raises the question whether the sleep disorder may be a cause of the depression, whether the depression leads to a secondary sleep disorder, or whether both disorders have a common link to a problem in timing. Agomelatine and other melatonergic agents that are under development should help to clarify these issues. Whatever the case may be, agents such agomelatine are active against both the depressive and sleep disorders.

In SAD there is also an association of depression and sleep disorder. The linkage of SAD to an alteration in hours of illumination makes it likely that the underlying mechanism is similar to that of seasonality in animals. This relationship to illumination has been very clearly established by the proven efficacy of light therapy in this disorder. The question of the role of melatonin, however, is unresolved. In seasonal animals alteration in the pattern of nocturnal melatonin secretion mediates the effects of light in seasonality. The role of such alterations in melatonin in SAD is not yet clear and awaits further study.

In Alzheimer's disease there is a disturbance in body rhythms that is related to a disruption of linkage between the SCN and the pineal gland. Moreover, there is a well documented decrease in melatonin along with alterations in membrane melatonin receptors in several regions. It is possible that treatment with a potent melatonin agonist such as ramelteon could be beneficial in controlling the sleep and rhythm disruption.

Melatonin has also been shown to have a neuroprotective effect at levels that are reported to be supraphysiologic. However, it has also been postulated that this neuroprotective effect may be at least in part via the enzyme QR2, which in addition to being a target for melatonin also interacts with resveratrol which has been shown to have neuroprotective, cardioprotective, and anti-aging properties. Melatonin and resveratrol also prevent damage to mitochondria possibly via the same enzyme. However, at this time there are many unanswered questions about QR2 [95]. Melatonin is clearly neuroprotective at supraphysiologic doses but whether it is protective at physiologic levels is unanswered although it has been speculated that low levels of melatonin during development may be a risk factor for autism spectrum disorder. Agents targeting the enzyme QR2 (as well as QR1) are currently under active investigation as possible future neuroprotective treatment agents.

References

1. Wetterberg L, Beck-Friis J, Aperia B, Petterson U. Melatonin/cortisol ratio in depression [letter]. *Lancet.* 1979;**2**:1361.

2. Karasek M, Winczyk K. Melatonin in humans. *J Physiol Pharmacol.* 2006;**57** Suppl 5:19–39.

3. Grof E, Grof P, Brown GM, Arato M, Lane J. Investigations of melatonin secretion in man. *Prog Neuropsychopharmacol Biol Psychiatry.* 1985;**9**:609–12.

4. Moore RY. Suprachiasmatic nucleus in sleep–wake regulation. *Sleep Med.* 2007;**8** Suppl 3:27–33.

5. Lee HS, Billings HJ, Lehman MN. The suprachiasmatic nucleus: a clock of multiple components. *J Biol Rhythms.* 2003;**18**:435–49.

6. Chik CL, Ho AK, Klein DC. Dual receptor regulation of cyclic nucleotides: alpha 1-adrenergic potentiation of vasoactive intestinal peptide stimulation of pinealocyte adenosine $3',5'$-monophosphate. *Endocrinol.* 1988;**122**:1646–51.

7. Klein DC. Arylalkylamine N-acetyltransferase: "the Timenzyme". *J Biol Chem.* 2007;**282**:4233–7.

8. Waldhauser F, Waldhauser M, Lieberman HR, *et al.* Bioavailability of oral melatonin in humans. *Neuroendocrinol.* 1984;**39**:307–13.

9. Ceinos RM, Chansard M, Revel F, *et al.* Analysis of adrenergic regulation of melatonin synthesis in Siberian hamster pineal emphasizes the role of HIOMT. *Neurosignals.* 2004;**13**:308–17.

10. Liu T, Borjigin J. N-acetyltransferase is not the rate-limiting enzyme of melatonin synthesis at night. *J Pineal Res.* 2005;**39**:91–6.

11. Arendt J, Broadway J. Light and melatonin as zeitgebers in man. *Chronobiol Int.* 1987;**4**:273–82.

12. Arendt J, Aldhous M, Wright J. Synchronisation of a disturbed sleep-wake cycle in a blind man by melatonin treatment [letter]. *Lancet.* 1988;**1**:772–3.

13. McArthur AJ, Lewy AJ, Sack RL. Non-24-hour sleep-wake syndrome in a sighted man: circadian rhythm studies and efficacy of melatonin treatment. *Sleep.* 1996;**19**:544–53.

14. Reppert SM, Weaver DR, Ebisawa T. Cloning and characterization of a mammalian melatonin receptor that mediates reproductive and circadian responses. *Neuron.* 1994;**13**:1177–85.

15. Reppert SM, Godson C, Mahle CD, *et al.* Molecular characterization of a second melatonin receptor expressed in human retina and brain: the Mel1b melatonin receptor. *Proc Natl Acad Sci USA.* 1995;**92**:8734–8.

16. Reppert SM, Weaver DR, Ebisawa T, Mahle CD, Kolakowski LJ. Cloning of a melatonin-related receptor from human pituitary. *FEBS Lett.* 1996;**386**:219–24.

17. Pickering DS, Niles LP. Pharmacological characterization of melatonin binding sites in Syrian hamster hypothalamus. *Eur J Pharmacol.* 1990;**175**:71–7.

18. Dubocovich ML, Cardinali DP, Delagrange P, *et al.* Melatonin receptors. In: IUPHAR, ed., *The IUPHAR Compendium of Receptor Characterization and Classification*, 2nd edn. (London: IUPHAR Media, 2000; 271–7).

19. Nosjean O, Ferro M, Coge F, *et al.* Identification of the melatonin-binding site MT3 as the quinone reductase 2. *J Biol Chem.* 2000;**275**:31311–17.

20. Liu C, Weaver DR, Jin X, Shearman LP, *et al.* Molecular dissection of two distinct actions of melatonin on the suprachiasmatic circadian clock. *Neuron.* 1997;**19**:91–102.

21. Wan Q, Man HY, Liu F, *et al.* Differential modulation of GABAA receptor function by Mel1a and Mel1b receptors. *Nature Neuroscience.* 1999;**2**:401–3.

22. Daulat AM, Maurice P, Froment C, *et al.* Purification and identification of G protein-coupled receptor protein complexes under native conditions. *Mol Cell Proteomics.* 2007;**6**:835–44.

23. Levoye A, Dam J, Ayoub MA, *et al.* The orphan GPR50 receptor specifically inhibits MT1 melatonin receptor function through heterodimerization. *EMBO J.* 2006;**25**:3012–23.

24. Dubocovich ML. Melatonin receptors: role on sleep and circadian rhythm regulation. *Sleep Med.* 2007; 8 Suppl 3:34–42.

25. Wu YH, Zhou JN, Balesar R, *et al.* Distribution of MT1 melatonin receptor immunoreactivity in the human hypothalamus and pituitary gland: colocalization of MT1 with vasopressin, oxytocin, and corticotropin-releasing hormone. *J Compar Neurol.* 2006;**499**:897–910.

26. Savaskan E, Olivieri G, Meier F, *et al.* Increased melatonin 1a-receptor immunoreactivity in the hippocampus of Alzheimer's disease patients. *J Pineal Res.* 2002;**32**:59–62.

27. Savaskan E, Ayoub MA, Ravid R, *et al.* Reduced hippocampal MT2 melatonin receptor expression in Alzheimer's disease. *J Pineal Res.* 2005;**38**:10–16.

28. Brunner P, Sozer-Topcular N, Jockers R, *et al.* Pineal and cortical melatonin receptors MT1 and MT2 are decreased in Alzheimer's disease. *Eur J Histochem.* 2006;**50**:311–16.

29. Uz T, Arslan AD, Kurtuncu M, *et al.* The regional and cellular expression profile of the melatonin receptor MT1 in the central dopaminergic system. *Brain Res Mol Brain Res.* 2005;**136**:45–53.

30. Imbesi M, Uz T, Yildiz S, Arslan AD, Manev H. Drug- and region-specific effects of protracted antidepressant and cocaine treatment on the content of melatonin MT(1) and MT(2) receptor mRNA in the mouse brain. *Int J Neuroprot Neuroregener.* 2006;**2**:185–9.

31. Lam RW. Sleep disturbances and depression: a challenge for antidepressants. *Int Clin Psychopharmacol.* 2006;**21** Suppl 1:S25–S29.

32. American Psychiatric Association. *Diagnostic and Statistical Manual of Mental Disorders*, 4th edn (DSM-IV-TR). (Washington, DC: American Psychiatric Press, 2000).

33. Srinivasan V, Smits M, Spence W, *et al.* Melatonin in mood disorders. *World J Biol Psychiatry.* 2006;**7**:138–51.

34. Hirsch-Rodriguez E, Imbesi M, Manev R, Uz T, Manev H. The pattern of melatonin receptor expression in the brain may influence antidepressant treatment. *Med Hypotheses.* 2007;**69**:120–4.

35. Yous S, Andrieux J, Howell HE, *et al.* Novel napthalenic ligands with high affinity for the melatonin receptor. *J Med Chem.* 1992;**35**:1484–6.

36. Millan MJ, Gobert A, Lejeune F, *et al.* The novel melatonin agonist agomelatine (S20098) is an antagonist at 5-hydroxytryptamine 2C receptors, blockade of which enhances the activity of frontocortical dopaminergic and adrenergic pathways. *J Pharmacol Exp Ther.* 2003;**306**:954–64.

37. Loo H, Hale A, D'haenen H. Determination of the dose of agomelatine, a melatoninergic agonist and selective 5-HT(2C) antagonist, in the treatment of major depressive disorder: a placebo-controlled dose range study. *Int Clin Psychopharmacol.* 2002;**17**:239–47.

38. Lopes MC, Quera-Salva MA, Guilleminault C. Non-REM sleep instability in patients with major depressive disorder: subjective improvement and

improvement of non-REM sleep instability with treatment (Agomelatine). *Sleep Med.* 2007;**9**:33–41.

39. Rouillon F. Efficacy and tolerance profile of agomelatine and practical use in depressed patients. *Int Clin Psychopharmacol.* 2006;**21** Suppl 1:S31–S35.

40. Olie JP, Kasper S. Efficacy of agomelatine, a MT1/MT2 receptor agonist with 5-HT2C antagonistic properties, in major depressive disorder. *Int J Neuropsychopharmacol.* 2007;**10**:661–73.

41. Kennedy SH, Emsley R. Placebo-controlled trial of agomelatine in the treatment of major depressive disorder. *Eur Neuropsychopharmacol.* 2006;**16**:93–100.

42. Kennedy SH, Rizvi S, Fulton K, Rasmussen J. A double-blind comparison of sexual functioning, antidepressant efficacy, and tolerability between agomelatine and venlafaxine XR. *J Clin Psychopharmacol.* 2008;**28**:329–33.

43. Montgomery SA, Kasper S. Severe depression and antidepressants: focus on a pooled analysis of placebo-controlled studies on agomelatine. *Int Clin Psychopharmacol.* 2007;**22**:283–91.

44. Kennedy SH, Kutcher SP, Ralevski E, Brown GM. Nocturnal melatonin and 24-hour 6-sulphatoxymelatonin levels in various phases of bipolar affective disorder. *Psychiatry Res.* 1996;**63**:219–22.

45. Kennedy SH, Tighe S, McVey G, Brown GM. Melatonin and cortisol "switches" during mania, depression, and euthymia in a drug-free bipolar patient. *J Nerv Ment Dis.* 1989;**177**:300–3.

46. Thomson PA, Wray NR, Thomson AM, *et al.* Sex-specific association between bipolar affective disorder in women and GPR50, an X-linked orphan G protein-coupled receptor. *Mol Psychiatry.* 2005;**10**:470–8.

47. Praschak-Rieder N, Willeit M, Winkler D, *et al.* Role of family history and 5-HTTLPR polymorphism in female seasonal affective disorder patients with and without premenstrual dysphoric disorder. *Eur Neuropsychopharmacol.* 2002;**12**:129–34.

48. Calabrese JR, Guelfi JD, Perdrizet-Chevallier C. Agomelatine adjunctive therapy for acute bipolar depression: preliminary open data. *Bipolar Disord.* 2007;**9**:628–35.

49. Parry BL, Meliska CJ, Sorenson DL, *et al.* Increased melatonin and delayed offset in menopausal depression: role of years past menopause, follicle-stimulating hormone, sleep end time, and body mass index. *J Clin Endocrinol Metab.* 2008;**93**:54–60.

50. Bartness TJ, Goldman BD. Mammalian pineal melatonin: a clock for all seasons. *Experientia.* 1989;**45**:939–45.

51. Checkley SA, Murphy DG, Abbas M, *et al.* Melatonin rhythms in seasonal affective disorder. *Br J Psychiatry.* 1993;**163**:332–7.

52. Partonen T. Involvement of melatonin and serotonin in winter depression. *Medical Hypotheses.* 1994;**43**:165–6.

53. Thompson C, Franey C, Arendt J, Checkley SA. A comparison of melatonin secretion in depressed patients and normal subjects. *Br J Psychiatry.* 1988;**152**:260–5.

54. Wehr TA, Duncan WC, Jr., Sher L, *et al.* A circadian signal of change of season in patients with seasonal affective disorder. *Arch Gen Psychiatry.* 2001;**58**:1108–14.

55. Sack RL, Lewy AJ, White DM, *et al.* Morning vs evening light treatment for winter depression. Evidence that the therapeutic effects of light are mediated by circadian phase shifts [published erratum appears in *Arch Gen Psychiatry.* 1992;**49**(8):650]. *Arch Gen Psychiatry.* 1990;**47**:343–51.

56. Terman JS, Terman M, Lo ES, Cooper TB. Circadian time of morning light administration and therapeutic response in winter depression. *Arch Gen Psychiatry.* 2001;**58**:69–75.

57. Eastman CI, Young MA, Fogg LF, Liu L, Meaden PM. Bright light treatment of winter depression: a placebo-controlled trial. *Arch Gen Psychiatry.* 1998;**55**:883–9.

58. Lewy AJ, Lefler BJ, Emens JS, Bauer VK. The circadian basis of winter depression. *Proc Natl Acad Sci USA.* 2006;**103**:7414–19.

59. Lewy AJ. Melatonin and human chronobiology. *Cold Spring Harb Symp Quant Biol.* 2007;**72**:623–36.

60. Pjrek E, Winkler D, Konstantinidis A, *et al.* Agomelatine in the treatment of seasonal affective disorder. *Psychopharmacology (Berl).* 2007;**190**:575–79.

61. Ancoli-Israel S. Sleep and aging: prevalence of disturbed sleep and treatment considerations in older adults. *J Clin Psychiatry.* 2005;**66** Suppl 9:24–30.

62. Bliwise DL, Hughes M, McMahon PM, Kutner N. Observed sleep/wakefulness and severity of dementia in an Alzheimer's disease special care unit. *J Gerontol A Biol Sci Med Sci.* 1995;**50**:M303–M306.

63. Van Someren EJ, Hagebeuk EE, Lijzenga C, *et al.* Circadian rest-activity rhythm disturbances in Alzheimer's disease. *Biol Psychiatry.* 1996;**40**:259–70.

64. Ancoli-Israel S, Ayalon L, Salzman C. Sleep in the elderly: normal variations and common sleep disorders. *Harv Rev Psychiatry.* 2008;**16**:279–86.

65. Finocchiaro L, Callebert J, Launay JM, Jallon JM. Melatonin biosynthesis in *Drosophila*: its nature and its effects. *J Neurochem.* 1988;**50**:382–7.

127

66. Skene DJ, Swaab DF. Melatonin rhythmicity: effect of age and Alzheimer's disease. *Exp Gerontol.* 2003; **38**:199–206.

67. Mishima K, Tozawa T, Satoh K, *et al.* Melatonin secretion rhythm disorders in patients with senile dementia of Alzheimer's type with disturbed sleep-waking. *Biol Psychiatry.* 1999;**45**:417–21.

68. Ferrari E, Arcaini A, Gornati R, *et al.* Pineal and pituitary-adrenocortical function in physiological aging and in senile dementia. *Exp Gerontol.* 2000;**35**:1239–50.

69. Luboshitzky R, Shen-Orr Z, Tzischichinsky O, *et al.* Actigraphic sleep-wake patterns and urinary 6-sulfatoxymelatonin excretion in patients with Alzheimer's disease. *Chronobiol Int.* 2001;**18**:513–24.

70. Mahlberg R, Walther S, Kalus P, *et al.* Pineal calcification in Alzheimer's disease: an in vivo study using computed tomography. *Neurobiol Aging.* 2008;**29**:203–9.

71. Wu YH, Fischer DF, Kalsbeek A, *et al.* Pineal clock gene oscillation is disturbed in Alzheimer's disease, due to functional disconnection from the "master clock". *FASEB J.* 2006;**20**:1874–6.

72. Hofman MA, Swaab DF. Alterations in circadian rhythmicity of the vasopressin-producing neurons of the human suprachiasmatic nucleus (SCN) with aging. *Brain Res.* 1994;**651**:134–42.

73. Liu RY, Zhou JN, Hoogendijk WJ, *et al.* Decreased vasopressin gene expression in the biological clock of Alzheimer disease patients with and without depression. *J Neuropathol Exp Neurol.* 2000;**59**:314–22.

74. Wu YH, Zhou JN, Van HJ, Jockers R, Swaab DF. Decreased MT1 melatonin receptor expression in the suprachiasmatic nucleus in aging and Alzheimer's disease. *Neurobiol Aging.* 2007;**28**:1239–47.

75. Wu YH, Swaab DF. Disturbance and strategies for reactivation of the circadian rhythm system in aging and Alzheimer's disease. *Sleep Med.* 2007;**8**:623–36.

76. Singer C, Tractenberg RE, Kaye J, *et al.* A multicenter, placebo-controlled trial of melatonin for sleep disturbance in Alzheimer's disease. *Sleep.* 2003;**26**:893–901.

77. Richardson GS, Zee PC, Wang-Weigand S, Rodriguez L, Peng X. Circadian phase-shifting effects of repeated ramelteon administration in healthy adults. *J Clin Sleep Med.* 2008;**4**:456–61.

78. Johnson MW, Suess PE, Griffiths RR. Ramelteon: a novel hypnotic lacking abuse liability and sedative adverse effects. *Arch Gen Psychiatry.* 2006;**63**:1149–57.

79. Sateia MJ, Kirby-Long P, Taylor JL. Efficacy and clinical safety of ramelteon: an evidence-based review. *Sleep Med Rev.* 2008;**12**:319–32.

80. Asayama K, Yamadera H, Ito T, Suzuki H, Kudo Y, Endo S. Double blind study of melatonin effects on the sleep-wake rhythm, cognitive and non-cognitive functions in Alzheimer type dementia. *J Nippon Med Sch.* 2003;**70**:334–41.

81. Dowling GA, Burr RL, Van Someren EJ, *et al.* Melatonin and bright-light treatment for rest-activity disruption in institutionalized patients with Alzheimer's disease. *J Am Geriatr Soc.* 2008; **56**:239–46.

82. Riemersma-van der Lek RF, Swaab DF, Twisk J, *et al.* Effect of bright light and melatonin on cognitive and noncognitive function in elderly residents of group care facilities: a randomized controlled trial. *JAMA.* 2008;**299**:2642–55.

83. Delagrange P, Boutin JA. Therapeutic potential of melatonin ligands. *Chronobiol Int.* 2006;**23**:413–18.

84. Buryanovskyy L, Fu Y, Boyd M, *et al.* Crystal structure of quinone reductase 2 in complex with resveratrol. *Biochem.* 2004;**43**:11417–26.

85. Hsieh TC, Lu X, Wang Z, Wu JM. Induction of quinone reductase NQO1 by resveratrol in human K562 cells involves the antioxidant response element ARE and is accompanied by nuclear translocation of transcription factor Nrf2. *Med Chem.* 2006;**2**:275–85.

86. Kirimlioglu H, Ecevit A, Yilmaz S, Kirimlioglu V, Karabulut AB. Effect of resveratrol and melatonin on oxidative stress enzymes, regeneration, and hepatocyte ultrastructure in rats subjected to 70% partial hepatectomy. *Transplant Proc.* 2008;**40**:285–9.

87. Mancuso C, Bates TE, Butterfield DA, *et al.* Natural antioxidants in Alzheimer's disease. *Expert Opin Investig Drugs.* 2007;**16**:1921–31.

88. Milne JC, Lambert PD, Schenk S, *et al.* Small molecule activators of SIRT1 as therapeutics for the treatment of type 2 diabetes. *Nature.* 2007;**450**:712–16.

89. Arendt J, Bhanji S, Franey C, Mattingly D. Plasma melatonin levels in anorexia nervosa. *Brit J Psychiatry.* 1992;**161**:361–4.

90. Chik CL, Ho AK, Brown GM. Effect of food restriction on 24-h serum and pineal melatonin content in male rats. *Acta Endocrinol.* 1987;**115**:507–13.

91. Melke J, Goubran BH, Chaste P, *et al.* Abnormal melatonin synthesis in autism spectrum disorders. *Mol Psychiatry.* 2008;**13**:90–8.

92. Harada S, Fujii C, Hayashi A, Ohkoshi N. An association between idiopathic Parkinson's disease and polymorphisms of phase II detoxification enzymes: glutathione S-transferase M1 and quinone oxidoreductase 1 and 2. *Biochem Biophys Res Commun.* 2001;**288**:887–92.

93. Harada S, Tachikawa H, Kawanishi Y. A possible association between an insertion/deletion polymorphism of the NQO2 gene and schizophrenia. *Psychiatr Genet.* 2003;**13**:205–9.

94. Ostrousky O, Meged S, Loewenthal R, *et al.* NQO2 gene is associated with clozapine-induced agranulocytosis. *Tissue Antigens.* 2003;**62**:483–91.

95. Vella F, Ferry G, Delagrange P, Boutin JA. NRH:quinone reductase 2: an enzyme of surprises and mysteries. *Biochem Pharmacol.* 2005;**71**:1–12.

Chapter 12

Dim light melatonin onset in psychiatric disorders

Marcel G. Smits, D. Warren Spence, S. R. Pandi-Perumal, and Gregory M. Brown

Introduction

In 1999, Lewy proposed that the dim light melatonin onset (DLMO) was the most useful marker for human circadian phase position and that the DLMO was optimally obtained by sampling blood or saliva in the evening at intervals of 30 minutes or less under conditions of less than 30 to 50 lux. The DLMO is now commonly used both experimentally and in clinical practice for objectively assessing the functioning of the body's biological clock. Biological clock disturbances are reflective of more general sleep–wake rhythm disturbances, but are being increasingly used for diagnosing broader conditions, such as several psychiatric disorders, that are associated with it. Furthermore, DLMO has been used for identifying optimal application times for treatments, such as bright light therapy and exogenous melatonin treatment. In this chapter the role of DLMO in the diagnosis and treatment of psychiatric disorders is discussed.

Circadian pacemaker and dim light melatonin onset

Circadian pacemaker

Molecular mechanisms regulating the mammalian biological clock are present in all cells. These mechanisms consist of gene–protein–gene feedback loops in which proteins downregulate their own transcription and stimulate the transcription of other clock proteins. The mammalian biological clock consists of a hierarchy of oscillators, the central coordinator of which is found in the brain, formed by the cells of the suprachiasmatic nuclei (SCN) within the anterior hypothalamus [1]. The pacemaker in these nuclei generates and maintains circadian rhythms in many physiological and psychological processes, including the sleep–wake cycle, core body temperature, blood pressure, task performance, metabolic cycles, and synthesis and secretion of several hormones, such as melatonin and cortisol [2].

Although anchored genetically, circadian rhythms are synchronized (entrained) by exogenous factors (time cues, or *zeitgebers*), especially the light–dark (LD) cycle coordinating the cycles with solar time. When external time cues are suppressed or removed, e.g., in constant darkness, the rhythms will persist with a period deviating slightly from the 24-hour diurnal cycle [3]. In a controlled laboratory environment the intrinsic period of the human biological clock is approximately 24.2 hours, with quite small inter- and intra-individual variances [4]. However, a large-scale epidemiologic study in the community revealed that in this population the clock follows a Gaussian curve so that extreme early types wake up when extreme late types fall asleep [5].

It is now well established that light is the predominant synchronizer of circadian rhythms [6]. Light shifts human circadian rhythms according to a phase response curve so that exposure in the early subjective night delays the timing of the circadian clock, while exposure in the late subjective night delays the clock [7–11]. Light signals from the retina act on a population of sensitive cells in the SCN, which in turn acts both on other areas of the SCN and via an indirect pathway to influence the pineal gland [12, 13]. The pineal enzyme, arylalkylamine N-acetyltransferase (AA-NAT), which is rate limiting for melatonin synthesis, is acutely suppressed by this light signal so that melatonin levels drop very rapidly [14]. Under normal conditions, melatonin secretion increases

Sleep and Mental Illness, eds. S. R. Pandi-Perumal and M. Kramer. Published by Cambridge University Press.
© Cambridge University Press 2010.

soon after the onset of darkness, peaks in the middle of the night (between 02:00 and 04:00 hours), and gradually falls during the second half of the night reaching basal levels in the morning. Peak levels can be more than 100 times basal levels. Melatonin, however, is acutely suppressed under low levels of light exposure with as little as 300 lux being capable of decreasing melatonin levels in blood or saliva [15–17].

While the 24-hour melatonin rhythm is strongly suppressed by bright light, unlike other rhythms, it remains generally uninfluenced by the other external factors [18]. The measurement of circulating melatonin levels in dim light (<10 lux) is therefore preferred for assessing circadian phase.

Similar to the effects of light, exogenous administration of the pineal hormone melatonin induces phase changes in circadian rhythms, either by accelerating (phase advance) or slowing them down (phase delay). The direction of the shift depends on the time that exogenous melatonin is administered: when administered five hours before DLMO the melatonin rhythm is maximally advanced, while administrations made ten hours after DLMO will maximally delay the melatonin rhythm, thus the phase response curve is about twelve hours out of phase with that to light [19, 20].

Several physiological 24-hour rhythms, including those of cortisol, melatonin, temperature, and sleep–wake rhythm, have been used as markers of the circadian phase. All are influenced to some extent and can even be masked by external factors such as food, exercise, and temperature and the sleep–wake cycle itself, which has a weak synchronizing effect [18]. In a comparison of temperature, cortisol and eight different analysis methods for melatonin, the variability of melatonin as a marker for circadian rhythms was superior [21].

Dim light melatonin onset

The 24-hour melatonin rhythm can be assessed by measuring melatonin in blood or saliva at regular intervals, and usually this is done hourly. While measurement of the entire 24-hour rhythm of melatonin is thought to be the most robust phase marker, it is also time consuming and inconvenient for the patient, and therefore this protocol is not frequently employed in clinical studies. The DLMO, the time at which melatonin levels start to rise in dim light, is considered a reliable marker of circadian phase [21]. Typically, in clinical studies, the moment at which melatonin production starts increasing in the evening (the DLMO) is used as an indication of the circadian phase.

Dim light melatonin onset was initially defined as the time at which a melatonin concentration of 10 pg/ml was reached in blood. This level was chosen in an era when blood melatonin levels of less than 10 pg/ml could not be detected. Later, when new quantification technology became available, it was possible to detect lower melatonin levels both in blood and saliva. It is currently possible to measure salivary melatonin levels of about 0.5 pg/ml. This enhanced measurement capability demonstrated that salivary melatonin levels have a correlation of about 0.93 with their concentration in blood although levels are about 40% as high [22, 23]. Consequently salivary DLMO has been defined by several authors as the time at which 4 pg/ml was reached in saliva [24]. Because of the convenience to both researchers and patients of measuring melatonin levels in saliva rather than blood, this has become a widely used technique both in research and clinical practice.

An alternate method proposed for establishing the DLMO is calculation of the interpolated time point where the melatonin level exceeds the mean of a number of previous samples by two standard deviations [25]. More recently, a method has been described that is reported to make it possible to assess the 24-hour melatonin rhythm by fitting a predetermined curve through a reduced number of measurements [22]. This method has been proposed not only as a means of estimating the DLMO, but also the melatonin offset time, the melatonin peak, and the peak width.

A group of workshop leaders came together on their own following a 2005 Associated Professional Sleep Societies workshop, assessed benefits and disadvantages of current methods of collecting and analyzing melatonin and concluded that although a single method of analysis would be the most effective way to compare studies, limitations of current methods preclude this possibility [26]. Given that the best analysis method for use under multiple conditions is not established, this group recommended that one of the established low threshold measures of DLMO (e.g., 2 SD, or <10 pg/ml for plasma or <3 pg/ml for saliva) be included in any published report to facilitate comparison between studies.

It is known that activity and postural changes increase melatonin levels and that these effects are reversed rapidly [27]. Thus postural changes should be minimized just prior to and during collection of blood or saliva samples.

However, despite these recommendations it is known that there can be a huge difference between individuals in the peak melatonin levels whether studied by measuring blood levels or urinary output, and that this difference is stable within individuals [28–30]. Thus one person may have a peak blood level around 10 pg/ml and another person a peak that exceeds 100 pg/ml. This can provide such great difficulty in using a fixed level for the DLMO that an alternate marker may be preferable [31]. To ensure that low melatonin levels are not a problem it would be advisable to obtain a measure of peak melatonin, whether by sampling blood, saliva, or urine.

In healthy adults and children (aged 6 to 12 years) with a normally functioning biological clock, DLMO usually occurs between 19:30 and 21:30 hours and between 19:00 and 21:00 hours respectively [32].

Clinical significance of DLMO

Since DLMO is a reliable phase marker of the biological clock [21], its measurement helps considerably in the diagnosis of circadian rhythm disorders. The measurement of DLMO has helped to clarify certain poorly understood signs and symptoms of several disorders that are thought to result from disturbed circadian rhythms. Treatment of the underlying circadian rhythm disorder has often been shown to produce remarkable clinical improvement. Among the disorders that have been shown by DLMO measurement to involve disruptions to circadian rhythms are chronic sleep onset insomnia in children with [33] and without [34, 35] attention-deficit/hyperactivity disorder (ADHD), chronic whiplash syndrome [36], and chronic fatigue syndrome [37, 38].

Dim light melatonin onset is not only important for diagnosing circadian rhythm disorders, it is also important for the adequate timing of their treatment. As noted above, bright light delays melatonin (and other associated biological clock rhythms, such as the sleep–wake rhythm) if it is applied during the rising part of the 24-hour melatonin curve but advances biological clock rhythms if applied during the decreasing part of the melatonin curve. Similar but inverse effects can be induced with exogenous melatonin. When administered five hours before the DLMO, exogenous melatonin advances biological rhythms

maximally, and, conversely, when administered ten hours after the DLMO, it produces a maximal delay in these rhythms [19, 20].

A meta-analysis of studies of melatonin's effects in insomniac patients with delayed DLMO concluded that melatonin evidently advances sleep onset and other sleep–wake rhythm parameters but that the treatment must be strategically timed [39]. A study by Mundey et al. found that melatonin shifts circadian rhythms most when administered five to six hours before DLMO, thus demonstrating the importance of measuring the timing of DLMO as a guide for therapy [40]. Buscemi et al. concluded that the administration of exogenous melatonin in patients with insomnia was generally ineffective, but their meta-analysis did not take into account the timing of the DLMO [41].

A study in children with idiopathic chronic sleep onset insomnia and late DLMO showed that the earlier melatonin was administered before DLMO, the more advanced DLMO and sleep onset time [42]. This finding was confirmed in a study with children with ADHD and chronic sleep onset insomnia [43]. Taken together these studies support the conclusion that measurement of the DLMO not only aids the diagnosis and treatment of circadian rhythm sleep–wake disorders, it also helps to predict treatment effects.

Measurement of DLMO

Dim light melatonin onset can be measured by sampling blood or saliva at regular intervals: at least once every hour although some authors use more frequent sampling [31]. In clinical practice DLMO is often measured in saliva, since saliva can be collected easily at home. In the Dutch national referral center of sleep–wake disturbances and chronobiology, headed by one of the authors of this chapter, the parents of children who are suspected of having delayed circadian rhythms are asked to assist in this process. Parents of children aged 6 to 12 years are asked to collect saliva hourly between 19:00 and 23:00 hours. For adolescents aged 13 to 16 the recommended saliva collection schedule is hourly between 20:00 and 24:00 hours, while patients over 16 years are asked to make saliva collections hourly between 21:00 and 01:00 hours [32]. The saliva is then sent to the laboratory by regular mail and reaches the laboratory within three to five days. We have found this home collection procedure to be effective in determining DLMO in about 80% of patients. In the remaining 20%, saliva has to be collected additionally at other times.

Dim light melatonin onset in psychiatric and medical disorders

The measurement of DLMO in medical or psychiatric conditions that are often associated with biological clock disorders can often clarify whether these rhythmic disturbances are present and, if so, the degree of their severity. These medical and psychiatric conditions are summarized here.

Delayed sleep phase syndrome

Delayed sleep phase syndrome (DSPS) is one of the most frequently occurring circadian rhythm disorders. It is characterized by an abnormally delayed sleep–wake rhythm. The major symptoms are extreme difficulty in initiating sleep at a conventional hour of the night and great difficulty in waking up on time in the morning for school or work. Most patients are tired during the day [44]. In a sleep disorder clinic population, DSPS is often associated with major depression [45]. Delayed sleep phase syndrome patients may present with chronic sleep onset insomnia, difficulty in waking up in the morning, tiredness during the day, sleepiness during the day, and symptoms sometimes mimicking narcolepsy, or depression.

Delayed sleep phase syndrome is associated with a polymorphism of the PER3 clock gene [46, 47]. An association with the arylalkylamine N-acetyltransferase (AA-NAT) gene has also been reported [48].

Chronotherapy was the first treatment described for this circadian rhythm disorder [49]. However, long-term results usually are poor [50]. Another treatment for delayed sleep phase syndrome is bright light in the morning [51]. The most frequently reported treatment is melatonin, administered five hours before DLMO [52, 53]. This treatment is reported to both advance the phase of melatonin and to improve symptoms.

Advanced sleep phase syndrome

Advanced sleep phase syndrome (ASPS) is the counterpart of DSPS. It is characterized by extreme sleepiness in the evening or early at night and early morning awakenings.

Many patients say that they cannot go to the theater in the evening because they always fall asleep or else complain that they awaken early in the morning (say 3:00 hours) and cannot sleep any more.

Advanced sleep phase syndrome is associated with a polymorphism of the Per2 clock gene within the casein kinase I (CKI)-binding domain [54, 55]. Extreme morning preference is also associated with a mis-sense of this gene [56]. A mis-sense mutation (T44A) in the human CKI delta gene, which results in ASPS, has also been reported [57]. The preferred treatments for ASPS are administration of bright light in the evening, or administration of exogenous melatonin ten hours after DLMO [58].

Seasonal affective disorder

Seasonal affective disorder (SAD) is characterized by recurrent episodes of depression during winter months, and euthymia or hypomania in spring or summer. The leading hypothesis of SAD is the phase shift hypothesis (PSH). According to this hypothesis the melatonin rhythm in SAD patients during the winter is either advanced (mimicking ASPS), or delayed (mimicking DSPS). The PSH was recently given support by a study in which SAD patients were given low-dose melatonin in the afternoon/evening to promote phase advances, or in the morning to promote phase delays, or placebo. The prototypical phase-delayed patient, as well as the smaller subgroup of phase-advanced patients, optimally responded to melatonin given at the correct time. Symptom severity improved as circadian misalignment was corrected. Circadian misalignment is best measured as the time interval between the DLMO and mid-sleep. The average interval between DLMO and mid-sleep in healthy controls is six hours, which is associated with optimal mood in SAD patients [59].

Bipolar affective disorder

Bipolar affective disorder is characterized by the occurrence of mania or hypomania either preceded or followed by episodes of depression. Three studies have demonstrated that the phase of melatonin secretion varies systematically with mood changes in bipolar affective disorder [60–62]. Hypersensitivity to light may be a major trait marker [63, 64] although one study failed to confirm supersensitivity [62]. There is evidence that melatonin supersensitivity to light is an inherited trait suggesting its usefulness as a potential endophenotypic marker of bipolar affective disorder [65].

Several studies have shown that phototherapy and chronotherapy are effective treatments in bipolar illness. Exposure to morning sunlight has been reported to reduce the length of hospitalization in bipolar patients [66]. In a single case study, a rapid cycling bipolar patient was successfully treated using an extended controlled dark period combined with morning light treatment [67]. There is also evidence that light therapy causes a rapid antidepressant response in bipolar illness when combined with sleep deprivation [68, 69] and that this effect is more marked in homozygotes for the long variant of the serotonin transporter (5-HTTLPR) [70]. In one study, bipolar type 1 patients were reported to respond best when treatment was given at midday [71]. In contrast there are few studies supporting the use of melatonin in bipolar affective disorder [72, 73]. A pilot study of manic patients with treatment-resistant insomnia reported a significant improvement in both sleep and mania following melatonin add-on treatment [74]. Whether DLMO would be useful in studies of these patients has yet to be determined.

Major depressive disorder

The diagnosis of major depressive disorder is made when patients suffer for more than two weeks from depressed mood, markedly diminished interest in work, significant weight loss, insomnia or hypersomnia, psychomotor agitation, fatigue or loss of energy, feelings of worthlessness, diminished ability to concentrate, or recurrent thoughts of death [75].

The nature and extent of disruption of melatonin secretion in major depressive disorder has been under intense investigation during the last few decades, ever since Wetterberg and coworkers formulated the "low melatonin syndrome" hypothesis in 1984 [76]. It has been suggested that the low melatonin levels seen in depressives might be due to reduced norepinephrine and serotonin levels in the brain [77]. Unipolar patients with low melatonin syndrome are reported to differ clinically from patients with normal or high melatonin secretion in having low psychomotor retardation [78]. Proper identification of these subgroups of patients may be helpful for optimal pharmacotherapy.

Agomelatine is a novel melatonergic antidepressant drug. Agomelatine combines antidepressant efficacy, including quality and efficiency of sleep, with a more favorable side-effect profile than current antidepressant treatments, including neutral effects on sexual function, body weight, and the absence of discontinuation symptoms. These positive features provide a novel approach to the treatment of depression and the attainment of high-quality remission in major depressive disorder [79].

Future studies will reveal if patients with a low melatonin syndrome or with altered DLMO respond better than other patients.

Attention-deficit/hyperactivity disorder and chronic insomnia

About 30% of medication-free children with ADHD suffer from chronic sleep onset insomnia [80, 81]. Van der Heijden reported that this insomnia is caused by a circadian rhythm disorder, characterized by a delayed DLMO [82]. A regimen of 3 or 6 mg melatonin taken at 19:00 hours for four weeks was found to advance sleep onset but did not improve behavior [42].

At the Dutch referral center for sleep–wake disorders and chronobiology, about 500 children with ADHD and chronic insomnia are treated every year with melatonin. Many caregivers report that behavior improves after two or three months of melatonin treatment.

Also, in adults with ADHD and chronic insomnia, DLMO often is delayed. Well timed treatment with melatonin improves sleep and enhances the effectiveness of methylphenidate on behavior (S. Kooij, personal communication).

Chronic fatigue syndrome

Chronic fatigue syndrome (CFS) is characterized by chronic fatigue of unknown cause [83]. A subset of CFS patients may possibly be classified as having DSPS, with chronic fatigue as their main problem [38, 84]. It has been suggested that in other CFS patients the main difficulty may be a disruption of the neuronal connection between SCN and pineal gland, possibly due to an infection. As a consequence of these disorders melatonin production starts later rather than at the normal time. A third explanation is that daily activity of CFS patients changes so that a delay in the sleep–wake rhythm occurs, mimicking DSPS [38, 84].

Open-label studies using administration of exogenous melatonin timed using DLMO, have shown that melatonin rhythm can be advanced, health status improved, and fatigue decreased [38, 84].

Chronic whiplash syndrome and mild cerebral trauma

Chronic whiplash syndrome (CWS) is characterized by symptoms of fatigue and impaired memory. Many CWS patients suffer from insomnia [85]. In some CWS patients DLMO is delayed indicating that melatonin production starts later than normal [86–88].

As in patients with mild cerebral trauma, damage may occur in the neuronal connections between the SCN and the pineal gland, resulting in delayed DLMO and sleep–wake rhythm disturbances [89].

At the Dutch referral center for sleep–wake disorders and chronobiology, every year about 50 CWS patients with delayed DLMO are treated with melatonin. We have found that most sleep better and in about half of these patients daily functioning improves.

Conclusion

DLMO measurements are not generally available. Therefore many patients with circadian rhythm disorders are treated without confirmation of their DLMO. When therapy is successful, there is no problem. However, when it does not work, optimal treatment is unnecessarily delayed. This is because it may take several months after stopping the treatment before the pretreatment melatonin rhythm is reached again and a proper diagnosis can be made. The Dutch referral center for sleep–wake disorders and chronobiology recommends that the timing of DLMO be measured before undertaking therapy, especially if this involves melatonin [90].

To prevent unnecessary "doctor delay" Dutch chronobiologists have facilitated access to DLMO measurements. The referring doctor sends information to a central laboratory. The laboratory dispatches salivettes to the patient. The patient sends these to the laboratory and the lab informs the referring doctor about the results.

This method is going to be made available to other countries in the world. Facilitating DLMO measurements will increase awareness of circadian rhythm disorders in an increasing number of diseases, and will help their optimal treatment. A list of laboratories where DLMO can be measured is published at www.dlmo.org.

There is still no internationally agreed method of analysis and definitions for DLMO, and the issue of the huge variability in profiles and peaks between individuals are unresolved. It is recommended that activity and postural changes be minimized just prior to and during collection of blood or saliva samples. It is recommended that anyone using and reporting on DLMO use one of the established methods when reporting results and be aware of the possible limitations of current procedures [26].

References

1. Hastings M, O'Neill JS, Maywood ES. Circadian clocks: regulators of endocrine and metabolic rhythms. *J Endocrinol.* 2007;**195**:187–98.

2. Hastings MH, Maywood ES, Reddy AB. Two decades of circadian time. *J Neuroendocrinol.* 2008;**20**:812–19.

3. Saper CB, Scammell TE, Lu J. Hypothalamic regulation of sleep and circadian rhythms. *Nature.* 2005;**437**:1257–63.

4. Czeisler CA, Duffy JF, Shanahan TL, *et al.* Stability, precision, and near-24-hour period of the human circadian pacemaker. *Science.* 1999;**284**:2177–81.

5. Roenneberg T, Kuehnle T, Juda M, *et al.* Epidemiology of the human circadian clock. *Sleep Med Rev.* 2007;**11**:429–38.

6. Czeisler CA, Gooley JJ. Sleep and circadian rhythms in humans. *Cold Spring Harb Symp Quant Biol.* 2007;**72**:579–97.

7. Czeisler CA, Kronauer RE, Allan JS, *et al.* Bright light induction of strong (type 0) resetting of the human circadian pacemaker. *Science.* 1989;**244**:1328–33.

8. Khalsa SB, Jewett ME, Cajochen C, Czeisler CA. A phase response curve to single bright light pulses in human subjects. *J Physiol.* 2003;**549**:945–52.

9. Skene DJ. Optimization of light and melatonin to phase-shift human circadian rhythms. *J Neuroendocrinol.* 2003;**15**:438–41.

10. Lewy AJ, Sack RA, Singer CL. Assessment and treatment of chronobiologic disorders using plasma melatonin levels and bright light exposure: the clock-gate model and the phase response curve. *Psychopharmacol Bulletin.* 1984;**20**:561–5.

11. Zeitzer JM, Dijk DJ, Kronauer R, Brown E, Czeisler C. Sensitivity of the human circadian pacemaker to nocturnal light: melatonin phase resetting and suppression. *J Physiol.* 2000;**526** Pt 3:695–702.

12. Lee HS, Billings HJ, Lehman MN. The suprachiasmatic nucleus: a clock of multiple components. *J Biol Rhythms.* 2003;**18**:435–49.

13. Moore RY. Suprachiasmatic nucleus in sleep-wake regulation. *Sleep Med.* 2007;**8** Suppl 3:27–33.

135

14. Klein DC. Arylalkylamine N-acetyltransferase: "the Timenzyme". *J Biol Chem.* 2007;**282**:4233–7.

15. Aoki H, Yamada N, Ozeki Y, Yamane H, Kato N. Minimum light intensity required to suppress nocturnal melatonin concentration in human saliva. *Neurosci Lett.* 1998;**252**:91–4.

16. McIntyre IM, Norman TR, Burrows GD, Armstrong SM. Human melatonin suppression by light is intensity dependent. *J Pineal Res.* 1989;**6**:149–56.

17. Lewy AJ, Wehr TA, Goodwin FK, Newsome DA, Markey SP. Light suppresses melatonin secretion in humans. *Science.* 1980;**210**:1267–9.

18. Mistlberger RE, Skene DJ. Nonphotic entrainment in humans? *J Biol Rhythms.* 2005;**20**:339–52.

19. Lewy AJ, Ahmed S, Jackson JM, Sack RL. Melatonin shifts human circadian rhythms according to a phase-response curve. *Chronobiol Int.* 1992;**9**:380–92.

20. Lewy AJ, Bauer VK, Ahmed S, *et al.* The human phase response curve (PRC) to melatonin is about 12 hours out of phase with the PRC to light. *Chronobiol Int.* 1998;**15**:71–83.

21. Klerman EB, Gershengorn HB, Duffy JF, Kronauer RE. Comparisons of the variability of three markers of the human circadian pacemaker. *J Biol Rhythms.* 2002;**17**:181–93.

22. Van Someren EJ, Nagtegaal E. Improving melatonin circadian phase estimates. *Sleep Med.* 2007;**8**:590–601.

23. Leibenluft E, Feldman-Naim S, Turner EH, Schwartz PJ, Wehr TA. Salivary and plasma measures of dim light melatonin onset (DLMO) in patients with rapid cycling bipolar disorder. *Biol Psychiatry.* 1996;**40**:731–5.

24. Nagtegaal E, Peeters T, Swart W, *et al.* Correlation between concentrations of melatonin in saliva and serum in patients with delayed sleep phase syndrome. *Ther Drug Monit.* 1998;**20**:181–3.

25. Voultsios A, Kennaway DJ, Dawson D. Salivary melatonin as a circadian phase marker: validation and comparison to plasma melatonin. *J Biol Rhythms.* 1997;**12**:457–66.

26. Benloucif S, Burgess HJ, Klerman EB, *et al.* Measuring melatonin in humans. *J Clin Sleep Med.* 2008;**4**:66–9.

27. Deacon S, Arendt J. Posture influences melatonin concentrations in plasma and saliva in humans. *Neurosci Lett.* 1994;**167**:191–4.

28. Bergiannaki JD, Soldatos CR, Paparrigopoulos TJ, Syrengelas M, Stefanis CN. Low and high melatonin excretors among healthy individuals. *J Pineal Res.* 1995;**18**:159–64.

29. Grof E, Grof P, Brown GM, Arato M, Lane J. Investigations of melatonin secretion in man. *Prog Neuropsychopharmacol Biol Psychiat.* 1985;**9**:609–12.

30. Travis RC, Allen NE, Peeters PH, van Noord PA, Key TJ. Reproducibility over 5 years of measurements of 6-sulphatoxymelatonin in urine samples from postmenopausal women. *Cancer Epidemiol Biomarkers Prev.* 2003;**12**:806–8.

31. Lewy AJ, Cutler NL, Sack RL. The endogenous melatonin profile as a marker for circadian phase position. *J Biol Rhythms.* 1999;**14**:227–36.

32. Pandi-Perumal SR, Smits M, Spence W, *et al.* Dim light melatonin onset (DLMO): a tool for the analysis of circadian phase in human sleep and chronobiological disorders. *Prog Neuropsychopharmacol Biol Psychiatry.* 2007;**31**:1–11.

33. Van der Heijden KB, Smits MG, Van Someren EW, Gunning WB. Reply to Jenni. Childhood chronic sleep onset insomnia and late sleep onset: What's the difference? *J Sleep Res.* 2005;**14**:197–9.

34. Smits MG, Nagtegaal EE, van der HJ, Coenen AM, Kerkhof GA. Melatonin for chronic sleep onset insomnia in children: a randomized placebo-controlled trial. *J Child Neurol.* 2001;**16**:86–92.

35. Smits MG, van Stel HF, van der HK, *et al.* Melatonin improves health status and sleep in children with idiopathic chronic sleep-onset insomnia: a randomized placebo-controlled trial. *J Am Acad Child Adolesc Psychiatry.* 2003;**42**:1286–93.

36. Smits MG. Whiplash injury may deregulate the biological clock. *J Neurol Neurosurg Psychiatry.* **2005**;76:1044.

37. Nagtegaal JE, Laurant MW, Kerkhof GA, *et al.* Effects of melatonin on the quality of life in patients with delayed sleep phase syndrome. *J Psychosom Res.* 2000;**48**:45–50.

38. van Heukelom RO, Prins JB, Smits MG, Bleijenberg G. Influence of melatonin on fatigue severity in patients with chronic fatigue syndrome and late melatonin secretion. *Eur J Neurol.* 2006;**13**:55–60.

39. Smits MG, Geijlswijk I. Exogenous melatonin for delayed sleep phase syndrome: meta-analysis. *J Sleep Res.* 2008;**17**:1.

40. Mundey K, Benloucif S, Harsanyi K, Dubocovich ML, Zee PC. Phase-dependent treatment of delayed sleep phase syndrome with melatonin. *Sleep.* 2005;**28**:1271–8.

41. Buscemi N, Vandermeer B, Hooton N, *et al.* Efficacy and safety of exogenous melatonin for secondary sleep disorders and sleep disorders accompanying sleep restriction: meta-analysis. *BMJ.* 2006;**332**:385–93.

42. Van der Heijden KB, Smits MG, Van Someren EJ, Boudewijn GW. Prediction of melatonin efficacy by pretreatment dim light melatonin onset in children

with idiopathic chronic sleep onset insomnia. *J Sleep Res.* 2005;**14**:187–94.

43. Van der Heijden KB, Smits MG, Van Someren EJ, Ridderinkhof KR, Gunning WB. Effect of melatonin on sleep, behavior, and cognition in ADHD and chronic sleep-onset insomnia. *J Am Acad Child Adolesc Psychiatry.* 2007;**46**:233–41.

44. Weitzman ED, Czeisler CA, Coleman RM, *et al.* Delayed sleep phase syndrome. A chronobiological disorder with sleep-onset insomnia. *Arch Gen Psychiatry.* 1981;**38**:737–46.

45. Regestein QR, Monk TH. Delayed sleep phase syndrome: a review of its clinical aspects. *Am J Psychiatry.* 1995;**152**:602–8.

46. Archer SN, Robilliard DL, Skene DJ, *et al.* A length polymorphism in the circadian clock gene Per3 is linked to delayed sleep phase syndrome and extreme diurnal preference. *Sleep.* 2003;**26**:413–15.

47. Pereira DS, Tufik S, Louzada FM, *et al.* Association of the length polymorphism in the human Per3 gene with the delayed sleep-phase syndrome: does latitude have an influence upon it? *Sleep.* 2005;**28**:29–32.

48. Hohjoh H, Takasu M, Shishikura K, Takahashi Y, Honda Y, Tokunaga K. Significant association of the arylalkylamine N-acetyltransferase (AA-NAT) gene with delayed sleep phase syndrome. *Neurogenetics.* 2003;**4**:151–3.

49. Czeisler CA, Richardson GS, Coleman RM, *et al.* Chronotherapy: resetting the circadian clocks of patients with delayed sleep phase insomnia. *Sleep.* 1981;**4**:1–21.

50. Wagner DR. Disorders of the circadian sleep–wake cycle. *Neurologic Clinics.* 1996;**14**:651–70.

51. Cole RJ, Smith JS, Alcala YC, Elliott JA, Kripke DF. Bright-light mask treatment of delayed sleep phase syndrome. *J Biol Rhythms.* 2002;**17**:89–101.

52. Nagtegaal JE, Kerkhof GA, Smits MG, Swart AC, van der Meer YG. Delayed sleep phase syndrome: A placebo-controlled cross-over study on the effects of melatonin administered five hours before the individual dim light melatonin onset. *J Sleep Res.* 1998;**7**:135–43.

53. Mundey K, Benloucif S, Harsanyi K, Dubocovich ML, Zee PC. Phase-dependent treatment of delayed sleep phase syndrome with melatonin. *Sleep.* 2005;**28**:1271–8.

54. Toh KL, Jones CR, He Y, *et al.* An hPer2 phosphorylation site mutation in familial advanced sleep phase syndrome. *Science.* 2001;**291**:1040–3.

55. Vanselow K, Vanselow JT, Westermark PO, *et al.* Differential effects of PER2 phosphorylation: molecular basis for the human familial advanced sleep phase syndrome (FASPS). *Genes Dev.* 2006;**20**:2660–72.

56. Carpen JD, Archer SN, Skene DJ, Smits M, von SM. A single-nucleotide polymorphism in the 5′-untranslated region of the hPER2 gene is associated with diurnal preference. *J Sleep Res.* 2005;**14**:293–7.

57. Xu Y, Padiath QS, Shapiro RE, *et al.* Functional consequences of a CKIdelta mutation causing familial advanced sleep phase syndrome. *Nature.* 2005;**434**:640–4.

58. Pandi-Perumal SR, Trakht I, Spence DW, *et al.* The roles of melatonin and light in the pathophysiology and treatment of circadian rhythm sleep disorders. *Nat Clin Pract Neurol.* 2008;**4**:436–47.

59. Lewy AJ, Rough JN, Songer JB, *et al.* The phase shift hypothesis for the circadian component of winter depression. *Dialogues Clin Neurosci.* 2007;**9**:291–300.

60. Lewy AJ, Wehr TA, Gold PW, Goodwin FK. Melatonin secretion in manic-depressive illness. In: Obiols J, Ballus C, Gonzalez E, Pujol J, eds. *Biological Psychiatry Today.* (Amsterdam: Elsevier/North-Holland Biomedical Press, 1979; 563–5).

61. Kennedy SH, Tighe S, McVey G, Brown GM. Melatonin and cortisol "switches" during mania, depression, and euthymia in a drug-free bipolar patient. *J Nervous and Mental Disease.* 1989;**177**:300–3.

62. Nurnberger JI, Jr., Adkins S, Lahiri DK, *et al.* Melatonin suppression by light in euthymic bipolar and unipolar patients. *Arch Gen Psychiatry.* 2000;**57**:572–9.

63. Lewy AJ, Nurnberger JI, Jr., Wehr TA, *et al.* Supersensitivity to light: possible trait marker for manic-depressive illness. *Am J Psychiatry.* 1985;**142**:725–7.

64. Nathan PJ, Burrows GD, Norman TR. Melatonin sensitivity to dim white light in affective disorders. *Neuropsychopharmacology.* 1999;**21**:408–13.

65. Hallam KT, Olver JS, Chambers V, *et al.* The heritability of melatonin secretion and sensitivity to bright nocturnal light in twins. *Psychoneuroendocrinol.* 2006;**31**:867–75.

66. Benedetti F, Colombo C, Barbini B, Campori E, Smeraldi E. Morning sunlight reduces length of hospitalization in bipolar depression. *J Affect Disord.* 2001;**62**:221–3.

67. Wirz-Justice A, Quinto C, Cajochen C, Werth E, Hock C. A rapid-cycling bipolar patient treated with long nights, bedrest, and light. *Biol Psychiatry.* 1999;**45**:1075–7.

68. Benedetti F, Dallaspezia S, Fulgosi MC, *et al.* Phase advance is an actimetric correlate of antidepressant

response to sleep deprivation and light therapy in bipolar depression. *Chronobiol Int.* 2007;**24**:921–37.

69. Colombo C, Lucca A, Benedetti F, *et al.* Total sleep deprivation combined with lithium and light therapy in the treatment of bipolar depression: replication of main effects and interaction. *Psychiatry Res.* 2000;**95**:43–53.

70. Benedetti F, Colombo C, Serretti A, *et al.* Antidepressant effects of light therapy combined with sleep deprivation are influenced by a functional polymorphism within the promoter of the serotonin transporter gene. *Biol Psychiatry.* 2003;**54**:687–92.

71. Sit D, Wisner KL, Hanusa BH, Stull S, Terman M. Light therapy for bipolar disorder: a case series in women. *Bipolar Disord.* 2007;**9**:918–27.

72. Tuunainen A, Kripke DF, Endo T. Light therapy for non-seasonal depression. *Cochrane Database Syst Rev.* 2004;**2**:CD004050.

73. Grunhaus L, Hirschman S, Dolberg OT, Schreiber S, Dannon PN. Coadministration of melatonin and fluoxetine does not improve the 3-month outcome following ECT. *J ECT.* 2001;**17**:124–8.

74. Bersani G, Garavini A. Melatonin add-on in manic patients with treatment resistant insomnia. *Prog Neuropsychopharmacol Biol Psychiatry.* 2000;**24**:185–91.

75. American Psychiatric Association. *Diagnostic and Statistical Manual of Mental Disorders,* 4th edn (*DSM-IV-TR*). (Washington, DC: American Psychiatric Press, 2000).

76. Beck-Friis J, von Rosen D, Kjellman BF, Ljunggren J-G, Wetterberg L. Melatonin in relation to body size measures, sex, age, season and the use of drugs in patients with major affective disorders and healthy subjects. *Psychoneuroendocrinol.* 1984;**9**:261–77.

77. Arendt J. Melatonin: a new probe in psychiatric investigation? *Br J Psychiatry.* 1989;**155**:585–90.

78. Wahlund B, Grahn H, Saaf J, Wetterberg L. Affective disorder subtyped by psychomotor symptoms, monoamine oxidase, melatonin and cortisol: identification of patients with latent bipolar disorder. *Eur Arch Psychiatry Clin Neurosci.* 1998;**248**:215–24.

79. Lam R. Addressing circadian rhythm disturbances in depressed patients. *J Psychopharmacol.* 2008;**22**:13–18.

80. Stein MA. Unravelling sleep problems in treated and untreated children with ADHD. *J Child Adolesc Psychopharmacol.* 1999;**9**:157–68.

81. Corkum P, Moldofsky H, Hogg-Johnson S, Humphries T, Tannock R. Sleep problems in children with attention-deficit/hyperactivity disorder: impact of subtype, comorbidity, and stimulant medication. *J Am Acad Child Adolesc Psychiatry.* 1999;**38**:1285–93.

82. Van der Heijden KB, Smits MG, Van Someren EJ, Gunning WB. Idiopathic chronic sleep onset insomnia in attention-deficit/hyperactivity disorder: a circadian rhythm sleep disorder. *Chronobiol Int.* 2005;**22**:559–70.

83. Wyller VB. The chronic fatigue syndrome – an update. *Acta Neurol Scand Suppl.* 2007;**187**:7–14.

84. Smits MG, Rooij RV, Nagtegaal JE. Influence of melatonin on quality of life in patients with chronic fatigue and late melatonin onset. *JCFS.* 2000;**48**:45–50.

85. Schlesinger I, Hering-Hanit R, Dagan Y. Sleep disturbances after whiplash injury: objective and subjective findings. *Headache.* 2001;**41**:586–9.

86. Nagtegaal JE, Kerkhof GA, Smits MG, Swart AC, van der Meer YG. Traumatic brain injury-associated delayed sleep phase syndrome. *Funct Neurol.* 1997;**12**:345–8.

87. Smits MG, Nagtegaal JE. Post-traumatic delayed sleep phase syndrome. *Neurology.* 2000;**55**:902–3.

88. Wieringen SV, Jansen T, Smits MG, Nagtegaal JE, Coenen AML. Melatonin for chronic whiplash syndrome with delayed melatonin onset. Randomised, placebo-controlled trial. *Clin Drug Invest.* 2001;**21**:813–20.

89. Ayalon L, Borodkin K, Dishon L, Kanety H, Dagan Y. Circadian rhythm sleep disorders following mild traumatic brain injury. *Neurology.* 2007;**68**:1136–40.

90. Smits M. Measure dim light melatonin onset before prescribing melatonin treatment. *J Sleep Res.* 2008;**17**:1.

Classification of sleep disorders

Imran M. Ahmed and Michael J. Thorpy

Introduction

The International Classification of Sleep Disorders (ICSD-2) [1] classification lists 85 sleep disorders in eight major categories, each presented in detail with a descriptive diagnostic text that includes specific diagnostic criteria: (1) the *insomnias*; (2) the *sleep-related breathing disorders*; (3) the *hypersomnias not due to a breathing disorder*; (4) the *circadian rhythm sleep disorders*; (5) the *parasomnias*; (6) *the sleep-related movement disorders;* (7) *other sleep disorders*; and (8) *isolated symptoms, apparently normal variants and unresolved issues.* The ICSD-2 also includes in its appendices: *Sleep disorders that are associated with conditions classifiable elsewhere* (Appendix A); as well as *Other psychiatric and behavioral disorders frequently encountered in the differential diagnosis of sleep disorders* (Appendix B) (see Table 13.1).

Insomnias

The insomnias are defined by the symptom of difficulty with sleep initiation and/or maintenance, and final awakenings that occur earlier than the desired wake-up time. There can also be a complaint of non-restorative sleep or poor sleep quality. Such symptoms occur despite adequate time and opportunity for sleep and result in some form of daytime impairment. The insomnias can be either primary or secondary. Secondary forms of insomnia can occur when insomnia is a symptom of a medical or psychiatric illness, other sleep disorders, or substance abuse. Primary sleep disorders are those that can have both intrinsic and extrinsic factors involved in their etiology but are not regarded as having causes secondary

to those disorders that can result in (secondary) insomnia. Although not specifically discussed in the ICSD-2, the term *comorbid insomnia* is now championed by many sleep experts as the more appropriate term to describe many secondary insomnias. In comorbid insomnia, the insomnia is usually associated with an underlying psychiatric or medical disorder and it can be difficult to discern whether the insomnia preceded or resulted from the psychiatric or medical condition. In either case, when the underlying medical or psychiatric disorder remits, the insomnia often will persist. Accordingly, for optimal patient care, it is essential to treat both the underlying psychiatric or medical disorder as well as the insomnia at the same time.

The ICSD-2 classifies six main types of insomnia and three secondary forms of insomnia; however, *primary insomnia* as described in the *Diagnostic and Statistical Manual of Mental Disorders*, 4th edition, text revision (DSM IV-TR) [36], subsumes these six main insomnia diagnoses (namely, adjustment insomnia, behavioral insomnia of childhood, psychophysiological insomnia, paradoxical insomnia, idiopathic insomnia, and inadequate sleep hygiene).

Psychophysiological insomnia [2, 3, 4] is a common form of insomnia that is present for at least one month and characterized by a heightened level of arousal with learned sleep-preventing associations. Such sleep-preventing associations may be learned during episodes of insomnia associated with conditions such as depression, shift work, or environmental noise. The insomnia is then sustained by the learned behavior in the absence of the triggers. There is usually an overconcern with the inability to sleep. Frequently, an associated mood or anxiety disturbance

Table 13.1 International Classification of Sleep Disorders – ICSD 2; International Classification of Diseases (ICD); and the Diagnostic and Statistical Manual of Mental Disorders, 4th edition, text revision (DSM IV-TR)

ICD-9-CM	DSM IV-TR	Classification
Insomnia (adapted from the International Classification of Sleep Disorders, second edition)		
307.42	307.42	Psychophysiological insomnia
307.42	307.42	Paradoxical insomnia
307.41	307.42	Adjustment insomnia
V69.4	307.42	Inadequate sleep hygiene
307.42	307.42	Idiopathic insomnia
327.02	327.02	Insomnia due to mental disorder
V69.5	307.42	Behavioral insomnia of childhood
327.01	327.01	Insomnia due to a medical condition
292.85	291.85	Insomnia due to a drug or substance
291.82	291.82	Insomnia due to alcohol
327.00		Physiologic (organic) insomnia, unspecified
780.52.1.1		Insomnia not due to a substance or known physiological condition, unspecified

ICD-9-CM	DSM IV-TR	Classification
Sleep-related breathing disorders		
327.21	780.57	Primary central sleep apnea
786.04	780.57 or 327.xx	Central sleep apnea, including Cheyne–Stokes breathing pattern
327.22	780.57 or 327.xx	Central sleep apnea, including high altitude periodic breathing
327.27	327.xx	Central sleep apnea due to medical condition not Cheyne–Stokes breathing pattern
327.28		Central sleep apnea due to a drug or substance
770.81		Primary sleep apnea of infancy
327.23	780.57	Obstructive sleep apnea, adult
327.23	780.57	Obstructive sleep apnea, pediatric
327.24	780.57	Sleep-related non-obstructive alveolar hypoventilation, idiopathic
327.26		Sleep-related hypoventilation/hypoxemia due to lower airways obstruction
327.26		Sleep-related hypoventilation/hypoxemia due to neuromuscular and chest wall disorders
327.26		Sleep-related hypoventilation/hypoxemia due to pulmonary parenchymal or vascular pathology
327.25		Congenital central alveolar hypoventilation syndrome
327.20	780.57	Sleep apnea/sleep-related breathing disorder, unspecified

Table 13.1 (*cont.*)

ICD-9-CM	DSM IV-TR	Classification
Hypersomnia not due to a sleep-related breathing disorder		
347.01		Narcolepsy with cataplexy
347.00		Narcolepsy without cataplexy
347.11		Narcolepsy due to medical condition with cataplexy
347.10		Narcolepsy due to medical condition without cataplexy
347.00	347.00	Narcolepsy unspecified
327.13	307.44	Recurrent hypersomnia
327.11	307.44	Idiopathic hypersomnia with long sleep time
327.12	307.44	Idiopathic hypersomnia without long sleep time
307.44		Behaviorally induced insufficient sleep syndrome
327.14	327.14	Hypersomnia due to medical condition
292.85	292.85	Hypersomnia due to a drug or substance
291.82	291.82	Hypersomnia due to alcohol
327.15	327.15	Hypersomnia not due to a substance or known physiological condition
327.10		Physiological (organic) hypersomnia, unspecified

ICD-9-CM	DSM IV-TR	Classification
Circadian rhythm sleep disorder		
327.31	307.45	Delayed sleep phase type
327.32	307.45	Advanced sleep phase type
327.33		Irregular sleep–wake type
327.34		Non-entrained type (free running)
327.37.1.1		Circadian rhythm sleep disorder due to medical condition
327.39	307.45	Other circadian rhythm sleep disorder
327.35	307.45	Jet-lag type
327.36	307.45	Shift-work type
292.85	292.85	Circadian rhythm sleep disorders due to a drug or substance
291.82	291.82	Circadian rhythm sleep disorders due to alcohol

ICD-9-CM	ICD 10	Classification
Parasomnia		
327.41		Confusional arousals
307.46	307.46	Sleepwalking
307.46	307.46	Sleep terrors
327.42	307.47	REM sleep behavior disorder
327.43		Recurrent isolated sleep paralysis

Table 13.1 (cont.)

ICD-9-CM	DSM IV-TR	Classification
307.47	307.47	Nightmare disorder
300.15	300.15	Sleep-related dissociative disorders
788.36	307.6	Sleep enuresis
327.49		Catathrenia (sleep-related groaning)
327.49		Exploding head syndrome
368.16		Sleep-related hallucinations
327.49	307.50	Sleep-related eating disorder
327.40	307.47	Parasomnia, unspecified
292.85	292.85	Parasomnia due to a drug or substance
291.82	291.82	Parasomnia due to alcohol
327.44	327.44	Parasomnia due to medical condition

ICD-9-CM	DSM IV-TR	Classification
Sleep-related movement disorder		
333.99		Restless legs syndrome
327.51		Periodic limb movement disorder
327.52		Sleep-related leg cramps
327.53		Sleep-related bruxism
327.59		Sleep-related rhythmic movement disorder
327.59		Other sleep-related movement disorder, unspecified
327.59	292.85	Sleep-related rhythmic movement disorder
292.85		Sleep-related rhythmic movement disorder due to drug or substance
327.59		Sleep-related rhythmic movement disorder due to medical condition

ICD-9-CM	DSM IV-TR	Classification
Isolated symptoms, apparently normal variants and unresolved issues		
307.49	307.47	Long sleeper
307.49	307.47	Short sleeper
786.09		Snoring
307.49		Sleep talking
307.47		Sleep starts, hypnic jerks
781.01		Benign sleep myoclonus of infancy
781.01		Hypnagogic foot tremor and alternating leg muscle activation
781.01	307.47	Propriospinal myoclonus at sleep onset
781.01	307.47	Excessive fragmentary myoclonus

Table 13.1 *(cont.)*

ICD-9-CM	DSM IV-TR	Classification
Other sleep disorder		
307.48	F51.8	Environmental sleep disorder
327.8	G47.9	Physiological sleep disorder, unspecified

ICD-9-CM	Classification
Appendix A: Sleep disorders associated with conditions classifiable elsewhere	
046.8	Fatal familial insomnia
729.1	Fibromyalgia
345	Sleep-related epilepsy
784.0	Sleep-related headaches
530.1	Sleep-related gastroesophageal reflux
411.8	Sleep-related coronary artery ischemia
787.2	Sleep-related abnormal swallowing, choking, and laryngospasm

DSM IV-TR	Mood disorders
Appendix B: Other psychiatric/behavioral disorders frequently encountered in the differential diagnosis of sleep disorders (DSM IV-TR codes are utilized here) classification	
296.xx	Major depressive disorder, bipolar I and II disorder, bipolar disorder not otherwise specified, mood disorder not otherwise specified
300.4	Dysthymic disorder
311	Depressive disorder not otherwise specified
301.13	Cyclothymic disorder
293.83	Mood disorder due to … (general medical condition)
29x.xx	Substance induced mood disorder
Anxiety disorders	
300.xx	Panic disorder w/ or w/o agoraphobia
309.81	Post-traumatic stress disorder
308.3	Acute stress disorder
300.02	Generalized anxiety disorder
Schizophrenia	
295.xx	
Selected somatoform disorders	
300.8x	Somatization disorder, undifferentiated somatization disorder, somatoform disorder not otherwise specified
307.8x	Pain disorder
300.11	Conversion disorder
Selected disorders usually diagnosed in infancy	
317	Mild mental retardation

Table 13.1 (cont.)

ICD-9-CM	DSM IV-TR	Classification
318.x	Moderate, severe, profound mental retardation	
319	Mental retardation, severity unspecified	
299.00	Autistic disorder	
299.80	Rett's disorder, Asperger's disorder, pervasive developmental disorder NOS	
Attention-deficit/hyperactivity disorder		
	314.xx	

Source: Adapted from ICSD 2 and DSM IV-TR.

that is not severe enough to be diagnosed as a separate psychiatric disorder is present with psychophysiologic insomnia. It is, therefore, difficult at times to distinguish between psychophysiologic insomnia and insomnia due to a mental disorder or even insomnia due to a drug or substance. A diagnosis of psychophysiologic insomnia is usually not made in the context of drug or substance use unless the insomnia preceded the use of the drug or substance. Psychophysiologic insomnia is most descriptive of the primary insomnia defined in the DSM IV-TR in terms of conditioning factors and arousals. *Paradoxical insomnia* [5] (previously known as sleep state misperception) is a complaint of severe insomnia that occurs without evidence of objective sleep disturbance and without daytime impairment of the extent that would be suggested by the amount of sleep disturbance reported. The patient often reports little or no sleep on most nights and may indicate nearly continuous awareness of environmental stimuli throughout most nights. It is thought to occur in up to 5% of insomniac patients. Disorders that result in significant sleep fragmentation, e.g., heart disease, bipolar disorder, depression, etc., may also cause the misperception of inadequate total sleep time; however, unlike these disorders, paradoxical insomnia does not have features of mood disturbance or cannot be explained by other medical conditions resulting in disrupted sleep. *Adjustment insomnia* [6] is insomnia that is associated with a specific psychological, physiological, environmental, or physical stressor. This disorder exists for a short period, usually days to weeks, and usually resolves when the stressor is no longer present. The type of stressor present and the severity of the sleep disturbance determine whether adjustment sleep disorder can be diagnosed. If the stressor is a medical condition or a psychiatric disorder, then adjustment sleep disorder is diagnosed only if the acute sleep disturbance is more than typically experienced by an individual stressor. *Inadequate sleep hygiene* is a disorder associated with common daily activities that are inconsistent with good quality sleep and full daytime alertness. Such activities include irregular sleep onset and wake times, stimulating and alerting activities before bedtime, substances ingested around sleep including alcohol, or caffeine, and smoking cigarettes. These practices do not necessarily cause a sleep disturbance in everyone. For example, an irregular bedtime or wake time that might be instrumental in producing insomnia in one person may not be important in another. *Idiopathic insomnia* [7] is a chronic form of insomnia that usually has an insidious onset during childhood and has a persistent course without periods of remission. *Behavioral insomnia of* childhood [8, 9] includes *limit-setting sleep disorder* and *sleep-onset association disorder*. Limit-setting sleep disorder is stalling or refusing to go to sleep that is eliminated once a caretaker enforces limits on sleep times and other sleep-related behaviors. Sleep-onset association disorder occurs when there is reliance on inappropriate sleep associations such as rocking, watching television, or holding a toy, or requiring environmental conditions such as a lighted room. The child is unable to fall asleep in the absence of these circumstances. Anxiety disorders frequently manifest during the night and may be confused with behavioral insomnia of childhood; however, these disorders usually do not respond to the typical treatments for behavioral insomnia of childhood and they usually also have daytime anxiety symptoms.

Several secondary insomnias are listed. As mentioned above, the term comorbid insomnia may be more appropriate when the insomnia is due to psychiatric or medical conditions. *Insomnia due to a medical condition* applies when medical or neurological disorders give rise to the insomnia. The medical disorder and the insomnia type are given when a patient is diagnosed. Features associated with this type of insomnia vary as a function of the medical condition causing the insomnia. *Insomnia due to a drug or substance* is applied when there is suppression or disruption of sleep caused by consumption of a medication, recreational drug, caffeine, alcohol, or food. It is also applicable when sleep is disrupted by exposure to an environmental toxin. The insomnia may occur during use or exposure of the substance or after its discontinuation. It is important to note that alcohol is commonly used as a sleep aid as it initially may reduce sleep onset latency; however, it also may result in increased sleep fragmentation and restless sleep. In addition, tolerance to alcohol may develop after chronic use and withdrawal results in an exacerbation of the insomnia. *Insomnia not due to a substance or known physiological condition, unspecified or non-organic insomnia not otherwise specified* is the diagnosis applied when an underlying mental disorder, psychological factors, or sleep-disruptive practices are suspected to be related to the insomnia, but further evaluation is required to identify which specific disorder. *Physiologic (organic) insomnia, unspecified* is applied to forms of insomnia that cannot be classified elsewhere and is suspected to be associated with an underlying medical condition, physiological state, or substance use or exposure.

Sleep-related breathing disorders

The disorders characterized in this group have disordered respiration during sleep. *Central apnea disorders* [10, 11] include disorders resulting in the cessation of breathing and are associated with diminished or absent respiratory effort in an intermittent or cyclical fashion due to cardiac or central nervous system dysfunction. *Other central sleep apnea* forms are associated with underlying pathologic or environmental causes, such as *Cheyne–Stokes breathing* or *high-altitude periodic breathing*.

Primary central sleep apnea is a sleep-related breathing disorder of unknown cause. A complaint of excessive daytime sleepiness, insomnia, or difficulty breathing during sleep is often reported. The patient must not be hypercapnic ($PaCO_2$ greater than 45 mmHg). Usually these patients have a $PaCO_2$ that is less than 40 mmHg during wakefulness. Five or more apneic episodes per hour of sleep are required for a diagnosis by polysomnography. Many experts in the field do not make this diagnosis unless at least 50% of the scored apneas in the polysomnogram record are central events. *Central sleep apnea due to Cheyne–Stokes breathing pattern* is characterized by recurrent central apnea and/or hypopneas alternating with prolonged hyperpnea in which tidal volume waxes and wanes in a crescendo–decrescendo pattern. Each ventilatory-apneic cycle is typically longer than 45 seconds duration and is characteristically seen only in NREM sleep. It occurs in medical disorders such as heart failure, cerebrovascular disorders, and renal failure. *Central sleep apnea due to high-altitude periodic breathing* is characterized by central apnea–hyperpnea cycle that is due to acute mountain sickness. Five or more central apneas per hour of sleep with a typical apnea–hyperpnea cycle length between 12 and 34 seconds in people with a recent ascent to an altitude of at least 4,000 m is diagnostic.

A secondary form of *central sleep apnea due to a drug or substance* is most commonly associated with users of long-term (at least two months) opioid use. The substance causes respiratory depression by acting on the mu-receptors of the ventral medulla. Opioids may also result in ataxic breathing, periodic breathing similar to Cheynes–Stokes, obstructive respiratory events, or hypoventilation. A central apnea index of five or more or episodes of periodic breathing is required for the diagnosis. *Primary sleep apnea of infancy* is a disorder of respiratory control most often seen in preterm infants (apnea of prematurity) and is believed to be due to a developmental pattern (immaturity), or secondary to other medical disorders. Apnea of infancy may occur in infants, usually younger than six months, who have medical conditions (such as infection, anemia, and gastroesophageal reflux) or have drug or anesthesia exposure. The *obstructive sleep apnea disorders* are characterized by an obstruction in the airway resulting in increased breathing effort and inadequate ventilation. Adult and pediatric forms of obstructive sleep apnea syndrome are defined separately because of the notable differences in diagnosis and management between the two.

Obstructive sleep apnea, Adult [12, 13, 14] involves repetitive episodes of cessation of breathing (apneas) or partial upper airway obstruction (hypopneas) that last a minimum of ten seconds. These events are often associated with reduced blood oxygen saturation, snoring, and sleep disruption. Excessive daytime sleepiness or insomnia is the common clinical complaint. Five or more respiratory events (apneas, hypopneas, or respiratory effort related arousals [RERAs]) per hour of sleep are required for diagnosis. Upper airway resistance syndrome (UARS) has been included under the heading of obstructive sleep apnea disorders. It usually presents with excessive daytime somnolence but does not meet the standard criteria (in terms of desaturations, apneas, or hypopneas) for obstructive sleep apnea syndrome. Frequent arousals are noted in UARS that are attributed to increased respiratory effort (RERAs) and are best seen using esophageal balloon manometry. *Obstructive sleep apnea, Pediatric* [15, 16, 17] is characterized by similar features to those seen in the adult form, but cortical arousals may not occur, possibly because of a higher arousal threshold. Some children display a pattern of obstructive hypoventilation that consists of long periods of persistent partial upper airway obstruction associated with hypercarbia, arterial oxygen desaturation, or hypercarbia and desaturation. At least one obstructive event of at least two respiratory cycles duration per hour of sleep is required for diagnosis. Sleep apnea syndrome may be confused with other disorders. For instance, panic attacks may consist of nocturnal awakenings due to episodes of choking or gasping for air or a sensation of loss of breath. Symptoms of attention-deficit/hyperactivity disorder [18] may be clinically similar to those of sleep apnea, both manifesting inattention, irritability, and hyperactivity (especially in children with OSA). A polysomnogram is necessary to differentiate sleep apnea from other mimickers.

Hypoventilation/hypoxemic disorders are related to elevated arterial carbon dioxide tension (PaCO$_2$). The disorder, *sleep-related non-obstructive alveolar hypoventilation syndrome, idiopathic* is not common. It consists of diurnal and nocturnal hypoventilation that is usually associated with hypercapnia and hypoxemia, and is without an identifiable medical or neurologic cause. A polysomnogram usually demonstrates decreased tidal volume lasting up to several minutes with sustained arterial oxygen desaturation that is often worse during REM sleep. *Congenital central alveolar hypoventilation syndrome* is a failure of automatic central control of breathing in infants who do not breathe spontaneously, or breathe shallowly and erratically. Most of these patients

demonstrate hypoventilation during sleep and many also hypoventilate during wakefulness. Hypoventilation with the associated hypoxemia and hypercapnia are usually more severe during slow-wave sleep than during REM sleep. If poorly controlled (especially during infancy), this disorder may result in, among other things, mental retardation, seizures, and growth failure. Of interest to note is the theory that individuals who cannot perceive elevations of CO$_2$ will be less anxious than individuals with intact CO$_2$ perception. Accordingly, patients with alveolar hypoventilation will tend to be less anxious [19].

Sleep-related hypoventilation/hypoxemia due to a medical condition includes the sleep disorders due to pulmonary parenchymal or vascular pathology (e.g., cystic fibrosis, interstitial lung disease, and hemoglobinopathies), due to lower airway obstruction (e.g., emphysema, bronchiectasis, or cystic fibrosis), and due to neuromuscular and chest wall disorders (e.g., neuromuscular diseases, "obesity-hypoventilaton syndrome", and kyphoscoliosis).

Hypersomnia not due to a sleep-related breathing disorder

The hypersomnia disorders are those in which the primary complaint is daytime sleepiness (the inability to stay alert and awake during the major waking episodes of the day) and the cause of the primary symptom is not disturbed nocturnal sleep or misaligned circadian rhythms. Other sleep disorders, that may be present, must first be treated effectively prior to giving this additional diagnosis.

Narcolepsy with cataplexy [20, 21] requires the documentation of a definite history of cataplexy in conjunction with excessive daytime somnolence. Cataplexy is defined as a sudden onset of temporary loss of muscle tone provoked by emotion. *Narcolepsy without cataplexy* is diagnosed when there is daytime sleepiness in the absence of cataplexy. Other associated features of narcolepsy including sleep paralysis, hypnagogic hallucinations, and automatic behaviors may also be present. Supportive evidence of daytime somnolence in the form of a positive MSLT with a mean sleep latency of less than eight minutes as well as two or more sleep onset REM periods is necessary to make this diagnosis. *Narcolepsy due to a medical condition* is the diagnosis applied to a patient with sleepiness who has a significant neurological or medical disorder (e.g., tumor, neurosarcoidosis,

Niemann–Pick type C) that accounts for the daytime sleepiness and/or cataplexy. Narcolepsy with cataplexy is extremely rare prior to the age of four. In children, the daytime sleepiness may present with the reappearance of regular daytime naps in a child who had previously discontinued regular napping, has behavioral problems, or has decreased school performance. Genetic disorders (e.g., Niemann–Pick type C disease) should be considered in children (especially those under five years of age) suspected of narcolepsy [22, 23]. *Recurrent hypersomnia* [24] includes both Kleine–Levin syndrome and menstrual-related hypersomnia. Episodes of sleepiness associated with binge eating, hypersexuality, and/or behavioral abnormalities (e.g., aggression, irritability, confusion) typify Klein–Levin syndrome. Menstrual-related hypersomnia consists of recurrent episodes of sleepiness associated with the menstrual cycle. These disorders require episodes of hypersomnia of two days to four weeks in duration and the time in between these episodes demonstrates normal cognition and behaviors. *Idiopathic hypersomnia with and without long sleep time* [25, 26] are characterized by a major sleep episode that is at least ten hours or between six and ten hours duration, respectively. Patients take unintended naps that are typically unrefreshing. Idiopathic hypersomnia is rarely seen prior to adolescence. These two diagnoses are made only after excluding other causes of hypersomnia. *Behaviorally induced insufficient sleep syndrome* occurs in patients who habitually sleep deprive themselves; however, these patients sleep considerably longer when their "habit" is not maintained.

Hypersomnia due to a medical condition is hypersomnia that is caused by a medical or neurological disorder (e.g., Parkinson's disease, post-traumatic hypersomnia, hypothyroidism). Cataplexy or other diagnostic features of narcolepsy are not present. *Hypersomnia due to a drug or substance* is diagnosed when the complaint is believed to be secondary to current use, past use, or recent discontinuation of drugs or alcohol. Recent discontinuation of stimulants or a past history of stimulant abuse may result in hypersomnia. Use of benzodiazepines, barbiturates, neuroleptics, or antiepileptics also often results in hypersomnia. *Hypersomnia not due to a substance or known physiological condition* is excessive sleepiness that is temporally associated with a psychiatric diagnosis. For example, bipolar disorder or seasonal affective disorder may manifest with recurrent episodes of sleepiness; conversion disorder may be difficult to differentiate from narcolepsy with or without cataplexy; and some mood disorders may present with episodes of excessive sleepiness that vary on a daily basis. *Physiologic (organic) hypersomnia, unspecified* is usually a temporary diagnosis made when a physiologic condition is responsible for hypersomnia and the patient's symptoms do not meet the criteria for other hypersomnolence conditions.

Circadian rhythm sleep disorders

The circadian rhythm sleep disorders [27, 28, 29] share a common underlying chronophysiological basis. The major feature of these disorders is a persistent or recurrent misalignment between the patient's sleep pattern and the pattern that is desired or regarded as the societal norm. Maladaptive behaviors influence the presentation and severity of the circadian rhythm sleep disorders. The underlying problem in the majority of the circadian rhythm sleep disorders is that the patient cannot sleep when sleep is desired. The wake episodes can occur at undesired times as a result of sleep episodes that occur at inappropriate times; therefore, the patient may complain of insomnia or excessive sleepiness. For several of the circadian rhythm sleep disorders, once sleep is initiated, the major sleep episode is of normal duration and sleep architecture.

Delayed sleep phase type, more commonly seen in adolescents, is characterized by a delay in the phase of the major sleep period in relation to the desired sleep time and wake time. A*dvanced sleep phase type,* on the other hand is more commonly seen in the elderly and is characterized by an advance in the phase of the major sleep period in relation to the desired sleep time and wake-up time. The *irregular sleep–wake type,* a disorder that has a lack of a clearly defined circadian rhythm of sleep and wakefulness, is most often seen in the institutionalized elderly and is associated with a lack of synchronizing agents such as light, activity, and social activities. The *free-running type* occurs because there is a lack of entrainment to the 24-hour period and the sleep pattern often follows that of the underlying free-running pacemaker with a sequential shift in the daily sleep pattern. The free-running type is most commonly seen in completely blind individuals and occasionally in patients being treated with chronotherapy for delayed sleep phase type.

Shift-work sleep type is characterized by complaints of insomnia or excessive sleepiness that occur in relation to work hours that are scheduled during the usual sleep period. *Circadian rhythm sleep disorders due to a medical condition* are abnormal sleep–wake patterns that are related to an underlying primary medical or neurological disorder. A disrupted sleep–wake pattern leads to complaints of insomnia or excessive daytime sleepiness. The *jet lag type* (*jet lag disorder*) is related to a mismatch between the timing of the sleep–wake cycle generated by the endogenous circadian clock and the common sleep–wake schedule of the new time zone. The number of time zones crossed and the direction of travel, with eastward travel usually being more disruptive, influence the severity of the disorder. Travel across at least two time zones with the associated complaint of hypersomnia or insomnia is required to make this diagnosis.

Other circadian rhythm sleep disorders due to a drug or substance refers to those conditions that are due to a drug, alcohol, or other substance. *Other circadian rhythm sleep disorders* (unspecified) identifies disorders of circadian rhythm that cannot be classified in the above headings.

Patients with mood disorders or psychoses can, at times, have a sleep pattern similar to that of delayed sleep phase type. A second diagnosis of a circadian rhythm disorder should be avoided unless the disorder is unrelated to the psychiatric diagnosis.

Parasomnias

The parasomnias [30, 31] are disorders of arousal and sleep-stage transition that consist of abnormal sleep-related movements, behaviors, emotions, perceptions, dreaming, and autonomic nervous system functioning that accompany sleep. The parasomnias often occur in the setting of disturbed or fragmented sleep and thus may be seen in conjunction with other sleep disorders (such as obstructive sleep apnea syndrome or narcolepsy), medical disorders (e.g., febrile illness), or psychiatric disorders (e.g., anxiety disorders). Occasionally, several parasomnias may occur in the same patient.

There are three parasomnias that are typically associated with arousal from non-REM sleep. *Confusional arousals* are characterized by confusion and/or disorientation following arousal from sleep (usually slow-wave sleep). The patient may be slow in speech and mentation as well as slow in response to questioning. These arousals are common in children and

can occur not only from nocturnal sleep but also from daytime naps. *Sleepwalking* is a series of complex behaviors that occur from sudden arousals from slow-wave sleep and result in walking behavior during a state of altered consciousness. *Sleep terrors* also occur primarily from slow-wave sleep and are associated with a cry or piercing scream accompanied by autonomic system activation and behavioral manifestation of intense fear. A common feature in these NREM parasomnias is that individuals may be difficult to arouse from the episode and when aroused can be confused and/or aggressive with subsequent amnesia for the episode. Usually there is no dreaming reported during these events; however, occasionally individuals may recollect vague and fragmented dreams. These three disorders can often coexist and sometimes one form may blend into the other or be difficult to distinguish from the other.

There are several parasomnias that are typically associated with the REM sleep stage. *REM sleep behavior disorder* [32, 33] (RBD) has dream enactment behaviors that occur from REM sleep and can cause injury or sleep disruption. The behaviors are often violent and/or are action filled. This disorder often precedes the development of a neurodegenerative disorder, such as Parkinson's disease or diffuse Lewy body dementia by up to 20 years or so, and is especially common in men over the age of 50 years. *Recurrent isolated sleep paralysis* is atonia of REM sleep that intrudes into wakefulness. The paralysis occurs at sleep onset or upon awakening and is characterized by an inability to perform voluntary movements. Auditory, visual, or tactile hallucinatory experiences often accompany the paralysis. The episodes last seconds to minutes and resolve spontaneously, but may also be terminated by sensory stimulation. *Nightmare disorder* is characterized by recurrent nightmares that occur primarily from REM sleep, and result in an awakening with intense anxiety, fear, or other negative feelings. There is usually a delay in returning to sleep. In people with acute stress disorder or post-traumatic stress disorders, nightmares may arise out of stage 2 sleep.

There are other parasomnias, such as *sleep enuresis* (recurrent involuntary voiding during sleep) and *sleep-related groaning* (catathrenia) that may be associated with either REM or NREM sleep. Also in this group is *sleep-related dissociative disorder*, which is a disorder that involves a disruption of the integrative features of consciousness, memory, identity, or perception of the environment. This disorder can occur in the transition from wakefulness to sleep, after an awakening from stages 1 or 2 sleep, or from REM sleep. A history of physical or sexual abuse is common in such patients. These patients fulfill the DSM-IV-TR criteria for a dissociative disorder. *Sleep-related hallucinations* are visual, tactile, vestibular, or auditory hallucinations that occur at sleep onset (hypnagogic) or on awakening from sleep (hypnapompic). They may be simple or complex (vivid images of people or animals). *Exploding head syndrome* is characterized by a perceived loud noise, sense of a violent explosion with or without a flash of light, inside the head as the patient is falling asleep or during waking in the night. *Sleep-related eating disorder* involves recurrent eating and drinking episodes during arousals or partial arousals from nocturnal sleep. The eating behavior is uncontrollable and often the patient is unaware of the behavior until the next morning. In addition, the behavior may have adverse health consequences (e.g., consumption of inedible or toxic substances, obesity). It can be associated with sleepwalking and can be medication induced.

Parasomnia, unspecified applies to parasomnias that are believed to be due to an undetermined psychiatric disorder. *Parasomnias due to drug or substance* are parasomnias that have a close temporal relationship between exposure to a drug, medication, or biological substance. For instance, somnambulism may result from the use of non-benzodiazepine receptor agonists and REM sleep behavior disorder may result from the use of tricyclic antidepressants. *Parasomnias due to a medical condition* are the manifestation of a parasomnia associated with an underlying medical or neurological disorder.

Sleep-related movement disorders

The sleep-related movement disorders comprise disorders with relatively simple, usually stereotyped, movements that disturb sleep. Restless legs syndrome [34, 35], although not exactly a movement disorder, is included here because of its high association with periodic limb movements during sleep. *Restless legs syndrome* is typified by a complaint of a nearly irresistible urge to move the legs. This sensation tends to have a circadian pattern, usually occurring more frequently in the evening or during the night. It is also worse when at rest and relieved with walking or moving the legs. Children who are unable to

communicate a description of their leg discomfort may meet diagnostic criteria for RLS with the demonstration of sleep disruption, having a family member with definite RLS, and/or having polysomnographically documented periodic limb movements during sleep. Periodic limb movements during sleep are often associated with restless legs syndrome but can occur as an independent disorder, *periodic limb movement disorder* [36]. In this condition repetitive, highly stereotyped limb movements occur during sleep that are associated with clinical sleep disturbance or daytime consequences (e.g., fatigue). *Sleep-related leg cramps* are painful sensations that result from sudden intense muscle contractions usually of the calves or small muscles of the feet. Episodes commonly occur during the sleep period and can lead to disrupted sleep. Relief is usually obtained by stretching the affected muscle. *Sleep-related bruxism,* characterized by clenching or grinding of the teeth during sleep, occurs in two types: sustained jaw clenching (tonic contractions) or a series of phasic contractions (rhythmic masticatory muscle activity). Both types are often associated with arousals. The activity may be severe or frequent enough to result in symptoms of temporomandibular joint pain or wearing down of the teeth. Bruxism is often associated with anxiety or stress. *Sleep-related rhythmic movement disorder* is a stereotyped, repetitive rhythmic motor behavior that occurs during drowsiness or light sleep and results in large movements of the head, body, or limbs. Typically seen in children, the disorder can also be seen in adults. Rhythmic movement disorder can also occur during full wakefulness and alertness, particularly in individuals who are mentally retarded. It is only diagnosed if there is an associated sleep disturbance, impairment in daytime function, or significant self-injury from violent movements. Children who are able to communicate are unaware of their sleep-related rhythmic movements. Stereotypic rhythmic movements that occur mostly during wakefulness are common in children with certain developmental disorders (e.g., autism or pervasive developmental disorder); however, a diagnosis of sleep-related movement disorder is only given to these patients if the abnormal movements occur predominantly during sleep.

Sleep-related movement disorders, unspecified are movement disorders that occur during sleep that are diagnosed before a psychiatric disorder can be ascertained. *Sleep-related movement disorder due to a medical condition* is a sleep disorder not specified elsewhere that appears to have a medical/neurologic basis. Often, this is a temporary diagnosis until the underlying medical/neurologic condition can be identified; it is then given the diagnosis of the identified medical/neurologic condition. *Sleep-related movement disorders due to a drug or substance* are sleep disorders not specified elsewhere that appear to have a drug or toxin or bioactive substance as their basis.

Other sleep disorders

The ICSD-2 has categorized three disorders that were difficult to fit into any other classification section under this heading. *Environmental sleep disorder* is a sleep disturbance that is caused by a disturbing environmental factor that disrupts sleep and leads to a complaint of insomnia, hypersomnia, or parasomnias. For example, a person who is unable to sleep because of passing traffic outside her home has an environmental sleep disorder. The two remaining disorders in this category, namely *Other physiological (organic) sleep disorder* and *Other sleep disorder not due to substance or known physiological condition,* are intended to be a temporary diagnosis. The former is given the label when a sleep disorder is believed to be due to a medical or neurologic condition that has not yet been ascertained. The latter is temporarily diagnosed when it is suspected of being due to psychiatric or behavioral factors.

Isolated symptoms, apparently normal variants, and unresolved issues

This section lists sleep-related symptoms that are on the borderline between normal and abnormal sleep.

A *long sleeper* is a person who sleeps ten hours or longer in a 24-hour day. Symptoms of excessive sleepiness occur if the person does not get that amount of sleep. In children, the age-appropriate sleep needs should be considered before making this diagnosis. A *short sleeper,* on the other hand, is a person who requires five hours or less of sleep in the 24-hour day. Long and short sleepers' sleep is normal in architecture and quality. *Snoring* is diagnosed when a respiratory sound during sleep is audible to the patient, a bed partner, or others and is not associated with insomnia, excessive sleepiness, or obstructive sleep apnea syndrome. *Sleep talking* can be either idiopathic or associated with other disorders such as REM sleep behavior disorder, or sleep-related

eating disorder. It can occur during any sleep stage. *Sleep starts* (*hypnic jerks*) are sudden brief contractions of the body or part of the body that occur at sleep onset. These movements are associated either with a sensation of falling, a sensory flash, or a sleep-onset dream. These events occur in almost everyone at some point in their life, but occasionally may result in sleep onset insomnia or chronic anxiety. *Benign sleep myoclonus of infancy* is a benign disorder of myoclonic jerks that occur only during sleep in infants. It typically occurs from birth to age six months and resolves spontaneously. The movements may be provoked or exacerbated by gentle rocking of the infant or gentle restraints. The events invariably end with the infant awaking. *Hypnagogic foot tremor and alternating leg muscle activation* are two disorders that are considered together in the ISCD-2 because the similarities between them suggest that they may represent the same condition. The former has clinical symptoms of rhythmic movement of the feet during sleep and is associated with recurrent foot EMG potentials in the myoclonic range. The latter is a polysomnographic diagnosis demonstrated by alternating left and right anterior tibialis muscle activation. They occur at the transition between wake and sleep or during light NREM sleep. *Propriospinal myoclonus at sleep onset* is a disorder of recurrent sudden muscular jerks (involving abdominal, truncal, proximal limbs, and neck muscles) in the transition from wakefulness to sleep. The episodes cease when mental activity or sleep occurs. The disorder may be associated with severe sleep-onset insomnia. *Excessive fragmentary myoclonus* is a finding during polysomnography, characterized by small muscle twitches in the fingers, toes, or the corner of the mouth that do not cause actual movements across a joint. This is usually asymptomatic; however, it can be associated with daytime sleepiness or fatigue.

Appendices A and B: other organic disorders frequently encountered in the differential diagnosis of sleep disorders; and other psychiatric/behavioral disorders frequently encountered in the differential diagnosis of sleep disorders

The ICSD-2 has two appendices that list some common medical/neurologic and psychiatric diagnoses that are often encountered during an evaluation of sleep complaints. These disorders are associated with disturbances of sleep and wakefulness. Some of these disorders have been briefly described in the above text.

Psychiatric diagnoses [37] that are discussed include: mood disorders; anxiety disorders; somatoform disorders; schizophrenia and other psychotic disorders; disorders first diagnosed in childhood or adolescence; and personality disorders. The reader is referred to the DSM-IV for a detailed discussion of the diagnostic criteria for these disorders. Some of the associations of these disorders to sleep are discussed here. As a group, a common symptom of psychiatric diagnoses discussed in the ICSD-2 is difficulty with sleep initiation, sleep maintenance, or early morning awakening. Circadian rhythm disorders and parasomnias are also described in some of the disorders.

Typical depressive episodes usually result in insomnia. Frequent nocturnal awakenings and early morning awakenings are common; occasionally, sleep onset difficulty may occur. Sleep disturbances in an atypical depressive episode, representing about 15 to 20% of cases, on the other hand, are defined by excessive daytime sleepiness or prolonged nocturnal sleep as well as excessive eating. Manic episodes are usually accompanied by a decrease amount of sleep and/or a decreased need for sleep. Individuals with mania often do not volunteer a sleep disturbance complaint; however, they may identify a history of insomnia preceding their manic episode. The insomnia may represent a prodrome or a provocative factor of manic episodes in these patients.

The insomnia associated with mood disorders is differentiated from primary insomnias in that with a primary insomnia complaints are more focused on their sleep disturbance. Conversely, other symptoms of mood disorders, e.g., feelings of hopelessness in depression, predominate over the sleep disturbance in insomnias associated with mood disorders.

The anxiety disorders described in the ICSD-2 include panic disorder, post-traumatic stress disorder, acute stress disorder, and generalized anxiety disorder. They usually present with sleep initiation and maintenance problems. In post-traumatic stress disorder and occasionally in acute stress disorder, nocturnal awakenings are often due to nightmares of the traumatic event. These nightmares may persist in post-traumatic stress disorder even when other symptoms of the disorder have remitted. In about two thirds of patients with panic disorder (with or without agoraphobia), sleep initiation and maintenance

disturbances are present. Occasionally, episodes of awakening from sleep, choking or shortness of breath with associated anxiety that is typical of nocturnal panic attacks may be confused with similar symptoms of obstructive sleep apnea.

Schizophrenia [38] has been described to have a number of associated sleep disturbances. Sleep onset and sleep maintenance insomnia are well reported in this disorder and have been correlated with the severity of symptoms, such as hallucinations, delusions, and disorganized thoughts. The insomnia is believed to be due to a number of factors, including inadequate sleep hygiene, medication effects, or a conditioned behavioral response (i.e., psychophysiologic). A circadian rhythm disorder, delayed sleep phase type, is also commonly reported in schizophrenia. Occasionally, a complete reversal of the day–night sleep pattern may occur. An acute onset or exacerbation of the sleep disturbance may be a marker for the onset of an acute psychotic episode.

Compared to the above-described psychiatric disorders, there are significantly fewer studies describing the sleep disturbances present in somatoform disorders, disorders first diagnosed in childhood or adolescence (e.g., mental retardation, Asperger's disease, autism, Rett's disorder), and personality disorders. In somatoform disorders, some reports suggest the occurrence of sleep initiation and maintenance problems as well as daytime fatigue. People with mental retardation or Asperger's disease also have similar problems and/or early morning awakenings. In general, the lower the IQ the worse the possible sleep disturbance. Early morning awakenings as well as rhythmic movements (e.g., body rocking) also occur in autism. If these movements meet the diagnostic criteria for rhythmic movement disorder described earlier then it is assigned this separate diagnosis, otherwise it is considered as part of the primary disorder. Stereotyped movements, such as hand wringing, are typical in Rett's disorder; however, it is usually not considered a rhythmic movement disorder as it fails to satisfy the aforementioned criteria. A number of the disorders first diagnosed during childhood have other associated abnormalities that predispose them to certain sleep disturbances or disorders. For instance, people with Down's syndrome have hypotonia, midfacial hypoplasia, obesity, glossoptosis/macroglossia, and/or hypothyroidism that place them at a much higher risk for the development of obstructive sleep apnea.

Medical and neurologic diagnoses that are described in the ICSD-2 include: *fatal familial insomnia; fibromyalgia; sleep-related epilepsy; sleep-related headaches; sleep-related gastroesopheageal reflux; sleep-related coronary artery ischemia*; and *sleep-related abnormal swallowing, choking, and laryngospasm*. Fatal familial insomnia and fibromyalgia will be briefly discussed here.

Fatal familial insomnia [39, 40] is an autosomal dominantly inherited prion disease that is localized to the PRNP gene. It usually becomes symptomatic around 35 to 60 years of age, beginning with a progressively worsening insomnia and autonomic hyperactivity. Agitation, ataxia, dysarthria, myoclonus, tremor-like activity, and memory loss are also characteristic. Polysomnographic testing may show loss of spindles, loss of slow-wave sleep, and/or dissociated REM sleep. The pathology reveals degeneration of the anterior and dorsomedial thalamus.

Fibromyalgia [41, 42] is a disorder that involves pain affecting multiple parts of the body. It is characterized by tender points at up to 18 (11 of 18 required for diagnosis) specific anatomic sites located bilaterally throughout the body. Patients typically report daytime fatigue and non-restorative sleep. Polysomnograms and EEGs often demonstrate alpha intrusion into sleep.

Conclusion

There is often considerable overlap between symptoms of primary sleep disorders and medical or psychiatric disorders. Symptoms of insomnia, excessive sleepiness, or abnormal behaviors/movements during sleep can result from medical, psychiatric, or primary sleep disorders. The co-occurrence of sleep disorder symptoms can make it more difficult to manage the underlying medical or psychiatric disorder. If the sleep symptom is a prominent focus of the patient's presentation, then a separate sleep disorder diagnosis should be assigned and treated independently of the underlying medical or psychiatric disorder.

References

1. American Academy of Sleep Medicine. *International Classification of Sleep Disorders – 2*. (Chicago, IL: American Academy of Sleep Medicine; 2005).

2. Nino-Murcia G. Diagnosis and treatment of insomnia and risks associated with lack of treatment. *J Clin Psychiatry*. 1992;**53** Suppl:43–7;discussion 48–9.

3. Hauri PJ, Esther MS. Insomnia. *Mayo Clin Proc*. 1990;**65**(6):869–82.

4. Hauri PJ, Fischer J. Persistent psychophysiological (learned) insomnia. *Sleep*. 1986;**9**:38–53.

5. Edinger JD, Fins A. The distribution and clinical significance of sleep time misperceptions. *Sleep*. 1995;**18**:232–9.

6. Morin CM, Rodriquez S, Ivers H. Role of stress, arousal and coping skills in primary insomnia. *Psychosomatic Medicine*. 2003;**65**(2):259–67.

7. Hauri PJ, Olmsted E. Childhood onset insomnia. *Sleep*. 1980;359–65.

8. Heussler HS. Common causes of sleep disruption and daytime sleepiness: childhood sleep disorders II. *Med J Aust*. 2005;**182**(9):484–9.

9. Gaylor EE, Goodlin-Jones BL, Anders TF. Classification of young children's sleep problems. *J Am Acad Child Adolesc Psychiatry*. 2001;**40**:60–7.

10. Arzt M, Bradley TD. Treatment of sleep apnea in heart failure. *Am J Respir Crit Care Med*. 2006;**173**(12):1300–8.

11. Guilleminault C, Robinson A. Central sleep apnea. *Neurol Clin*. 1996;**14**:611–28.

12. McNicholas WT, Ryan S. Obstructive sleep apnoea syndrome: translating science to clinical practice. *Respirology*. 2006;**11**(2):136–44.

13. White DP. Sleep apnea. *Proc Am Thorac Soc*. 2006;**3**(1):124–8.

14. Ancoli-Israel S, Ayalon L. Diagnosis and treatment of sleep disorders in older adults. *Am J Geriatr Psychiatry*. 2006;**14**(2):95–103.

15. Gozal D, Kheirandish-Gozal L. Sleep apnea in children: treatment considerations. *Paediatr Respir Rev*. 2006;7 Suppl 1:S58–61.

16. Ray RM, Bower CM. Pediatric obstructive sleep apnea: the year in review. *Curr Opin Otolaryngol Head Neck Surg*. 2005;**13**(6):360–5.

17. Brouillette RT, Fernbach SK, Hunt CE. Obstructive sleep apnea in infants and children. *J Pediatr*. 1982;**100**:31–40.

18. Owens JA. The ADHD and sleep conundrum redux: moving forward. *Sleep Med Rev*. 2006;**10**(6):377–9.

19. Pine DS, Weese-Mayer DE, Silvestri JM, *et al.* Anxiety and congenital central hypoventilation syndrome. *Am J Psychiatry*. 1994;**151**(6):864–70.

20. Dyken ME, Yamada T. Narcolepsy and disorders of excessive somnolence. *Prim Care*. 2005; **32**(2):389–413.

21. Overeem S, Mignot E, van Dijk JG, Lammers GJ. Narcolepsy: clinical features, new pathophysiologic

insights, and future perspectives. *J Clin Neurophysiol.* 2001;**18**(2):78–105.

22. Vankova J, Stepanova I, Jech R, *et al.* Sleep disturbances and hypocretin deficiency in Niemann-Pick disease type C. *Sleep.* 2003;**26**(4):427–30.

23. Stores G. The protean manifestations of childhood narcolepsy and their misinterpretation. *Dev Med Child Neurol.* 2006;**48**(4):307–10.

24. Dauvilliers Y. Differential diagnosis in hypersomnia. *Curr Neurol Neurosci Rep.* 2006;**6**(2):156–62.

25. Billiard M, Dauvillier Y. Idiopathic hypersomnia. *Sleep Medicine Reviews.* 2001;**5**:351–60.

26. Reid KJ, Burgess HJ. Circadian rhythm sleep disorders. *Prim Care.* 2005;**32**(2):449–73.

27. Klerman EB. Clinical aspects of human circadian rhythms. *J Biol Rhythms.* 2005;**20**(4):375.

28. Thorpy MJ, Korman E, Spielman AJ, *et al.* Delayed sleep phase syndrome in adolescents. *J Adolesc Health Care.* 1988;**9**:22–7.

29. Capp PK, Pearl PL, Lewin D. Pediatric sleep disorders. *Prim Care.* 2005;**32**(2):549–62.

30. Malow BA. Paroxysmal events in sleep. *J Clin Neurophysiol.* 2002;**19**(6):522–34.

31. Ferini-Strambi L, Fantini ML, Zucconi M, *et al.* REM sleep behaviour disorder. *Neurol Sci.* 2005;**26** Suppl 3:s186–92.

32. Olson E, Boeve B, Silber M. Rapid eye movement sleep behavior disorder: demographic, clinical, and laboratory findings in 93 cases. *Brain.* 2000;**123**:331–9.

33. Chahine LM, Chemali ZN. Restless legs syndrome: a review. *CNS Spectr.* 2006;**11**(7):511–20.

34. Ekbom KA. Restless legs syndrome. *Neurology.* 1960;**10**:868–73.

35. Mazza M, Della Marca G, De Risio S, Mennuni GF, Mazza S. Sleep disorders in the elderly. *Clin Ter.* 2004;**155**(9):391–4.

36. American Psychiatric Association. *Diagnostic and Statistical Manual of Mental Disorders,* 4th edn, *Text Revision.* (Washington, DC: American Psychiatric Association, 1994).

37. Benca RM. Sleep in psychiatric disorders. *Neurol Clin.* 1996;**14**(4):739–64.

38. Benson KL. Sleep in schizophrenia: impairments, correlates, and treatment. *Psychiatr Clin North Am.* 2006;**29**(4):1033–45.

39. Montagna P. Fatal familial insomnia: a model disease in sleep physiopathology. *Sleep Med Rev.* 2005;**9**(5):339–53.

40. Montagna P, Gambetti P, Cortelli P, Lugaresi E. Familial and sporadic fatal insomnia. *Lancet Neurol.* 2003;**2**(3):167–76.

41. Abad VC, Sarinas PS, Guilleminault C. Sleep and rheumatologic disorders. *Sleep Med Rev.* 2008;**12**(3):211–28.

42. Menefee LA, Cohen MJ, Anderson WR, *et al.* Sleep disturbance and nonmalignant chronic pain: a comprehensive review of the literature. *Pain Med.* 2000;**1**(2):156–72.

Insomnia: a risk for future psychiatric illness

Matthew R. Ebben and Lina Fine

Abstract

Insomnia is the most common sleep disorder and significantly impacts quality of life for millions of sufferers worldwide. Often insomnia is a symptom of another mental disorder, and when the underlying psychiatric condition is treated, the insomnia dissipates. However, there is a growing body of evidence that treatment of insomnia can lead to a better management of mental illness and that insomnia can be predictive of onset and relapse of multiple psychiatric problems. This chapter aims to review the evidence for insomnia as a predictor of mental illness.

Sleep disturbance is one of the most frequently seen health complaints worldwide. Estimates indicate that 6 to 15% of the population suffers from insomnia [1]. Among demographic characteristics, female gender and older age appear to impart greater risk for insomnia [2]. The most commonly accepted definition for insomnia is the one taken from the *International Classification of Sleep Disorders* [3]. In this text, insomnia is defined as a complaint of difficulty initiating or maintaining sleep, waking up too early, or as sleep that is consistently unrefreshing. This definition assumes that the individual has set aside ample opportunity to sleep. If this is not the case, it is possible that the individual is suffering from behaviorally induced sleep deprivation, not insomnia. Daytime impairment should also be associated with the difficulty sleeping; daytime symptoms commonly include fatigue, stomach problems, difficulty concentrating, memory difficulties, irritability, and/or reduced motivation. Insomnia has been shown to be associated with higher absenteeism, impaired job performance, and higher healthcare utilization [4, 5].

Although the focus of this chapter is not treatment of insomnia, in the course of discussing the association between insomnia and psychiatric illness treatments will be mentioned. With mounting evidence for the efficacy of cognitive–behavioral treatments for insomnia (CBT-I), these techniques have progressively received more attention. A recent National Institutes of Health State-of-the-Science Conference recognized CBT-I therapies to be effective for the treatment of chronic insomnia [6].

A number of studies on treatment efficacy have shown that behavioral treatments for insomnia could help around 70 to 80% of patients with insomnia [7–11]. These techniques were also found useful for elderly patients, as well as patients with comorbid medical and psychiatric conditions [7]. Studies comparing behavioral strategies with pharmacological approaches have shown that behavioral interventions were as effective as hypnotics during short-term treatment [12], and might generate more long-lasting outcomes in long-term follow-up [13, 14]. CBT-I for insomnia is fairly well standardized and effective for a wide range of insomnia problems including primary as well as comorbid insomnia. This chapter's bias toward CBT-I stems from this extensive body of evidence.

In order to understand the development and progression of insomnia over time, it is helpful to consider the 3Ps model of insomnia (see Figure 14.1) [15]. The 3Ps in this model stand for predisposing, precipitating, and perpetuating factors. Predisposing factors may be genetic or underlying personality traits such as basal level of anxiety or hyperarousal. This latter factor deserves closer attention given its significant role in the development of insomnia. Individuals who are hyperaroused can be recognized by their stronger than normal startle response. Family members and friends often describe these individuals

Sleep and Mental Illness, eds. S. R. Pandi-Perumal and M. Kramer. Published by Cambridge University Press.

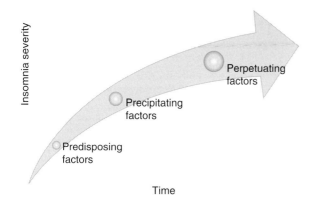

Figure 14.1 The role of the 3Ps in the increase of insomnia severity over time.

as being "on edge." The term hyperarousal is used to describe an amalgamation of both physiological and behavioral components of arousal [16]. The behavioral traits of hyperarousal commonly involve strong reaction to loud noises, tendency towards rumination, conscientiousness, predictability, and negative response to unexpected events. Sensitivity to the effects of caffeine and bright lights, prolonged sleep latency, increased cortisol levels and metabolic rate, and cortical activation are among the most common physiologic qualifiers of hyperaroused individuals. In one study, patients with primary insomnia suffered from increased daytime hyperarousal and also had higher evoked potential responses to auditory stimuli than normal controls [16]. Insomniacs were found to have higher 24-hour mean plasma cortisol levels, and a higher whole-body metabolic rate compared to controls [17, 18]. In addition, it has been observed that insomniacs have an altered pattern of release of proinflammatory and fatigue inducing cytokines, interleukin-6 (Il-6) and TNF alpha. Hypothalamic–pituitary–adrenal (HPA) axis activation may lead to circadian alteration and elevation in the level of these cytokines that causes fatigue and poor sleep of the insomniacs [19]. One neuro-imaging study comparing glucose metabolism in 7 patients with major depressive disorder (MDD) and 20 healthy subjects by positron emission tomography (PET) scan found increased metabolism in the ascending reticular activating system, hypothalamus, thalamus, insular cortex, amygdala, and hippocampus and in part of the prefrontal cortex during non-REM stages, but reduced metabolism while awake. The investigators suggested that patients' hyperarousal was due to the poor decline in arousal system that is

expected in transition to sleep [20–22]. Interestingly, although, by definition, insomniacs have difficulty sleeping at night, they have higher mean sleep latency scores during the day on the multiple sleep latency test [18, 23–25]. Therefore, even though insomniacs subjectively report less sleep at night, they continue to be less sleepy during the day than individuals without insomnia. Hyperarousal may be the cause for this increased daytime activation.

Although no definitive pathways have been established to account for the close relationship between insomnia and psychiatric illness, several possible interactions have been postulated. Insomnia may cause the individual to experience a greater sense of stress that would lead to the elevation of corticotropin-releasing factor (CRF) and cortisol. The same hypothalamic axis is implicated in depression and anxiety, as increased levels of CRF have been observed in these conditions. In turn, CRF may disrupt both REM and non-REM sleep and contribute to frequent arousals. Vgontzas et al. [17] found significantly higher levels of cortisol and ACTH in insomniacs when compared with subjects without insomnia. The degree of cortisol elevation correlated directly with higher measures of insomnia. One study reported elevated blood levels of norepinephrine in patients with primary insomnia when compared with healthy or depressed individuals [26].

Genetic links play a powerful role in determining one's predisposition to insomnia as the following data demonstrate. Recently, a questionnaire (Ford Insomnia Response to Stress Test [FIRST]) was developed to identify individuals who have an increased risk of developing sleep difficulty when confronted with a stressor [27]. This questionnaire consists of nine items that ask the respondent to rate the likelihood that various stressful events would disturb their sleep. Although individuals with insomnia tended to score higher than those without insomnia on this test, this test was not developed to screen for insomnia. It was designed to screen for those at increased risk of developing transient insomnia. In a sense, one could say that this test measures the predisposition to develop insomnia. This test was used to look at familial aggregation in terms of vulnerability to insomnia [28]. In this study, siblings' scores on the FIRST were significantly correlated (r = 0.61). In addition, familial aggregation accounted for 37% of the variance in FIRST scores. This suggests that there may be a genetic component to an individual's predisposition to develop insomnia.

According to the 3Ps model, predisposing traits place individuals who carry them at a higher risk of developing chronic insomnia [27]. Precipitating events such as stress at home or work as well as health and/or emotional problems can induce periods of difficulty sleeping [29]. Maladaptive habits, practices, and worrying about sleep can then cause the transient insomnia to become chronic. Common perpetuating activities include prolonged time in bed, eating, surfing the web and/or watching television in bed, and drinking alcohol to help promote sleep. Other perpetuating factors include daytime activities aimed at reducing tiredness associated with insomnia, such as drinking more caffeine-containing beverages or napping.

Commonly, a mood disorder such as major depression, bipolar disorder, or an anxiety disorder can serve as a precipitating event, and through maladaptive practices insomnia can become long-lasting. The perpetuating component of the 3Ps model of insomnia draws attention to habits and practices that maintain insomnia and make it chronic regardless of its initial trigger. Therefore, in cases in which acute insomnia is secondary to a mood disorder, once the mood disorder is adequately treated, if sleep disturbance continues to be present, treatment must focus on insomnia, not the mood disorder. As illustrated in Figure 14.1, over time, the importance of each of these three factors can change with perpetuating habits and practices frequently gaining in importance. The non-pharmacological treatments often target these perpetuating features in order to alleviate the sleep disturbance.

Depression and insomnia

Psychiatric disorders frequently co-occur with insomnia in clinical practice. In fact, the most common diagnosis pattern in sleep centers is the comorbidity of insomnia and mental illness [30]. The prevalence rate for major depression in any given year in adults in the United States is approximately 7% [31]. In patients with major depression, sleep disturbance is present in nearly 80% of cases [32, 33]. Moreover, 91% of patients with primary insomnia have either depressive and/or anxiety symptoms that are significant but do not fulfill the DSM-IV criteria for a full affective disorder diagnosis [30] in the appropriate category. In insomniacs, the prevalence of depression is nearly ten times greater than in those without

insomnia [34]. Interestingly, insomniacs who report difficulty with both sleep onset and maintenance are at a higher risk for depression than those with either sleep onset or maintenances problems alone [34]. Moreover, 90% of patients with depression complain of difficulty with both sleep onset and maintenance [30]. Patients with depression and insomnia also report more severe daytime impairment than individuals with anxiety and insomnia [30].

Ford and Kamerow [35] found that subjects who had insomnia on two consecutive interviews had a 35 times greater risk of developing depression. In addition, among adolescents, 69% report insomnia before the onset of depression [36]. In another study looking at young adults, insomnia lasting two weeks or longer predicted depression in 17 to 50% of cases [37]. This study also found that women have a two times greater risk of developing insomnia compared to men. Looking at individuals 50 years of age or older, sleep difficulties were found to predict depression one year later [38]. In another study, insomnia was found to predict depression in middle-aged women 12 years later, but not in men [39]. Buyesse et al. [37] have reviewed and analyzed the insomnia and depression data available as part of the Zurich Study (a prospective epidemiological study of depressive, neurotic, and psychosomatic syndromes), a longitudinal study of a sample of subjects residing in the canton of Zurich, Switzerland over a period of 20 years. They found pure insomnia as well as insomnia comorbid with depression to be predictive of future episodes of depression in young adults. A review by Riemann and Voderholzer assessed the value of insomnia as a determinant of the future development of depression [40]. Evaluating eight epidemiological studies, they concluded that insomnia predicted depression in nearly every reviewed study. In general, worsening health contributes significantly to depression in older persons, and, conversely, improved health was a factor in remission of depression [41]. Therefore, overall health status is an important consideration in patients with comorbid sleep disturbance and depression because both conditions are commonly associated with a variety of health conditions.

Functional neuroimaging also allows for a glimpse into the interaction between insomnia and depression. One study found depressed patients to have greater activation of anterior paralimbic structures when compared with healthy individuals. The brains of depressed patients showed greater activation of the midbrain reticular formation and the executive cortex. The interplay between these regions may be the potential causal link between depression and insomnia [20–22].

Traditionally, treatment has focused on the assumed cause of the insomnia, the mood disorder. However, the most typical residual symptoms following a successful treatment of depression are disturbed sleep and fatigue [42, 43]. Conversely, patients with insomnia are two to four times more likely to remain depressed even when treatment of the depression is attempted [44]. As mentioned above, a number of studies have shown a common sequence of insomnia preceding the development of depression. These studies have also shown that insomnia is a risk factor for depression. Insomnia not only precedes depression, but successful treatment of the sleep problem lessened the risk of future depression [35, 45]. A recent study investigating the relationship between insomnia and depression targeted both insomnia and depression from the beginning of treatment [46]. A selective serotonin reuptake inhibitor (SSRI) medication was combined with either a hypnotic or placebo in patients with major depression. In the group taking hypnotic medication, both depression and sleep disturbance were improved. In a similar study investigating comorbid depression and insomnia, antidepressant medication was supplemented with CBT-I [47]. This study found that medication + CBT-I had a greater improvement on both depression and insomnia than antidepressant medication alone. These studies indicate that insomnia should not be considered secondary to depression, but rather a significant interdependent condition to be diagnosed and treated as aggressively as the underlying depression.

As a side note, in the past few decades sleep has been thoroughly investigated to identify objective measures of depression through the use of polysomnography. The most consistent objective findings on sleep architecture in depressed patients include reduced REM latency, total sleep time and sleep efficiency, and increased REM density [48]. Other changes in sleep architecture of depressed patients include reduction of slow-wave sleep and a disinhibition of REM sleep [49]. However, these finding are not specific to depression, and similar changes in sleep architecture can be found in bipolar disorder and schizophrenia. Therefore, sleep studies are not typically performed to evaluate patients for depression.

Bipolar disorder

Bipolar illness is characterized by significant shifts in sleep patterns that are tied closely to impairments in behavior and judgment. The one-year prevalence rate for bipolar disorder in adults in the United States is approximately 3% [31]. The most striking examples of sleeplessness are frequently observed in bipolar patients who are in the midst of a manic episode. These patients frequently report a total lack of sleep for days on end. During these episodes not only is there a lack of sleep, but often the patients feel as though they have freed themselves from the need for sleep. This phenomenon is quite different from the experience of patients with primary insomnia, who complain of daytime consequences of insufficient sleep. These periods of sleeplessness are commonly punctuated by prolonged bouts of sleep, suggesting that sleep need is not reduced, but is simply delayed. Objective measures of sleep utilizing polysomnography in manic patients found sleep quality to be very similar to patients with major depression, with increased sleep fragmentation and stage 1 sleep, and a shortened latency to REM sleep [50].

The direction of causality between sleeplessness and bipolar disorder has long been an area of debate. Is sleeplessness a risk factor for a manic episode or a direct cause for a relapse? In a comprehensive review in the early 1990s, Wu and Bunney found that not only does total sleep deprivation have an antidepressive effect in patients suffering from depression, but that, frequently, total sleep deprivation can precipitate manic or hypomanic episodes in bipolar patients [51, 52]. More recent studies have found the risk of a manic relapse after sleep deprivation to be between 5 and 7%, and the risk for hypomania to be between 6 and 12% [53, 54]. Interestingly, other causes of sleep fragmentation such as obstructive sleep apnea have been associated with treatment-resistant mania [55]. Moreover, treatment of obstructive sleep apnea has been associated with an improvement in manic symptoms [56].

A few studies have looked at the role of sleep in predicting mood changes in bipolar illness. Some of these studies have found sleep fluctuation to be a predictor of the subsequent mood change [52, 57]. Yet reports in the literature have varied as other studies have not confirmed the predictive value of reduced sleep for future bouts of mania [58].

However, when patients are asked what symptoms are most commonly associated with a future episode of mania, sleep disturbance is by far the most robust and consistent symptom reported [59]. Harvey reviewed a number of studies investigating the association between bipolar disorder and sleep problems. Based on the literature, she came to the conclusion that although sleep appears to be disturbed throughout the entire course of bipolar disorder, sleep disturbance is greatly exacerbated both before and during manic episodes [60].

Anxiety and difficulty sleeping

Anxiety is a term that includes a heterogeneous group of disorders with a broad range of epidemiology and symptomatology. In any given year, the prevalence rate for an anxiety disorder for individuals over 18 years of age is approximately 18% [31]. This statistic makes it the most common type of DSM-IV diagnosis in the United States. Moreover, the general prevalence rate for insomnia related to anxiety disorders has been estimated to be approximately 8% [30]. The relationship between anxiety and insomnia has been explored empirically since the late 1960s. Many of the studies at that time investigated the relationship between anxiety and sleep disturbance using subjective rating measures without accompanying objective scales. These studies regularly demonstrated a link between anxiety and subjective reports of sleep disturbance [61, 62]. However, when the relationship between anxiety and sleep disturbance was investigated using both subjective and objective measures (e.g., EEG), the results were less consistent. Many of these studies induced anxiety or measured situational anxiety in subjects using a variety of techniques such as electric shock [63], traumatic films [64], exams [65], and anticipation of a first attempt at skydiving [66]. Overall, these studies showed a moderate relationship between anxiety and sleep disturbance. Other studies investigating chronic anxiety in poor sleepers did not find a consistent relationship between poor sleep and anxiety level [67–69]. However, one of the early well controlled studies selecting subjects on the basis of high scores on measures of chronic anxiety, while parceling out the confounding influence of depression, found a statistically significant relationship between anxiety and a variety of sleep measures including total sleep time (TST), latency to REM

sleep, and amount of delta sleep [70]. Moreover, when partial correlations were performed (controlling for depression) significant relationships were found between level of anxiety and number of awakenings (positive), sleep latency (positive), REM sleep percentage (negative), and percent of delta or slow-wave sleep (negative).

More recently, Benca [71] performed a meta-analysis (with a combined $N = 7,151$) investigating the relationship between psychiatric illness and sleep disruption. In this study it was found that anxiety level was associated with a reduction in total sleep time, and sleep efficiency (the ratio of total sleep time over time in bed), as well as an increase in sleep latency. In the case of anxiety and insomnia the vital question is whether insomnia preceded or followed the development of anxiety. Ohayon and Roth [72] found that anxiety appeared before insomnia in 43% of cases and that insomnia co-occurred with anxiety in 39% of cases. In his 1997 meta-analysis investigating this issue, Ohayon came to the conclusion that insomnia is mostly an associated symptom of another psychiatric disorder [73]. Given the relatively high estimated lifetime prevalence rate of 15 to 25% of anxiety disorders in the general population, the comorbidity with insomnia underlines the significance of sleep disturbance in patients with this spectrum of mental illness [74]. Moreover, 44% of insomniacs report a history of generalized anxiety [72], with an estimated prevalence of insomnia ranging from 6 to 15% depending on the definition used [1]. These compelling statistics are suggestive of the contributing role of anxiety to patients' insomnia and the close interplay between these two conditions.

Ohayon and Roth's findings in adults are consistent with a recent study of adolescents, which found that insomnia manifested before anxiety in 16% of cases, and that anxiety occurred before insomnia in 73% of cases [36]. This study also found that in 11% of cases, insomnia and anxiety occurred at the same time. In general, insomniacs have a 17 times greater risk of suffering from anxiety than those without insomnia [34]. Interestingly, even though women have higher rates of insomnia, at least one study found that anxiety levels in women are not necessarily higher than in men [34]. The causal link between anxiety and insomnia is not definitive, but the investigations point to a strong correlation between these prevalent conditions.

Post-traumatic stress disorder and insomnia

Post-traumatic stress disorder (PTSD) is an important condition that is often accompanied by significant sleep disruption. However, unlike in the generalized anxiety disorders, insomnia does not follow, but instead co-occurs, with the other symptoms consistent with PTSD. The prevalence rate for PTSD in adults 18 years old and older for any given year is approximately 5% [31]. The majority of individuals who experience traumatic events recover their sleep quality with time. However, a subset of trauma victims develop PTSD, which frequently involves persistent deficits in sleep quality [75]. One hypothesis suggests that persons with PTSD become hypervigilant to protect against external threats and this hyperarousal prevents restful sleep [76]. Studies on the prevalence of sleep disturbance in PTSD have found that 70 to 87% of people with PTSD also have sleep difficulties [77–80]. It appears that there is a direct relationship between severity of PTSD and sleep quality. Worsening sleep disturbance correlates with the severity of PTSD. One study found a statistically significant relationship between moderate and severe PTSD and subjective sleep quality, sleep duration, and daytime dysfunction [81]. Other important variables such as age, gender, and psychiatric comorbidity were found to correlate with the development of PTSD [80, 82, 83]. In addition to co-occurring sleep disturbance and PTSD, there is some evidence that sleep disturbance can be prognostic for the development of PTSD. A study by Koren *et al.* [84] found that sleep disturbance as early as one month after trauma predicted PTSD one year later.

There is evidence that even individuals who cannot be formally diagnosed with PTSD, but were exposed repeatedly to traumatic events, are at higher risk for insomnia than those not exposed to persistent trauma. In a large study of Vietnam veterans, even veterans that did not meet the full criteria for PTSD had a higher frequency of sleep disturbance compared to non-military controls; veterans with PTSD had a higher proportion of sleep disturbance than either the non-PTSD veteran or civilian groups [85]. In terms of objective measures of sleep architecture in PTSD, the results have been mixed. Some studies investigating sleep efficiency have found a decrease in sleep efficiency [86, 87]; however, others have found no decrease [88–90]. Studies investigating REM sleep variables are also not definitive. Some investigators have found more REM sleep in PTSD [89, 91], but other studies have not confirmed this finding [87, 92, 93]. REM latency findings have also been contradictory, with some studies showing shorter REM latencies [94] and others showing longer latencies [95, 96]. One consistent REM finding is an increase in REM density in PTSD [87, 91, 97]; moreover, it appears that REM density is positively correlated with severity of PTSD [86].

Sleep disturbance and psychosis

Patients with schizophrenia frequently complain of difficulty sleeping. This is particularly true during active periods of psychosis during which schizophrenics can go for days without sleep [98]. The one-year prevalence rate for schizophrenia in adults in the United States is approximately 1% [31]. In a meta-analysis performed in 2004 of 60 different studies looking at objective sleep quality in untreated schizophrenics by analyzing polysomnographic measures, it was found that these patients tend to have increased sleep latency, and decreased total sleep time and sleep efficiency compared to normal subjects [99]. In terms of sleep architecture, there has been a lot of interest in the REM sleep of psychotics because of the similarity of dreams during REM episodes in healthy individuals and hallucinations in wakefulness during periods of active psychosis. Some studies show that REM sleep is unaffected by schizophrenia [100]. However, REM latency in schizophrenics is consistently found to be shorter than that of unaffected subjects [98].

There exists good evidence that sleep disturbance is a predictor of a psychotic relapse in schizophrenia. In a questionnaire study of patients and family members of schizophrenics, sleep disturbance was reported to be one of the most common prodromes of an active psychotic phase [101]. In a prospective study by Chemerinski *et al.*, schizophrenics were evaluated during a three-week wash-out period from antipsychotic medication [102]. Insomnia before the wash-out period was a good predictor of both psychotic and disorganized thought process symptom severity at the end of the medication wash-out period. In addition, during the medication wash-out period insomnia progressively became worse in the early, middle, and late portions of the night.

Insomnia is a common residual symptom in psychotic patients treated with medication. Rates of residual insomnia range from 16 to 30% depending on the specific medication used [98]. In an attempt to manage the insomnia clinicians frequently choose a more sedating antipsychotic agent. Subsequent over-sedation due to these agents may be an important reason why some patients discontinue drug treatment [103], increasing the rates of non-compliance that lead to faster relapses. On measures of objective sleep quality, antipsychotics have been shown to improve sleep latency, REM latency, and sleep efficiency in schizophrenics [104].

Alcoholism and insomnia

Alcoholics report high rates of insomnia, ranging from 36 to 72%. In addition, subjects with insomnia have a significantly increased likelihood of developing alcohol abuse compared with adults without insomnia [105]. Patients with alcohol dependence are also twice as likely to report symptoms of insomnia prior to alcohol dependence [106]. Polysomnographic studies revealed that alcoholics over the age of 55 had higher sleep latency, lower sleep efficiency, and less slow-wave sleep when compared with younger alcoholics and with non-alcoholics of both age groups [107]. For many alcoholics, insomnia was exacerbated by the drinking habit. The relationship between sleep disruption and alcohol dependence is bidirectional because a number of alcoholics report that their sleep difficulty preceded their alcohol dependence [106]. In fact, 50% of alcoholics reported sleep problems before the onset of alcohol dependence [106]. Sleep disruption commonly continues in alcoholics long after they stop drinking and may predict relapse [108].

Borderline personality disorder

It is of interest to note briefly that insomnia appears to also play an important role in axis II disorders such as borderline personality disorder (BPD). Patients with BPD have more reports of poor quality sleep, with polysomnography studies revealing shortened REM latency, and significantly reduced REM sleep when compared with age and gender-matched controls, without comorbid substance abuse or affective illness. These subjects also have significantly higher delta power in total REM [109]. Future research may determine the underlying pathophysiological and neuroendocrine pathways that may account for this relationship.

Summary

In summary, insomnia appears to be an important predictor for a variety of mental disorders. As stated above, in cases of depression insomnia is a prodromal symptom in 17 to 69% of cases [36, 37]. In bipolar disorder, manic and hypomanic episodes can be anticipated in certain cases by sleep difficulties. In anxiety disorders, insomnia comes before anxiety in a number of cases. However, anxiety pre-dates sleep problems in the majority of cases [36]. The connection is more robust in the case of PTSD, as insomnia one month after a traumatic event has been shown to predict PTSD one year later [84]. In schizophrenia, multiple studies uncovered the predictive value of sleep disturbance before periods of active psychosis [101, 102]. Together the data show that insomnia should be seen not only as an important quality of life issue that should be treated, but also as possible harbinger of mental health issues.

References

1. Ohayon MM. [Prevalence and comorbidity of sleep disorders in general population]. *La Revue du Praticien.* 2007;**57**(14):1521–8.

2. Klink ME, Quan SF, Kaltenborn WT, Lebowitz MD. Risk factors associated with complaints of insomnia in a general adult population. Influence of previous complaints of insomnia. *Arch Intern Med.* 1992;**152**(8):1634–7.

3. American Academy of Sleep Medicine. *The International Classification of Sleep Disorders: Diagnostic and Coding Manual,* 2nd edn. (Westchester, IL: American Academy of Sleep Medicine, 2005).

4. Kuppermann M, Lubeck DP, Mazonson PD, *et al.* Sleep problems and their correlates in a working population. *J Gen Intern Med.* 1995;**10**(1):25–32.

5. Simon GE, VonKorff M. Prevalence, burden, and treatment of insomnia in primary care. *Am J Psychiatry.* 1997;**154**(10):1417–23.

6. National Institues of Health. National Institutes of Health State of the Science Conference statement on Manifestations and Management of Chronic Insomnia in Adults, June 13–15, 2005. *Sleep.* 2005;**28**:1049–57.

7. Morin CM, Bootzin RR, Buysse DJ, *et al.* Psychological and behavioral treatment of insomnia: update of the recent evidence (1998–2004). *Sleep.* 2006;**29**(11):1398–414.

8. Lacks P, Morin CM. Recent advances in the assessment and treatment of insomnia. *J Consult Clin Psychol.* 1992;**60**(4):586–94.

9. Morin CM, Culbert JP, Schwartz SM. Nonpharmacological interventions for insomnia: a meta-analysis of treatment efficacy. *Am J Psychiatry.* 1994;**151**(8):1172–80.

10. Morin CM, Hauri PJ, Espie CA, *et al.* Nonpharmacologic treatment of chronic insomnia. An American Academy of Sleep Medicine review. *Sleep.* 1999;**22**(8):1134–56.

11. Murtagh DR, Greenwood KM. Identifying effective psychological treatments for insomnia: a meta-analysis. *J Consult Clin Psychol.* 1995;**63**(1):79–89.

12. Smith MT, Perlis ML, Park A, *et al.* Comparative meta-analysis of pharmacotherapy and behavior therapy for persistent insomnia. *Am J Psychiatry.* 2002;**159**(1):5–11.

13. Jacobs GD, Pace-Schott EF, Stickgold R, Otto MW. Cognitive behavior therapy and pharmacotherapy for insomnia: a randomized controlled trial and direct comparison. *Arch Int Med.* 2004;**164**(17):1888–96.

14. Morin CM, Colecchi C, Stone J, Sood R, Brink D. Behavioral and pharmacological therapies for late-life insomnia: a randomized controlled trial. *JAMA.* 1999;**281**(11):991–9.

15. Yang CM, Spielman AJ, Glovinsky P. Nonpharmacologic strategies in the management of insomnia. *Psychiatr Clin North Am.* 2006;**29**(4):895–919; abstract viii.

16. Regestein QR, Dambrosia J, Hallett M, Murawski B, Paine M. Daytime alertness in patients with primary insomnia. *Am J Psychiatry.* 1993;**150**(10):1529–34.

17. Vgontzas AN, Bixler EO, Lin HM, *et al.* Chronic insomnia is associated with nyctohemeral activation of the hypothalamic-pituitary-adrenal axis: clinical implications. *J Clin Endocrinol Metab.* 2001;**86**(8):3787–94.

18. Bonnet MH, Arand DL. 24-Hour metabolic rate in insomniacs and matched normal sleepers. *Sleep.* 1995;**18**(7):581–8.

19. Basta M, Chrousos GP, Vela-Bueno A, Vgontzas AN. Chronic insomnia and the stress system. *Sleep Med. Clin.* 2007;**2**:279–91.

20. Nofzinger EA, Buysse DJ, Germain A, *et al.* Increased activation of anterior paralimbic and executive cortex from waking to rapid eye movement sleep in depression. *Arch General Psychiatry.* 2004;**61**(7):695–702.

21. Nofzinger EA, Buysse DJ, Germain A, *et al.* Functional neuroimaging evidence for hyperarousal in insomnia. *Am J Psychiatry.* 2004;**161**(11):2126–8.

22. Riemann D, Berger M, Voderholzer U. Sleep and depression – results from psychobiological studies: an overview. *Biol Psychol.* 2001;**57**(1–3):67–103.

23. Stepanski E, Zorick F, Roehrs T, Young D, Roth T. Daytime alertness in patients with chronic insomnia compared with asymptomatic control subjects. *Sleep.* 1988;**11**(1):54–60.

24. Schneider-Helmert D. Twenty-four-hour sleep–wake function and personality patterns in chronic insomniacs and healthy controls. *Sleep.* 1987;**10**(5):452–62.

25. Haynes SN, Fitzgerald SG, Shute GE, Hall M. The utility and validity of daytime naps in the assessment of sleep-onset insomnia. *J Behav Med.* 1985;**8**(3):237–47.

26. Irwin M, Clark C, Kennedy B, Christian Gillin J, Ziegler M. Nocturnal catecholamines and immune function in insomniacs, depressed patients, and control subjects. *Brain Behav Immun.* 2003;**17**(5):365–72.

27. Drake C, Richardson G, Roehrs T, Scofield H, Roth T. Vulnerability to stress-related sleep disturbance and hyperarousal. *Sleep.* 2004;**27**(2):285–91.

28. Drake CL, Scofield H, Roth T. Vulnerability to insomnia: the role of familial aggregation. *Sleep Med.* 2008;**9**(3):297–302.

29. Bastien CH, Vallieres A, Morin CM. Precipitating factors of insomnia. *Behav Sleep Med.* 2004;**2**(1):50–62.

30. Ohayon MM, Caulet M, Lemoine P. Comorbidity of mental and insomnia disorders in the general population. *Compr Psychiatry.* 1998;**39**(4):185–97.

31. Kessler RC, Chiu WT, Demler O, Merikangas KR, Walters EE. Prevalence, severity, and comorbidity of 12-month DSM-IV disorders in the National Comorbidity Survey Replication. *Arch Gen Psychiatry.* 2005;**62**(6):617–27.

32. Ohayon MM, Shapiro CM, Kennedy SH. Differentiating DSM-IV anxiety and depressive disorders in the general population: comorbidity and treatment consequences. *Can J Psychiatry.* 2000;**45**(2):166–72.

33. Weissman MM, Bland RC, Canino GJ, *et al.* Cross-national epidemiology of major depression and bipolar disorder. *JAMA.* 1996;**276**(4):293–9.

34. Taylor DJ, Lichstein KL, Durrence HH, Reidel BW, Bush AJ. Epidemiology of insomnia, depression, and anxiety. *Sleep.* 2005;**28**(11):1457–64.

35. Ford DE, Kamerow DB. Epidemiologic study of sleep disturbances and psychiatric disorders. An opportunity for prevention? *JAMA.* 1989;**262**(11):1479–84.

36. Ford DE, Kamerow DB. Epidemiologic study of sleep: exploration of the direction of risk. *J Psychiatric Res.* 2006;**40**(8):700–8.

37. Buysse DJ, Angst J, Gamma A, *et al*. Prevalence, course, and comorbidity of insomnia and depression in young adults. *Sleep*. 2008;**31**(4):473–80.

38. Roberts RE, Shema SJ, Kaplan GA, Strawbridge WJ. Sleep complaints and depression in an aging cohort: A prospective perspective. *Am J Psychiatry*. 2000;**157**(1):81–8.

39. Mallon L, Broman JE, Hetta J. Relationship between insomnia, depression, and mortality: a 12-year follow-up of older adults in the community. *Int Psychogeriatr*. 2000;**12**(3):295–306.

40. Riemann D, Voderholzer U. Primary insomnia: a risk factor to develop depression? *J Affect Disord*. 2003;**76**(1–3):255–9.

41. Kennedy GJ, Kelman HR, Thomas C, *et al*. Hierarchy of characteristics associated with depressive symptoms in an urban elderly sample. *Am J Psychiatry*. 1989;**146**(2):220–5.

42. Nierenberg AA, Keefe BR, Leslie VC, *et al*. Residual symptoms in depressed patients who respond acutely to fluoxetine. *J Clin Psychiatry*. 1999;**60**(4):221–5.

43. Carney CE, Segal ZV, Edinger JD, Krystal AD. A comparison of rates of residual insomnia symptoms following pharmacotherapy or cognitive-behavioral therapy for major depressive disorder. *J Clin Psychiatry*. 2007;**68**(2):254–60.

44. Pigeon WR, Hegel M, Unutzer J, *et al*. Is insomnia a perpetuating factor for late-life depression in the IMPACT cohort? *Sleep*. 2008;**31**(4):481–8.

45. Breslau N, Roth T, Rosenthal L, Andreski P. Sleep disturbance and psychiatric disorders: a longitudinal epidemiological study of young adults. *Biol Psychiatry*. 1996;**39**(6):411–18.

46. Fava M, McCall WV, Krystal A, *et al*. Eszopiclone co-administered with fluoxetine in patients with insomnia coexisting with major depressive disorder. *Biol Psychiatry*. 2006;**59**(11):1052–60.

47. Manber R, Edinger JD, Gress JL, *et al*. Cognitive behavioral therapy for insomnia enhances depression outcome in patients with comorbid major depressive disorder and insomnia. *Sleep*. 2008;**31**(4):489–95.

48. Wooten V, Buysse D. Sleep in psychiatric disorders. In: Chokroverty S, ed. *Sleep Disorders Medicine: Basic Science, Technical Considerations, and Clinical Aspects*, 2nd edn. (Boston: Butterworth-Heinemann, 1999; xxiii).

49. Riemann D. Insomnia and comorbid psychiatric disorders. *Sleep Med*. 2007;**8** Suppl 4:S15–20.

50. Hudson JI, Lipinski JF, Keck PE, *et al*. Polysomnographic characteristics of young manic patients. Comparison with unipolar depressed patients

51. Wu JC, Bunney WE. The biological basis of an antidepressant response to sleep deprivation and relapse: review and hypothesis. *Am J Psychiatry*. 1990;**147**(1):14–21.

52. Wehr TA, Goodwin FK, Wirz-Justice A, Breitmaier J, Craig C. 48-hour sleep-wake cycles in manic-depressive illness: naturalistic observations and sleep deprivation experiments. *Arch Gen Psychiatry*. 1982;**39**(5):559–65.

53. Kasper S, Wehr TA. The role of sleep and wakefulness in the genesis of depression and mania. *L'Encephale*. 1992;**18** Spec No 1:45–50.

54. Colombo C, Benedetti F, Barbini B, Campori E, Smeraldi E. Rate of switch from depression into mania after therapeutic sleep deprivation in bipolar depression. *Psychiatry Res*. 1999;**86**(3):267–70.

55. Strakowski SM, Hudson JI, Keck PE, *et al*. Four cases of obstructive sleep apnea associated with treatment-resistant mania. *J Clin Psychiatry*. 1991;**52**(4):156–8.

56. Fleming JA, Fleetham JA, Taylor DR, Remick RA. A case report of obstructive sleep apnea in a patient with bipolar affective disorder. *Can J Psychiatry*. 1985;**30**(6):437–9.

57. Leibenluft E, Albert PS, Rosenthal NE, Wehr TA. Relationship between sleep and mood in patients with rapid-cycling bipolar disorder. *Psychiatry Res*. 1996;**63**(2–3):161–8.

58. Perlman CA, Johnson SL, Mellman TA. The prospective impact of sleep duration on depression and mania. *Bipolar Disord*. 2006;**8**(3):271–4.

59. Jackson A, Cavanagh J, Scott J. A systematic review of manic and depressive prodromes. *J Affect Disord*. 2003;**74**(3):209–17.

60. Harvey AG. Sleep and circadian rhythms in bipolar disorder: seeking synchrony, harmony, and regulation. *American J Psychiatry*. 2008;**165**(7):820–9.

61. Haynes SN, Follingstad DR, McGowan WT. Insomnia: sleep patterns and anxiety level. *J Psychosom Res*. 1974;**18**(2):69–74.

62. Kazarian SS, Howe MG, Merskey H, Deinum EJ. Insomnia: anxiety, sleep-incompatible behaviors and depression. *J Clin Psychology*. 1978;**34**(4):865–9.

63. Bonnet MH, Webb WB. Effect of two experimental sets on sleep structure. *Percept Mot Skills*. 1976;**42**(2):343–50.

64. Baekland F, Koulack E, Lasky R. Effects of a stressful presleep experience on electroencephalograph-recorded sleep. *Psychophysiology*. 1968;**4**:443–63.

and normal control subjects. *Arch Gen Psychiatry*. 1992;**49**(5):378–83.

65. Lester BK, Burch NR, Dossett RC. Nocturnal EEG-GSR profiles: the influence of presleep states. *Psychophysiology*. 1967;**3**(3):238–48.

66. Beaumaster EJ, Knowles JB, MacLean AW. The sleep of skydivers: a study of stress. *Psychophysiology*. 1978;**15**(3):209–13.

67. Freedman R, Papsdorf JD. Biofeedback and progressive relaxation treatment of sleep-onset insomnia: a controlled, all-night investigation. *Biofeedback Self Regul*. 1976;**1**(3):253–71.

68. Karacan I, Orr WC, Roth T, *et al.* Establishment and implementation of standardized sleep laboratory data collection and scoring procedures. *Psychophysiology*. 1978;**15**(2):173–9.

69. Monroe LJ. Psychological and physiological differences between good and poor sleepers. *J Abnormal Psychol*. 1967;**72**(3):255–64.

70. Rosa RR, Bonnet MH, Kramer M. The relationship of sleep and anxiety in anxious subjects. *Biol Psychol*. 1983;**16**(1–2):119–26.

71. Benca RM, Obermeyer WH, Thisted RA, Gillin JC. Sleep and psychiatric disorders. A meta-analysis. *Arch General Psychiatry*. 1992;**49**(8):651–68; discussion 69–70.

72. Ohayon MM, Roth T. Place of chronic insomnia in the course of depressive and anxiety disorders. *J Psychiatr Res*. 2003;**37**(1):9–15.

73. Ohayon MM. Prevalence of DSM-IV diagnostic criteria of insomnia: distinguishing insomnia related to mental disorders from sleep disorders. *J Psychiatr Res*. 1997;**31**(3):333–46.

74. Kessler RC, McGonagle KA, Zhao S, *et al.* Lifetime and 12-month prevalence of DSM-III-R psychiatric disorders in the United States. Results from the National Comorbidity Survey. *Archives Gen Psychiatry*. 1994;**51**(1):8–19.

75. Lavie P. Sleep disturbances in the wake of traumatic events. *N Eng J Med*. 2001;**345**(25):1825–32.

76. Krakow B, Germain A, Warner TD, *et al.* The relationship of sleep quality and posttraumatic stress to potential sleep disorders in sexual assault survivors with nightmares, insomnia, and PTSD. *J Trauma Stress*. 2001;**14**(4):647–65.

77. Leskin GA, Woodward SH, Young HE, Sheikh JI. Effects of comorbid diagnoses on sleep disturbance in PTSD. *J Psychiatr Res*. 2002;**36**(6):449–52.

78. Foa EB, Riggs DS, Gershuny BS. Arousal, numbing, and intrusion: symptom structure of PTSD following assault. *Am J Psychiatry*. 1995;**152**(1):116–20.

79. Kilpatrick KL, Williams LM. Potential mediators of post-traumatic stress disorder in child witnesses to domestic violence. *Child Abuse Negl*. 1998;**22**(4):319–30.

80. Ohayon MM, Shapiro CM. Sleep disturbances and psychiatric disorders associated with posttraumatic stress disorder in the general population. *Compr Psychiatry*. 2000;**41**(6):469–78.

81. Germain A, Nielsen TA. Sleep pathophysiology in posttraumatic stress disorder and idiopathic nightmare sufferers. *Biol Psychiatry*. 2003;**54**(10):1092–8.

82. Doi Y, Minowa M, Uchiyama M, Okawa M. Subjective sleep quality and sleep problems in the general Japanese adult population. *Psychiatry Clin Neurosci*. 2001;**55**(3):213–15.

83. Kessler RC, Sonnega A, Bromet E, Hughes M, Nelson CB. Posttraumatic stress disorder in the National Comorbidity Survey. *Arch Gen Psychiatry*. 1995;**52**(12):1048–60.

84. Koren D, Arnon I, Lavie P, Klein E. Sleep complaints as early predictors of posttraumatic stress disorder: a 1-year prospective study of injured survivors of motor vehicle accidents. *Am J Psychiatry*. 2002;**159**(5):855–7.

85. Neylan TC, Marmar CR, Metzler TJ, *et al.* Sleep disturbances in the Vietnam generation: findings from a nationally representative sample of male Vietnam veterans. *Am J Psychiatry*. 1998;**155**(7):929–33.

86. Mellman TA, Kulick-Bell R, Ashlock LE, Nolan B. Sleep events among veterans with combat-related posttraumatic stress disorder. *Am J Psychiatry*. 1995;**152**(1):110–5.

87. Mellman TA, Nolan B, Hebding J, Kulick-Bell R, Dominguez R. A polysomnographic comparison of veterans with combat-related PTSD, depressed men, and non-ill controls. *Sleep*. 1997;**20**(1):46–51.

88. Mellman TA, David D, Kulick-Bell R, Hebding J, Nolan B. Sleep disturbance and its relationship to psychiatric morbidity after Hurricane Andrew. *Am J Psychiatry*. 1995;**152**(11):1659–63.

89. Engdahl BE, Eberly RE, Hurwitz TD, Mahowald MW, Blake J. Sleep in a community sample of elderly war veterans with and without posttraumatic stress disorder. *Biol Psychiatry*. 2000;**47**(6):520–5.

90. Hurwitz TD, Mahowald MW, Kuskowski M, Engdahl BE. Polysomnographic sleep is not clinically impaired in Vietnam combat veterans with chronic posttraumatic stress disorder. *Biol Psychiatry*. 1998;**44**(10):1066–73.

91. Ross RJ, Ball WA, Dinges DF, *et al.* Rapid eye movement sleep disturbance in posttraumatic stress disorder. *Biol Psychiatry*. 1994;**35**(3):195–202.

92. Dow BM, Kelsoe JR, Jr., Gillin JC. Sleep and dreams in Vietnam PTSD and depression. *Biol Psychiatry*. 1996;**39**(1):42–50.

163

93. Lavie P, Hefez A, Halperin G, Enoch D. Long-term effects of traumatic war-related events on sleep. *Am J Psychiatry.* 1979;**136**(2):175–8.

94. Schlosberg A, Benjamin M. Sleep patterns in three acute combat fatigue cases. *J Clin Psychiatry.* 1978;**39**(6):546–9.

95. Greenberg R, Pearlman CA, Gampel D. War neuroses and the adaptive function of REM sleep. *Br J Med Psychol.* 1972;**45**(1):27–33.

96. Reist C, Kauffmann CD, Chicz-Demet A, Chen CC, Demet EM. REM latency, dexamethasone suppression test, and thyroid releasing hormone stimulation test in posttraumatic stress disorder. *Prog Neuropsychopharmacol Biol Psychiatry.* 1995;**19**(3):433–43.

97. Ross RJ, Ball WA, Sanford LD, *et al.* Rapid eye movement sleep changes during the adaptation night in combat veterans with posttraumatic stress disorder. *Biol Psychiatry.* 1999;**45**(7):938–41.

98. Benson KL. Sleep in schizophrenia: impairments, correlates, and treatment. *Psychiatr Clin North Am.* 2006;**29**(4):1033–45; abstract ix–x.

99. Chouinard S, Poulin J, Stip E, Godbout R. Sleep in untreated patients with schizophrenia: a meta-analysis. *Schizophr Bull.* 2004;**30**(4):957–67.

100. Lauer CJ, Schreiber W, Pollmacher T, Holsboer F, Krieg JC. Sleep in schizophrenia: a polysomnographic study on drug-naive patients. *Neuropsychopharmacology.* 1997;**16**(1):51–60.

101. Herz MI, Melville C. Relapse in schizophrenia. *Am J Psychiatry.* 1980;**137**(7):801–5.

102. Chemerinski E, Ho BC, Flaum M, *et al.* Insomnia as a predictor for symptom worsening following antipsychotic withdrawal in schizophrenia. *Compr Psychiatry.* 2002;**43**(5):393–6.

103. Hofer A, Kemmler G, Eder U, *et al.* Attitudes toward antipsychotics among outpatient clinic attendees with schizophrenia. *J Clin Psychiatry.* 2002;**63**(1):49–53.

104. Taylor SF, Tandon R, Shipley JE, Eiser AS. Effect of neuroleptic treatment on polysomnographic measures in schizophrenia. *Biol Psychiatry.* 1991;**30**(9):904–12.

105. Weissman MM, Greenwald S, Nino-Murcia G, Dement WC. The morbidity of insomnia uncomplicated by psychiatric disorders. *Gen Hosp Psychiatry.* 1997;**19**(4):245–50.

106. Currie SR, Clark S, Rimac S, Malhotra S. Comprehensive assessment of insomnia in recovering alcoholics using daily sleep diaries and ambulatory monitoring. *Alcohol Clin Exp Res.* 2003;**27**(8):1262–9.

107. Brower KJ, Aldrich MS, Hall JM. Polysomnographic and subjective sleep predictors of alcoholic relapse. *Alcohol Clin Exp Res.* 1998;**22**(8):1864–71.

108. Brower KJ, Aldrich MS, Robinson EA, Zucker RA, Greden JF. Insomnia, self-medication, and relapse to alcoholism. *Am J Psychiatry.* 2001;**158**(3):399–404.

109. Philipsen A, Feige B, Al-Shajlawi A, *et al.* Increased delta power and discrepancies in objective and subjective sleep measurements in borderline personality disorder. *J Psychiatr Res.* 2005;**39**(5):489–98.

The association between sleep disorders and depression: implications for treatment

Negar Ahmadi, Philip Saleh, and Colin M. Shapiro

Sleep and psychiatric disorders

Sleep disturbances and psychiatric disorders are closely related. Sleep disturbances of various forms are present in many psychiatric disorders such as mood disorders, anxiety disorders, post-traumatic stress disorders, substance abuse, and schizophrenia [1]. Some of the most common sleep disturbances among patients suffering from psychiatric disorders are: difficulty initiating sleep, frequent awakenings, early morning awakenings, daytime sleepiness, fatigue, nightmares, and disrupted sleep–wake cycle. Furthermore, polysomnography (PSG) studies have reported sleep architectural changes among patients with various psychiatric disorders. For instance, many patients suffering from anxiety disorders complain of difficulty initiating and maintaining sleep and polysomnographic studies of these patients show longer sleep latency, increased time awake, and reduced sleep efficiency compared to normal individuals [2]. Moreover, several studies have supported the association between specific sleep disturbances such as shortened rapid eye movement (REM) latencies in patients suffering from a variety of psychiatric disorders including schizophrenia [3, 4], borderline personality disorder [5], anxiety disorder [6], anorexia nervosa [7], panic disorder [8], and depression [9, 10].

The association between sleep disturbances and mood disorders, in particular, has been studied extensively. Traditionally, sleep disturbances have been considered as a consequence of mood disorders and even to this date sleep disturbances are listed as symptoms of mood disorders in the *Diagnostic and Statistical Manual of Mental Disorders* (4th edition) (DSM-IV). However, there has been a recent shift of perspective in that sleep disturbances are beginning to be viewed as comorbid conditions or even underlying conditions of mood disorders [11–15]. This shift in perspective has come about through some of the recent literature on the association between sleep disturbances and mood disorders. First, studies have shown that for many patients treatment of their mood disorder does not resolve the sleep issues [16–19]. In other words, patients continue to report sleep disturbances even after they have been treated for their mood disorder. Second, sleep disturbances such as insomnia or sleep apnea have been shown to be risk factors for onset or recurrence of mood disorders [20–22]. Third, a few studies have reported better treatment outcomes for patients receiving simultaneous mood and sleep treatments [15, 23]. Therefore, more recent evidence is emerging to suggest that sleep disturbances are not merely symptoms of mood disorders but in many cases are the comorbid or the underlying causes of mood disorders. The aim of this review is to survey the existing literature on the issue of the association between sleep and mood disorders as well as the treatment of comorbid sleep disorders and mood disorders.

Sleep in depressed patients
Sleep complaints in depressed patients

A recent review of epidemiological studies done in the area of sleep and psychiatric disorders found that depression has the highest rate of comorbidity with sleep disorders where 50 to 90% of depressed patients complain of poor sleep [24]. It is also reported that about 80% of hospitalized depressed patients and 70% of outpatients with major depression complain of difficulties initiating and maintaining sleep, as well as early morning awakening and maintaining wakefulness during the day [25]. A recent study of 3,051 community dwelling older men reported a stronger

---

association between self-reported sleep disturbance and depression measures [26]. Depressed patients also report high levels of daytime sleepiness [27, 28]. Furthermore, fatigue is recognized as one of the prominent symptoms of depression [29, 30] and several studies have found that the majority of depressed patients have significant levels of fatigue prior to treatment [31–33].

Polysomnographic features of depression

In addition to shortened REM latencies mentioned above, many EEG studies have identified other unique sleep alterations when comparing the polysomnographic recordings of depressed patients to those of healthy controls. Depressed patients are found to have reduced amounts of slow-wave sleep (SWS), increased duration of REM sleep, and increased number of eye movements during REM sleep [24, 34, 35]. Hatzinger and colleagues have found that patients with reduced amounts of SWS and increased REM density, especially in the first part of the night, experienced recurrences of depression over the following years [36]. Apart from alterations in sleep architecture, reduced sleep efficiency and decreased total sleep time have also been reported in depressed patients [37].

Depression in sleep-disordered patients

Conversely, sleep disturbances and changes in sleep have been shown to influence the development, onset and course of psychiatric disorders [38–43]. Prolonged untreated sleep disorders such as difficulty initiating and maintaining sleep as well as restless and non-restorative sleep could cause low mood and therefore trigger a state of depression. Indeed, a Japanese nationwide study [44] found that those with greater sleep complaints (such as difficulty initiating sleep, difficulty maintaining sleep, early morning awakening, and daytime sleepiness) were more likely to score higher on a depression scale (Center for Epidemiological Studies Depression Scale, CES-D).

Depression and insomnia share a number of symptoms such as cognitive difficulties, reduced sleep, and fatigue [45]. An epidemiological study done by Ford and Kamerow [42] found that 40% of those with insomnia and 46.5% with hypersomnia had a psychiatric disorder compared to 16.4% of those with no sleep disturbance. This study also investigated the risk of new onset of depression and found that individuals who had untreated insomnia

for one year had a much higher risk of developing depression (odds ratio (OR): 39.8; 95% CI: 19.8–80) compared to those whose insomnia had been resolved by the one-year follow-up interview (OR: 1.6; 95% CI: 0.5–5.3). In a longitudinal study of young adults, Breslau and colleagues [39] found that insomnia significantly increased the risk of new onset of depression and reported an odds ratio of 3.95 (95% CI: 2.22–7.00) for new onset of major depression among a group of patients with a prior history of insomnia. In other words, future incidence of depression was almost four-fold in patients with a history of insomnia. Similarly, another longitudinal study of adults over 17 years has found insomnia as a risk factor for depression [46]. Other studies have also suggested an increased rate of depression onset in patients with insomnia [47–49]. Therefore, as suggested by Shapiro and colleagues [43], insomnia might actually be an underlying cause of depression.

Although the majority of depressed patients complain of insomnia, a significant proportion of them present with excessive daytime sleepiness (EDS) [27, 28, 50, 51]. In fact, Chellapa and Araujo [27] have reported a strong association between EDS and suicidal ideations among depressed patients. For some depressed patients, EDS might be consequence of an untreated sleep disorder such as sleep apnea or circadian rhythm disorder [50]. However, very few studies have evaluated objective EDS, using a physiologic measure such as the multiple sleep latency test (MSLT), in depressed patients. Despite subjective complaints of EDS, in one study [52] depressed patients were found to have MSLT scores within the normal range. However, the issue of EDS in depressed patients needs further research and the underlying cause of the relationship is still not clear.

Moreover, obstructive sleep apnea (OSA, a disorder of breathing in sleep) has been found to be associated with an increased prevalence of depression [53–58]. According to a recent review of literature 16 to 41% of patients with mild OSA had depression [59]. Peppard and colleagues [60] reported that within a four-year longitudinal study, those patients who developed sleep-related breathing disorders (including OSA) were at 80% greater odds for developing depression. Furthermore, another study of 157 obese OSA patients found that 33% of their study group had high to severe depression [61]. In many studies, the depression reported seems to be secondary to the OSA and is improved with treatment of OSA [59]. Furthermore, women with untreated OSA have higher risks of having depression than men with untreated OSA [62]. However, it is worth mentioning here that even though treatment of OSA with continuous positive airway pressure (CPAP) would improve depressive symptoms, patients who score high on measures of depression are also likely to be less compliant with CPAP treatment [63]. Thus, it is possible that patients with OSA who are also depressed will require extra measures to ensure proper CPAP compliance in order to treat both their OSA and depressive symptoms. On the other hand, strong support from the sleep laboratory team [64] has been shown to improve CPAP compliance.

Restless legs syndrome (RLS) is another sleep disorder found to be associated with depression [65–67]. Although, the relationship between RLS and depression is rather complex as there is some limited evidence suggesting antidepressants might cause or exacerbate RLS symptoms [68–72]. However, a number of studies [73–75] have found that patients with RLS are more likely to have been diagnosed with depression prior to receiving treatment for their depression. In fact, according to Partinen [65], RLS can cause four of the nine DSM-IV criteria for major depression including insomnia or hypersomnia, fatigue/loss of energy, diminished concentration, and psychomotor retardation or agitation.

Additionally, a number of studies have found a strong association between depression and a disturbed circadian rhythm [76–80]. In fact, some of the common symptoms of depression including difficulty falling asleep or early morning awakenings are also features of a delayed or advanced circadian rhythm. The shortening of REM latency in depressed patients is taken as further evidence for an advanced circadian phase [76, 79]. Furthermore, some studies have reported lower blood concentrations of melatonin in depressed patients compared to controls [81–83]. Melatonin is a hormone involved in the sleep–wake cycle as well as many other circadian-regulated cycles in the body [81]. Furthermore, studies of patients with delayed sleep phase syndrome (DSPS) have found a high prevalence of depression in patients suffering from DSPS [80, 84]. Therefore, the association between circadian rhythm and depression has been clearly established. Depressive symptoms have also been identified in approximately one in five patients with narcolepsy [85, 86]. A cohort study of 866 sleep clinic patients has found an association between depressive symptoms and sleep paralysis as well as self-reported cataplexy [87]. There appears to be a clear association between sleep disorders and depression and the two conditions often coexist.

Underlying mechanism of relationship between sleep and depression

Depression entails several biological changes involving the hormones and neurotransmitters in the body. Many antidepressants work by restoring the balance of neurotransmitters in depressed patients. Indeed, some of the neurotransmitters and hormones that are found to be involved with mood also affect sleep. One might argue that biological changes in the endocrine or the nervous system might be responsible for both disturbed sleep and depressed mood. However, not all those with such altered biological systems will develop both mood disorders and sleep disorders. Among neurotransmitters, diminished serotonin levels have often been associated with depressed mood [88]. Serotonin is involved in a number of bodily functions including sleep. Therefore, imbalance in serotonin levels not only disrupts mood but may also affect sleep.

The dysregulation of the hypothalamic–pituitary–adrenocortical (HPA) system, which results in elevated cortisol levels, has been found to be one of the most robust biological markers of depression [89]. The HPA system is also known to influence sleep. Hatzinger and colleagues have found a strong association between dysregulated HPA system and disturbed sleep [36]. Furthermore, studies have found overactivity in the HPA system among patients with primary insomnia (without depression) [90–92]. Based on these observations, it is likely that for some insomnia patients and depressed patients, the underlying neurophysiology might be very similar. Moreover, Buckley and Schatzberg [93] have proposed that untreated OSA causes nocturnal awakening and autonomic activations that are associated with elevated cortisol levels and a disturbed HPA system. One could argue that the untreated sleep disorder might cause elevated cortisol levels, disrupt the HPS system, and eventually cause depressed mood.

Treatment of depression and sleep disorders

The close association between sleep disorders and depression would have significant implications for treatment of either of the conditions. When faced with the issue of treatment of comorbid sleep disorders and depression, it is important to understand which disorder came first. There are a number of studies suggesting that in a significant proportion of patients with comorbid sleep disorders and depression, it was the sleep disorder that preceded depression. In particular, insomnia, sleep apnea, and circadian rhythm disturbances have been shown to precede the onset of depression in many patients [15, 48, 79, 94, 95]. Therefore, one argument is that if the sleep disorders are left untreated, depression may develop. As Meerlo and colleagues suggest, untreated sleep disorders can sensitize individuals to develop depression [95]. Once depression develops, the underlying sleep disorder might simply appear to be a symptom of depression and may be resolved when the depression is treated.

As noted above, insomnia is the most common sleep complaint among depressed patients. Treatment of depression with certain antidepressants is known to increase insomnia in depressed patients [76]. Insomnia has been shown to hinder treatment of depression with antidepressants and further influence the course of treatment [15, 23]. A randomized control trial by Manber and colleagues showed that augmenting antidepressant treatment with cognitive behavioral therapy (CBT) for insomnia improves both sleep and depression [23]. However, studies have shown that early treatment of insomnia might even prevent the onset of depression or prevent the recurrence of a depressive episode [46, 96]. Furthermore, untreated insomnia can increase the relapse rate among depressed patients. Pigeon and colleagues [15] studied a large group of elderly patients treated for their depression and found that those with persistent insomnia were three times less likely to remit from their depression within a six-month period compared to those without persistent insomnia. Indeed, rates of relapse of depression increase dramatically when any of the vegetative symptoms of depression (including poor sleep) remain following treatment [97]. Therefore, treatment of insomnia can prevent the onset of depression, improve response to depression treatment, and further reduce recurrences of depression.

Breathing-related sleep disorder in depressed patients is often unrecognized and untreated. Research has shown that as many as 18% of depressed patients have an undiagnosed breathing-related sleep disorder [98]. However, the study by Ohayon [98] used DSM-IV criteria to diagnose breathing-related sleep disorder as opposed to PSG, which is the gold standard method of diagnosis of breathing-related sleep disorders including sleep apnea. Research has shown that women with sleep apnea are at a greater risk of having comorbid depression [51]. Moreover, sleep apnea is more likely to be undiagnosed or misdiagnosed with depression among women [62]. Although, the estimates of undiagnosed sleep apnea among depressed patients are high, there is limited research to utilize PSGs to investigate the proportion of undiagnosed sleep apnea cases among depressed patients. However, once diagnosed, studies have shown that treatment of sleep apnea improves mood and alleviates symptoms of depression [54, 94, 99–101]. Improvements in depressive symptoms have been shown to be apparent not only after treatment with CPAP [102, 103] but also after treatment with mandibular repositioning appliances (MRA) [104]. However, once again, the studies that have investigated the effect of treatment of sleep apnea on depression are either limited in the number of participants or are restricted to the use of self-reports to measure depressive symptoms.

The issue of treatment of RLS comorbid with depression is somewhat more complex due to the fact that some studies have suggested that some antidepressants could exacerbate RLS symptoms [66, 67, 69]. However, the evidence is limited and there is further evidence suggesting that RLS could in fact be the cause of depression [65]. Picchietti and Winkelman have proposed a specific treatment approach for patients with comorbid RLS and depression [105]. According to this approach, patients suffering from chronic mild depression (without risk of suicide) comorbid with RLS should have their RLS treated first followed by depression treatment [105]. The approach proposed by Picchietti and Winkelman [105] seems to be more effective than initial treatment of depression followed by RLS treatment. Therefore, RLS comorbid with depression should be considered independent of depression and be treated as such. Similarly, treatment of disturbed circadian rhythm by restoring the normal circadian cycle can enhance mood and alleviate depressive symptoms [77]. One may anticipate that treatment of other sleep disorders such as EDS or narcolepsy would also improve depression, or reduce relapse rates.

Conclusion

Sleep disorders and depression are clearly associated in that sleep disorders are often present in patients with depression who present to mood disorder clinics and depression is often found as a comorbid condition in sleep clinic patients with sleep disorders. Sleep disturbances have traditionally been viewed as merely symptoms of depression. However, the emerging literature supports the notion that sleep disturbances could be an underlying cause or a comorbid condition and should be investigated independent of depression. Furthermore, research studies over the past decades have shown that untreated sleep disorders such as insomnia, OSA, or DSPS can cause depression, act as a barrier to treatment of depression, and further increase relapse rates. Furthermore, there is some evidence to suggest that treatment of sleep disorders can prevent the onset of depression or enhance the effectiveness of depression treatment. However, the studies that have investigated the effect of treatment of sleep disorders on depression have often been limited in terms of the number of patients, and many studies either did not use PSGs to diagnose sleep disorders or lacked proper assessment of depression through clinical interviews. Therefore, future studies should focus on investigating the effect of treatment of sleep disorders on depression.

References

1. Benca RM, Obermeyer WH, Thisted RA, Gillin JC. Sleep and psychiatric disorders. A meta-analysis. *Arch Gen Psychiatry.* 1992;**49**:651–68.

2. Papadimitriou GN, Linkowski P. Sleep disturbance in anxiety disorders. *Int Rev Psychiatry.* 2005;**17**:229–36.

3. Reich L, Weiss BL, Coble P, McPartland R, Kupfer DJ. Sleep disturbance in schizophrenia. A revisit. *Arch Gen Psychiatry.* 1975;**32**:51–55.

4. Zarcone VP Jr, Benson KL, Berger PA. Abnormal rapid eye movement latencies in schizophrenia. *Arch Gen Psychiatry.* 1987;**44**:45–8.

5. Philipsen A, Feige B, Al-Shajlawi A, *et al.* Increased delta power and discrepancies in objective and subjective sleep measurements in borderline personality disorder. *J Psychiatr.Res.* 2005;**39**:489–98.

6. Rotenberg VS, Arshavsky VV. REM sleep, stress and search activity. A short critical review and a new conception. *Waking Sleeping.* 1997;**3**:235–44.

7. Neil JF, Merikangas JR, Foster FG, *et al.* Waking and all-night sleep EEG's in anorexia nervosa. *Clin Electroencephalogr.* 1980;**11**:9–15.

8. Uhde TW, Roy-Byrne P, Gillin JC, *et al.* The sleep of patients with panic disorder: a preliminary report. *Psychiatry Res.* 1984;**12**:251–9.

9. Stefos G, Staner L, Kerkhofs M, *et al.* Shortened REM latency as a psychobiological marker for psychotic depression? An age-, gender-, and polarity-controlled study. *Biol. Psychiatry.* 1998;**44**:1314–20.

10. Berger M, van Calker D, Riemann D. Sleep and manipulations of the sleep-wake rhythm in depression. *Acta Psychiatr Scand Suppl.* 2003;**418**:83–91.

11. Buysse DJ, Angst J, Gamma A, *et al.* Prevalence, course, and comorbidity of insomnia and depression in young adults. *Sleep.* 2008;**31**:473–80.

12. Krahn LE. Psychiatric disorders associated with disturbed sleep. *Semin Neurol.* 2005;**25**:90–6.

13. Krystal AD. Sleep and psychiatric disorders: future directions. *Psychiatr Clin North Am.* 2006;**29**:1115–30.

14. Krystal AD, Thakur M, Roth T. Sleep disturbance in psychiatric disorders: effects on function and quality of life in mood disorders, alcoholism, and schizophrenia. *Ann Clin Psychiatry.* 2008;**20**:39–46.

15. Pigeon WR, Hegel M, Unutzer J, *et al.* Is insomnia a perpetuating factor for late-life depression in the IMPACT cohort? *Sleep.* 2008;**31**:481–8.

16. Fava M. Daytime sleepiness and insomnia as correlates of depression. *J Clin Psychiatry.* 2004;**65** (Suppl 16):27–32.

17. Becker PM. Treatment of sleep dysfunction and psychiatric disorders. *Curr Treat Options Neurol.* 2006;**8**:367–75.

18. Nierenberg AA, Keefe BR, Leslie VC, *et al.* Residual symptoms in depressed patients who respond acutely to fluoxetine. *J Clin Psychiatry.* 1999;**60**:221–5.

19. Giglio LM, Andreazza AC, Andersen M, *et al.* Sleep in bipolar patients. *Sleep Breath.* 2008;**13**(2):169–73.

20. Moller HJ. Outcomes in major depressive disorder: the evolving concept of remission and its implications for treatment. *World J Biol Psychiatry.* 2008;**9**:102–14.

21. Cho HJ, Lavretsky H, Olmstead R, *et al.* Sleep disturbance and depression recurrence in community-dwelling older adults: a prospective study. *Am J Psychiatry.* 2008;**165**(12):1543–50.

22. Dombrovski AY, Cyranowski JM, Mulsant BH, *et al.* Which symptoms predict recurrence of depression in women treated with maintenance interpersonal psychotherapy? *Depress Anxiety.* 2008;**25**(12):1060–6.

23. Manber R, Edinger JD, Gress JL, *et al.* Cognitive behavioral therapy for insomnia enhances depression outcome in patients with comorbid major depressive disorder and insomnia. *Sleep.* 2008;**31**:489–95.

24. Tsuno N, Besset A, Ritchie K. Sleep and depression. *J Clin Psychiatry.* 2005;**66**:1254–69.

25. Ohayon MM, Shapiro CM. Sleep disturbances and psychiatric disorders associated with posttraumatic

stress disorder in the general population. *Compr Psychiatry*. 2000;**41**:469–78.

26. Paudel ML, Taylor BC, Diem SJ, *et al*. Association between depressive symptoms and sleep disturbances in community-dwelling older men. *J Am Geriatr Soc*. 2008;**56**:1228–35.

27. Chellappa SL, Araujo JF. Excessive daytime sleepiness in patients with depressive disorder. *Rev Bras Psiquiatr*. 2006;**28**:126–9.

28. Lundt L. Use of the Epworth Sleepiness Scale to evaluate the symptom of excessive sleepiness in major depressive disorder. *Gen Hosp Psychiatry*. 2005;**27**:146–8.

29. Menza M, Marin H, Opper RS. Residual symptoms in depression: can treatment be symptom-specific? *J Clin Psychiatry*. 2003;**64**:516–23.

30. Hossain JL, Ahmad P, Reinish LW, *et al*. Subjective fatigue and subjective sleepiness: two independent consequences of sleep disorders? *J Sleep Res*. 2005;**14**:245–53.

31. Moos RH, Cronkite RC. Symptom-based predictors of a 10-year chronic course of treated depression. *J Nerv Ment Dis*. 1999;**187**:360–8.

32. Tylee A, Gastpar M, Lepine JP, Mendlewicz J. DEPRES II (Depression Research in European Society II): a patient survey of the symptoms, disability and current management of depression in the community. DEPRES Steering Committee. *Int Clin Psychopharmacol*. 1999;**14**:139–51.

33. Baker M, Dorzab J, Winokur G, Cadoret RJ. Depressive disease: classification and clinical characteristics. *Compr Psychiatry*. 1971;**12**:354–65.

34. Arriaga F, Rosado P, Paiva T. The sleep of dysthymic patients: a comparison with normal controls. *Biol Psychiatry*. 1990;**27**:649–56.

35. Reynolds CF III, Newton TF, Shaw DH, Coble PA, Kupfer DJ. Electroencephalographic sleep findings in depressed outpatients. *Psychiatry Res*. 1982;**6**:65–75.

36. Hatzinger M, Hemmeter UM, Brand S, Ising M, Holsboer-Trachsler E. Electroencephalographic sleep profiles in treatment course and long-term outcome of major depression: association with DEX/CRH-test response. *J Psychiatr Res*. 2004;**38**:453–65.

37. Benca RM, Obermeyer WH, Thisted RA, Gillin JC. Sleep and psychiatric disorders. A meta-analysis. *Arch Gen Psychiatry*. 1992;**49**:651–68.

38. Monti JM, Monti D. Sleep disturbance in generalized anxiety disorder and its treatment. *Sleep Med Rev*. 2000;**4**:263–76.

39. Breslau N, Roth T, Rosenthal L, Andreski P. Sleep disturbance and psychiatric disorders: a longitudinal epidemiological study of young adults. *Biol Psychiatry*. 1996;**39**:411–18.

40. Lustberg L, Reynolds CF. Depression and insomnia: questions of cause and effect. *Sleep Med Rev*. 2000;**4**:253–62.

41. Aikens JE, Vanable PA, Tadimeti L, Caruana-Montaldo B, Mendelson WB. Differential rates of psychopathology symptoms in periodic limb movement disorder, obstructive sleep apnea, psychophysiological insomnia, and insomnia with psychiatric disorder. *Sleep*. 1999;**22**:775–80.

42. Ford DE, Kamerow DB. Epidemiologic study of sleep disturbances and psychiatric disorders. An opportunity for prevention? *JAMA*. 1989;**262**:1479–84.

43. Shapiro GK, Shen J, Shapiro CM. Sleep changes in the depressed older adults: implications for management. *Geriatric and Aging Supplement*. 2004;**7**:25–31.

44. Kaneita Y, Ohida T, Uchiyama M, *et al*. The relationship between depression and sleep disturbances: a Japanese nationwide general population survey. *J Clin Psychiatry*. 2006;**67**:196–203.

45. Moul DE, Nofzinger EA, Pilkonis PA, *et al*. Symptom reports in severe chronic insomnia. *Sleep*. 2002;**25**:553–63.

46. Colman I, Croudace TJ, Wadsworth ME, Jones PB. Factors associated with antidepressant, anxiolytic and hypnotic use over 17 years in a national cohort. *J Affect Disord*. 2008;**110**:234–40.

47. Taylor DJ. Insomnia and depression. *Sleep*. 2008;**31**:447–8.

48. Ohayon MM. Insomnia: a ticking clock for depression? *J Psychiatr Res*. 2007;**41**:893–4.

49. Roth T. Insomnia: definition, prevalence, etiology, and consequences. *J Clin Sleep Med*. 2007;**3**:S7–10.

50. Chellappa SL, Schroder C, Cajochen C. Chronobiology, excessive daytime sleepiness and depression: Is there a link? *Sleep Med*. 2009;**10**(5):505–14.

51. Basta M, Lin HM, Pejovic S, *et al*. Lack of regular exercise, depression, and degree of apnea are predictors of excessive daytime sleepiness in patients with sleep apnea: sex differences. *J Clin Sleep Med*. 2008;**4**:19–25.

52. Nofzinger EA, Thase ME, Reynolds CF III, *et al*. Hypersomnia in bipolar depression: a comparison with narcolepsy using the multiple sleep latency test. *Am J Psychiatry*. 1991;**148**:1177–81.

53. Aikens JE, Vanable PA, Tadimeti L, Caruana-Montaldo B, Mendelson WB. Differential rates of psychopathology symptoms in periodic limb movement disorder, obstructive sleep apnea, psychophysiological insomnia, and insomnia with psychiatric disorder. *Sleep*. 1999;**22**:775–80.

54. El-Ad B, Lavie P. Effect of sleep apnea on cognition and mood. *Int Rev Psychiatry*. 2005;**17**:277–82.

55. McCall WV, Harding D, O'Donovan C. Correlates of depressive symptoms in patients with obstructive sleep apnea. *J Clin Sleep Med*. 2006;**2**:424–6.

56. Andrews JG, Oei TP. The roles of depression and anxiety in the understanding and treatment of Obstructive Sleep Apnea Syndrome. *Clin Psychol Rev*. 2004;**24**:1031–49.

57. Baran AS, Richert AC. Obstructive sleep apnea and depression. *CNS Spectr*. 2003;**8**:128–34.

58. Millman RP, Fogel BS, McNamara ME, Carlisle CC. Depression as a manifestation of obstructive sleep apnea: reversal with nasal continuous positive airway pressure. *J Clin Psychiatry*. 1989;**50**:348–51.

59. Saunamaki T, Jehkonen M. Depression and anxiety in obstructive sleep apnea syndrome: a review. *Acta Neurol Scand*. 2007;**116**:277–88.

60. Peppard PE, Szklo-Coxe M, Hla KM, Young T. Longitudinal association of sleep-related breathing disorder and depression. *Arch Intern Med*. 2006;**166**:1709–15.

61. Pierobon A, Giardini A, Fanfulla F, Callegari S, Majani G. A multidimensional assessment of obese patients with obstructive sleep apnoea syndrome (OSAS): A study of psychological, neuropsychological and clinical relationships in a disabling multifaceted disease. *Sleep Med*. 2008;**9**(8):882–9.

62. Wahner-Roedler DL, Olson EJ, Narayanan S, *et al.* Gender-specific differences in a patient population with obstructive sleep apnea-hypopnea syndrome. *Gend Med*. 2007;**4**:329–38.

63. Kjelsberg FN, Ruud EA, Stavem K. Predictors of symptoms of anxiety and depression in obstructive sleep apnea. *Sleep Med*. 2005;**6**:341–6.

64. Brin YS, Reuveni H, Greenberg S, Tal A, Tarasiuk A. Determinants affecting initiation of continuous positive airway pressure treatment. *Isr Med Assoc J*. 2005;**7**:13–18.

65. Partinen M. Challenging issues: sleep-wake, augmentation and quality of life. *Sleep Med*. 2007;**8** (Suppl 2):S19–24.

66. Baumann CR, Marti I, Bassetti CL. Restless legs symptoms without periodic limb movements in sleep and without response to dopaminergic agents: a restless legs-like syndrome? *Eur J Neurol*. 2007;**14**:1369–72.

67. Page RL, Ruscin JM, Bainbridge JL, Brieke AA. Restless legs syndrome induced by escitalopram: case report and review of the literature. *Pharmacotherapy*. 2008;**28**:271–80.

68. Prospero-Garcia KA, Torres-Ruiz A, Ramirez-Bermudez J, *et al.* Fluoxetine-mirtazapine interaction may induce restless legs syndrome: report of 3 cases from a clinical trial. *J Clin Psychiatry*. 2006;**67**:1820.

69. Perroud N, Lazignac C, Baleydier B, *et al.* Restless legs syndrome induced by citalopram: a psychiatric emergency? *Gen Hosp Psychiatry*. 2007;**29**:72–4.

70. Chang CC, Shiah IS, Chang HA, Mao WC. Does domperidone potentiate mirtazapine-associated restless legs syndrome? *Prog Neuropsychopharmacol Biol Psychiatry*. 2006;**30**:316–18.

71. Yang C, White DP, Winkelman JW. Antidepressants and periodic leg movements of sleep. *Biol Psychiatry*. 2005;**58**:510–14.

72. Novak M, Shapiro CM. Drug-induced sleep disturbances. Focus on nonpsychotropic medications. *Drug Saf*. 1997;**16**:133–49.

73. Banno K, Delaive K, Walld R, Kryger MH. Restless legs syndrome in 218 patients: associated disorders. *Sleep Med*. 2000;**1**:221–9.

74. Hornyak M, Kopasz M, Berger M, Riemann D, Voderholzer U. Impact of sleep-related complaints on depressive symptoms in patients with restless legs syndrome. *J Clin Psychiatry*. 2005;**66**:1139–45.

75. Sevim S, Dogu O, Kaleagasi H, *et al.* Correlation of anxiety and depression symptoms in patients with restless legs syndrome: a population based survey. *J Neurol Neurosurg Psychiatry*. 2004;**75**:226–30.

76. Germain A, Kupfer DJ. Circadian rhythm disturbances in depression. *Hum Psychopharmacol*. 2008;**23**:571–85.

77. Lader M. Limitations of current medical treatments for depression: disturbed circadian rhythms as a possible therapeutic target. *Eur Neuropsychopharmacol*. 2007;**17**:743–55.

78. Monteleone P, Maj M. The circadian basis of mood disorders: recent developments and treatment implications. *Eur Neuropsychopharmacol*. 2008;**18**:701–11.

79. Turek FW. From circadian rhythms to clock genes in depression. *Int Clin Psychopharmacol*. 2007;**22** (Suppl 2):S1–8.

80. Regestein QR, Monk TH. Delayed sleep phase syndrome: a review of its clinical aspects. *Am J Psychiatry*. 1995;**152**:602–8.

81. Srinivasan V, Smits M, Spence W, *et al.* Melatonin in mood disorders. *World J Biol Psychiatry*. 2006;**7**:138–51.

82. Tuunainen A, Kripke DF, Elliott JA, *et al.* Depression and endogenous melatonin in postmenopausal women. *J Affect Disord*. 2002;**69**:149–58.

83. Claustrat B, Chazot G, Brun J, Jordan D, Sassolas G. A chronobiological study of melatonin and cortisol

secretion in depressed subjects: plasma melatonin, a biochemical marker in major depression. *Biol Psychiatry.* 1984;**19**:1215–28.

84. Kripke DF, Rex KM, Ancoli-Israel S, *et al.* Delayed sleep phase cases and controls. *J Circadian Rhythms.* 2008;**6**:6.

85. Roth B, Nevsimalova S. Depresssion in narcolepsy and hypersommia. *Schweiz Arch Neurol Neurochir Psychiatr.* 1975;**116**:291–300.

86. Adda C, Lefevre B, Reimao R. Narcolepsy and depression. *Arq Neuropsiquiatr.* 1997;**55**:423–6.

87. Szklo-Coxe M, Young T, Finn L, Mignot E. Depression: relationships to sleep paralysis and other sleep disturbances in a community sample. *J Sleep Res.* 2007;**16**:297–312.

88. Cleare AJ, Murray RM, O'Keane V. Assessment of serotonergic function in major depression using d-fenfluramine: relation to clinical variables and antidepressant response. *Biol Psychiatry.* 1998;**44**:555–61.

89. Hatzinger M, Hemmeter UM, Baumann K, Brand S, Holsboer-Trachsler E. The combined DEX-CRH test in treatment course and long-term outcome of major depression. *J Psychiatr Res.* 2002;**36**:287–97.

90. Richardson GS, Roth T. Future directions in the management of insomnia. *J Clin Psychiatry.* 2001;**62** (Suppl 10):39–45.

91. Vgontzas AN, Tsigos C, Bixler EO, *et al.* Chronic insomnia and activity of the stress system: a preliminary study. *J Psychosom Res.* 1998;**45**:21–31.

92. Vgontzas AN, Bixler EO, Lin HM, *et al.* Chronic insomnia is associated with nyctohemeral activation of the hypothalamic-pituitary-adrenal axis: clinical implications. *J Clin Endocrinol Metab.* 2001;**86**:3787–94.

93. Buckley TM, Schatzberg AF. On the interactions of the hypothalamic-pituitary-adrenal (HPA) axis and sleep: normal HPA axis activity and circadian rhythm, exemplary sleep disorders. *J Clin Endocrinol Metab.* 2005;**90**:3106–14.

94. Schroder CM, O'Hara R. Depression and obstructive sleep apnea (OSA). *Ann Gen Psychiatry.* 2005;**4**:13.

95. Meerlo P, Sgoifo A, Suchecki D. Restricted and disrupted sleep: Effects on autonomic function, neuroendocrine stress systems and stress responsivity. *Sleep Med Rev.* 2008;**12**(3):197–210.

96. Jindal RD, Thase ME. Treatment of insomnia associated with clinical depression. *Sleep Med Rev.* 2004;**8**:19–30.

97. Kennedy S, Parikh SV, Shapiro CM. *Defeating Depression.* (Thornhill, ON: Joli Joco Publications Inc., 1998).

98. Ohayon MM. The effects of breathing-related sleep disorders on mood disturbances in the general population. *J Clin Psychiatry.* 2003;**64**:1195–200.

99. Schwartz DJ, Kohler WC, Karatinos G. Symptoms of depression in individuals with obstructive sleep apnea may be amenable to treatment with continuous positive airway pressure. *Chest.* 2005;**128**:1304–9.

100. Yamamoto H, Akashiba T, Kosaka N, Ito D, Horie T. Long-term effects of nasal continuous positive airway pressure on daytime sleepiness, mood and traffic accidents in patients with obstructive sleep apnoea. *Respir Med.* 2000;**94**:87–90.

101. Kawahara S, Akashiba T, Akahoshi T, Horie T. Nasal CPAP improves the quality of life and lessens the depressive symptoms in patients with obstructive sleep apnea syndrome. *Intern Med.* 2005;**44**:422–7.

102. Krahn LE, Miller BW, Bergstrom LR. Rapid resolution of intense suicidal ideation after treatment of severe obstructive sleep apnea. *J Clin Sleep Med.* 2008;**4**:64–5.

103. Hirshkowitz M. The clinical consequences of obstructive sleep apnea and associated excessive sleepiness. *J Fam Pract.* 2008;**57**:S9–16.

104. Saletu A, Anderer P, Parapatics S, *et al.* Effects of a mandibular repositioning appliance on sleep structure, morning behavior and clinical symptomatology in patients with snoring and sleep-disordered breathing. *Neuropsychobiology.* 2007;**55**:184–93.

105. Picchietti D, Winkelman JW. Restless legs syndrome, periodic limb movements in sleep, and depression. *Sleep.* 2005;**28**:891–8.

Sleep in late-life depression

Wilfred R. Pigeon and Sara Matteson-Rusby

Introduction

Both sleep disorders and mood disorders are significant public health issues in the geriatric population. Sleep disturbance is a symptom criterion across a number of psychiatric illnesses in the Diagnostic and Statistical Manual of Mental Disorders, 4th Revision (DSM) including major depressive disorder (MDD), which will be the primary focus of this chapter [1]. In MDD, the sleep disturbance may be either in the form of insomnia or hypersomnia, where the latter is also known as excessive daytime sleepiness (EDS) and is most often associated with the presence of sleep-disordered breathing conditions such as obstructive sleep apnea. The most common sleep disorders in the general population are, in fact, insomnia and sleep-disordered breathing, each of which increase rather dramatically in prevalence across the lifespan [2–4]. The prevalence of mood disorders remains somewhat constant from middle to old age [5].

This chapter will review literature from older populations, but supplemented by extrapolation of findings from non-elder populations where appropriate. Especially with respect to epidemiologic data, the definition of sleep disturbance varies. Such investigations often report on one or more single item measures of sleep complaints either developed for the study or embedded within other instruments. For instance, the Hamilton Rating Scale for Depression [6] has three items related respectively to early, middle, and late night insomnia. These items have been validated as an insomnia subscale [7–9]. For this chapter we have adopted the convention of using the term "insomnia" in such cases and "sleep disturbance" when a more general assessment of sleep difficulties was made. Finally, the chapter will focus on describing the extent of sleep disturbances and their consequences in late-life depression and the possible role of sleep disturbances as risk factors for depression. We only address issues of sleep architecture and pathophysiology when these are specific to older cohorts, as these topics are well covered elsewhere in this volume.

Sleep disturbance and depression

The association between disturbed sleep in the elderly, in general, and depression, in particular, has been the focus of several investigations and a significant relationship between the two has been found regarding some specific sleep disorders. In fact, depression has been found to be significantly and negatively associated with sleep satisfaction in community-dwelling older adults ($r = 0.47$; $p < 0.001$) [10].

Data from the National Institute of Aging's EPESE study was used to assess the sleep–depression relationship in 9,282 people aged 65 and older in three community-based cohorts. During in-person interviews, participants were asked about the frequency of five different sleep complaints (trouble falling asleep, staying asleep, waking up too early, needing to nap, and not feeling rested). Over half of the participants reported at least one sleep complaint occurring most of the time; 13% reported chronically waking up not rested and 7 to 15% rarely or never felt rested when waking up in the morning. Depressive symptomatology was the strongest correlate of both this complaint and of insomnia. Those in the top two quartiles of the depression scores were 2.5 times more likely to wake not feeling rested compared to those with lower scores with an odds ratio (OR) of 2.45 [2.11–2.85] [11]. Sleep quality, as assessed by the Pittsburgh Sleep Quality Index (PSQI) [12], along

Sleep and Mental Illness, eds. S. R. Pandi-Perumal and M. Kramer. Published by Cambridge University Press.
© Cambridge University Press 2010.

Table 16.1 Association of sleep complaints with depression

Sleep complaint (n = 1,506)	Odds ratio [95% CI]
Difficulty falling asleep	2.44 [1.59–3.73]
Awake a lot during the night	1.59 [1.14–2.22]
Waking up too early	2.21 [1.49–3.29]
Waking feeling not refreshed	2.18 [1.53–3.13]
Daytime sleepiness	2.19 [1.36–3.55]
Breathing pauses during sleep	2.84 [1.76–4.57]
Unpleasant feelings in legs	1.64 [1.07–2.56]

Notes: Data from Foley *et al.* [14].
CI = confidence interval.

with residual anxiety, independently predicted early recurrence of depression in a study of 116 patients aged 70 and older [13]. Thus, there appears to be a relationship between symptoms of depression and poor sleep quality in this age group.

This association was also found in a study conducted via telephone interviews with 1,506 community-dwelling men and women aged 55 to 84 [14]. Depression was among the conditions most associated with a number of sleep complaints (see Table 16.1), though other conditions commonly diagnosed in the elderly were also associated with sleep-related problems. Thus, sleep complaints in the elderly appear to be related to a variety of comorbid conditions, including depression, rather than to aging, per se. Roberts and colleagues [15] also found sleep problems were the best predictor of depression over a one-year period (OR 6.84 [4.27–10.97]). Although this type of relationship between sleep complaints and depression is increasingly well established, as in the prior study, several other factors including older age and female gender were also significant predictors of depression among this elderly sample. In respect to sleep disturbance and depression, therefore, there is some evidence to suggest that sleep disturbance is associated with, and in some cases is a risk factor for, late-life depression.

Insomnia and depression

The extant literature on the relationship between insomnia and depression is fairly large and includes cross-sectional and longitudinal data as well as data from depression treatment trials. Several large studies with stratified age samples bear out that insomnia is about twice as prevalent as depression. The National

Institute of Mental Health Epidemiologic Catchment Area study (N = 7,954) found prevalence rates of 10% for insomnia and 5% for depression [16]. An automated telephone screening of the general population of France (N = 5,622), found prevalence rates of 17% for insomnia and 6% for depression [17]. In a United States community sample of 772 individuals, the prevalence rates were 20% and 10% respectively for insomnia and depression [18]. When more stringent diagnostic criteria were applied to data from the Second National Survey of Psychiatric Morbidity conducted in the United Kingdom (N = 8,580), prevalence rates of 5% for insomnia and 3% for depression were observed [19].

Two large-scale studies have been conducted in older populations. Foley *et al.* assessed data from 9,282 elderly community dwellers and found prevalence rates of 28% for insomnia and 20% for depression [4]. In a longitudinal study of community residents aged 50 and over in Alameda County, CA (N = 2,272), baseline estimates for the prevalence of insomnia and depression were 24% and 9% respectively [15]. Two studies in primary care samples [20, 21] have found prevalence rates of 16 to 19% for insomnia and 7 to 8% for depression.

An interesting addition to the findings from the above studies can be derived by looking at the subsamples of participants who were determined to report both insomnia and depression. Overall, in a combined sample of 37,367 respondents, 4% had comorbid depression and insomnia. Moreover, of those with depression, 48% had insomnia, whereas in those with insomnia, 27% were depressed (see Table 16.2). Taken together, these findings make clear that both insomnia and depression are highly prevalent in the elderly and that it is more likely that insomnia occurs in the context of depression as opposed to depression occurring in the context of insomnia.

Longitudinal studies provide some additional information about the relationship between insomnia and depression. For instance, when patients with remitted, but recurrent MDD were followed weekly for up to 42 weeks or until a recurrent episode, those who experienced a recurrence of depression (compared to those with no recurrence) exhibited an increased level of sleep disturbance consistent with insomnia that began five weeks prior to and peaked at recurrence, and was of highest severity at the week of recurrence [22]. This suggests that insomnia is

Table 16.2 Prevalence rates of comorbid depression and insomnia

Study	Sample size	Comorbid, %	In depressed, % with insomnia	In insomnia, % with depression
[4] Foley	9,282	10%	49%	34%
[17] Ohayon	5,622	3%	57%	18%
[19] Stewart	8,580	1%	40%	21%
[18] Taylor	772	4%	41%	20%
[42] Simon	373	5%	58%	31%
[16] Ford	7,954	2%	42%	23%
[15] Roberts	2,272	5%	50%	19%
[20] Hohagen	2,512	4%	52%	18%
Total N:	37,367	4%	48%	27%

a prodromal sign of an impending depressive episode, albeit this finding was not in an elderly cohort.

Longitudinal studies in mixed-age cohorts have found that insomnia predicts subsequent depression. Three studies have evaluated the onset of new depression over a one-year time period. Two of these have found that insomnia posed an increased risk for the development of depression [16, 23], while the third found an increased risk for depression in women only [24]. In a study that began with college-aged men, insomnia conferred a relative risk of 2.0 (1.2–3.3) for developing depression at some point during the following 30 years [25].

When longitudinal studies have been conducted in older cohorts, the findings have been similar, but mixed. Among 524 community-dwelling elders, persistent insomnia across three years was associated with depression at the three-year time point. [26]. In a subsample who had activity limitations, but no psychiatric morbidity at baseline, baseline insomnia was not associated with depression three years later [27]. Others have found that insomnia at a baseline assessment and persistent insomnia across one year are each associated with depression at one year, the latter being associated with an eight-fold risk [15]. In another study, initial insomnia, but not middle of the night insomnia or early morning awakening, was associated with the development of new depression at three years [28]. A study assessing these factors over 12 years again found that insomnia was an independent predictor of later depression, but in women only [29]. Finally, in a meta-analysis of studies conducted in older adults, sleep disturbance was

second to recent bereavement as an independent risk factor for late-life depression [30]. In summary, there is a good body of evidence that suggests that both incident and persistent insomnia are risk factors for new onset depression, although the findings are not unanimous across all studies. Appropriate caution is warranted given the variety of study designs and manners in which insomnia is operationalized.

Additional information comes to us from treatment trials for depression. In antidepressant medication trials, insomnia is often a residual symptom in 30 to 50% of participants [31–35]. For instance, in a fluoxetine trial, disturbed sleep was the most common residual symptom, occurring in 44% of depression remitters [34]. In a trial of nortriptyline, depression remitters had significant decreases in mean sleep disturbance scores on the Pittsburgh Sleep Quality Index (PSQI) [36], but their mean global PSQI score remained above the clinical cut-off for disturbed sleep and higher than that of healthy controls [37]. Interestingly, the treatment of depression with targeted behavioral interventions mirrors some of the outcomes observed following pharmacotherapy for depression [38, 39]. In a trial comparing cognitive and behavioral therapy (CBT) for depression to antidepressant medication, residual insomnia was evenly distributed between intervention groups and occurred in approximately 50% of those with remitted depression [40]. Similar findings were observed in a trial comparing CBT to nefazadone [41]. Finally, in a trial of stepped care depression management in depressed elders presenting to primary care, participants with persistent insomnia were two to four times more likely to remain depressed at later time points than patients with no insomnia [42]. Together this set of findings from treatment trials suggests that insomnia (for some individuals) may persist despite a seeming resolution of depression. This is in addition to empirical evidence that insomnia is a risk factor for the onset and recurrence of late-life depression.

Treating insomnia in the context of depression

Some promising options have begun to emerge for the treatment of insomnia in depression at the comorbid phase (as opposed to waiting for the residual phase). A recent co-administration study found that eszopiclone with fluoxetine resulted in sustained sleep improvements as well as a faster and more robust antidepressant effect than fluoxetine alone [43]. In a unique co-administration study highlighting the importance of behavioral interventions for sleep, the combined use of escitilopram and cognitive behavioral therapy for insomnia (CBT-I) resulted in larger improvements in both sleep and depression outcomes than escitilopram and a control therapy [44]. There are also two uncontrolled studies that have shown that patients presenting with insomnia and depression who completed only a course of CBT-I had improvements in both sleep and depression [45, 46]. No such data are available with respect to late-life depression, but it is not unreasonable to expect that the above findings would generalize to the elderly given the success of both hypnotics and CBT-I in older patients with primary insomnia.

Insomnia and bereavement

Bereavement refers to the emotion that occurs in response to the loss of a loved one by death and since 75% of all deaths occur in persons 65 years of age and older [47], it is a condition whose incidence and prevalence increases across the lifespan. In addition, a meta-analysis of studies in community-dwelling elders found that recent bereavement was the biggest risk factor for depression [30], making this an important topic to address. In several smaller scale studies, sleep disturbance and/or insomnia have been reported in one third to one half of subjects with bereavement [48–53] and the level of sleep disturbance was higher than in that of control groups without bereavement [50–52]. In an epidemiologic study of 2,121 subjects with insomnia, bereavement along with stress and loneliness were the most often cited precipitants of insomnia [54]. There are no data to suggest whether or not sleep disturbance or insomnia are associated with complicated grief reactions that do occur in 10 to 20% of persons experiencing bereavement [55] or whether sleep disturbances in the context of bereavement may give rise to MDD. These latter questions do seem worthy of study.

Depression and other sleep disorders

It is important to note that although insomnia represents the most commonly occurring sleep disorder in depression, two additional sleep disturbances have been investigated. Hypersomnia (or excessive daytime sleepiness) has not always been included in epidemiologic studies, but when included has been found to have a prevalence rate of 5 to 10% and to be associated with depression [15, 16]. In both epidemiologic and clinical studies, depression is also associated with obstructive sleep apnea. In a large sample of the general population, Ohayon reported that approximately 18% of subjects with a sleep-related breathing disorders also met criteria for MDD and similarly, approximately 18% of subjects with MDD also met criteria for a sleep-related breathing disorder [56]. A recent review indicated that the prevalence of depression ranges from 20 to 60% in clinic patients with obstructive sleep apnea (OSA), with some evidence that depression increases with OSA severity [57]. These data suggest that the presence of either OSA or MDD may be a clinical indication to assess for the other disorder.

Sleep-disordered breathing and depression

Sleep-disordered breathing (SDB) comprises a number of related conditions, the most common of which include obstructive sleep apnea (OSA), central sleep apnea (CSA), and upper airway resistance syndrome (UARS). As has been reviewed elsewhere in this volume, OSA involves obstruction of the airway during sleep, and is the most common form of this family of disorders with prevalence rates rising to as high as 20 to 30% in middle age and 50 to 70% in the elderly [58–60]. Breathing alterations may include apneas (nearly full to full cessation of breathing), hypopneas (partial cessation of breathing), and respiratory events related to arousals that are observed in UARS. Severity is measured in terms of the number of breathing disturbances occurring per hour of sleep and reported either as a respiratory disturbance index (RDI) that includes all breathing events or an apnea–hypopnea index (AHI) that includes apneas and hypopneas only. Most clinicians consider an AHI or RDI ≥ 5 and <15 represents mild apnea or SDB, while an AHI ≥ 15 represents a very clearcut indication of SDB. In an epidemiologic sample, including but not limited to older adults, approximately 18% of subjects with SDB met criteria for MDD; similarly approximately 18% of subjects with MDD also met criteria for SDB [56].

While the majority of the literature on SDB is related to OSA, hypersomnia is worthy of review as well. As a symptom hypersomnia is, of course, one form of sleep disturbance that may present in depression. It is also a very common symptom of OSA, where it is typically referred to as excessive daytime sleepiness (EDS).

Hypersomnia and depression

The prevalence of hypersomnia (i.e., EDS) has been assessed in some epidemiologic studies. The findings include prevalence rates of 5 to 10% in mixed-age cohorts [15, 16, 61], 20% in a sample of 4,578 Medicare enrollees [62], and 19% among 1,050 rural community dwellers [63].

Two of these studies also found depression to be more strongly associated with EDS scores than with other variables consistent with SDB (e.g., snoring, gasping/snorting, and trouble breathing) [61, 62]. One of these studies also found a significant relationship between EDS and use of antidepressant medication (OR 3.3 [2.9–3.8]; $p <0.0001$), although this was in the mixed-age sample. The authors did find, however, a significant association between depression and EDS in those younger than 30 and in those ≥ 75 years of age [61]. In longitudinal studies, EDS has been found to be associated with the development of depression, though it was a less robust predictor than insomnia [15, 16]. Excessive daytime sleepiness was also associated with all cause mortality in one elderly sample [63]. In summary, there is a high prevalence of hypersomnia in the elderly population and there is limited, but positive, evidence that the presence of hypersomnia is a risk factor for subsequent late-life depression.

Obstructive sleep apnea and depression

Obstructive sleep apnea has also been found to be associated with depression in a variety of small studies, although only a handful have been conducted in the elderly. Data include findings from one small comparison of elders with and without OSA in which those with OSA were found to have higher levels of EDS, depression, and cognitive impairment than those without OSA [64]. In a larger study of 427 randomly selected older adults, apnea severity was found to be significantly and positively correlated with depression severity [65]. A recent review indicated that the prevalence of depression ranges from 20 to 60% in clinic patients with obstructive sleep apnea (OSA), with some evidence that depression increases with OSA severity [57]. Other factors, however, have been found to partially account for the severity of depression among OSA patients such as age, BMI, hypertension, and fatigue [66, 67]. Thus, while depression has been found to occur at higher rates among those with OSA compared to matched controls and the severity of OSA is correlated with depression, there is limited empirical evidence on which to assess whether OSA is a risk factor for late-life depression.

Treating SDB in the context of depression

The treatment of sleep apnea with nasal administration of continuous positive airway pressure (CPAP) has been shown to reverse the depression associated with sleep apnea in some, but not all studies [68–80]. These studies have tended to be small in size and the findings mixed, so that larger, well controlled studies are needed to fully address whether CPA therapy may improve depression in general, or late-life depression in particular. There are no data that we are aware of with respect to other therapeutic interventions for SDB and their effect on depression.

Other sleep disorders and depression

There is scant empirical data when it comes to other sleep disorders or conditions and late-life depression. While narcolepsy is characterized by EDS, little is known about its association with depression in patients with narcolepsy. In a UK sample with a median age of 56 years, 57% of 305 narcolepsy patients responding had some degree of depression (BDI ≥ 10) and 15% scored 20 or above, suggesting the presence of moderate to severe depression [81]. Thus, although not focusing exclusively on the elderly, this study included a good number of older respondents with the results suggesting that this condition is associated with depressed mood.

Restless legs syndrome (RLS) and periodic limb movement disorder are also common in the elderly, but in our review they have not been found to be associated/correlated with late-life depression. Youngstedt and colleagues sought to describe the frequency of periodic limb movements (PLMs) during the sleep of 22 elders who complained of insomnia and/or depression [82]. In their sample, where participants underwent five nights of polysomnography, all complained of disturbed sleep and 12 reported depressed mood. Despite a high mean myoclonus index of 34.5 (SD 31.6) per hour, no significant associations were found between this index of PLMs and either depression or EDS. Similar findings were observed in a sample of 39 elderly subjects diagnosed with RLS who did not undergo polysomnography but had disease severity measured by an RLS scale [83]. In this study, depression was not significantly different in a mild/moderate RLS group compared to a severe RLS group. At present, these findings suggest that RLS severity is not associated with depression.

Two additional areas of concern regarding sleep and the elderly are the potential for falls and hypnotic use/abuse in the elderly with poor sleep. Hill and colleagues assessed 150 adults in assisted living (mean age = 81) and 150 elders (mean age = 70) completing internet-administered questionnaires [84]. Falling in the preceding year was reported by 44% and 41% of assisted living and internet respondents, respectively. Falls were associated with self-reported poor sleep quality, elevated depression scores, and pain ratings. Surprisingly, there was no association between falls and either the use of hypnotics or EDS. Among the internet responders, falls were associated with poor health, visual impairment, and the use of walking aids. No association between falls and any measure of sleep disturbance or depression was found in this group except that fewer falls were reported by those without any sleep disturbances. Thus, in this sole study assessing both sleep and depression, falls among assisted-living residents were associated with both depression and poor sleep quality.

The second area of concern, particularly by prescribing physicians, is hypnotic use. One investigation of 129 older outpatients who received a new prescription for benzodiazepines found that only a minority of patients (30%) were using these medications on a daily basis after two months. Of note, only 15% of the sample had depression at baseline [85]. Kripke analyzed data from a large mixed-age cohort study assessing risk factors for smoking in 1982 and reported increased mortality risk associated with taking older generation "sleep prescription pills" [86]. More recently, data from FDA clinical trials of the modern hypnotics were examined and it was found that the incidence of new depression in medication arms was twice the incidence in placebo conditions [87]. Thus, while the newer hypnotics are generally viewed as having fewer side effects and less abuse potential than older hypnotic medications, these data suggest that they may be associated with depression, if not necessarily late-life depression.

As this review indicates, there are many possible connections between depression and disturbed sleep in the elderly. Disturbed sleep in general is a concern as is sleep disordered breathing. However, RLS/PLMS do not appear to be related to depression in this population. It is important to be cognizant of the many medical, medication, social, and psychological factors that can be interacting to create not only the disturbed mood but the disturbed sleep experienced by many elderly individuals.

Summary and conclusions

Sleep disturbances are a common feature of late-life depression and come in a variety of forms. The most common sleep disturbances are insomnia and sleep-disordered breathing, which both have a high prevalence of co-occurrence in late-life depression. Approximately 50% of depressed older adults have comorbid insomnia. Moreover, insomnia has been shown to be not only highly comorbid with depression, but to also serve as a risk factor for the development of new and recurrent episodes of depression and to serve as a barrier to complete recovery from depression in many individuals treated with a variety of antidepressant interventions. The emerging data that treating insomnia in the context of ongoing depression (either as an adjuvant or monotherapy) can also produce improvements in mood is not only encouraging, but further solidifies the possibility of insomnia existing as a variable in depression's causal chain. While some of the empirical evidence in elderly samples mirrors that found in mixed-age cohorts, we await further data from intervention studies in the elderly to fully conclude that all these statements apply to late-life depression. In comparison, the evidence with respect to the role of hypersomnia/excessive daytime sleepiness and sleep-disordered breathing conditions is less convincing. It is safe to say that depression is a common feature of both EDS and SDB (as well as in other sleep disorders reviewed, though these data are even more limited). It will be difficult to describe or establish the full relationship between OSA, for example, and late-life depression in the absence of large and lengthy epidemiologic studies. As reviewed, well powered and well designed interventional studies that measure depression as an outcome are also needed. To date, there is only a modest suggestion that depression is reversed following treatment of OSA. Similar data are needed for other SDB conditions, EDS, and the other sleep disorders. Nonetheless, the prevalence of late-life depression in each of these conditions is such that a depression screen is warranted in the presence of any sleep disturbance. Conversely, a sleep history/assessment is clearly indicated in the presence of late-life depression. When a sleep disturbance is identified in the context of late-life depression, consideration should be given to treating the sleep disturbance immediately and not waiting for the possibility that it will abate following resolution of the mood disorder.

References

1. American Psychiatric Association. *Diagnostic and Statistical Manual of Mental Disorders*, 4th edn, Revised (DSM-IV-TR). (Washington DC: APA, 2000).

2. Ancoli-Israel S, Kripke DF. Prevalent sleep problems in the aged. *Biofeedback Self Regul.* 1991;**16**(4):349–59.

3. Carskadon MA, van den Hoed J, Dement WC. Insomnia and sleep disturbances in the aged: Sleep and daytime sleepiness in the elderly. *J Geriatr Psychiatry.* 1980;**13**:135–51.

4. Foley DJ, Monjan AA, Brown SL, *et al.* Sleep complaints among elderly persons: an epidemiologic study of three communities. *Sleep.* 1995;**18**(6):425–32.

5. Lyness JM, Caine ED, King DA, *et al.* Depressive disorders and symptoms in older primary care patients: one-year outcomes. *Am J Geriatr Psychiatry.* 2002;**10**(3):275–82.

6. Hamilton M. Development of a rating scale for primary depressive illness. *Br J Soc Clin Psychol.* 1967;**6**:278–96.

7. Fleck MPA, Poirierlittre MF, Guelfi JD, Bourdel MC, Loo H. Factorial structure of the 17-item Hamilton Depression Rating-Scale. *Acta Psychiatr Scand.* 1995;**92**(3):168–72.

8. Thase ME, Rush AJ, Manber R, *et al.* Differential effects of nefazodone and cognitive behavioral analysis system of psychotherapy on insomnia associated with chronic forms of major depression. *J Clin Psychiatry.* 2002;**63**(6):493–500.

9. Manber R, Blasey C, Arnow B, *et al.* Assessing insomnia severity in depression: comparison of depression rating scales and sleep diaries. *J Psychiatr Res.* 2005;**39**(5):481–8.

10. Ouellet N, Morris DL. Sleep satisfaction of older adults living in the community: identifying associated behavioral and health factors. *J Gerontol Nurs.* 2006;**32**(10):5–11.

11. Foley D, Monjan AA, Brown SL, *et al.* Sleep complaints among elderly persons: an epidemiologic study of three communities. *Sleep.* 1995;**18**(6):425–32.

12. Buysse DJ, Reynolds CF, Monk TH, Berman SR, Kupfer DJ. The Pittsburgh Sleep Quality Index: a new instrument for psychiatric practice and research. *Psychiatry Res.* 1989;**28**(2):193–213.

13. Dombrovski AY, Mulsant BH, Houck PR, *et al.* Residual symptoms and recurrence during maintenance treatment of late-life depression. *J Affect Disdord.* 2007;**103**:77–82.

14. Foley D, Ancoli-Israel S, Britz P, Walsh J. Sleep disturbances and chronic disease in older adults: results of the 2003 National Sleep Foundation Sleep in America Survey. *J Psychosom Res.* 2004;**56**(5):497–502.

15. Roberts RE, Shema SJ, Kaplan GA, Strawbridge WJ. Sleep complaints and depression in an aging cohort: A prospective perspective. *Am J Psychiatry.* 2000;**157**(1):81–8.

16. Ford DE, Kamerow DB. Epidemiologic study of sleep disturbances and psychiatric disorders. An opportunity for prevention? *JAMA.* 1989;**262**(11):1479–84.

17. Ohayon MM, Caulet M, Lemoine P. Comorbidity of mental and insomnia disorders in the general population. *Comp Psychiatry.* 1998;**39**(4):185–97.

18. Taylor DJ, Lichstein KL, Durrence HH, Reidel BW, Bush AJ. Epidemiology of insomnia, depression, and anxiety. *Sleep.* 2005;**28**(11):1457–64.

19. Stewart R, Besset A, Bebbington P, *et al.* Insomnia comorbidity and impact and hypnotic use by age group in a national survey population aged 16 to 74 years. *Sleep.* 2006;**29**(11):1391–7.

20. Hohagen F, Rink K, Kappler C, Schramm E. Prevalence and treatment of insomnia in general

practice: A longitudinal study. *Eur Arch Psychiatry Clin Neurosci.* 1993;**242**(6):329–36.

21. Simon GE, VonKorff M. Prevalence, burden, and treatment of insomnia in primary care. *Am J Psychiatry.* 1997;**154**(10):1417–23.

22. Perlis ML, Buysse D, Giles DE, Tu X, Kupfer DJ. Sleep disturbance may be a prodromal symptom of depression. *J Affect Disord.* 1997;**42**(2–3):209–12.

23. Weissman MM, Greenwald S, Nino-Murcia G, Dement WC. The morbidity of insomnia uncomplicated by psychiatric disorders. *Gen Hosp Psychiatry.* 1997;**19**(4):245–50.

24. Dryman A, Eaton WW. Affective symptoms associated with the onset of major depression in the community: findings from the US National Institute of Mental Health Epidemiologic Catchment Area Program. *Acta Psychiatr Scand.* 1991;**84**(1):1–5.

25. Chang PP, Ford DE, Mead LA, Cooper-Patrick L, Klag MJ. Insomnia in young men and subsequent depression. The Johns Hopkins Precursors Study. *Am J Epidemiol.* 1997;**146**(2):105–14.

26. Livingston G, Blizard B, Mann A. Does sleep disturbance predict depression in elderly people? A study in inner London. *Br J Gen Pract.* 1993;**43**(376):445–8.

27. Livingston G, Watkin V, Milne B, Manela MV, Katona C. Who becomes depressed? The Islington community study of older people. *J Affect Disord.* 2000;**58**(2):125–33.

28. Brabbins CJ, Dewey ME, Copeland JR, Davidson IA. Insomnia in the elderly: Prevalence, gender differences and relationships with morbidity and mortality. *Int J Geriatr Psychiatry.* 1993;**8**(6):473–80.

29. Mallon L, Broman JE, Hetta J. Relationship between insomnia, depression, and mortality: a 12-year follow-up of older adults in the community. *Int Psychogeriatr.* 2000;**12**(3):295–306.

30. Cole MG, Dendukuri N. Risk factors for depression among elderly community subjects: A systematic review and meta-analysis. *Am J Psychiatry.* 2003;**160**(6):1147–56.

31. Hauri P, Chernik D, Hawkins D, Mendels J. Sleep of depressed patients in remission. *Arch Gen Psychiatry.* 1974;**31**(3):386–91.

32. Karp JF, Buysse DJ, Houck PR, *et al.* Relationship of variability in residual symptoms with recurrence of major depressive disorder during maintenance treatment. *Am J Psychiatry.* 2004;**161**(10):1877–84.

33. Opdyke KS, Reynolds CF, III, Frank E, *et al.* Effect of continuation treatment on residual symptoms in late-life depression: how well is "well"? *Depress Anxiety.* 1996;**4**(6):312–19.

34. Nierenberg AA, Keefe BR, Leslie VC, *et al.* Residual symptoms in depressed patients who respond acutely to fluoxetine. *J Clin Psychiatry.* 1999;**60**(4):221–5.

35. Paykel ES, Ramana R, Cooper Z, *et al.* Residual symptoms after partial remission: an important outcome in depression. *Psychol Med.* 1995;(25):1171–80.

36. Buysse DJ, Reynolds CF, Monk TH, Berman SR, Kupfer DJ. The Pittsburgh Sleep Quality Index: a new instrument for psychiatric practice and research. *Psychiatry Res.* 1989;**28**(2):193–213.

37. Reynolds CF, Hoch CC, Buysse DJ, *et al.* Sleep in late-life recurrent depression. Changes during early continuation therapy with nortriptyline. *Neuropsychopharmacology.* 1991;**5**(2):85–96.

38. Simons AD, Murphy GE, Levine JL, Wetzel RD. Cognitive therapy and pharmacotherapy for depression: Sustained improvement over one year. *Arch Gen Psychiatry.* 1986;**43**:43–8.

39. Thase ME, Simons AD, Cahalane JF, McGeary J. Cognitive behavior therapy of endogenous depression: I. An outpatient clinical replication series. *Behav Ther.* 1991;**22**(4):457–67.

40. Carney CE, Segal ZV, Edinger JD, Krystal AD. A comparison of rates of residual insomnia symptoms following pharmacotherapy or cognitive-behavioral therapy for major depressive disorder. *J Clin Psychiatry.* 2007;**68**(2):254–60.

41. Manber R, Rush J, Thase ME, *et al.* The effects of psychotherapy, Nefazodone, and their combination on subjective assessment of disturbed sleep in chronic depression. *Sleep.* 2003;**26**(2):130–6.

42. Pigeon WR, Hegel MT, Unutzer J, *et al.* Is insomnia a perpetuating factor for late-life depression in the IMPACT cohort? *Sleep.* 2008;**31**(4):481–8.

43. Fava M, McCall WV, Krystal A, *et al.* Eszopiclone co-administered with fluoxetine in patients with insomnia coexisting with major depressive disorder. *Biol Psychiatry.* 2006;**59**(11):1052–60.

44. Manber R, Edinger J, San Pedro M, Kuo T. Combining escitalopram oxalate (ESCIT) and individual cognitive behavioral therapy for insomnia (CBTI) to improve depression outcome. *Sleep.* 2007;**30**:A232.

45. Morawetz D. Behavioral self-help treatment for insomnia: a controlled evaluation. *Behav Ther.* 1989; **20**:365–79.

46. Taylor DJ, Lichstein K, Weinstock J, Temple J, Sanford S. A pilot study of cognitive-behavioral therapy of insomnia in people with mild depression. *Behav Ther.* 2007; **38**:49–57.

47. Hamilton BE, Minino AM, Martin JA, *et al.* Annual summary of vital statistics: 2005. *Pediatrics.* 2007;**119**(2):345–60.

48. Prigerson HG, Frank E, Kasl SV, *et al*. Complicated grief and bereavement-related depression as distinct disorders: preliminary empirical validation in elderly bereaved spouses. *Am J Psychiatry*. 1995;**152**(1):22–30.

49. Germain A, Caroff K, Buysse DJ, Shear MK. Sleep quality in complicated grief. *J Trauma Stress*. 2005;**18**(4):343–6.

50. Richardson SJ, Lund DA, Caserta MS, Dudley WN, Obray SJ. Sleep patterns in older bereaved spouses. *Omega J Death Dying*. 2003;**47**(4):361–83.

51. Valdimarsdottir U, Helgason AR, Furst CJ, Adolfsson J, Steineck G. Long-term effects of widowhood after terminal cancer: a Swedish nationwide follow-up. *Scand J Pub Health*. 2003;**31**(1):31–6.

52. Beem EE, Maes S, Cleiren M, Schut HAW, Garssen B. Psychological functioning of recently bereaved middle-aged women: the first 13 months. *Psychol Rep*. 2000;**87**(1):243–54.

53. Horowitz MJ, Siegel B, Holen A, *et al*. Diagnostic criteria for complicated grief disorder. *Am J Psychiatry*. 1997;**154**(7):904–10.

54. Allaert FA, Urbinelli R. Sociodemographic profile of insomniac patients across national surveys. *CNS Drugs*. 2004;**18**:3–7.

55. Prigerson HG. When the path of adjustment leads to a dead-end. *Bereavement Care*. 2004;**23**:38–40.

56. Ohayon MM. The effects of breathing-related sleep disorders on mood disturbances in the general population. *J Clin Psychiatry*. 2003;**64**(10):1195–200.

57. Schroder CM, O'Hara R. Depression and obstructive sleep apnea (OSA). *Ann Gen Psychiatry* 2005;**4**(13):1–8.

58. Bixler EO, Kales A, Soldatos CR, Kales JD, Healey S. Prevalence of sleep disorders in the Los Angeles metropolitan area. *Am J Psychiatry*. 1979;**136**:1257–62.

59. Shapiro CM, Dement WC. ABC of sleep disorders. Impact and epidemiology of sleep disorders. *BMJ*. 1993;**306**(6892):1604–7.

60. Young T, Peppard PE, Gottlieb DJ. Epidemiology of obstructive sleep apnea: a population health perspective. *Am J Respir Crit Care Med*. 2002;**165**(9):1217–39.

61. Bixler EO, Vgontzas AN, Lin HM, *et al*. Excessive daytime sleepiness in a general population sample: the role of sleep apnea, age, obesity, diabetes, and depression. *J Clin Endocrinol Metab*. 2005;**90**(8):4510–15.

62. Whitney CW, Enright PL, Newman AB, *et al*. Correlates of daytime sleepiness in 4578 elderly persons: the cardiovascular health study. *Sleep*. 1998;**21**(1):27–36.

63. Ganguli M, Reynolds CF, Gilby JE. Prevalence and persistence of sleep complaints in a rural elderly community sample: the MoVIES project. *J Am Geriatr Soc*. 1996;**44**(7):778–84.

64. Berry DT, Phillips BA, Cook YR, *et al*. Geriatric sleep apnea syndrome: a preliminary description. *J Gerontol*. 1990;**45**(5):M169–M174.

65. Ancoli-Israel S, Kripke DF, Klauber MR, *et al*. Sleep-disordered breathing in community-dwelling elderly. *Sleep*. 1991;**14**(6):486–95.

66. Bardwell WA, Berry CC, Ancoli-Israel S, Dimsdale JE. Psychological correlates of sleep apnea. *J Psychosom Res*. 1999;**47**(6):583–96.

67. Bardwell WA, Moore P, Ancoli-Israel S, Dimsdale JE. Fatigue in obstructive sleep apnea: driven by depressive symptoms instead of apnea severity? *Am J Psychiatry*. 2003;**160**(2):350–5.

68. Engleman HM, Cheshire KE, Deary IJ, Douglas NJ. Daytime sleepiness, cognitive performance and mood after continuous positive airway pressure for the sleep apnoea/hypopnoea syndrome. *Thorax*. 1993;**48**(9):911–14.

69. Yu BH, Ancoli-Israel S, Dimsdale JE. Effect of CPAP treatment on mood states in patients with sleep apnea. *J Psychiatr Res*. 1999;**33**(5):427–32.

70. Cooke JR, Amador X, Lawton S, *et al*. Long-term CPAP may improve cognition, sleep, and mood in patients with Alzheimer's disease and SDB. *Sleep*. 2006;**29**:A103–A104.

71. Schwartz DJ, Kohler WC, Karatinos G. Symptoms of depression in individuals with, obstructive sleep apnea may be amenable to treatment with continuous positive airway pressure. *Chest*. 2005;**128**(3):1304–9.

72. Kawahara S, Akashiba T, Akahoshi T, Horie T. Nasal CPAP improves the quality of life and lessens the depressive symptoms in patients with obstructive sleep apnea syndrome. *Intern Med*. 2005;**44**(5):422–7.

73. Engleman HM, Asgari-Jirhandeh N, McLeod AL, *et al*. Self-reported use of CPAP and benefits of CPAP therapy: a patient survey. *Chest*. 1996;**109**(6):1470–6.

74. Borak J, Cieslicki JK, Koziej M, Matuszewski A, Zielinski J. Effects of CPAP treatment on psychological status in patients with severe obstructive sleep apnoea. *J Sleep Res*. 1996;**5**(2):123–7.

75. Derderian SS, Bridenbaugh RH, Rajagopal KR. Neuropsychologic symptoms in obstructive sleep apnea improve after treatment with nasal continuous positive airway pressure. *Chest*. 1988;**94**(5):1023–7.

76. Millman RP, Fogel BS, McNamara ME, Carlisle CC. Depression as a manifestation of obstructive sleep apnea: reversal with nasal continuous positive

181

airway pressure. *J Clin Psychiatry.* 1989;
50(9):348–51.

77. Henke KG, Grady JJ, Kuna ST. Effect of nasal continuous positive airway pressure on neuropsychological function in sleep apnea-hypopnea syndrome: a randomized, placebo-controlled trial. *Am J Respir Crit Care Med.* 2001;**163**(4):911–17.

78. Munoz A, Mayoralas LR, Barbe F, Pericas J, Agusti AGN. Long-term effects of CPAP on daytime functioning in patients with sleep apnoea syndrome. *Eur Respir J.* 2000;**15**(4):676–81.

79. Edinger JD, Carwile S, Miller P, Hope V, Mayti C. Psychological status, syndromatic measures, and compliance with nasal CPAP therapy for sleep-apnea. *Percep Mot Skills.* 1994;**78**(3):1116–18.

80. Lewis KE, Seale L, Bartle IE, Watkins AJ, Ebden P. Early predictors of CPAP use for the treatment of obstructive sleep apnea. *Sleep.* 2004;**27**(1):134–8.

81. Daniels E, King MA, Smith IE, Shneerson JM. Health-related quality of life in narcolepsy. *J Sleep Res.* 2001;**10**:75–81.

82. Youngstedt SD, Kripke DF, Klauber MR, Sepulveda RS, Mason WJ. Periodic leg movements during sleep and sleep disturbances in elders. *J Gerontol A Biol Sci Med Sci.* 1998;**53**(5):391–4.

83. Cuellar NG, Strumpf NE, Ratcliffe SJ. Symptoms of restless leg syndrome in older adults: outcomes on sleep quality, sleepiness, fatigue, depression, and quality of life. *JAGS.* 2007;**55**:1387–92.

84. Hill EL, Cumming RJ, Lewis R, Carrington S, Le Couteur DG. Sleep disturbances and falls in older people. *J Gerontol.* 2007;**62A**(1):62–6.

85. Simon GE, Ludman EJ. Outcome of new benzodiazepine prescriptions to older adults in primary care. *Gen Hosp Psychiatry.* 2006;**28**:374–8.

86. Kripke DF, Klauber MR, Wingard DL, *et al.* Mortality hazard associated with prescription hypnotics. *Biol Psychiatry.* 1998;**43**(9):687–93.

87. Kripke DF. Greater incidence of depression with hypnotic use than with placebo. *BMC Psychiatry.* 2007;**7**:42.

Long-term effects of antidepressants on sleep

Marie E. Beitinger and Stephany Fulda

Introduction

Many antidepressants have a pronounced effect on sleep EEG, and this effect can often be observed after the very first administration [1] (see also Chapter 18 in this volume). In general, the effects of antidepressants on sleep occur distinctly earlier than the effects on mood, which may take two to four weeks to develop [2]. These rapid effects may also be substantial, for example a complete elimination of REM sleep, which has been observed with monoamine oxidase inhibitors (MAOIs) [3]. This raises the question whether these changes in sleep EEG can really be sustained over weeks and months. In 2001, Landolt and de Boer [4] reported on three depressed patients who had been treated with phenelzine, a non-selective MAOI, for several months. Polysomnographies were conducted at two- to four-week intervals throughout treatment, and all patients were clinically remitted from depression after five weeks. The repeated sleep EEG demonstrated a complete absence of REM sleep for three to six months in each of the three patients. It was only after several months that very low amounts of REM sleep reappeared, and in the case of discontinuation in two of the patients, a massive REM rebound was observed. This suggests that the effect of an antidepressant can indeed be sustained over long periods of time. At the same time, small amounts of REM sleep reappearing after several months point to some development of tolerance of only minor magnitude – at least with this substance. Furthermore, the massive REM rebound after withdrawal also suggests that no long-term loss of effect had occurred. That this effect is not restricted to patients with depression has been shown by Wyatt and coworkers [5] in a long-term observation in narcolepsy patients, in one of whom the dramatic

and nearly complete reduction of REM sleep after administration of phenelzine was documented for over a year. The longest study to date has been undertaken by Kupfer and coworkers [6] from the University of Pittsburgh who followed a group of 27 depressed patients on imipramine treatment for about four years. During the last three years, in the maintenance phase, sleep EEG was obtained every three months. Compared to a drug-free baseline in the depressed state, imipramine significantly reduced the amount of REM sleep and increased REM density (REMD) at every time point during this three-year period. The only sleep parameters that showed a significant time-related trend were slow-wave sleep and stage 1 sleep, which decreased over the years. Taken together, these studies suggest a long-term effect of antidepressants on sleep with little indication of developing tolerance or decreasing effects on sleep.

In the following we review these long-term effects of antidepressants – both with and without REM suppressing properties – on sleep EEG. We conducted a systematic literature search and considered all studies that assessed the effects of antidepressants on sleep for six weeks or longer. Although the cut-off of six weeks was chosen arbitrarily, it reflects the time point at which most of the clinical improvement has occurred [2].

Long-term effects of antidepressants on sleep
Tricyclic antidepressants

In the short run, tricyclic antidepressants (TCAs) have pronounced effects on polysomnographic sleep. With the exception of trimipramine [7–10], TCAs suppress REM sleep as evidenced by substantially

Sleep and Mental Illness, eds. S. R. Pandi-Perumal and M. Kramer. Published by Cambridge University Press.
© Cambridge University Press 2010.

reduced REM sleep and increased REM latencies [1]. Rapid eye movement activity, i.e., the total number of rapid eye movements during REM sleep, is reduced in the acute treatment but returns to baseline values within four weeks, while at the same time REM density (number of rapid eye movements per minute of REM sleep) is consistently increased [1].

For *imipramine*, as mentioned above, Kupfer and coworkers have conducted a seminal long-term study recording sleep throughout an approximate four-year period of treatment with about 200 mg of imipramine in 27 patients with depression [6]. In essence, both after about eight months and after four years REM sleep was significantly suppressed with reduced amounts of REM sleep, a reduced number of REM episodes, and increased REM latencies and REM density (Table 17.1). Rapid eye movement activity remained unchanged at both time points. Kupfer *et al.* explicitly analyzed whether sleep parameters differed across the last three years of the treatment period in which sleep was recorded every three months. During these three years, slow-wave sleep and stage 1 sleep decreased, while REM sleep parameters showed no evidence of systematic variation over time. In addition, a smaller study has recorded sleep parameters in 12 patients with sleep apnea who responded to imipramine in dosages between 25 and 50 mg [11]. After four months of treatment, the apnea index and the number of apneas decreased and slow-wave sleep increased; however, there was no change in REM sleep. Potential explanations for this negative finding were the low percentage of REM sleep at baseline (12.5%) and the low dosage of imipramine (25–50 mg).

For *nortriptyline* three long-term studies recorded sleep after three to fifteen months of treatment [12–15]. All studies included elderly patients with depression. After three to five months the studies report consistently reduced REM sleep and increased REM density (Table 17.1). No change in REM activity was observed. In addition, increases in sleep stage 2 [15] and slow-wave sleep as well as reduced wake during sleep were reported [12]. One of the studies followed a group of 21 patients over a 15-month double-blind maintenance treatment with nortriptyline [13]. Compared to a placebo group nortriptyline reduced the amount of REM sleep and increased REM density even after 15 months. However, effects on other sleep stages and sleep continuity measures as well as on REM latency, which were observed after a three-month

open-label treatment (Table 17.1) [12], were not sustained one year later, indication a diminishing effect at least for non-REM (NREM) sleep parameters.

For *amitriptyline* effects on polysomnographically recorded sleep have been documented for six to seven weeks in patients with major depression [16–19]. All four studies [16–19] showed consistently that REM-suppressing effects are still observable after this time span (Table 17.1). Effects on other sleep stages or sleep continuity have been found in some of the studies, mostly as a decrease in wake time [18] and the number of awakenings [16, 17] or as an increase in sleep stage 2 [17, 19]. Only one study [16] assessed acute (three days), short-term (fourteen days) as well as long-term effects (six weeks) and found no systematic change in REM sleep parameters over time. Sleep onset latencies, however, that were significantly shortened after acute amitriptyline treatment returned to baseline values after six weeks. In addition, Linkowski and coworkers recorded sleep in a single patient after approximately one year of amitriptyline intake and found no evidence that the REM-suppressing effect had diminished over time [18]. Finally, two studies explored sleep EEG in patients with fibromyalgia and after eight weeks of low-dose treatment with amitriptyline [20, 21]. Both studies did not find any changes in REM sleep parameters when comparing a drug-free baseline to sleep after eight weeks of amitriptyline treatment. However, dosages of 25 mg and 50 mg of amitriptyline may have been too low to have exerted any effects on REM sleep.

For *protriptyline*, interestingly, no studies documenting the effects on sleep EEG in depressed patients have been conducted. Instead, protriptyline has been repeatedly applied in patients with sleep-related breathing disorders (SRBD) or chronic obstructive pulmonary disease (COPD). In patients with obstructive sleep apnea (OSAS) protriptyline in dosages between 20 and 30 mg reduced REM sleep after three to six months in two [22, 23] out of three studies [22–24]. None of these studies has reported other REM parameters such as REM latencies or REM density. A consistent reduction of REM sleep has also been observed for patients with COPD and 15 to 20 mg of protriptyline for six weeks to three months [25–28]. In a further study, reduced REM sleep was still observed after an average of three years of treatment [29]. Again, other parameters of REM sleep were not reported.

Table 17.1 Long-term effects of tricyclic antidepressants (TCAs) on sleep EEG

Drug, reference	No. patients, condition, study design	Study duration, drug dosage	Findings[a]
Imipramine			
Kupfer et al. 1994 [6]	27 MD	~8.5 m	↓REM$_{m\%}$ NoREM ↑REML REMD = REM act
	DB PC PG	~210 mg	↑S1$_{\%}$, ↑S2$_{\%}$
		~4 y	↓REM$_{m\%}$ NoREM ↑REML
		~200 mg	REMD = REM act ↑S2$_{\%}$
			Changes across the last three years:
			No changes in REM sleep; ↓SWS$_{\%}$ S1$_{\%}$
Rubin et al. 1986 [11]	12 SRBD	~4 m	= REM$_m$ REML
	OL	25–50 mg	↑SWS$_{\%}$ ↓apnea index
Nortriptyline			
Buysse et al. 1996 [13]	30 elderly MD	~3.5 m	↓REM$_{m\%}$ NoREM ↑REML REMD = REM act
Reynolds et al. 1991 [12]	OL	~80 mg	↓SOL WASOm W% SWS% ↑S1% S2%
	DB PC PG	~15 m	vs. placebo group (n = 10):
		~85 mg	↓REM$_{\%}$ ↑REMD = REML
			↑DSR
Taylor et al. 1999 [14]	18 elderly MD	~4 m	↓REM$_{m\%}$ ↑REML REMD = REM act
	DB PC PG	~70 mg	
Pasternak et al. 1994 [15]	10 elderly MD	~4.9 m	↓REM$_{\%}$ ↑REML REMD = REM act
	OL	~50 mg	↑S2$_{\%}$ DSR
Amitriptyline			
Hubain et al. 1990 [17]	4 MD	42 d	vs. single-blind placebo baseline:
	DB AC PG	~170 mg	↑REML = REM$_{m\%}$
			↓NoW S4$_{m\%}$ ↑S2$_m$
Kerkhofs et al. 1990 [19]	10 MD	42 d	↓REM$_{\%}$ ↑REML
	DB AC PG	150 mg	↑S2$_{\%}$
Scharf et al. 1986 [16]	10 MD	44 d	↓REM$_{\%}$ ↑REML = REMD
	SB PC	~120 mg	↓NoW ↑SE
			Change across days 3, 14, and 44: ↑SOL
Linkowski et al. 1987 [18]	5 MD	~49 d	↓REM$_m$ ↑REML
	OL	~200 mg	↓W$_m$
Kempenaers et al. 1994 [20]	6 fibromyalgia	56 d	= REM$_m$ REML
	DB PC PG	50 mg	↑arousal index
Carette et al. 1995 [21]	22 fibromyalgia	56 d	= REM$_{\%}$ REML
	DB PC CO	25 mg	↑S2$_{\%}$

Table 17.1 (cont.)

Drug, reference	No. patients, condition, study design	Study duration, drug dosage	Findings[a]
Protriptyline			
Conway et al. 1982 [22]	6 OSAS	~3 m/20 mg	= REM$_\%$
	OL		↓TST
Smith et al. 1983 [23]	12 OSAS	~4 m/20 mg	↓REM$_\%$
	OL		↑S2$_\%$
Brownell et al. 1982 [24]	3 OSAS	~6 m/30 mg	↓REM$_\%$
	OL		↓arousal index
Carroll et al. 1990 [27]	18 COPD	42 d/10 mg	↓REM$_\%$
	DB PC CO		
Series et al. 1989 [25]	11 COPD/OL	70 d/20 mg	↓REM$_\%$
Series & Cormier 1990 [26]	11 COPD	70 d/20 mg	↓REM$_\%$
	SB PC		↓NoSS/h
Lin 1993 [28]	10 COPD/OL	~3 m/~15 mg	↓REM$_\%$
Series et al. 1993 [29]	9 COPD/OL	~37 m/~20 mg	↓REM$_\%$
Clomipramine			
Guilleminault et al. 1976 [30]	7 narcolepsy	42 d	↓REM$_\%$
	OL	100 mg	
	11 narcolepsy	42 d	↓REM$_\%$
	OL	75 mg	
		126 d/75 mg	↓REM$_\%$

Notes: [a]Compared to drug-free baseline unless otherwise specified.
↓ decreased; ↑ increased; = unchanged.
AC: active controlled; AHI: apnea hypopnea index; CO: cross-over; COPD: chronic obstructive pulmonary disease; DB: double-blind; DSR: delta sleep ratio; MD: major depression; MSLT: multiple sleep latency test; NoREM: number of REM episodes; NoSS/h: number of stage shifts per hour; NoW: number of awakenings; OL: open-label; PC: placebo-controlled; PTSD: post-traumatic stress disorder; OSAS: obstructive sleep apnea syndrome; PG: parallel-group; PLMD: periodic limb movement disorder; PLMI: number of periodic limb movements/hour; REM$_m$: minutes of REM sleep; REM$_\%$: percentage of REM sleep; REM act: REM activity; REMD: REM density; REML: REM latency; S1/S2/S3/S4/SWS/W$_m$: minutes of sleep stage 1/2/3/4/slow-wave sleep/wake; S1/S2/S3/S4/SWS/W$_\%$: percentage of sleep stage 1/2/3/4/slow-wave sleep/wake; SAD: seasonal affective disorder; SE: sleep efficiency; SOL: sleep onset latency; SWS: slow-wave sleep; TST: total sleep time; WASOm: minutes of wake after sleep onset.

Finally, there is only one study that documented the effects of *clomipramine* in two groups of patients with narcolepsy [30]. In these groups 75 and 100 mg of clomipramine reduced REM sleep after six weeks (Table 17.1). In one group sleep was also measured again after three months and REM sleep was still reduced. Although the authors noted an increase in REM sleep compared to the six-week polysomnography, the change was not statistically significant. Other measures of REM sleep, such as REM density or REM latencies, were not reported.

In summary, TCAs suppressing REM sleep in the short run also exert these effects in the long run. There is little indication that the magnitude of REM suppression diminishes over periods of up to four years although some slight attenuation may be possible. The effects on other NREM sleep parameters are less consistent across studies in the long run and seem to occur mainly after acute or short-term administration. It must be stressed, however, that only one of the reviewed studies actually compared the long-term effects to acute effects after one to three days.

Table 17.2 Long-term effects of monoamine oxidase inhibitor (MAOI) antidepressants on sleep EEG

Drug, reference	No. patients, condition, study design	Study duration, drug dosage	Findings[a]
Phenelzine			
Gillin & Wyatt 1975 [32]	7 MD	~42 d	vs. single-blind placebo baseline:
	SB PC	~75 mg	↓REM$_{m\%}$
Landolt & de Boer 2001 [4]	3 MD	~126 d	↓REM$_\%$
	OL	~65 mg	↑WASO$_\%$ S2$_\%$
		~210–525 d	↓REM$_\%$
		~60 mg	↑WASO$_\%$ S2$_\%$
Wyatt *et al.* 1971 [5]	7 narcolepsy	up to ~3 y	vs. single-blind placebo baseline:
	SB PC	~60 mg	↓REM$_\%$ NoREM
Tranylcypromine			
Jindal *et al.* 2003 [96]	23 bipolar dis.	42 d	↓REM$_{m\%}$ NoREM REMact ↑REML = REMD
	DB AC PG	~37 mg	↓TST ↑S1$_\%$ S2$_\%$
Moclobemide			
Mann *et al.* 2001 [33]	6 psychogenic erectile dysfunction	56 d	↑REML = REM$_m$
	DB PC PG	600 mg	

Note: [a]Compared to drug-free baseline unless otherwise specified.
For abbreviations see Table 17.1.

Therefore, it cannot be ruled out that the very acute effects are of greater magnitude than the long-term effects.

Monoamine oxidase inhibitors

Just like TCAs, monoamine oxidase inhibitors (MAOIs) suppress REM sleep [1, 3]. Rapid eye movement sleep suppression appears to be more complete with MAOIs, in particular the non-selective MAOIs, where a total elimination of REM sleep has been observed, but complete suppression occurs with a longer latency, i.e., a time lag of about five to ten days [1, 4, 31]. Long-term studies assessing sleep EEG have been reported for phenelzine, tranylcypromine, and moclobemide.

Phenelzine, a non-selective MAOI, reduced REM sleep to zero or near zero values in a small group of depressed patients after six weeks [32] (Table 17.2). After discontinuation, a pronounced and long-lasting

(>14 days) rebound of REM sleep was observed. This concurs with the long-term study of Landolt and de Boer [4], mentioned in the introduction, where phenelzine completely eliminated REM sleep in three patients with depression after about six weeks and for time spans of three to five months. After about six months, very low amounts of REM sleep reappeared, which at least in one patient were reduced again by increasing phenelzine dosage. Very low amounts of REM sleep were sustained for up to three years. Reduction of dosage during that time predictably resulted in a substantial rebound of REM sleep, arguing against the existence of a long-term loss of effect. In addition, increases in sleep stage 2 and wake after sleep onset were also observed throughout the entire period of time. A drastic reduction in REM sleep has also been reported for a small group of narcolepsy patients and time periods of up to three years [5]. In particular, details of one female patient were reported whose REM sleep was absent for more than a year before small amounts reappeared during nocturnal polysomnographies.

For *tranylcypromine*, another non-selective MAOI, only one study recorded sleep in patients with bipolar disorder over a longer period of time and found that after six weeks REM sleep was reduced and REM latencies were increased. Interestingly, and in contrast to TCAs, REM activity was reduced but REM density was unchanged (Table 17.2). As with phenelzine, an increase in sleep stages 1 and 2 and a reduction of total sleep time were observed.

Finally, the only long-term study with *moclobemide*, a selective MAO-A inhibitor, was conducted with patients suffering from psychogenic erectile dysfunction [33]. Interestingly, in this population REM latencies were prolonged but the amount of REM sleep was unchanged after treatment with 600 mg for about eight weeks (Table 17.2). Existing studies show, however, that the effects of moclobemide on REM sleep are small and/or inconsistent across studies even with acute administration [34–37].

In summary, only a few studies have recorded sleep in long-term treatment with MAOIs. For the non-selective MAOIs, phenelzine and tranylcypromine, a complete REM sleep suppressing effect has been documented for at least several months. Although REM sleep reappears again after this time, the amount can be substantially decreased for years with continuing treatment. Information about REM activity or REM density has not been systematically reported. In addition, the sleep-disturbing effects such as an increase in wake after sleep onset or a decrease in total sleep time may also persist over time. Selective MAOIs seem to have a lesser effect on sleep and specifically REM sleep, and accordingly, the one long-term study with moclobemide found little or no effect on REM sleep.

Selective serotonin reuptake inhibitors

Selective serotonin reuptake inhibitors (SSRIs) are another class of antidepressants that have REM-suppressing effects [1] and in many cases are also associated with insomnia [38]. *Fluoxetine* is the SSRI for which the most long-term studies are available (Table 17.3). In patients with depression, daily treatment with dosages between 20 and 60 mg for six to eight weeks had mild to moderate REM-suppressing effects with either a decrease in REM time or an increase in REM latency [19, 39, 40]. Only one of the four studies, the largest one with more than 50 patients, reported a change in both parameters at the same time [41]. All four, however, showed evidence of a sleep-disturbing effect with increased wake, light sleep stage 1, or reduced sleep efficiency (Table 17.3). Three further studies confirmed these REM-suppressing effects for periods of ten weeks to four months [42–44] and two of them reported REM densities that were also increased during fluoxetine treatment [42, 43], while the third one reported no changes in REM activity [44]. Two of the studies also reported a sleep-disturbing effect with increased sleep stage 1 [42, 43]. Among the studies, four recorded sleep at several time points allowing for direct within-study comparisons. Comparing sleep after two- and eight-week administration of fluoxetine, Winokur *et al.* [39] found that sleep stage 1 increased between both time points while REM sleep parameters did not change. In another study [40], no changes in REM or NREM sleep parameters were observed between four and eight weeks of treatment. However, Trivedi and coworkers [42] assessed sleep after one, five, and ten weeks of fluoxetine treatment, and within this time span, REM suppressing effects lessened with both time spent in REM and REM density increasing and sleep stage 2 decreasing over time. In the same study [42], a subgroup of 12 patients was additionally followed up for another 20 weeks. In this group, the amount of REM sleep increased significantly between week 10 and week 30. The longest study to date has been undertaken by Haro and Drucker-Colin [45] who reported the effects of 20 mg of fluoxetine given three to five times per week for eight months in twelve patients with depression. Starting with the first month, polysomnography was conducted every two months. At any time – in comparison with the drug-free baseline – minutes spent in REM sleep were reduced and REM latencies increased. In addition, sleep-disturbing effects such as reduced sleep efficiency and increased sleep stage 1 were observed throughout the entire study. Across these seven months, there was a linear increase in REM latency and in time spent awake. Taken together, these studies suggest that fluoxetine has long-lasting effects on both REM and NREM sleep. There is also some indication, however, that the REM-suppressing effect may diminish over time.

Single long-term studies on the effects of *paroxetine* (20 mg in each study) have been conducted with depressed patients [46], insomniacs [47], and patients with OSAS [48]. In depressed patients, eight weeks of paroxetine use were associated with decreased

Table 17.3 Long-term effects of selective serotonin reuptake inhibitor (SSRIs) antidepressants on sleep EEG

Drug, reference	No. patients, condition, study design	Study duration, drug dosage	Findings[a]
Fluoxetine			
Kerkhofs et al. 1990 [19]	9 MD	42 d	↓REM% = REML
	DB AC PG	60 mg	↑NoSS NoW S1%
Rush et al. 1998 [41]	57 MD	56 d	↓REM% ↑REML
	DB AC PG	~32 mg	↓SE SWS% ↑NoW S1%
Winokur et al. 2003 [39]	13 MD	56 d	↑REML = REM$_m$
	DB AC PG	40 mg	↑S1$_m$
			Across days 7, 14, and 56: ↑S1$_m$
Levitan et al. 2000 [40]	15 MD	56 d	↑REML = REM%
	DB AC PG	20 mg (+ placebo)	↓SWS%
			Across days 28 and 56: no changes
Trivedi et al. 1999 [42]	36 MD	70 d	↓REM% ↑REML REMD
	OL	~25 mg	↓SWS$_{m\%}$ S2$_{m\%}$ SOL ↑S1$_{m\%}$
			Across days 7, 35, and 70:
			↑REMD REM% ↓S2$_{m\%}$
	12 MD	210 d	↑REML REMD = REM%
	OL	~25 mg	↑S1$m\%$
			Across weeks 10 and 30: ↑REM%
Hendrickse et al. 1994 [43]	9 MD	~83 d	↓REM% ↑REML REMD
	OL	~37 mg	↑S1$_m$
Nofzinger et al. 1995 [44]	11 MD	~122 d	↑REML = REM$_{m\%}$ REM act
	OL	~25 mg	
Haro & Drucker-Colin 2004 [45]	12 MD	3 m	↓REM$_m$ ↑REML
	DB AC PG	100 mg/w	↓TST SE S2$_m$ S3$_m$ S4$_m$ ↑W$_m$ S1$_m$
		5 m	↓REM$_m$ ↑REML
		100 mg/w	↓TST SE S2$_m$ ↑W$_m$ S1$_m$ SOL
		7 m	↓REM$_m$ ↑REML
		60 mg/w	↓TST SE S2$_m$ S4$_m$ ↑W$_m$ S1$_m$
			Across 7 months: ↑REML
Paroxetine			
Hicks et al. 2002 [46]	16 MD	56 d	↓REM% ↑REML
	DB AC PG	20 mg	↑NoW
			across days 1, 10, and 56:
			↑NoW SE S1% ↓REML

Table 17.3 (cont.)

Drug, reference	No. patients, condition, study design	Study duration, drug dosage	Findings[a]
Nowell et al. 1999 [47]	13 insomnia	42 d	= REM$_m$ REML
	OL	~20 mg	
Kraiczi et al. 1999 [48]	18 OSAS	42 d	↑REML = REM$_%$
	DB PC CO	20 mg	↓AHI
Citalopram			
Van Bemmel et al. 1993a, 1993b [51, 52]	16 MD	42 d	↓REM$_{m%}$ ↑REML
	SB PC	40 mg	↑S2$_%$
			Across days 1 and 42: no changes
Sertraline			
Jindal et al. 2003 [49]	25 MD	84 d	↓NoREM ↑REML = REM% REMD REM act
	DB PC PG	~142 mg	↑SOL Delta sleep ratio
Fluvoxamine			
Wilson et al. 2000 [50]	12 MD	~3 m	↑REML = REM$_m$ ↓SWS$_%$
	OL	~130 mg	Across days 2, 21, and month 3: ↓SWS$_{m%}$

Note: [a]Compared to drug-free baseline unless otherwise specified.
For abbreviations see Table 17.1.

REM time, increased REM latency, and an increased number of awakenings [46]. In this study sleep was recorded also after three and ten days of paroxetine treatment and the sleep-disturbing effects such as decreased sleep time and sleep efficiency and increased wake were observed after acute treatment and returned to baseline values in the course of eight weeks. While REM sleep amount continued on a low level during the eight weeks there was also a time-related decrease in REM latency. Paroxetine was also employed in a six-week open-label treatment of patients with insomnia [47]. Here, REM sleep decreased (from 94 to 58 minutes) and REM latencies increased numerically (from 67 to 170 minutes) but the difference between baseline and treatment was not statistically significant. Finally, paroxetine was also given to 18 OSAS patients for six weeks and resulted in prolonged REM latencies [48]. At the same time the REM sleep amount was unaffected, which might have been due to the low REM sleep amount at baseline in this group (12%).

For three other SSRIs, fluvoxamine, sertraline, and citalopram, single studies have reported long-term effects on sleep in patients with depression [49–52]. Six weeks of *citalopram* reduced the amount of REM sleep, increased REM latency, and increased sleep stage 2 [51, 52]. Comparison of sleep after acute (one day) and long-term treatment did not reveal any systematic changes. *Sertraline* given for 12 weeks increased REM latencies and decreased the number of REM episodes but had no effect on the amount of REM sleep, REM density, or REM activity [49]. In addition, the delta sleep ratio and the sleep onset latency were increased. Finally, one study applied *fluvoxamine* in a small group of depressed patients and recorded sleep at baseline, after two days, three weeks and about three months of treatment [50]. In this study, the amount of REM sleep was decreased after two days and three weeks but returned to baseline values after three months. On the contrary, REM latencies did not differ from baseline after two days but were prolonged after longer term administration. In addition, an increase in slow-wave sleep was observed after acute administration but no longer apparent after three weeks or three months.

In summary, SSRIs tend to suppress REM sleep and many show sleep-disturbing properties. Significant effects on sleep are also observed after longer periods of time and seem to be at least moderately stable for sleep disturbing NREM effects. There is also converging evidence that the REM-suppressing effect although still evident may diminish over time.

Norepinephrine reuptake inhibitors

There are only a limited number of studies that have explored the long-term effects of norepinephrine reuptake inhibitors (NRIs) on sleep.

For *reboxetine*, two acute studies with depressed patients showed that reboxetine increased REM latency [53, 54], but only in one of the two studies a reduced amount of REM sleep was observed [54]. In patients with dysthymia, Ferini-Strambi and coworkers documented sleep after 1, 7, and 120 days of treatment with 4 mg of reboxetine [55]. After three months and compared to a drug-free baseline the amount of REM sleep was decreased and REM latencies were increased. In addition, the number of awakenings was reduced, too. Compared to the acute effects over time the amount of REM sleep increased and sleep in general improved (Table 17.4).

Bupropion inhibits the reuptake of norepinephrine but also dopamine. Bupropion has been applied in several long-term studies in small groups of depressed patients (Table 17.4). While the first study that explored the effects of bupropion on sleep patterns reported an REM-enhancing effect [44], this could not be replicated and later studies mostly found no effect on REM parameters [56–58]. This first study by Nofzinger and coworkers recorded sleep in seven patients with depression before and after about three months of bupropion intake [44]. They found that, on average, REM latencies decreased and time spent in REM increased during treatment. However, in later studies administration of bupropion for seven weeks had no effect on REM or NREM sleep parameters [56]. Three other studies have explored the long-term effect of a sustained-release preparation of bupropion for 8 to 11 weeks [57–59], and in none of them effects on REM sleep were observed with the exception of Ott [59] who reported a moderate increase in REM

latency from about 50 minutes to 75 minutes after 8 weeks of treatment. This last study also found that the number of awakenings was increased with bupropion [59].

Viloxazine, another putative norepinephrine reuptake inhibitor, reduced the amount of REM sleep and increased REM latencies during short-term application and in healthy subjects [60, 61]. In a small study with six depressed patients, however, viloxazine had no effect on REM, and with the exception of an increase in wake after four weeks, no effect on NREM sleep [62]. There is only one long-term study that has explored the effects of viloxazine on daytime and nocturnal sleep patterns in patients with narcolepsy [63]. After seven weeks of 50 to 100 mg of viloxazine, Guilleminault and coworkers found no effect on REM or NREM sleep parameters during the night. Rapid eye movement sleep during the daytime multiple sleep latency test, however, was reduced.

In summary, for reboxetine and viloxazine, there is some weak evidence from single studies that the effects on sleep may diminish over time. For bupropion, no consistent or significant effects have been reported for the short-term use and none are evident in the long-term application.

Other antidepressants

Other antidepressants for which long-term effects on sleep have been reported include nefazodone, mirtazapine, trazodone, clovoxamine, and agomelatine (Table 17.5). For each of the last three substances only a single study was available.

Trazodone is a serotonin antagonist for which in short-term studies inconsistent effects have been reported for REM and NREM sleep parameters [64–68]. The only study of longer duration has been undertaken by Parrino and coworkers who treated six patients with dysthymia and insomnia with 150 mg of trazodone CR for six weeks [69]. Trazodone had no effect on REM sleep but increased slow-wave sleep and reduced various parameters of the cyclic alternating pattern, which is consistent with a sleep-improving effect of trazodone. No systematic changes in sleep parameters between days 4, 14, and 42 were observed.

Clovoxamine, which has reuptake inhibiting effects for both norepinephrine and serotonin, has so far only been employed in two studies. In healthy subjects, acute administration of 150 rather than 50 mg reduced the amount of REM sleep and the

Table 17.4 Long-term effects of selective norepinephrine reuptake inhibitors (NRI) antidepressants on sleep EEG

Drug, reference	No. patients, condition, study design	Study duration, drug dosage	Findings[a]
Reboxetine			
Ferini-Strambi et al. 2004 [55]	12 dysthymia	120 d	↓REM% ↑REML
	SB PC	4 mg	↓NoW
			Across days 3, 7, and 120 d:
			↑REM% SE SWS%
			↓SOL WASO$_m$ S1%
Bupropion			
Evans et al. 2002 [56]	8 MD	~49 d	= REMm% REML REMD
	OL	~170 mg	
Nofzinger et al. 1995 [44]	7 MD	~115 d	↓REML ↑REM$_{m\%}$
	OL	~429 mg	
Bupropion SR			
Ott et al. 2004 [59]	20 MD	~56 d	↑REML REMD = REM$_{m\%}$ REM act NoREM
	OL	~290 mg	↑NoW
Nofzinger et al. 2000 [57]	5MD & PLMD	~70 d	= REM$_m$ REM
	OL	~400 mg	↓PLMI
Nofzinger et al. 2001 [58]	9 MD	~77 d	= REM$_{m\%}$ REML REMD
	OL	~400 mg	↑SOL
Viloxazine			
Guilleminault et al. 1986 [63]	22 narcolepsy	49 d	vs. single-blind placebo baseline:
	SB PC	~50 mg	= REM% REML
			MSLT: ↓REM$_m$

Note: [a]Compared to drug-free baseline unless otherwise specified. For abbreviations see Table 17.1.

amount of REM episodes [70]. Indeed, four of the twelve subjects had no REM sleep at all. In addition, 150 mg reduced slow-wave sleep and total sleep time, while the number of awakenings in sleep stage 1 was increased. The only long-term study was conducted in a small group of five patients with depression and insomnia where 240 mg of clovoxamine was applied for 90 days [71]. After four weeks, clovoxamine increased REM latency and total sleep time, while after 90 days REM latency was still increased, as

was slow-wave sleep. The amount of REM sleep was not affected by clovoxamine either after 4 or after 13 weeks [71].

Nefazodone operates by blocking postsynaptic serotonin type 2A receptors and, to a lesser extent, by inhibiting presynaptic serotonin and norepinephrine reuptake. In the short run, it has been shown to increase REM sleep in healthy subjects [72–74]. Long-term administration in depressed patients showed no effect on REM sleep parameters in three out of

Table 17.5 Long-term effects of other antidepressants on sleep EEG

Drug, reference	No. patients, condition, study design	Study duration, drug dosage	Findings[a]
Trazodone			
Parrino et al. 1994 [69]	6 dysthymia	42 d	= REML REM$_{m\%}$
	SB PC	150 mg	↓S2$_{m\%}$ ↑SWS$_{m\%}$
			Across days 4, 14, and 42: no changes
Clovoxamine			
Minot et al. 1985 [71]	5 MD	90 d	↑REML = REM$_m$
	OL	240 mg	↑SWS$_m$
Nefazodone			
Armitage et al. 1994 [75]	10 MD	~42 d	= REM$_{m\%}$ REML REMD
	OL	~520 mg	↓S1$_{m\%}$ W$_{m\%}$ ↑S2$_{m\%}$
Scharf et al. 1999 [76]	16 MD	42 d	= REM$_\%$ REML
	SB PC	~340 mg	↓S1$_\%$
Hicks et al. 2002 [46]	14 MD	56 d	= REM$_\%$ REML
	DB AC PG	200 mg	Across days 3, 10, and 56: ↑WASO$_m$
Rush et al. 1998 [41]	59 MD	56 d	↓REML ↑REM$_\%$
	DB AC PG	~420 mg	↓NoW SWS$_\%$ ↑SE S2$_\%$
			Across week 2, 4, and 8: ↑SE
Gillin et al. 2001 [78]	12 PTSD	84 d	= REM$_\%$ REML REMD
	OL	~440 mg	Across weeks 2, 4, 8, and 12: no changes
Neylan et al. 2003 [77]	10 PTSD	84 d	= REM$_{m\%}$ REML REM act REMD
	OL	~570 mg	↑TST SE S2$_m$
Shen et al. 2005 [79]	9 SAD	56 d	= REM$_\%$ REML
	OL	~400 mg	↓SOL S1$_\%$ ↑SE
			Across weeks 4 and 8: ↓SOL ↑SE
Mirtazapine			
Shen et al. 2006 [84]	16 MD	58 d	= REM$_\%$ ↓No REM ↑REML
	OL	30 mg	↑S3$_\%$
			Across days 2, 9, 16, 30, and 58: no changes
Winokur et al. 2003 [39]	9 MD	56 d	= REM$_m$ REML
	DB AC	~45 mg	↑SE TST ↓SOL WASO$_m$
			Across days 7, 14, and 56: ↑TST

Table 17.5 (*cont.*)

Drug, reference	No. patients, condition, study design	Study duration, drug dosage	Findings[a]
Schittecatte *et al.* 2002 [85]	17 MD	~42 d	↑REML = REMm
	OL	~45 mg	↑TST SE ↓W%
Agomelatine			
Quera Salva *et al.* 2007 [88]	15 MD	~42 d	= REM% REML REMD
	OL	25 mg	↓WASO ↑SE SWS%m
			across days 7, 14, and 42: ↓WASO ↑SE SWS%m

Note: [a]Compared to drug-free baseline unless otherwise specified.
For abbreviations see Table 17.1.

four studies over six to eight weeks [41, 46, 75, 76]. Only one study [41] found REM disinhibiting effects with a reduced REM latency and increased REM sleep after eight weeks. Most studies also reported some improvement of sleep such as a decrease in sleep stage 1 [75, 76], wake [41, 75], or an increased sleep efficiency [41] (Table 17.5). Two studies assessed sleep at multiple time points within the same study. In neither study [41, 46] did REM sleep parameters change over time. In one study, sleep efficiency improved over time [41], while in another study [46] wake after sleep onset decreased acutely but increased again to baseline values over time. In addition, in two studies nefazodone was given to patients with post-traumatic stress disorder (PTSD) [77, 78]; after 12 weeks, both found no effect on REM sleep parameters, while in one [77] of the two studies, total sleep times, sleep efficiency and sleep stage 2 were increased. Finally, a six-week treatment of patients with seasonal affective disorder (SAD) had no effect on REM sleep either; however, the beneficial effects with a decrease in sleep onset latency and an increase in sleep efficiency accumulated over time [79]. In summary, nefazodone has no short- or long-term effects on REM sleep but improves various NREM sleep parameters, and there is some indication that this sleep improvement increases over time.

Mirtazapine is a noradrenergic and specific serotonergic antagonist (NaSSA). It has no clear effect on REM sleep, but promotes slow-wave sleep and sleep continuity in the short run [80–83]. Mirtazapine has been employed in three studies with depressed patients for six to eight weeks (Table 17.5) [39, 84,

85]. In all three studies mirtazapine had no effect on the amount of REM sleep, while at dosages between 30 and 45 mg, REM latency was decreased in one study [84], increased in another [85], and unchanged in the third study [39]. Mirtazapine promoted sleep by increasing sleep efficiency [39, 85] or slow-wave sleep [84] (Table 17.5). With the exception of one study in which the increase in total sleep time appeared only after six weeks [85], no systematic changes of sleep parameters over time were reported [39, 84].

Finally, one of the most recent antidepressants is *agomelatine*, a melatonin agonist that has also 5-HT$_{2c}$ antagonist properties. The acute intake of both 5 mg and 100 mg leads to an increase in the percentage of REM sleep in young healthy subjects while REM latency and other sleep parameters were unaffected [86]. On the other hand, 15-day treatment with 50 mg of agomelatine in healthy elderly subjects did not affect sleep parameters [87]. Long-term experience is derived from the study of Quera Salva and coworkers who treated 15 patients with depression with 25 mg of agomelatine for six weeks [88]. Agomelatine had no effect on any REM parameter, but, interestingly, the sleep-promoting effects with increased sleep efficiency and slow-wave sleep as well as decreased wake after sleep onset became only apparent after six weeks rather than after one or two weeks.

In summary, also for diverse newer antidepressants the long-term effects on sleep mostly mirror the respective short-term effects. None of the five antidepressants reviewed here had a systematic effect on REM sleep either in the short or the long run.

For NREM parameters and especially sleep-promoting characteristics there is some indication that these start to emerge over longer time spans. This seems to be the case for nefazodone and mirtrazapine and possibly also for agomelatine. Whether this is a primary drug effect or secondary to the improvement of the mood disorder is unclear.

Summary, discussion, and conclusions

Reviewing the literature regarding the long-term effects of antidepressants on sleep, the first finding must be that of a general paucity of studies in this area. For the majority of antidepressants, no long-term studies were available. For several others such as imipramine, clomipramine, tranylcypromine, moclobemide, citalopram, sertraline, fluvoxamine, reboxetine, viloxazine, trazodone, clovoxamine, and agomelatine, only one or two studies at most could be located. Three or more studies were available for the TCAs nortriptyline, amitriptyline, and protriptyline, the MAOI phenelzine, the SSRIs fluoxetine and paroxetine, the NRI bupropion and for mirtazapine and nefazodone (see Table 17.6). Even for these substances, most of the long-term studies were conducted for only six to twelve weeks. Studies over longer periods of time (months, years) were only sporadically reported for nortriptyline, protriptyline, phenelzine, and fluoxetine.

Summarizing the evidence for the different drugs there is a distinction between the effects on REM sleep parameters and those on NREM parameters. For REM sleep, it is clear that those antidepressants that affect REM sleep acutely still exert systematic effects on sleep after six or more weeks. This is based on the repeated and converging evidence that after this time span there is still a significant difference in REM sleep patterns compared to a drug-free baseline in the depressed state. Furthermore, across the different drugs the presence and direction of the effect are congruent between short- and long-term administrations. Also, the magnitude of the specific long-term effects on sleep appears to roughly match that of the short-term effects. So far, the overall picture has been one where the acute and short-term effects are mirrored by the long-term effects: antidepressants suppressing REM sleep such as TCAs, MAOIs, or SSRIs, in the short run will also suppress REM sleep in the long-term studies. Antidepressants such as NRIs, NaSSAs, or nefazodone that do not affect

REM sleep in a systematic manner in the short run, also fail to do so in long-term administration. Across antidepressant drug classes, differences are also preserved in the long run. For example, REM-suppressing effects are largest with MAOIs, substantial with TCAs, and noticeable but moderate with SSRIs. These differences in the level of REM sleep suppression are also evident in the long-term studies. There were only a small number of studies that compared sleep at several time points and therefore allowed for a within-study comparison of the effects on sleep. The limited evidence nevertheless suggests that for TCAs and MAOIs there is no systematic change in the effect on REM sleep. For SSRIs, REM-suppressing effects are still observable in the long run; however, there appears to be some mild attenuation of the effect over longer – weeks to months – periods of time.

The long-term effects of antidepressants on NREM sleep are harder to summarize although we have tried to do so in Table 17.6. For one thing, even the acute effects on NREM sleep are not entirely consistent across studies. While a general sleep-disturbing or sleep-promoting effect is more consistently documented, this may manifest itself as an increase in the number of awakenings in one study, an increase in sleep stage 1 in another, and longer wake after sleep onset in a third study. One of the more consistent effects is an increase of sleep stage 2 in the case of TCAs and MAOIs, which seems to go hand in hand with the REM-suppressing effects. Nevertheless, while it seems that sleep-disturbing effects are rather stable over time, sleep-promoting effects appear to increase over extended periods of time (Table 17.6). Again, only a few studies measured sleep at multiple time points.

It has to be remembered, however, that especially in the long-term studies, only patients with full or partial remission have been included. Therefore, the generalizability of these findings might be limited. Especially in the light of the sleep promoting effects on NREM sleep, it must be questioned whether these effects reflect a primary or secondary effect of the antidepressant. In particular, the question is whether these long-term effects on sleep reflect (i) a continued pharmacological effect, (ii) a secondary effect based on the resolution of the mood disorder, and/or (iii) a normalization of the sleep pattern [89], potentially independent of the changes in mood.

For REM sleep, several arguments distinctly favor the assumption of a continued pharmacological effect: for

Table 17.6 Summary of effects of antidepressants on sleep (for drugs with three or more studies)

Drug	Acute effects	6–12 weeks	3–6 months	>6 months
TCA				
Nortriptyline	REM↓↓		REM↓↓	REM↓↓
	NREM↑		NREM↑	NREM↑–
Amitriptyline	REM↓↓	REM↓↓		
	NREM↑	NREM↑		
Protriptyline	REM↓	REM↓	REM↓	REM↓
	NREM=	NREM=	NREM=	NREM=
All studies conducted in patients with COPD or SRBD				
MAOI				
Phenelzine	REM↓↓↓	REM↓↓↓	REM↓↓↓	REM↓↓↓
	NREM↑	NREM↑	NREM↑	NREM↑
SSRI				
Fluoxetine	REM↓	REM↓	REM↓	REM↓
	NREM–	NREM–	NREM–	NREM–
Across weeks and months dimishing effects on REM sleep				
Paroxetine	REM↓	REM↓ =		
	NREM –	NREM –		
Across weeks diminishing effects on REM sleep				
NRI				
Bupropion/SR	REM=	REM=		
	NREM=	NREM=		
Other				
Nefazodone	REM↑	REM=		
	NREM+	NREM+		
Across weeks improved NREM sleep				
Mirtazapine	REM=	REM=		
	NREM+	NREM+		
Across weeks improved NREM sleep				

Notes: ↓decreased; ↑ increased; + improved; – impaired.
COPD: chronic obstructive pulmonary disease; SRBD: sleep-related breathing disorders; REM: rapid eye movement sleep; NREM: non-rapid eye movement sleep; TCA: tricyclic antidepressant; MAOI: monoamine oxidase inhibitor; SSRI: selective serotonin reuptake inhibitor; NRI: norepinephrine reuptake inhibitor.

one thing, even after prolonged use a massive rebound of REM sleep can be observed. In addition, REM sleep with TCAs, MAOIs, and partly SSRIs is suppressed to a level that is definitely below most age-related normative values, which argues against a mere normalization of REM sleep patterns. Furthermore, studies comparing changes in sleep patterns during non-pharmacological therapy, placebo, or in drug-free remission revealed only minor or no changes in REM sleep parameters [13, 90–92]. Indeed, it has been discussed whether certain abnormalities such as reduced REM latency or decreased SWS are trait-like features in depression [89, 91, 93]. Kupfer and Ehlers [94], for example, distinguished between trait-like sleep abnormalities including decreased SWS and a decreased delta sleep ratio and state-dependent characteristic features such as REM density and sleep efficiency. In this model, reduced REM latency was both a state and a trait marker for depression. Regarding changes in NREM sleep parameters some arguments can also be found for continuing drug effects. For one thing, changes in NREM sleep have been reported in the direction of both improvement and impairment of sleep quality, arguing against a uniform secondary effect on sleep. On the other hand, the delayed onset of sleep-promoting effects when using some of the antidepressants may parallel that of the clinical improvement. However, as with REM sleep, either no changes [13, 90] or deteriorations in sleep [91, 92] have been reported in other long-term observations.

The sleep abnormalities in depression encompass three general clusters: sleep continuity disturbances, slow-wave sleep deficits, and REM sleep abnormalities [95]. Although many antidepressants have systematic effects on sleep EEG, across the different substances there is no common cluster of effects. Some, but by no means all, antidepressants suppress REM sleep, some may improve sleep continuity measures and for some the exact opposite, i.e., a sleep-disturbing effect, has been reported. Therefore, although the effects of antidepressants on sleep are rapid, substantial, and long lasting they seem to be neither necessary nor sufficient [3] for the clinical improvement of the mood disturbances. Nevertheless, as we have reviewed here, sleep changes associated with antidepressants are robust and appear to be intrinsically intertwined with the pharmacological effect.

References

1. Mayers AG, Baldwin DS. Antidepressants and their effect on sleep. *Hum Psychopharmacol.* 2005;**20**:533–9.

2. Stassen HH, Delini-Stula A, Angst J. Time course of improvement under antidepressant treatment: a survival-analytical approach. *Eur Neuropsychopharmacol.* 1993;**3**(2):127–35.

3. Vogel GW, Buffenstein A, Minter K, Hennessey A. Drug effects on REM sleep and on endogenous depression. *Neurosci Biobehav Rev.* 1990;**14**:49–63.

4. Landolt HP, de Boer LP. Effect of chronic phenelzine treatment on REM sleep: report of three patients. *Neuropsychopharmacology.* 2001;**25** (5 Suppl):S63–S67.

5. Wyatt RJ, Fram DH, Buchbinder R, Snyder F. Treatment of intractable narcolepsy with a monoamine oxidase inhibitor. *N Engl J Med.* 1971; **285**(18):987–91.

6. Kupfer DJ, Ehlers CL, Frank E, *et al.* Persistent effects of antidepressants: EEG sleep studies in depressed patients during maintenance treatment. *Biol Psychiatry.* 1994;**35**(10):781–93.

7. Feuillade P, Pringuey D, Belugou JL, Robert P, Darcourt G. Trimipramine: acute and lasting effects on sleep in healthy and major depressive subjects. *J Affect Disord.* 1992;**24**(3):135–45.

8. Wiegand M, Berger M, Zulley J, Vonzerssen D. The effect of trimipramine on sleep in patients with major depressive disorder. *Pharmacopsychiatry.* 1986; **19**(4):198–9.

9. Wolf R, Dykierek P, Gattaz WF, *et al.* Differential effects of trimipramine and fluoxetine on sleep in geriatric depression. *Pharmacopsychiatry.* 2001; **34**(2):60–5.

10. Ware JC, Brown FW, Moorad PJ Jr., Pittard JT, Cobert B. Effects on sleep: a double-blind study comparing trimipramine to imipramine in depressed insomniac patients. *Sleep.* 1989;**12**(6):537–49.

11. Rubin AH, Alroy GG, Peled R, Lavie P. Preliminary clinical experience with imipramine HCl in the treatment of sleep apnea syndrome. *Eur Neurol.* 1986;**25**(2):81–5.

12. Reynolds CF III, Hoch CC, Buysse DJ, *et al.* Sleep in late-life recurrent depression. Changes during early continuation therapy with nortriptyline. *Neuropsychopharmacology.* 1991;**5**(2):85–96.

13. Buysse DJ, Reynolds CF III, Hoch CC, *et al.* Longitudinal effects of nortriptyline on EEG sleep and the likelihood of recurrence in elderly depressed patients. *Neuropsychopharmacology.* 1996; **14**(4):243–52.

14. Taylor MP, Reynolds CF III, Frank E, *et al.* EEG sleep measures in later-life bereavement depression. A randomized, double-blind, placebo-controlled evaluation of nortriptyline. *Am J Geriatr Psychiatry.* 1999;**7**(1):41–7.

15. Pasternak RE, Reynolds CF III, Houck PR, *et al.* Sleep in bereavement-related depression during and after pharmacotherapy with nortriptyline. *J Geriatr Psychiatry Neurol.* 1994;**7**(2):69–73.

16. Scharf MB, Hirschowitz J, Zemlan FP, Lichstein M, Woods M. Comparative effects of limbitrol and amitriptyline on sleep efficiency and architecture. *J Clin Psychiatry.* 1986;**47**(12):587–91.

17. Hubain PP, Castro P, Mesters P, de Maertelaer V, Mendlewicz J. Alprazolam and amitriptyline in the treatment of major depressive disorder: a double-blind clinical and sleep EEG study. *J Affect Disord.* 1990;**18**(1):67–73.

18. Linkowski P, Mendlewicz J, Kerkhofs M, *et al.* 24-hour profiles of adrenocorticotropin, cortisol, and growth hormone in major depressive illness: effect of antidepressant treatment. *J Clin Endocrinol Metab.* 1987;**65**(1):141–52.

19. Kerkhofs M, Rielaert C, de Maertelaer V, *et al.* Fluoxetine in major depression: efficacy, safety and effects on sleep polygraphic variables. *Int Clin Psychopharmacol.* 1990;**5**(4):253–60.

20. Kempenaers C, Simenon G, Vander EM, *et al.* Effect of an antidiencephalon immune serum on pain and sleep in primary fibromyalgia. *Neuropsychobiology.* 1994;**30**(2–3):66–72.

21. Carette S, Oakson G, Guimont C, Steriade M. Sleep electroencephalography and the clinical response to amitriptyline in patients with fibromyalgia. *Arthritis Rheum.* 1995;**38**(9):1211–17.

22. Conway WA, Zorick F, Piccione P, Roth T. Protriptyline in the treatment of sleep apnoea. *Thorax.* 1982;**37**(1):49–53.

23. Smith PL, Haponik EF, Allen RP, Bleecker ER. The effects of protriptyline in sleep-disordered breathing. *Am Rev Respir Dis.* 1983;**127**(1):8–13.

24. Brownell LG, West P, Sweatman P, Acres JC, Kryger MH. Protriptyline in obstructive sleep apnea: a double-blind trial. *N Engl J Med.* 1982;**307**(17):1037–42.

25. Series F, Cormier Y, La Forge J. Changes in day and night time oxygenation with protriptyline in patients with chronic obstructive lung disease. *Thorax.* 1989; **44**(4):275–9.

26. Series F, Cormier Y. Effects of protriptyline on diurnal and nocturnal oxygenation in patients with chronic obstructive pulmonary disease. *Ann Intern Med.* 1990;**113**(7):507–11.

27. Carroll N, Parker RA, Branthwaite MA. The use of protriptyline for respiratory failure in patients with chronic airflow limitation. *Eur Respir J.* 1990;**3**(7):746–51.

28. Lin CC. [Effects of protriptyline on day and night time oxygenation in patients with chronic obstructive pulmonary disease]. *J Formos Med Assoc.* 1993;**92** Suppl 4:S232–S236.

29. Series F, Marc I, Cormier Y, La Forge J. Long-term effects of protriptyline in patients with chronic obstructive pulmonary disease. *Am Rev Respir Dis.* 1993;**147**(6 Pt 1):1487–90.

30. Guilleminault C, Raynal D, Takahashi S, Carskadon M, Dement W. Evaluation of short-term and long-term treatment of the narcolepsy syndrome with clomipramine hydrochloride. *Acta Neurol Scand.* 1976;**54**(1):71–87.

31. Winokur A, Gary KA, Rodner S, *et al.* Depression, sleep physiology, and antidepressant drugs. *Depress Anxiety.* 2001;**14**(1):19–28.

32. Gillin JC, Wyatt RJ. Schizophrenia: perchance a dream? *Int Rev Neurobiol.* 1975;**17**:297–342.

33. Mann K, Pankok J, Leissner J, Benkert O. Effects of moclobemide on sexual performance and nocturnal erections in psychogenic erectile dysfunction. *Psychopharmacology (Berl).* 2001;**156**(1):86–91.

34. Monti JM. Effect of a reversible monoamine oxidase-A inhibitor (moclobemide) on sleep of depressed patients. *Br J Psychiatry Suppl.* 1989;**6**:61–5.

35. Monti JM, Alterwain P, Monti D. The effects of moclobemide on nocturnal sleep of depressed patients. *J Affect Disord.* 1990;**20**(3):201–8.

36. Minot R, Luthringer R, Macher JP. Effect of moclobemide on the psychophysiology of sleep/wake cycles: a neuroelectrophysiological study of depressed patients administered with moclobemide. *Int Clin Psychopharmacol.* 1993;**7**(3–4):181–9.

37. Hoff P, Golling H, Kapfhammer HP, *et al.* Cimoxatone and moclobemide, two new MAO-inhibitors: influence on sleep parameters in patients with major depressive disorder. *Pharmacopsychiatry.* 1986;**19**(4):249–50.

38. Anderson IM, Nutt DJ, Deakin JF. Evidence-based guidelines for treating depressive disorders with antidepressants: a revision of the 1993 British Association for Psychopharmacology guidelines. British Association for Psychopharmacology. *J Psychopharmacol.* 2000;**14**(1):3–20.

39. Winokur A, DeMartinis NA, III, McNally DP, *et al.* Comparative effects of mirtazapine and fluoxetine on sleep physiology measures in patients with major depression and insomnia. *J Clin Psychiatry.* 2003; **64**(10):1224–9.

40. Levitan RD, Shen JH, Jindal R, *et al.* Preliminary randomized double-blind placebo-controlled trial of tryptophan combined with fluoxetine to treat major depressive disorder: antidepressant and hypnotic effects. *J Psychiatry Neurosci.* 2000;**25**(4):337–46.

41. Rush AJ, Armitage R, Gillin JC, *et al.* Comparative effects of nefazodone and fluoxetine on sleep in outpatients with major depressive disorder. *Biol Psychiatry.* 1998;**44**(1):3–14.

42. Trivedi MH, Rush AJ, Armitage R, *et al.* Effects of fluoxetine on the polysomnogram in outpatients with major depression. *Neuropsychopharmacology.* 1999; **20**(5):447–59.

43. Hendrickse WA, Roffwarg HP, Grannemann BD, *et al.* The effects of fluoxetine on the polysomnogram of depressed outpatients: a pilot study. *Neuropsychopharmacology.* 1994;**10**(2):85–91.

44. Nofzinger EA, Reynolds CF III, Thase ME, *et al.* REM sleep enhancement by bupropion in depressed men. *Am J Psychiatry.* 1995;**152**(2):274–6.

45. Haro R, Drucker-Colin R. Effects of long-term administration of nicotine and fluoxetine on sleep in depressed patients. *Arch Med Res.* 2004;**35**(6):499–506.

46. Hicks JA, Argyropoulos SV, Rich AS, *et al.* Randomised controlled study of sleep after nefazodone or paroxetine treatment in out-patients with depression. *Br J Psychiatry.* 2002;**180**:528–35.

47. Nowell PD, Reynolds CF III, Buysse DJ, Dew MA, Kupfer DJ. Paroxetine in the treatment of primary insomnia: preliminary clinical and electroencephalogram sleep data. *J Clin Psychiatry.* 1999;**60**(2):89–95.

48. Kraiczi H, Hedner J, Dahlof P, Ejnell H, Carlson J. Effect of serotonin uptake inhibition on breathing during sleep and daytime symptoms in obstructive sleep apnea. *Sleep.* 1999;**22**(1):61–7.

49. Jindal RD, Friedman ES, Berman SR, *et al.* Effects of sertraline on sleep architecture in patients with depression. *J Clin Psychopharmacol.* 2003;**23**(6):540–8.

50. Wilson SJ, Bell C, Coupland NJ, Nutt DJ. Sleep changes during long-term treatment of depression with fluvoxamine: a home-based study. *Psychopharmacology (Berl).* 2000;**149**(4):360–5.

51. Van Bemmel AL, Beersma DG, Van Den Hoofdakker RH. Changes in EEG power density of NREM sleep in depressed patients during treatment with citalopram. *J Sleep Res.* 1993;**2**(3):156–62.

52. Van Bemmel AL, Van Den Hoofdakker RH, Beersma DG, Bouhuys AL. Changes in sleep polygraphic variables and clinical state in depressed patients during treatment with citalopram. *Psychopharmacology (Berl).* 1993;**113**(2):225–30.

53. Farina B, Della MG, Mennuni G, *et al.* The effects of reboxetine on human sleep architecture in depression: preliminary results. *J Affect Disord.* 2002;**71**(1–3):273–5.

54. Kuenzel HE, Murck H, Held K, Ziegenbein M, Steiger A. Reboxetine induces similar sleep-EEG changes like SSRIs in patients with depression. *Pharmacopsychiatry.* 2004;**37**(5):193–5.

55. Ferini-Strambi L, Manconi M, Castronovo V, Riva L, Bianchi A. Effects of reboxetine on sleep and nocturnal cardiac autonomic activity in patients with dysthymia. *J Psychopharmacol.* 2004;**18**(3):417–22.

56. Evans L, Golshan S, Kelsoe J, *et al.* Effects of rapid tryptophan depletion on sleep electroencephalogram

and mood in subjects with partially remitted depression on bupropion. *Neuropsychopharmacology.* 2002;**27**(6):1016–26.

57. Nofzinger EA, Fasiczka A, Berman S, Thase ME. Bupropion SR reduces periodic limb movements associated with arousals from sleep in depressed patients with periodic limb movement disorder. *J Clin Psychiatry.* 2000;**61**(11):858–62.

58. Nofzinger EA, Berman S, Fasiczka A, *et al.* Effects of bupropion SR on anterior paralimbic function during waking and REM sleep in depression: preliminary findings using. *Psychiatry Res.* 2001; **106**(2):95–111.

59. Ott GE, Rao U, Lin KM, Gertsik L, Poland RE. Effect of treatment with bupropion on EEG sleep: relationship to antidepressant response. *Int J Neuropsychopharmacol.* 2004;**7**(3):275–81.

60. Brezinova V, Adam K, Chapman K, Oswald I, Thomson J. Viloxazine, sleep, and subjective feelings. *Psychopharmacology (Berl).* 1977;**55**(2):121–8.

61. Wilson WH, Freemon FR, Ban TA, Petrie WM, Clinton CL. Acute effects of viloxazine HCl and flurazepam when given alone and in combination on sleep EEG: a double-blind interaction study with normals. *Pavlov J Biol Sci.* 1980;**15**(2):68–73.

62. Zung WWK. Comparison of the effects of viloxazine and placebo on the sleep of depressed patients. *Curr Ther Res Clin Exp.* 1980;**27**(2):152–6.

63. Guilleminault C, Mancuso J, Salva MA, *et al.* Viloxazine hydrochloride in narcolepsy: a preliminary report. *Sleep.* 1986;**9**(1 Pt 2):275–9.

64. Saletu-Zyhlarz GM, Abu-Bakr MH, Anderer P, *et al.* Insomnia related to dysthymia: polysomnographic and psychometric comparison with normal controls and acute therapeutic trials with trazodone. *Neuropsychobiology.* 2001;**44**(3):139–49.

65. Saletu-Zyhlarz GM, Abu-Bakr MH, Anderer P, *et al.* Insomnia in depression: differences in objective and subjective sleep and awakening quality to normal controls and acute effects of trazodone. *Prog Neuropsychopharmacol Biol Psychiatry.* 2002; **26**(2):249–60.

66. Montgomery I, Oswald I, Morgan K, Adam K. Trazodone enhances sleep in subjective quality but not in objective duration. *Br J Clin Pharmacol.* 1983; **16**(2):139–44.

67. Mouret J, Lemoine P, Minuit MP, Benkelfat C, Renardet M. Effects of trazodone on the sleep of depressed subjects: a polygraphic study. *Psychopharmacology (Berl).* 1988;**95** Suppl:S37–S43.

68. Van Bemmel AL, Havermans RG, van Diest R. Effects of trazodone on EEG sleep and clinical state in major

depression. *Psychopharmacology (Berl).* 1992;**107**(4):569–74.

69. Parrino L, Spaggiari MC, Boselli M, Di Giovanni G, Terzano MG. Clinical and polysomnographic effects of trazodone CR in chronic insomnia associated with dysthymia. *Psychopharmacology (Berl).* 1994;**116**(4):389–95.

70. Wilson WH, Ban T, Coleman B, Vause B, Papadatos J. The effects of clovoxamine on sleep of normal volunteers: a double-blind placebo-controlled study. *Drug Dev Res.* 1986;**9**(4):293–8.

71. Minot R, Crocq MA, Roussel B, Marie-Cardine M. [Action of clovoxamine on the sleep of depressed patients. "Polygraphic recordings"]. *Encephale.* 1985;**11**(2):65–70.

72. Sharpley AL, Williamson DJ, Attenburrow ME, *et al.* The effects of paroxetine and nefazodone on sleep: a placebo controlled trial. *Psychopharmacology (Berl).* 1996;**126**(1):50–4.

73. Sharpley AL, Walsh AE, Cowen PJ. Nefazodone – a novel antidepressant – may increase REM sleep. *Biol Psychiatry.* 1992;**31**(10):1070–3.

74. Ware JC, Rose FV, McBrayer RH. The acute effects of nefazodone, trazodone and buspirone on sleep and sleep-related penile tumescence in normal subjects. *Sleep.* 1994;**17**(6):544–50.

75. Armitage R, Rush AJ, Trivedi M, Cain J, Roffwarg HP. The effects of nefazodone on sleep architecture in depression. *Neuropsychopharmacology.* 1994;**10**(2):123–7.

76. Scharf MB, McDannold M, Zaretsky N, *et al.* Evaluation of sleep architecture and cyclic alternating pattern rates in depressed insomniac patients treated with nefazodone hydrochloride. *Am J Ther.* 1999;**6**(2):77–82.

77. Neylan TC, Lenoci M, Maglione ML, *et al.* The effect of nefazodone on subjective and objective sleep quality in posttraumatic stress disorder. *J Clin Psychiatry.* 2003;**64**(4):445–50.

78. Gillin JC, Smith-Vaniz A, Schnierow B, *et al.* An open-label, 12-week clinical and sleep EEG study of nefazodone in chronic combat-related posttraumatic stress disorder. *J Clin Psychiatry.* 2001;**62**(10):789–96.

79. Shen J, Kennedy SH, Levitan RD, Kayumov L, Shapiro CM. The effects of nefazodone on women with seasonal affective disorder: clinical and polysomnographic analyses. *J Psychiatry Neurosci.* 2005;**30**(1):11–16.

80. Winokur A, Sateia MJ, Hayes JB, *et al.* Acute effects of mirtazapine on sleep continuity and sleep architecture in depressed patients: a pilot study. *Biol Psychiatry.* 2000;**48**:75–8.

81. Aslan S, Isik E, Cosar B. The effects of mirtazapine on sleep: a placebo controlled, double-blind study in young healthy volunteers. *Sleep.* 2002;**25**:677–9.

82. Schmid DA, Wichniak A, Uhr M, *et al.* Changes of sleep architecture, spectral composition of sleep EEG, the nocturnal secretion of cortisol, ACTH, GH, prolactin, melatonin, ghrelin, and leptin, and the DEX-CRH test in depressed patients during treatment with mirtazapine. *Neuropsychopharmacology.* 2006;**31**:832–44.

83. Ruigt GS, Kemp B, Groenhout CM, Kamphuisen HA. Effect of the antidepressant Org 3770 on human sleep. *Eur J Clin Pharmacol.* 1990;**38**:551–4.

84. Shen J, Chung SA, Kayumov L, *et al.* Polysomnographic and symptomatological analyses of major depressive disorder patients treated with mirtazapine. *Can J Psychiatry.* 2006;**51**:27–34.

85. Schittecatte M, Dumont F, Machowski R, *et al.* Effects of mirtazapine on sleep polygraphic variables in major depression. *Neuropsychobiology.* 2002;**46**:197–201.

86. Cajochen C, Krauchi K, Mori D, Graw P, Wirz-Justice A. Melatonin and S-20098 increase REM sleep and wake-up propensity without modifying NREM sleep homeostasis. *Am J Physiol.* 1997;**272**(4 Pt 2):R1189–R1196.

87. Leproult R, Van Onderbergen A, L'hermite-Baleriaux M, Van Cauter E, Copinschi G. Phase-shifts of 24-h rhythms of hormonal release and body temperature following early evening administration of the melatonin agonist agomelatine in healthy older men. *Clin Endocrinol (Oxf).* 2005;**63**(3):298–304.

88. Quera Salva MA, Vanier B, Laredo J, *et al.* Major depressive disorder, sleep EEG and agomelatine: an open-label study. *Int J Neuropsychopharmacol.* 2007;**10**(5):691–6.

89. Thase ME, Fasiczka AL, Berman SR, Simons AD, Reynolds CF III. Electroencephalographic sleep profiles before and after cognitive behavior therapy of depression. *Arch Gen Psychiatry.* 1998;**55**(2):138–44.

90. Buysse DJ, Kupfer DJ, Frank E, Monk TH, Ritenour A. Electroencephalographic sleep studies in depressed outpatients treated with interpersonal psychotherapy: II. Longitudinal studies at baseline and recovery. *Psychiatry Res.* 1992;**42**(1):27–40.

91. Buysse DJ, Frank E, Lowe KK, Cherry CR, Kupfer DJ. Electroencephalographic sleep correlates of episode and vulnerability to recurrence in depression. *Biol Psychiatry.* 1997;**41**(4):406–18.

92. Steiger A, von Bardeleben U, Herth T, Holsboer F. Sleep EEG and nocturnal secretion of cortisol and growth hormone in male patients with endogenous depression before treatment and after recovery. *J Affect Disord.* 1989;**16**(2–3):189–95.

93. Reynolds CF III, Perel JM, Frank E, Imber S, Kupfer DJ. Open-trial maintenance nortriptyline in geriatric depression: survival analysis and preliminary data on the use of REM latency as a predictor of recurrence. *Psychopharmacol Bull.* 1989;**25**(1):129–32.

94. Kupfer DJ, Ehlers CL. Two roads to rapid eye movement latency. *Arch Gen Psychiatry.* 1989; **46**(10):945–8.

95. Benca RM, Obermeyer WH, Thisted RA, Gilllin JC. Sleep and psychiatric disorders. *Arch Gen Psychiatry.* 1992;**49**:651–68.

96. Jindal RD, Fasiczka AL, Himmelhoch JM, Mallinger AG, Thase ME. Effects of tranylcypromine on the sleep of patients with anergic bipolar depression. *Psychopharmacol Bull.* 2003; **37**(3):118–26.

Chapter

18

Antidepressant-induced alteration of sleep EEG

Luc Staner, Corinne Staner, and Remy Luthringer

Introduction

A large empirical data base supports the position that sleep dysregulation is closely linked to the underlying pathophysiology of depressive disorders. Depressed patients almost invariably complain about their sleep and changes in sleep patterns are included in the clinical diagnostic criteria for those illnesses. A close relationship between the regulation of mood and the regulation of sleep has been suggested by sleep deprivation studies showing that the procedure improves mood of depressed patients and can even trigger manic episodes in bipolar disorder [1–3]. Over the past 50 years, with the development of overnight laboratory sleep EEG studies, clinicians had available a powerful research tool that provides objective quantitative information on the nature of sleep disturbances. These studies brought evidence that the subjective sleep disturbances of depressed patients were linked to robust and relatively specific changes in sleep continuity and architecture that may relate to the underlying neurobiology of depression [4]. Characteristic sleep EEG changes reflect an increase of REM sleep propensity and an imbalance between sleep-promoting mechanisms and wake-promoting mechanisms [5]. It must be emphasized that nearly all antidepressants alter sleep in the opposite direction to these depression-related changes, even in non-depressed healthy subjects. Furthermore, there is evidence that depressed patients having those sleep changes are less likely to respond to non-pharmacological treatment than to antidepressant drugs [6–8]. If we assume a neurobiological link between mood and sleep, the recent advances in the field of functional neuroanatomy of sleep–wake regulation [9–12] should open new ways in our understanding of the interrelationship between sleep and depression. Moreover, it could bring new interpretation on the sleep effects of antidepressant drugs and how they relate to drug activity. Accordingly, the purpose of this chapter is to review studies investigating the effects of antidepressants on human sleep EEG and to discuss the possible pharmacological mechanisms involved in regard to proposed models of sleep dysregulation in depressive illness. Relevant effects of antidepressant drugs on the animal sleep EEG will be discussed but are not systematically reviewed here.

Sleep EEG in major depression

Sleep research over the past decades has primarily focused on major affective disorders such as depressive disorder or bipolar disorder, and minor affective conditions such as dysthymia or cyclothymia have been neglected in the research literature. Major affective disorders are recurrent illnesses characterized by episodes of major depression – and in cases of bipolar disorder, mania – that recur and remit repeatedly during the course of a patient's life. DSM-IV [13] diagnosis of a major depressive episode relies on the presence for a same two-week period of a series of at least five symptoms, one of them being either depressed mood or loss of interest or pleasure. Other symptoms include appetite disturbances (decrease or increase), sleep disturbances (insomnia or hypersomnia), psychomotor disturbances (agitation or retardation), decreased energy, feelings of worthlessness or guilt, poor concentration, and suicidal thoughts. It is worth noting that most of the sleep EEG studies were performed on patients with major depression, and for the last decade, on patients with moderate forms of depression. Ethical and safety issues in studying patients with greater symptoms severity, especially when patients are unmedicated, could explain the

202

Sleep and Mental Illness, eds. S. R. Pandi-Perumal and M. Kramer. Published by Cambridge University Press.
© Cambridge University Press 2010.

paucity of sleep EEG studies in more severely ill depressed patients [14].

Sleep EEG alterations in major depression

Characteristic sleep EEG disturbances associated with major depression have been consistently described in over 1,300 published reports [15]. Disruption of sleep continuity (lengthening of sleep latency and increased wake after sleep onset resulting in a decreased time spent asleep), deficit of slow-wave sleep (SWS), especially during the first sleep cycle, and dysregulation of REM sleep are the hallmarks of sleep EEG disturbances in major depression. Rapid eye movement sleep dysregulation, also known as an "increased REM sleep pressure" or as "REM sleep disinhibition" is characterized by a greater amount of REM sleep mostly in the beginning of the night (also reflected by a shortened REM onset latency) and an increase in actual number of rapid eye movements during this sleep stage (REM activity) or per minute of REM sleep (REM density) [16–17].

Rapid eye movement sleep abnormalities were first considered as pathognomonic of major depression [18] but many studies in the 1980s seriously questioned the specificity of this sleep EEG profile to depression. However, Benca et al. [19] who meta-analyzed sleep EEG studies performed in different groups of mental disorders mentioned that the most widespread and most severe disturbances are found in patients with depressive disorders. It has to be stressed that, beyond depression, evidence of REM sleep disinhibition conditions is more reliably reported in conditions comorbid with depression [20–21] or in antidepressant-responsive disorders such as obsessive–compulsive disorder [22], panic disorder [23], generalized anxiety disorder [24], or borderline personality disorder [25]. Accordingly, the lack of specificity of the REM sleep disinhibition profile to depression may relate to the fact that it could be linked to a biological endophenotype reflecting antidepressant-responsive conditions.

Studies using very large samples of depressed patients and multivariate statistics could investigate whether a particular sleep EEG profile could be specific to a subtype of depression (melancholic, psychotic, and bipolar), controlling for the effects of confounding factors such as age, gender, depressive symptom severity, or episode length [14]. The aim of these studies was to extract from the large sample

smaller groups of patients with a subtype and to match them for age and gender to patients without the subtype and between-group differences were further controlled for the effects of symptom severity and of other depressive subtypes. Results show that for most of the sleep EEG parameters the most important influences are those of age (all parameters) and of depression severity (duration of wake after sleep onset, of stage 2 and of REM sleep). After controlling for these effects, the melancholic/non-melancholic [26] and the bipolar/unipolar [27] distinctions could not be differentiated, whereas patients with the psychotic subtype had a shortest REM latency [28].

Depression and sleep–wake regulation mechanisms

Extensive description of the functional neuroanatomy of sleep and of its regulation mechanism has been recently reviewed elsewhere [9–11]. Briefly, the propensity to sleep or be awake at any given time is a consequence of a sleep need and its interaction with a wake-promoting system that includes the circadian clock located in the suprachiasmatic nucleus and different structures with widespread cortical projections located in the brainstem, the hypothalamus, and the basal forebrain. This wake-promoting system opposes the sleep need that progressively increases from morning awakening, ensuring an even degree of alertness throughout the day. At sleep onset, an imbalance between the two opposing influences favors sleep-promoting signals, and the sleep need and its electrophysiological signature, slow-wave activity (SWA), is at its higher level. Electrophysiological recordings have identified GABAergic SWS-active neurons in the ventrolateral preoptic nucleus located in the hypothalamus and lesions of this area produce insomnia in animals and humans. Rapid eye movement sleep results from bidirectional inhibitory influences between "REM-on" cholinergic neurons located in tegmentum nuclei and "REM-off" serotonergic (5-HT) and noradrenergic (NA) neurons respectively located in the dorsal raphe nuclei and the locus coeruleus. Transition from NREM to REM occurs when activity in the aminergic REM-off neurons ceases. We have recently suggested that a dysfunction of the interacting neuronal systems implicated in sleep–wake regulation (wake-promoting system, NREM-promoting system, and REM-promoting system) could

203

be implicated in the mechanisms of depressive-related sleep dysregulation [5].

Increased activity of wake-promoting mechanisms (or hyperarousal) in major depression is suggested by neuroimaging sleep studies showing a higher NREM whole brain glucose metabolism [29] and a smaller NREM cortical and thalamic deactivation [30–31] in major depression. Other evidence includes indices of sustained stress-induced arousal responses that implicate the corticotropin-releasing hormone (CRH) systems [32–33], the locus coeruleus [34–36], and the autonomic nervous system [37–39]. Another argument for the hyperarousal theory of depression lies on the demonstration that HPA hyperactivity is related to sleep continuity disturbances, SWS deficit, and shortened REM latency, particularly in the most severe subtypes of depression [40–42]. Rapid eye movement sleep could be indirectly influenced by CRH through its inhibitory effects on dorsal raphe 5-HT neurons [43–44] and, more specifically, by the corticosteroid-induced repression of the 5-HT_{1a} receptor gene [45–46]. Indeed, CNS acting drugs facilitating serotonin transmission at the level of the 5-HT_{1a} postsynaptic receptors have consistently been shown to decrease REM sleep propensity [47–48].

A deficient NREM promoting system may also underlie sleep disturbances in depressive disorder. This hypothesis, also known as "process S deficiency theory" [49] posits that the characteristic sleep disturbances of major depressive patients reflect a failure to accumulate sleep pressure during the daytime that results in a reduced amount of SWS/SWA in NREM sleep leading to sleep initiation and sleep maintenance difficulties and the early emergence of REM sleep. Studies investigating the first NREM period bring support to the theory by demonstrating lower SWA or decreased delta incidence in depressed patients [50–57]. Adenosine has been implicated in NREM sleep propensity because it both inhibits wake-promoting structures and activates sleep-promoting structures while its concentration increases with extended wakefulness and normalizes slowly during sleep [58–59]. There is little evidence for a deficit in adenosinergic transmission in depressive illness [60, 61], but there are some indications that adenosine could be implicated in mood regulation [62–66] and it has been suggested that the antidepressant effects of sleep deprivation or of electroconvulsive therapy could be mediated through an increase in adenosinergic transmission [67]. Brain-derived neurotrophic

factor (BDNF), that has been found reduced in depression [68, 69], could also be a good candidate as a recent study suggested a causal link between the cortical expression of BDNF during wakefulness and the level of SWA during the subsequent sleep period [70].

Rapid eye movement sleep disinhibition observed in major depression may directly relate to the monoamine hypothesis of depression that postulates a deficiency of NA and 5-HT neurotransmission because there is strong evidence that REM sleep generating neurons are under the opposite influence of inhibitory NA and 5-HT input and of excitatory cholinergic input [11, 71]. It has also been shown that, compared to healthy subjects, depressed patients display stronger signs of REM sleep disinhibition, as well as an increased rate of awakenings and arousals after administration of cholinergic enhancing drugs [14]. A neuroimaging sleep study [72] showing increased activation of REM-related structure in depressed patients brings further support to a cholinergic–aminergic imbalance in depression, a hypothesis originally proposed by Janowsky et al. [73]. It has to be stressed that hyperarousal, process S deficiency and cholinergic–aminergic imbalance could account for only a part of the picture and that they probably reflect different neurobiological mechanisms operating at various degree in depressed patients. In the next sections we will address how these different theories fit with experimental data coming from studies investigating the effects of antidepressant drugs on sleep.

Effects of antidepressant drugs on REM sleep

Changes in REM sleep variables are the best documented effects of most antidepressants on sleep EEG variables (Table 18.1). In the seminal paper of Vogel et al. [74] who reviewed 251 studies (from 1962 to 1989) on the influence of a variety of drugs (including antidepressants, antipsychotics, barbiturates, benzodiazepines, lithium, opioids, amine precursors, and ethanol) on REM sleep in animals, healthy controls and depressed patients, the authors concluded that all drugs producing large and sustained decrease of REM sleep time followed, on withdrawal, by a REM rebound, have demonstrated a significant clinical efficacy in treating endogenous depression.

Table 18.1 Overview of the antidepressant-induced sleep EEG alterations

Drug	EEG sleep effects		
	Continuity	SWS	REM
TCAs			
Amitriptyline	↑↑	↑	↓↓↓
Imipramine	↔	↔	↓↓↓
Trimipramine	↑↑↑	↔	↔
Doxepin	↑↑↑	↑↑	↓↓
Clomipramine	↑/↔	↑	↓↓↓
Nortriptyline	↔	↑	↓↓↓
Desipramine	↑/↔	↔	↓↓
MAOIs			
Phenelzine	↓	↔	↓↓↓
Tranylcypromine	↓	↔	↓↓↓
Moclobemide	↔	↔	↓
SSRIs			
Fluvoxamine	↓	↔	↓↓
Fluoxetine	↓	↔	↓↓
Paroxetine	↓	↔	↓↓
Citalopram	↓	↔	↓↓
Sertraline	↔	↔	↓↓
SNRIs			
Viloxazine	↓	↔/↓	↓↓
Reboxetine	↓	↔	↓↓
Dual NA/5-HT			
Venlafaxine	↓	↔	↓↓↓
Duloxetine	↓	↔	↓↓↓
Milnacipran	↑	↔	↓↓
Dual NA/DA			
Nomifensine	↓	↔	↔/↓
Bupropion	↔	↔	↑/↔
Others			
Trazodone	↑↑↑	↑↑↑	↔/↓
Nefazodone	↑	↑	↑/↔
Mianserin	↑↑	↑	↓
Mirtazapine	↑↑↑	↑↑↑	↔/↓
Agomelatine	↑↑	↑↑	↔
Tianeptine	↔	↔	↔

Notes: ↑ = increased; ↓ = decreased; ↔ = no change.
REM = rapid eye movement; SWS = slow-wave sleep.

Conversely, reserpine, an old antihypertensive agent that also leads to high rates of depression, causes dramatic increase in REM sleep and reduces REM latency [75]. In the same way, evidence of REM sleep disinhibition is observed after administration of a tryptophan-free amino acid drink, a procedure known to lower brain 5-HT level and to induce transient depressive relapse in remitted depressive patients [76–79]. A healthy volunteer study indicates that both tryptophan depletion and the SSRI fluvoxamine alter REM sleep but in an opposite fashion: tryptophan depletion disinhibits REM sleep whereas fluvoxamine inhibits REM sleep [5].

Classical antidepressants: tricyclic antidepressants and monoamine oxidase inhibitors

Most tricyclic antidepressants (TCAs) block both 5-HT and NA reuptake to some extent. Exceptions are trimipramine and iprindole [80, 81]. Some of the TCAs have much more potency for inhibition of the 5-HT reuptake pump (such as clomipramine), others are more selective for NE over 5-HT (such as desipramine and nortriptyline). Tricyclic antidepressants almost invariably decrease REM sleep and increase REM latency in healthy subjects, the sole exception being trimipramine [82]. This effect occurs from the first night, appears to persist during continued administration, though some tolerance phenomenon may occur, and is followed by REM rebound on withdrawal [83–85]. The REM suppressant effects of TCA are somewhat less pronounced in depressed patients. Although drugs such as clomipramine, amitriptyline, imipramine, and nortriptyline have clear REM suppressant effects [86–88], which have even been shown, for clomipramine, to persist after withdrawal [89–91] or, for imipramine and nortriptyline, to persist after long-term drug administration (up to two years) [92, 93] no such properties were observed for trimipramine [94–96] or iprindole [97]. Doxepin [98–100] and desipramine [101, 102] have also demonstrated milder REM suppressing effects.

Monoamine oxidases exist in two subtypes, A and B. Both forms are inhibited by the original irreversible monoamine oxidase inhibitors (MAOIs) such as phenelzine, isocarboxasid, and tranylcypromine.

Monoamine oxidase-A preferentially metabolizes NA and 5-HT and is inhibited by moclobemide, befloxatone, and clorgyline while both MAO-A and MAO-B metabolize dopamine (DA). Monoamine oxidase inhibitors are capable of virtually abolishing REM sleep in animals and humans [103–105]. As for TCAs, the initial large REM suppression persists for weeks and is followed by a rebound after withdrawal. This EEG sleep profile has been demonstrated in depressed patients for the non-selective phenelzine [106–109] and tranylcypromine [110] as well as for the type A MAOI clorgyline [105] and seems to be somewhat less marked with the reversible type A MAOI moclobemide [111–113] and toloxatone [114]. Interestingly, the REM-suppressant effects of phenelzine are reversed after the administration of a tryptophan-free amino acid drink [115].

Selective monoamine reuptake inhibitors

Healthy volunteer studies have clearly demonstrated that selective serotonin reuptake inhibitors (SSRIs) such as zimelidine, paroxetine, fluoxetine, fluvoxamine, and citalopram increase REM latency and decrease REM sleep [116–119]. In major depression, REM-suppressant effects of a single or repeated administration of zimelidine, citalopram, fluvoxamine, fluoxetine, and paroxetine have been confirmed [6, 102, 120–122]. A sustained REM sleep suppression was found after 6 to 12 weeks of treatment with fluoxetine, paroxetine, and sertraline but not following 12 weeks of fluvoxamine administration [123–126]. Fluoxetine has been shown to increase REM density in some studies, a finding that may relate to its paradoxical enhancing effect on REM density in depressive patients [127–129]. Studies investigating withdrawal effects of SSRIs demonstrated a REM sleep rebound about one to two days after paroxetine withdrawal [122], four to twelve days after fluoxetine withdrawal [130], and six days after citalopram withdrawal [121].

Selective noradrenalin reuptake inhibitors (SNRIs) induce similar REM sleep suppressant effects to SSRIs. This indicates that inhibiting at least one of the transporters of the two monoamines implicated in REM sleep regulation is a sufficient condition to lower REM sleep propensity. Accordingly, in healthy subjects, oxaprotiline, maprotiline, and viloxazine decreased REM sleep time and prolonged REM sleep latency [116, 131, 132]. The same picture was observed in major depressed patients with oxaprotiline and reboxetine [132, 133].

Selective multiple reuptake inhibitors

Selective multiple reuptake inhibitors combine two or more reuptake blocking properties. Sleep effects of selective triple monoamine reuptake inhibitors that are currently being developed for depression have, to our knowledge, not been published yet. Dual NA/5-HT reuptake blockers such as venlafaxine, milnacipran, and duloxetine have all shown potent REM sleep suppression effects both in healthy subjects [134, 135] and in major depressed patients [136–138]. The two dual NA/DA reuptake blockers bupropion and nomifensine differ from dual NA/5-HT reuptake blockers in terms of REM sleep effects. Bupropion was first reported to shorten REM latency and to increase REM sleep time in depressed patients [139]. Two subsequent studies in depressed patients did not replicate the finding and show that bupropion does not affect REM sleep [140, 141]. There is only one human sleep EEG study with nomifensine, which shows that the drug decreases REM sleep time in healthy subjects [142]. However, animal studies indicate that the REM sleep effect could be dose dependent, since lower doses of nomifensine promote REM sleep [143] whereas higher doses inhibit REM sleep [144].

Other antidepressant drugs

Trazodone and nefazodone share the ability to antagonize $5-HT_{2A}$ and $5-HT_{2C}$ receptors and to weakly inhibit 5-HT uptake. Nefazodone is also a weak NA reuptake inhibitor and trazodone antagonizes H_1 histaminergic receptors as well. Furthermore, the two drugs are thought to potentiate DA and NA transmission through their $5-HT_{2A/C}$ blocking properties [145]. Trazodone-induced alterations of REM sleep are inconsistent. Some studies in healthy subjects and in different clinical samples have shown evidence of REM sleep suppression [146–151], others were negative [152–155] and one study in depressive insomnia even evidenced REM-promoting effects [156]. Nefazodone was the first antidepressant drug reported to promote REM sleep [157]. This finding was replicated in healthy volunteers [150], in major depressive patients [158], and in primary insomniacs [159], but in most studies no effects of nefazodone on REM sleep could be evidenced [125, 160–165].

Mianserin and mirtazapine are tetracyclic compounds, devoided of monoamine reuptake abilities but having antagonist properties at a variety of monoamine receptors, including $5-HT_{2A/C}$ and $5-HT_3$ serotonergic receptors, α_2 adrenergic receptors and H_1 histaminergic receptors. In addition, unlike mirtazapine, mianserin antagonises α_1 adrenergic receptors [166]. The two drugs are thought to combine the $5-HT_{2A/C}$ effects of nefazodone and trazodone on NA, 5-HT, and DA transmission with the relief of α_2 presynaptic inhibitory influence on NA and 5-HT terminals [145]. Studies in healthy volunteers [167–169] and in major depressed patients [170] demonstrated a weak REM suppressant potency for mianserin, whereas reports on the effects of mirtazapine were contradictory. In healthy volunteers mirtazapine did not influence REM sleep parameters [171, 172] except for a prolongation of REM sleep latency in one study [171]. In depressed patients no REM sleep effect could be evidenced [173, 174] apart from a prolongation of REM sleep latency in one study [175] and an increase of REM sleep time in another one [176].

Agomelatine is a novel antidepressant drug that combines $5-HT_{2C}$ antagonism properties with agonist actions at melatonin receptors (MT1 and MT2). In healthy volunteers, agomelatine has been shown to increase REM sleep propensity, particularly during the first REM episode [177] whereas a study in major depressive disorder could not evidence any REM sleep effect of the compound [178]. Tianeptine is an antidepressant drug that enhances serotonin uptake and does not affect REM sleep parameters in healthy volunteers [179, 180] or in depressed patients [181, 182].

Pathophysiological mechanisms

The vast majority of sleep EEG studies investigating the effects of antidepressant drugs indicate that these drugs inhibit REM sleep. This is hardly surprising since, until recently, antidepressant drugs were developed in the frame of the monoaminergic hypothesis of depression, i.e., on the assumption that antidepressants are acting on abnormal brain monoaminergic systems in order to normalize their function. Accordingly, currently marketed antidepressant drugs are designed to facilitate at least one of the two neurotransmission systems supposed to be implicated in major depression, i.e., 5-HT and NA. Since there is mounting evidence to indicate that REM sleep generating neurons are under the influence of inhibitory NA and 5-HT input [9–11, 71], it is no wonder that drugs increasing 5-HT and NA transmission suppress REM sleep. Lack of REM-suppressant effect could indicate inefficient boost of 5-HT or NA transmission at the level of REM sleep generating neurons. It may relate to an insufficient *in situ* drug concentration or to an ineffective mechanism of action. The latter suggestion probably accounts for the doubtful (or the lack of) REM sleep suppression observed with trimipramine, iprindole, nefazodone, trazodone, mianserin, mirtazapine, agomelatine, and tianeptine. Alternatively, the 5-HT/NA mediated REM suppression is confounded by opposite drug effects on the REM sleep-regulating system. For instance, some recent evidence suggests that the DA system is implicated in REM sleep generation [183–185]. In this context, the atypical REM sleep effect of NA/5-HT reuptake blockers (bupropion and nomifensine) could result from a balance between DA-promoting influence and NA-inhibiting influence.

Effects of antidepressant drugs on NREM sleep

Since both hyperarousal and process S deficiency could account for the sleep continuity disturbances encountered in major depression, antidepressant drugs should reduce nocturnal wakefulness and increase duration of total sleep time. As antidepressants shorten REM sleep time, their effects on sleep continuity are generally linked to the way they affect NREM sleep (Table 18.1). Qualitative NREM sleep differences must to be taken into account, i.e., whether the drug enhances stage 1 or stage 2 sleep or deeper sleep stages (SWS, comprising stages 3 and 4). Besides enhancing sleep depth, increasing SWA during the first NREM period could be of particular therapeutic importance; for instance, it has been shown that the delta sleep ratio (i.e., the ratio of SWA in the first NREM period to that in the second NREM period) increased after antidepressant treatment [126, 186]. Notwithstanding, the effects of antidepressants on non-REM sleep variables are much less consistent than their effects on REM sleep. Quantitative EEG methods aimed at defining non-REM sleep

microarchitecture, such as period amplitude analysis and power spectral analysis, could represent more accurate tools to investigate the clinical significance of drug-induced non-REM sleep alterations. Accordingly, the few studies that used these techniques to characterize an antidepressant molecule are systematically discussed in the following sections.

Classical antidepressants: tricyclic antidepressants and monoamine oxidase inhibitors

Tricyclic antidepressants have various antagonism profiles at serotoninergic ($5\text{-}HT_{2A/C}$), muscarinic (M_1, M_3), histaminergic (H_1), and adrenergic (α_1) receptors that explain their different effects on NREM sleep propensity. Blockade of most of these receptors has NREM sleep-promoting properties since they control the post-synaptic effect of the major wake-promoting neurotransmitter systems. Tricyclic antidepressants, particularly tertiary amines such as amitriptyline and trimipramine, have been shown to increase sleep continuity in healthy volunteers with [83] or without [96] concomitant increase in SWS. In depressed patients, TCAs known as sedatives (trimipramine, doxepin, amitriptyline) also increase NREM sleep [95, 96, 99, 187] whereas imipramine [95] and nortriptyline [93] do not influence sleep continuity. Desipramine has been shown to disrupt sleep in healthy subjects [135] but to improve sleep continuity measures in depressed patients [102]. Regarding SWS, some TCAs have been reported to increase it, others to decrease it or to leave it unchanged either in healthy volunteers or in depressed patients. For instance, amitriptyline increases SWS in normal controls [83] but not in depressed subjects [87]. In major depression, imipramine was shown to decrease SWS [89, 95], whereas a SWS increase was observed with doxepin [98].

Electroencephalogram spectral analyses of the NREM sleep effects of TCAs indicate that acute administration of amitriptyline, clomipramine, imipramine, or nortriptyline increases SWA in the first non-REM period, i.e., it increased the delta-sleep ratio [90, 188, 189]. This redistribution of delta waves in the first part of the night was observed without an increase in the total amount of SWS throughout the night. It remains essentially unchanged thereafter, even as long as three years into maintenance treatment [189, 190].

Non-selective MAOIs, such as phenelzine and tranylcypromine, tend to impair sleep continuity of major depressed patients without producing consistent changes in SWS [107, 108, 110]. Moclobemide was shown to improve sleep continuity by decreasing awakenings in one study [111] but these findings were not replicated [113]. In the two studies, time spent in SWS appears to be unchanged by the treatment.

Selective monoamine reuptake inhibitors

Selective monoamine reuptake inhibitors generally exhibit alerting effects (i.e., tend to enhance vigilance/arousal and therefore to disturb sleep initiation and maintenance) on sleep continuity measures either in healthy controls or in depressed subjects. In healthy subjects, SSRIs like zimelidine, fluoxetine, paroxetine, fluvoxamine, and citalopram reduce total sleep time and sleep efficiency and increase wakefulness [116–119, 130, 160]. Impairment of sleep continuity has also been observed in depressed patients during acute or chronic (up to six weeks) treatment with zimelidine [120], fluvoxamine [102, 124], fluoxetine [123, 129], and paroxetine [122, 125]. A different sleep continuity profile for sertraline seems to emerge from a twelve-week study in depression [126] since only an effect on sleep initiation (i.e., a prolonged sleep onset latency) could be evidenced, the drug having no influence on sleep maintenance parameters (sleep efficiency, total sleep time, and wake after sleep onset). It has to be stressed that, as a general rule, the alerting effects of SSRIs are somewhat more marked after acute drug administration in healthy volunteer studies than after prolonged drug administration in depressed patients. For instance, the alerting effect of citalopram observed in a three-day administration study in healthy volunteer [119] was not evidenced in a five-week study in major depressed patients [121]. Another example is the prolonged (twelve weeks) fluvoxamine administration study in major depressed patients, which showed that sleep continuity disturbances were worsened after acute and subchronic (three weeks) administration but returned to their pretreatment baseline level at week twelve [124]. These results contrast with those obtained with prolonged administration of fluoxetine in depressed patients (ten weeks) or healthy subjects (three weeks) showing

a sustained sleep disruption effect of the drug on total sleep time and sleep efficiency [129–130].

No effects on SWS duration were evidenced for SSRIs either in normal volunteers [116–119, 130, 160] or in depressed patients [103, 120–126], the sole exception being a ten-week study with fluoxetine where SWS was found decreased [129]. Four studies investigated the effects of SSRIs on NREM quantitative EEG and brought somewhat contradictory results. In healthy controls, four weeks of paroxetine administration did not alter any of the EEG spectral power values, but significantly increased NREM delta to theta and delta to beta power correlations [191]. In another sample of healthy subjects [130], the single administration of fluoxetine 60 mg did not affect spectral EEG measurement. However the three-week administration of fluoxetine 40 mg induced a general increase of power values for the 12–32 Hz spectrum range (that includes sigma and beta bands) with a maximum of effect at the highest frequency (32 Hz). Interestingly all-night NREM SWA was only found slightly decreased but the delta sleep ratio increased. Of particular note is the persistent effect of fluoxetine on delta sleep ratio that was uncorrelated to the plasma drug concentration. Indeed the increase in delta ratio was prolonged up to the last sleep EEG recording after drug discontinuation (i.e., twelve days post-drug) and the authors suggest that delta sleep ratio could reflect secondary drug-induced brain adaptive processes [130]. Two spectral EEG studies were performed in depressed patients. The first study indicates that five weeks of citalopram treatment significantly decreases NREM power in the 8–9 Hz range (lower alpha waves) without changing the power of the delta frequency range [192]. The other study shows that a twelve-week administration of sertraline increases the delta sleep ratio of major depressed patients [126].

The effects of SNRIs on NREM sleep have been less reported than those observed with SSRIs although they seem comparable. In healthy subjects, maprotiline increased the duration of stage 2 sleep [116] and viloxazine has been shown to decrease both sleep continuity and SWS duration [131]. In major depressed patients, reboxetine increases intermittent wakefulness and sleep stage 2 and decreases sleep efficiency [133], and oxaprotiline produced a non-significant deterioration in sleep continuity without altering SWS [132]. A spectral EEG analysis of all-night NREM sleep did not reveal any significant effect of reboxetine in major depressed patients [133].

Selective multiple reuptake inhibitors

Discrepant sleep-promoting properties of NA/5-HT reuptake blockers have been reported. Milnacipran seems to have NREM-promoting properties. A four-week treatment in depressed patients shortened sleep onset latencies and increased total sleep time (through an increase of stage 2 sleep) and sleep efficiency [137]. Short-term duloxetine effects on NREM sleep, i.e., roughly after a one-week administration, seem to be dose related. In healthy volunteers, a 120 mg/day administration increases wake after sleep onset and stage 2 sleep and decreases SWS and sleep efficiency, whereas a 80 mg/day dose increased sleep efficiency [135]. In depressed patients administration of duloxetine 60 mg/day increases stage 3 sleep and tends to decrease the number of intrasleep awakenings [138]. Venlafaxine shows clear-cut alerting effects. In healthy subjects, it increases wake time and sleep stage 1 at the expense of stages 2 and 3 indicating sleep lightening [134]. These results are in accordance with a study in depressed patients showing that a five-week treatment with venlafaxine increases wake after sleep onset [136]. Although SWS duration was not significantly affected, all-night NREM spectral EEG analyses indicate that the drug decreased lower-frequency activities (delta to theta range) whereas fast beta activities were increased, further suggesting that venlafaxine lightens sleep intensity. As with other antidepressants, venlafaxine was found to increase the delta sleep ratio.

The only human sleep EEG study with nomifensine indicates that the dual NA/DA reuptake blocker increases wakefulness [142]. Bupropion does not impair sleep continuity parameters in major depressive patients but results on NREM sleep structure were divergent. Slow-wave sleep was found increased at the expense of stage 2 [140], unchanged [141], or decreased [139]. On basis of the findings by Monti *et al.* [193], who showed that a low dose of the D_2 receptor agonist apomorphine increased SWS in rats, while higher doses produced the opposite effect, it was suggested [140] that the different SWS responses to bupropion could relate to the different dosage used in the three studies (mean doses were 428 mg/day [139], 352 mg/day [141], and 290 mg/day [140]).

Other antidepressant drugs

As for TCAs, drugs discussed in this section have various antagonism profiles at serotoninergic (5-HT$_{2A/C}$), histaminergic (H$_1$), and adrenergic (α_1) receptors that may explain their different effects on NREM sleep propensity. The NREM sleep promoting effect of trazodone, a 5-HT$_{2A/C}$ and H$_1$ antagonist, is well documented in healthy subjects [146, 150, 153] and in various clinical samples including major depressed patients [147, 148, 151, 152, 154, 156]. Slow-wave sleep is generally found increased [146, 151, 153, 155, 156] and/or wakefulness decreased [146, 150, 154–156]. Spectral EEG analyses of all-night NREM sleep of depressed patients revealed that a five-week treatment with trazodone decreases EEG power in the 13 to 14 Hz (sigma) range without changing the power of the delta frequency range [149]. The NREM sleep-promoting effect of nefazodone, a 5-HT$_{2A/C}$ antagonist devoided of H$_1$ antagonist properties, is less well demonstrated. The three healthy volunteer studies did not document any effect of nefazodone on NREM sleep nor on sleep continuity parameters [150, 160–161]. However, four studies in depressed patients indicated that a six- to eight-week administration of nefazodone improved sleep continuity by decreasing sleep onset latency [162, 165] and wakefulness [125, 158], and by increasing total sleep time [125] and sleep efficiency [125, 158, 162, 165]. One of these four studies showed that when administration of nefazodone is prolonged up to twelve weeks, sleep continuity parameters return to their baseline pretreatment level [125]. The two twelve-week studies on the effects of nefazodone 400 to 600 mg/day in post-traumatic stress disorder brought conflicting results: one study did not evidence any change in NREM sleep and sleep continuity [163], the other showed increased total sleep time and improved sleep efficiency [164]. The latter study investigated NREM sleep microarchitecture by period amplitude analyses and showed that nefazodone increased delta sleep. Finally, an open pilot study in primary insomniacs reported that a two-week administration of nefazodone (400 mg) increases sleep onset latency and sleep stage 2 and decreases SWS [159].

Studies in healthy subjects [167–169] and depressed patients [170] investigating the effects of mianserin, a 5-HT$_{2A/C}$, H$_1$, and α_1 antagonist, on NREM sleep indicate that the drug promotes stage 2 [167, 170] or SWS [168] and increases total sleep time and sleep efficiency [170]. A very consistent NREM sleep promoting profile has been documented for mirtazapine, a 5-HT$_{2A/C}$ and H$_1$ antagonist devoided of α_1 antagonist properties, either in healthy subjects [171, 172] or in major depressed patients [173–176]. In all but one study [173] the drug increases SWS and generally improves sleep efficiency [172–174, 176] by decreasing wakefulness [172–175] and/or by increasing total sleep time [174, 176]. Two studies indicate that mirtazapine shortens sleep onset latency [173, 176]. One study confirmed that mirtazapine increased sleep depth with NREM spectral EEG analyses showing that a four-week administration of 15 to 45 mg/day of mirtazapine increased EEG power in a large low-frequency range (0.78–2.3 Hz and 3.9–10.9 Hz) that corresponds to slow delta, theta, and alpha activities. Interestingly, the study also demonstrated that the acute administration of mirtazapine (15 mg) did not influence sleep EEG spectral parameters [174].

The acute administration of agomelatine (which has 5-HT$_{2C}$ antagonism properties) in healthy volunteers (5 or 100 mg, five hours before bedtime) did not affect NREM sleep nor NREM EEG power densities [177] but a repeated administration (25 mg at 20:00 hours during five weeks) in major depressed patients improved sleep efficiency, decreased wake after sleep onset, and increased SWS. A spectral analysis of delta power shows an increased of the delta sleep ratio [178]. The latter finding indicates that delta sleep ratio increase is not necessarily linked to the REM suppressant effect of a drug that prolonged the duration of the first NREM period. Studies with tianeptine on healthy volunteers or on depressed patients did not evidence any NREM sleep effect [179–182].

Pathophysiological mechanisms

In summary, the reports on the effects of antidepressants on NREM sleep and sleep continuity are inconsistent. Non-REM sleep promoting effects and concomitant improvement of sleep maintenance are observed for most TCAs and some non-TCA antidepressants such as trazodone, nefazodone, mianserin, and mirtazapine, but on the contrary, MAOIs, SSRIs, SNRIs, and double reuptake inhibitors are rather sleep-disrupting drugs. These differences probably relate to inhibition or stimulation of key postsynaptic receptors of the monoaminergic wake-promoting system, i.e., serotonergic 5-HT$_{2A/C}$ receptors, histaminergic H$_1$ receptors, and adrenergic α_1 receptors. Indeed, monoaminergic transmission is largely implicated in the wake-promoting system and it has been shown that neuronal activities of 5-HT neurons in the dorsal raphe nuclei, NA neurons in the locus coeruleus, and histaminergic neurons in the posterior hypothalamus are inversely correlated to the degree of EEG synchronization. High neuronal activities are observed during wakefulness and a high synchronized (fast) EEG activity, and the progressive reduction of neuronal activities observed during NREM sleep is related to the progressive dominance of synchronized (slow) EEG activities [9–12].

Non-REM sleep promoting antidepressants improve sleep maintenance rather than sleep initiation, but studies were not statistically designed in terms of sample size to demonstrate such an effect. Therefore it is worth mentioning the improvement of sleep onset latency observed in major depression studies with doxepin [89], milnacipran [137], nefazodone [162, 165], and mirtazapine [171, 173]. Slow-wave sleep promoting effects of antidepressant drugs are largely attributable to blockade of the three aminergic receptors. The roles of H$_1$ and of α_1 are, however, less well established. Studies have shown that decreasing histaminergic function through the stimulation of H$_3$ autoreceptor increases SWS [194], an effect that seems mediated by H$_1$ receptors [195, 196]. In the same way, α_1 antagonists have shown SWS-promoting effects in the rat [197, 198]. In contrast, the role of 5-HT$_2$ receptors is well known since it was shown that ritanserin, a potent 5-HT$_{2A/C}$ antagonist, produces large dose-dependent increases in SWS in healthy controls [199–201] and in depressed patients [202]. Although a series of 5-HT$_{2A}$ antagonists or inverse agonists are currently being developed as hypnotic drugs for sleep maintenance difficulties [203], knockout studies in mice suggest that both 5-HT$_{2A}$ and 5-HT$_{2C}$ are implicated in SWS regulation [204]. Other arguments for a role of 5-HT$_{2C}$ receptors come from sleep studies with meta-chlorophenylpiperazine (mCPP) a 5-HT$_{2C}$ agonist that dose-dependently lowers SWS in healthy subjects [205], and with olanzapine, an antipsychotic drug with mixed 5-HT$_{2A/C}$ antagonistic properties, whose SWS promoting effect is linked to an allelic variant of the 5-HT$_{2C}$ receptor gene [206]. More generally, receptor $5\text{-HT}_{2A/C}$ gene polymorphisms could account for SWS responses obtained with drugs having $5\text{-HT}_{2A/C}$ blocking properties, including antidepressants. For instance, the SWS response to mirtazapine has recently been shown to be related to a 5-HT_{2A} polymorphism [207].

Studies investigating sleep microarchitecture are difficult to compare since different methodologies were used to record and analyze the data. The Pittsburgh group consistently reported that an increased delta sleep ratio characterizes the effects of antidepressant drugs [90, 188–190]. These findings were initially demonstrated in major depressed patients with TCAs. They have now been replicated in healthy subjects [130] and with non-TCA drugs with various mechanisms of action such as fluoxetine [130], sertraline [126], venlafaxine [136], and agomelatine [178]. The results of Feige *et al.* [130], showing that the increase of the delta sleep ratio is still present twelve days after drug discontinuation, suggest that it could reflect drug-induced brain plasticity mechanisms. Other quantitative sleep EEG studies reported earlier did not directly address the issue of the delta-shift hypothesis. One may summarize results obtained with spectral analyses as follows: NREM sleep promoting antidepressants such as mirtazapine and trazodone tend to increase slow-frequency activities [174] or to decrease fast-frequency activities [149] whereas, on the contrary, antidepressant drugs disrupting NREM such as fluoxetine, citalopram, or venlafaxine tend to lower slow-frequency activities [136, 192] and/or to increase fast-frequency activities [130, 136]. These findings are physiological correlates of the sedative versus alerting effects of these drugs.

Clinical significance

Clinical significance of antidepressant-induced alterations of the sleep EEG are manifold. First, the knowledge of the sleep EEG profile of an antidepressant drug is useful to the working out of major depression treatment strategies. Drugs having an NREM sleep-promoting profile tend to improve sleep continuity and are more helpful in depression with insomnia symptoms; however, it has to be kept in mind that studies investigating the effects of prolonged administration of antidepressant drugs in major depression showed that, at the end of the treatment (i.e., up to 12 weeks), NREM-promoting antidepressants such as nefazodone have only modest effects on

sleep continuity parameters [125] whereas the alerting effects of antidepressant drugs such as fluvoxamine are found attenuated [124].

Second, the amount of REM sleep suppression induced by an antidepressant drug could relate to its ability to facilitate 5-HT or NA neurotransmission and, eventually, to its clinical efficacy. Lack of REM suppressant effect could indicate inefficient boost of 5-HT or NA transmission. Since antidepressant drugs are supposed to act on abnormal brain 5-HT and/or NA systems in order to normalize their function, the amount of REM suppression induced by an antidepressant could more or less relate to its clinical efficacy. This view is supported by a recent meta-analytic study that compared effect sizes of published and non-published clinical trials regarding the 12 more recently launched antidepressant drugs. Results indicate that the three drugs with weak (mirtazapine) or no (bupropion and nefazodone) REM suppressant effects are among the four drugs for which the effect size has been mostly inflated by ignoring non-published trials. When considering published and non-published trials together, the effect sizes of bupropion (0.17) and nefazodone (0.26) were among the three lowest observed [208].

Third, sleep EEG alterations and particularly evidence of REM sleep disinhibition could indicate whether a depressed patient could respond to an antidepressant drug. Since REM sleep-generating neurons are under the inhibitory influence of NA and 5-HT inputs [9–11, 71], one may reasonably speculate that evidence of REM sleep disinhibition is a biological endophenotype reflecting an antidepressant-responsive condition. Accordingly several studies found a predictive value of a shortened REM latency or an increased REM density regarding response to an antidepressant treatment [209–211] or non-response to a non-pharmacological treatment [6–8, 212, 213]. Studies investigating the acute effect of antidepressant drugs on REM latency have less predictive value since the magnitude of the overall effect of antidepressant drug on this parameter overwhelms individual variability leading to a "ceiling" effect [140]. Delta sleep ratio, as discussed below, or REM density could be more relevant biomarkers of drug response, as shown by a study describing predictive value of REM density in patients taking either paroxetine or tianeptine [182].

Fourth, sleep EEG is a valuable tool to investigate the mechanism of action of antidepressant drugs and to further explore relationships between mood regulation and sleep regulation. At first glance, the efficacy of antidepressant drugs seems to be unrelated to their effects on sleep EEG. Studies showing that imipramine and trimipramine [95] or fluoxetine and nefazodone [158] have comparable efficacy despite different sleep EEG profile in terms of REM suppression and NREM promotion apparently indicate that multiple mechanisms are operating in the effects of antidepressant drugs. As discussed above, there are some arguments for the idea that drugs without clear-cut REM suppressant effect are less effective antidepressants in patients having evidence of REM sleep disinhibition, but this hypothesis has never been tested. Another point is whether NREM-promoting antidepressants are more effective in patients having severe insomnia symptoms. There are some reports that partially answer these issues. Studies with phenelzine, a drug that dramatically suppresses REM sleep, show that SWA during sleep was not affected by the drug [108]. This indicates that NREM sleep-regulating mechanisms are not related to the antidepressant efficacy of phenelzine. Another study showed that NREM EEG sigma and alpha activities predict clinical response to paroxetine and tianeptine in male but not in female depressed subjects [182]. This suggests that gender has to be taken into account when studying the effects of antidepressant drugs on quantitative EEG.

Fifth, sleep EEG is a valuable tool for the development of new antidepressant drugs and many pharmaceutical companies have been using it during the last four decades [214]. Moreover, evidence that REM sleep disinhibition is also observed in animal models of depression has led some authors to suggest that the REM disinhibition endophenotype could be a useful biomarker in translational medicine [215–217]. Correlations between pharmacokinetic data and sleep parameters as pharmacodynamic endpoints indicate that the most reliable markers of fluoxetine activity were REM latency and NREM EEG power densities in the 12 to 24 Hz frequency range (i.e., sigma and slow beta activities) [130]. These results were obtained after repeated administration and it is not clear if they can be generalized to acute administration or to other antidepressant drugs, particularly to those having an NREM sleep-promoting profile. The present review suggests that the delta sleep ratio could be a useful marker of drug activity since it has been shown to increase with various types of antidepressant drugs in depressed patients as well as in healthy volunteers [126, 130, 136, 178]. Further studies are needed in

order to delineate if delta sleep ratio is a class-specific marker or not. Finally, it has to be emphasized that, until now, marketed antidepressant drugs were designed to facilitate monoaminergic transmission. Whether the REM disinhibition phenotype remains valid for the development of antidepressant drugs that are not acting through the monoaminergic system is still an unanswered query.

Conclusions

To sum up, the studies reviewed in the present chapter could not provide clear evidence of a common and unique pharmaco–sleep EEG profile of antidepressant drugs that could account for their clinical efficacy in the treatment of major depression. Rather, the observed drug alteration in sleep EEG merely reflects the particular psychopharmacological properties of the molecule, i.e., its particular effects on serotonergic, noradrenergic, dopaminergic, or cholinergic transmission. Whether this influence of antidepressant drugs on sleep is related to clinical changes occurring in depressive patients during treatment is still unclear. The emergence of the concept of an antidepressant responsive REM sleep disinhibition endophenotype is discussed. More fundamental research on pharmaco–sleep EEG in terms of physiological processes is needed to interpret the relevance of antidepressant effects on sleep in major depression.

References

1. Wu JC, Bunney WE. The biological basis of an antidepressant response to sleep deprivation and relapse: review and hypothesis. *Am J Psychiatry.* 1990;**147**:14–21.

2. Wehr TA. Sleep-loss as a possible mediator of diverse causes of mania. *Br J Psychiatry.* 1991;**159**:576–8.

3. Barbini B, Bertelli S, Colombo C, *et al.* Sleep loss, a possible factor in augmenting manic episode. *Psychiatry Res.* 1996;**65**:121–5.

4. Benca R. Mood disorders. In: Kryger MH, Roth T, Dement WC, eds. *Principles and Practice of Sleep Medicine*, 4th edn. (Saunders, Philadelphia: Elsevier, 2005; 1311–26).

5. Staner L, Luthringer R, Le Bon O. Sleep disturbances in affective disorders. In: Pandi-Perumal SR, Monti JM, eds. *Clinical Pharmacology of Sleep.* (Basel: Birkhauser, 2006; 101–24).

6. Heiligenstein JH, Faries DE, Rush AJ, *et al.* Latency to rapid eye movement sleep as a predictor of treatment

response to fluoxetine and placebo in nonpsychotic depressed outpatients. *Psychiatry Res.* 1994;**52**:327–39.

7. Thase ME, Simons AD, Reynolds CF III. Abnormal electroencephalographic sleep profiles in major depression. Association with response to cognitive behavior therapy. *Arch Gen Psychiatry.* 1996;**53**:99–108.

8. Buysse DJ, Tu XM, Cherry CR *et al.* Pretreatment REM sleep and subjective sleep quality distinguish depressed psychotherapy remitters and nonremitters. *Biol Psychiatry.* 1999;**45**:205–13.

9. Saper CB, Scammell TE, Lu J. Hypothalamic regulation of sleep and circadian rhythms. *Nature.* 2005;**437**:1257–63.

10. Jones BE. From waking to sleeping: neuronal and chemical substrates. *Trends Pharmacol Sci.* 2005;**26**:578–86.

11. Datta S, Maclean RR. Neurobiological mechanisms for the regulation of mammalian sleep-wake behavior: reinterpretation of historical evidence and inclusion of contemporary cellular and molecular evidence. *Neurosci Biobehav Rev.* 2007;**31**:775–824.

12. Destexhe A, Hughes SW, Rudolph M, Crunelli V. Are corticothalamic 'up' states fragments of wakefulness? *Trends Neurosci.* 2007;**30**:334–42.

13. American Psychiatric Association (APA). *Diagnostic and Statistical Manual of Mental Disorder*, 4th edn. (Washington, DC: APA, 1994).

14. Riemann D, Berger M, Voderholzer U. Sleep and depression – results from psychobiological studies: an overview. *Biol Psychol.* 2001;**57**:67–103.

15. Armitage R, Cole D, Suppes T, Ozcan ME. Effects of clozapine on sleep in bipolar and schizoaffective disorder. *Progr Neuropsychopharm Biol Psychiatry.* 2004;**28**:1065–70.

16. Reynolds CF III, Kupfer DJ. Sleep research in affective illness: State of the art circa 1987. *Sleep.* 1987;**10**:199–215.

17. Buysse DJ, Kupfer DJ: Diagnostic and research applications of electroencephalographic sleep studies in depression: conceptual and methodological issues. *J Nerv Ment Dis.* 1990;**178**:405–14.

18. Kupfer DJ. REM latency: a psychobiological marker for primary depressive disease. *Biol Psychiatry.* 1976;**11**:159–74.

19. Benca RM, Obermeyer WH, Thisted RA, *et al.* Sleep and psychiatric disorders. A meta-analysis. *Arch Gen Psychiatry.* 1992;**49**:651–68.

20. Katz JL, Kuperberg A, Pollack CP, *et al.* Is there a relationship between eating disorder and affective disorder? New evidence from sleep recordings. *Am J Psychiatry.* 1984;**141**:753–9.

21. Moeller FG, Gillin JC, Irwin M, *et al.* A comparison of sleep EEGs in patients with primary major depression and major depression secondary to alcoholism. *J Affect Disord.* 1993;**27**:39–42.

22. Insel TR, Gillin JC, Moore A, *et al.* The sleep of patients with obsessive-compulsive disorder. *Arch Gen Psychiatry.* 1982;**39**:1372–7.

23. Uhde TW, Roy-Byrne P, Gillin JC, *et al.* The sleep of patients with panic disorder. A preliminary report. *Psychiatry Res.* 1984;**12**:251–9.

24. Rosa RR, Bonnet MH, Kramer M. The relationship of sleep and anxiety in anxious subjects. *Biol Psychol.* 1983;**16**:119–26.

25. Reynolds CF III, Soloff PH, Kupfer DJ, *et al.* Depression in borderline patients: a prospective EEG sleep study. *Psychiatry Res.* 1985;**14**:1–15.

26. Hubain P, Van Veeren C, Staner L, *et al.* Neuroendocrine and sleep variables in major depressed inpatients: role of severity. *Psychiatry Res.* 1996;**63**:83–92.

27. Fossion P, Staner L, Dramaix M, *et al.* Does sleep EEG data distinguish between UP, BPI or BPII major depressions? An age and gender controlled study. *J Affect Disord.* 1998;**49**:181–7.

28. Stefos G, Staner L, Kerkhofs M, *et al.* Shortened REM latency as a psychobiologic marker for psychotic depression? An age, gender and polarity controlled study. *Biol Psychiatry.* 1998;**44**:1314–20.

29. Ho AP, Gillin JC, Buchsbaum MS, *et al.* Brain glucose metabolism during non-rapid eye movement sleep in major depression. A positron emission tomography study. *Arch Gen Psychiatry.* 1996;**53**:645–52.

30. Germain A, Nofzinger EA, Kupfer DJ, Buysse DJ. Neurobiology of non-REM sleep in depression: further evidence for hypofrontality and thalamic dysregulation. *Am J Psychiatry.* 2004;**161**:1856–63.

31. Nofzinger EA, Price JC, Meltzer CC, *et al.* Toward a neurobiology of dysfunctional arousal in depression: the relationship between beta EEG power and regional cerebral glucose metabolism during NREM sleep. *Psychiatry Res Neuroimaging.* 2000;**98**:71–91.

32. Holsboer F. The corticosteroid receptor hypothesis of depression. *Neuropsychopharmacology.* 2000;**23**:477–501.

33. Müller MB, Wurst W. Getting closer to affective disorders: the role of the CRH receptor system. *Trends Mol Med.* 2004;**10**:409–15.

34. Arango V, Underwood MD, Mann JJ. Fewer pigmented locus coeruleus neurons in suicide victims: preliminary results. *Biol Psychiatry.* 1996;**39**:112–20.

35. Bissette G, Klimek V, Pan J, *et al.* Elevated concentrations of CRF in the locus coeruleus of

depressed subjects. *Neuropsychopharmacology.* 2003;**28**:1328–35.

36. Klimek V, Stockmeier C, Overholser J, *et al.* Reduced levels of norepinephrine transporters in the locus coeruleus in major depression. *J Neurosci.* 1997;**17**:8451–8.

37. Baumann B, Danos P, Diekman S, *et al.* Tyrosine hydroxylase immunoreactivity in the locus coeruleus is reduced in depressed non-suicidal patients but normal in depressed suicide patients. *Eur Arch Psychiatry Clin Neurosci.* 1999;**249**:212–19.

38. Agelink MW, Klimke A, Cordes J, *et al.* A functional-structural model to understand cardiac autonomic nervous system (ANS) dysregulation in affective illness and to elucidate the ANS effects of antidepressive treatment. *Eur J Med Res.* 2004;**9**:37–50.

39. Gorman JM, Sloan RP. Heart rate variability in depressive and anxiety disorders. *Am Heart J.* 2000; **140** (4 Suppl):77–83.

40. Hubain P, Staner L, Dramaix M, *et al.* The dexamethasone suppression test and sleep electroencephalogram in major depressed inpatients: a multivariate analysis. *Biol Psychiatry.* 1998;**43**:220–9.

41. Staner L, Duval F, Haba J, *et al.* Disturbances in hypothalamo pituitary adrenal and thyroid axis identify different sleep EEG patterns in major depressed patients. *J Psychiatry Res.* 2003;**37**:1–8.

42. Wong ML, Kling MA, Munson PJ, *et al.* Pronounced and sustained central hypernoradrenergic function in major depression with melancholic features: relation to hypercortisolism and corticotrophin-releasing-hormone. *Proc Natl Acad Sci USA.* 2000;**97**:325–30.

43. Ruggiero DA, Underwood MD, Rice PM, *et al.* Corticotropic-releasing hormone and serotonin interact in the human brainstem: behavioural implications. *Neuroscience.* 1999;**91**:1343–54.

44. Kirby LG, Rice KC, Valentino RJ. Effects of corticotropin-releasing factor on neuronal activity in the serotoninergic dorsal raphe nucleus. *Neuropsychopharmacology.* 2000;**22**:148–62.

45. Lopez JF, Chalmers DT, Little KY, Watson SJ. Regulation of serotonin 1a, glucocorticoid and mineralocorticoid receptor in rat and human hippocampus: implications for the neurobiology of depression. *Biol Psychiatry.* 1998;**43**:547–73.

46. Wissinski S, Meijer O, Pearce D, *et al.* Regulation of the rat serotonin-1A receptor gene by corticosteroids. *J Biol Chem.* 2000;**275**:1321–6.

47. Monti JM, Monti D. Role of the dorsal raphe nucleus serotonin 5-HT1A receptor in the regulation of sleep. *Life Sci.* 2000;**21**:1999–2012.

48. Staner L, Linker T, Toussaint M, *et al.* Effects of the selective activation of 5-HT3 receptors on sleep: a ploysomnographic study in healthy volunteers. *Eur Neuropsychopharmacol.* 2001;**11**:301–5.

49. Borbely AA, Wirz-Justice A. Sleep, sleep deprivation and depression. A hypothesis derived from a model of sleep regulation. *Hum Neurobiol.* 1982;**1**:205–10.

50. Borbely AA, Wirz-Justice A. Sleep, sleep deprivation and depression. A hypothesis derived from a model of sleep regulation. *Hum Neurobiol.* 1982;**1**:205–10.

51. Borbely AA, Tobler I, Loepfe M, *et al.* All-night spectral analysis of the sleep EEG in untreated depressives and normal controls. *Psychiatry Res.* 1984;**12**:27–33.

52. Kupfer DJ, Ulrich RF, Coble PA, *et al.* Applications of an automated REM and slow wave sleep analysis. II. Testing the assumptions of the two-process model of sleep regulation in normal and depressed subjects. *Psychiatry Res.* 1984;**13**:335–43.

53. Kupfer DJ, Frank E, Ehlers CL. EEG sleep in young depressives: first and second night effect. *Biol Psychiatry.* 1989;**25**:87–97.

54. Kupfer DJ, Frank E, Mc Eachran AB, Grochocinski VJ. Delta sleep ratio: a biological correlate of early recurrence in unipolar affective disorder. *Arch Gen Psychiatry.* 1990;**47**:1100–5.

55. Armitage R, Hoffmann RF, Trivedi M, Rush JA. Slow wave activity in NREM sleep: sex and age effects in depressed outpatients and healthy controls. *Psychiatry Res.* 2000;**95**:201–13.

56. Armitage R, Emslie GJ, Hoffmann RF, *et al.* Delta sleep EEG in depressed adolescent females and healthy controls. *J Affect Disord.* 2001;**63**:139–48.

57. Staner L, Cornette F, Maurice D, *et al.* Sleep microstructure around sleep onset differentiates major depressive insomnia from primary insomnia. *J Sleep Res.* 2003;**12**:319–30.

58. Basheer R, Strecker RE, Thakkar MM, Mc Carley RW. Adenosine and sleep–wake regulation. *Progr Neurobiol.* 2004;**73**:379–96.

59. Porkka-Heiskanen T, Strecker RE, Thakkar M, *et al.* Adenosine: a mediator of the sleep-inducing effects of prolonged wakefulness. *Science.* 1997;**276**:1265–8.

60. Berk M, Plein H, Ferreira D, Jersky B. Blunted adenosine A2a receptor function in platelets in patients with major depression. *Eur Neuropsychopharmacol.* 2001;**11**:183–6.

61. Elgun S, Keskinege A, Kumbasar H. Dipeptidyl peptidase IV and adenosine deaminase activity decrease in depression. *Psychoneuroendocrinology.* 1999;**24**:823–32.

62. Kaster MP, Rosa AO, Rosso MM, *et al*. Adenosine administration produces an antidepressant-like effect in mice: evidence for the involvement of A1 and A2A receptors. *Neurosci Lett*. 2004;**355**:21–4.

63. El Yacoubi M, Ledent C, Parmentier M, *et al*. Adenosine A2A receptor antagonists are potential antidepressants: evidence based on pharmacology and A2A receptor knockout mice. *Br J Pharmacol*. 2001;**134**:68–77.

64. Phillis JW, Wu PH. The effect of various centrally active drugs on adenosine uptake by the central nervous system. *Comp Biochem Physiol*. 1982;**72C**:179–87.

65. Phillis JW. Potentiation of the action of adenosine on cerebral cortical neurones by the tricyclic antidepressants. *Br J Pharmacol*. 1984;**83**:567–75.

66. Zahorodna A, Bijak M, Hess G. Differential effects of repeated imipramine on hippocampal responsiveness to adenosine and serotonin. *Eur Neuropsychopharmacol*. 2002;**12**:355–60.

67. Berger M, van Calker D, Riemann D. Sleep and manipulations of the sleep-wake rhythm in depression. *Acta Psychiatr Scand*. 2003;(suppl 418):83–91.

68. Castrén E, Rantamäki T. Neurotrophins in depression and antidepressant effects. *Novartis Found Symp*. 2008;**289**:43–52.

69. Duman RS, Monteggia LM. A neurotrophic model for stress-related mood disorders. *Biol Psychiatry*. 2006;**59**:1116–27.

70. Faraguna U, Vyazovskiy VV, Nelson AB, Tononi G, Cirelli C. A causal role for brain-derived neurotrophic factor in the homeostatic regulation of sleep. *J Neurosci*. 2008;**28**:4088–95.

71. Hobson JA, Pace-Schott EF, Stickgold R. Dreaming and the brain: toward a cognitive neuroscience of conscious states. In: Pace Schott EF, Solms M, Blagrove M, Harnad S, eds. *Sleep and Dreaming*. (Cambridge: Cambridge University Press, 2003; 1–50).

72. Nofzinger EA, Buysse DJ, Germain A, *et al*. Increased activation of anterior paralimbic and executive cortex from waking to rapid eye movement sleep in depression. *Arch Gen Psychiatry*. 2004;**61**:695–72.

73. Janowsky DS, El Youssef MK, Davis JM, Sekerke HJ. A cholinergic-adrenergic hypothesis of mania and depression. *Lancet*. 1972;**2**:632–5.

74. Vogel GW, Buffenstein A, Minter K, *et al*. Drug effects on REM sleep and on endogenous depression. *Neurosci Biobehav Rev*. 1990;**14**:49–63.

75. Hartmann E. Reserpine: its effect on the sleep-dream cycle in man. *Psychopharmacologia*. 1966;**9**:242.

76. Moore P, Gillin JC, Bhatti T, *et al*. Rapid tryptophan depletion, sleep electroencephalogram, and mood in men with remitted depression on serotonin reuptake inhibitors. *Arch Gen Psychiatry*. 1998;**55**:534–9.

77. Evans L, Golshan S, Kelsoe J, *et al*. Effects of rapid tryptophan depletion on sleep electroencephalogram and mood in subjects with partially remitted depression on bupropion. *Neuropsychopharmacology*. 2002;**27**:1016–26.

78. Landolt HP, Kelsoe JR, Rapaport MH, Gillin JC. Rapid tryptophan depletion reverses phenelzine-induced suppression of REM sleep. *J Sleep Res*. 2003;**12**:13–18.

79. Haynes PL, Mc Quaid JR, Kelsoe J, *et al*. Affective state and EEG sleep profile in response to rapid tryptophan depletion in recently recovered nonmedicated depressed individuals. *J Affect Disord*. 2004;**83**:253–62.

80. Pecknold JC, Luthe L. Trimipramine, anxiety, depression and sleep. *Drugs*. 1989;**38** Suppl 1:25–31.

81. Hindmarch I. Expanding the horizons of depression: beyond the monoamine hypothesis. *Hum Psychopharmacol*. 2001;**16**:203–18.

82. Nicholson AN, Pascoe PA, Turner C. Modulation of sleep by trimipramine in man. *Eur J Clin Pharmacol*. 1989;**37**:145–50.

83. Hartmann E, Cravens J. The effects of long-term administration of psychotropic drugs on human sleep. III. The effects of amitriptyline. *Psychopharmacologia*. 1974;**33**:185–202.

84. Passouant P, Cadhilac J, Billiard M. Withdrawal of the paradoxical sleep by clomipramine. An electrophysiological, histochemical and biochemical study. *Int J Neurol*. 1975;**10**:186–97.

85. Herdman JRE, Cowen PJ, Campling GM, *et al*. Effect of lofepramine on 5-HT function and sleep. *J Affect Disord*. 1993;**29**:63–72.

86. Kupfer DJ, Foster FG, Reich L, *et al*. EEG sleep changes as predictors in depression. *Am J Psychiatry*. 1976;**133**:622–6.

87. Gillin JC, Wyatt RJ, Fram D, *et al*. The relationship between changes in REM sleep and clinical improvement in depressed patients treated with amitriptyline. *Psychopharmacology*. 1978;**59**:267–72.

88. Mendlewicz J, Kempenaers C, De Martelaer V. Sleep EEG and amitriptyline treatment in depressed inpatients. *Biol Psychiatry*. 1991;**30**:691–702.

89. Hochli D, Riemann D, Zulley J, *et al*. Initial REM sleep suppression by clomipramine: a prognostic tool for treatment response in patients with major depressive disorder. *Biol Psychiatry*. 1986;**21**:1217–20.

90. Kupfer DJ, Ehlers CL, Pollock BJ, *et al*. Clomipramine and EEG sleep in depression. *Psychiatry Res*. 1989;**30**:165–80.

91. Chen CN. Sleep, depression and antidepressants. *Br J Psychiatry.* 1979;**135**:385–402.

92. Kupfer DJ, Coble P, Kane J, *et al.* Imipramine and EEG sleep in children with depressive symptoms. *Psychopharmacology.* 1979;**60**:117–23.

93. Kupfer DJ, Spiker DJ, Rossi A. *et al.* Nortriptyline and EEG sleep in depressed patients. *Biol Psychiatry.* 1982;**7**:535–46.

94. Wiegand M, Berger M, Zulley J, *et al.* The effect of trimipramine on sleep in patients with major depressive disorder. *Pharmacopsychiatry.* 1986;**19**:198–9.

95. Ware JC, Brown FW, Moorad PJ Jr., *et al.* Effects on sleep: a double-blind study comparing trimipramine to imipramine in depressed insomniac patients. *Sleep.* 1989;**12**:537–49.

96. Feuillade P, Pringuey D, Belogou JL, *et al.* Trimipramine: acute and lasting effects on sleep in healthy and major depressive subjects. *J Affect Disord.* 1992;**24**:135–46.

97. Baxter BL, Gluckman MI. Iprindole: an antidepressant which does not block REM sleep. *Nature.* 1969;**223**:750–2.

98. Blackburn AB, Karacan I, Salis PJ, *et al.* The effects of doxepin HCl on sleep patterns of neurotically depressed patients with sleep disturbances. *Sleep Res.* 1975;**4**:90.

99. Roth T, Zorick F, Wittig R, *et al.* The effect of doxepin HCl on sleep and depression. *J Clin Psychiatry.* 1982;**43**:366–8.

100. Roth T, Rogowski R, Hull S, *et al.* Efficacy and safety of doxepin 1 mg, 3 mg, and 6 mg in adults with primary insomnia. *Sleep,* 2007;**30**:1555–61.

101. Shipley JE, Kupfer DJ, Griffin SJ, *et al.* Comparison of effects of desipramine and amitriptyline on EEG sleep of depressed patients. *Psychopharmacology.* 1985;**85**:14–22.

102. Kupfer DJ, Perel JM, Pollock BG, *et al.* Fluvoxamine versus desipramine: comparative polysomnographic effects. *Biol Psychiatry.* 1991;**29**:23–40.

103. Jouvet M, Vimont P, Delorme F. Elective suppression of paradoxal sleep in the cat by monoamine oxidase inhibitors. *C R Seances Soc Biol Fil.* 1965;**159**:1595–9.

104. Cramer H, Kuhlo W. Effects of inhibitors of monoamine oxidase on sleep and the electroencephalogram in man. *Acta Neurol Psychiatr Belg.* 1967;**67**:658–69.

105. Cohen RM, Pickar D, Garnett, *et al.* REM sleep suppression induced by selective monoamine oxidase inhibitors. *Psychopharmacology.* 1982;**78**:137–40.

106. Wyatt RJ, Fram DH, Kupfer DJ. Total prolonged drug-induced REM sleep suppression in anxious-depressive patients. *Arch Gen Psychiatry.* 1971;**24**:145–55.

107. Kupfer DJ, Bowers MB Jr. REM sleep and central monoamine oxidase inhibitions. *Psychopharmacologia.* 1972;**27**:183–90.

108. Landolt HP, Raimo EB, Schnierow BJ, *et al.* Sleep and sleep electroencephalogram in depressed patients treated with phenelzine. *Arch Gen Psychiatry.* 2001;**58**:268–76.

109. Landolt HP, de Boer LP. Effect of chronic phenelzine treatment on REM sleep: report of three patients. *Neuropsychopharmacology.* 2001;**25**:S63–7.

110. Jindal RD, Fasiczka AL, Himmelhoch JM, *et al.* Effects of tranylcypromine on the sleep of patients with anergic bipolar depression. *Psychopharmacol Bull.* 2003;**37**:118–26.

111. Monti JM, Alterwain P, Monti D. The effects of moclobemide on nocturnal sleep of depressed patients. *J Affect Disord.* 1990;**20**:201–8.

112. Minot R, Luthringer R, Macher JP. Effect of moclobemide on the psychophysiology of sleep/wake cycles: a neuroelectrophysiological study of depressed patients administered with moclobemide. *Int Clin Psychopharmacol.* 1993;**7**:181–9.

113. Steiger A, Benkert O, Holsboer F. Effects of long-term treatment with the MAO-A inhibitor moclobemide on sleep EEG and nocturnal hormonal secretion in normal men. *Neuropsychobiology.* 1994;**30**:101–5.

114. Minot R, Luthringer R, Toussaint M, *et al.* Sleep/wake study of a selective IMAO antidepressant: Toloxatone. *Biol Psychiatry.* 1991;**29**:100.

115. Landolt HP, Kelsoe JR, Rapaport MH, Gillin JC. Rapid tryptophan depletion reverses phenelzine-induced suppression of REM sleep. *J Sleep Res.* 2003;**12**:13–18.

116. Nicholson AN, Pascoe PA. 5-hydroxytryptamine and noradrenaline uptake inhibitions. Studies on sleep in man. *Neuropharmacology.* 1986;**25**:1079–83.

117. Saletu B, Frey R, Krupka M, *et al.* Sleep laboratory studies on the single-dose effects of serotonin reuptake inhibitors paroxetine and fluoxetine on human sleep and awakening qualities. *Sleep.* 1991;**14**:439–47.

118. Wilson SJ, Bailey JE, Alford C, Nutt DJ. Sleep and daytime sleepiness the next day following single night-time dose of fluvoxamine, dothiepin and placebo in normal volunteers. *J Psychopharmacol.* 2000;**14**:378–86.

119. Wilson SJ, Bailey JE, Rich AS, *et al.* Using sleep to evaluate comparative serotonergic effects of paroxetine and citalopram. *Eur Neuropsychopharmacol.* 2004;**14**:367–72.

120. Shipley JE, Kupfer DJ, Dealy RS, *et al.* Differential effects of zimelidine on the sleep electroencephalogram of depressed patients. *Clin Pharmacol Ther.* 1984;**36**:251–9.

121. van Bemmel AL, van den Hoofdakker RH, Beersma DG, Bouhuys AL. Changes in sleep polygraphic variables and clinical state in depressed patients during treatment with citalopram. *Psychopharmacology.* 1993;**113**:225–30.

122. Staner L, Kerkhofs M, Detroux D, *et al.* Acute, subchronic, and withdrawal sleep EEG changes during treatment with paroxetine and amitriptyline: a double-blind randomized trial in major depression. *Sleep.* 1995;**18**:470–7.

123. Kerkhofs M, Rielaert C, De Martelaer V, *et al.* Fluoxetine in major depression: efficacy, safety and effects on sleep EEG variables. *Int Clin Psychopharmacol.* 1990;**5**:253–60.

124. Wilson SJ, Bell C, Coupland NJ, Nutt DJ. Sleep changes during long-term treatment of depression with fluvoxamine – a home-based study. *Psychopharmacology.* 2000;**149**:360–5.

125. Hicks JA, Argyropoulos SV, Rich AS, *et al.* Randomised controlled study of sleep after nefazodone or paroxetine treatment in out-patients with depression. *Br J Psychiatry.* 2002;**180**:528–35.

126. Jindal RD, Friedman ES, Berman SR, *et al.* Effects of sertraline on sleep architecture in patients with depression. *J Clin Psychopharmacol.* 2003;**23**:540–8.

127. Schenck CS, Mahowald MW, Kim SW, *et al.* Prominent eye movements during NREM sleep and REM sleep behavior disorder associated with fluoxetine treatment of depression and obsessive-compulsive disorder. *Sleep.* 1992;**15**:226–35.

128. Armitage R, Trivedi M, Rush AJ. Fluoxetine and oculomotor activity during sleep in depressed patients. *Neuropsychopharmacology.* 1995;**12**:159–65.

129. Trivedi MH, A John Rush AJ, Armitage R, *et al.* Effects of fluoxetine on the polysomnogram in outpatients with major depression. *Neuropsychopharmacology.* 1999;**20**:447–59.

130. Feige B, Voderholzer U, Riemann D, *et al.* Fluoxetine and sleep EEG: effects of a single dose, subchronic treatment, and discontinuation in healthy subjects. *Neuropsychopharmacology.* 2002;**26**:246–58.

131. Brezinova V, Adam K, Chapman K, *et al.* Viloxazine, sleep and subjective feelings. *Psychopharmacology.* 1977;**55**:121–8.

132. Steiger A, Gerken A, Benkert O, Holsboer F. Differential effects of the enantiomers R(–) and S(+) oxaprotiline on major endogenous depression, the sleep EEG and neuroendocrine secretion: studies on depressed patients and normal controls. *Eur Neuropsychopharmacol.* 1993;**3**:117–26.

133. Kuenzel HE, Murck H, Held K, *et al.* Reboxetine induces similar sleep-EEG changes like SSRIs in patients with depression. *Pharmacopsychiatry.* 2004;**37**:193–5.

134. Salín-Pascual RJ, Galicia-Polo L, Drucker-Colín R. Sleep changes after 4 consecutive days of venlafaxine administration in normal volunteers. *J Clin Psychiatry.* 1997;**58**:348–50.

135. Chalon S, Pereira A, Lainey E, *et al.* Comparative effects of duloxetine and desipramine on sleep EEG in healthy subjects. *Psychopharmacology.* 2005;**177**:357–65.

136. Luthringer R, Toussaint M, Schaltenbrand N, *et al.* A double-blind, placebo-controlled evaluation of the effects of orally administered venlafaxine on sleep in inpatients with major depression. *Psychopharm Bull.* 1996;**32**:637–46.

137. Lemoine P, Faivre T. Subjective and polysomnographic effects of milnacipran on sleep in depressed patients. *Hum Psychopharmacol.* 2004;**19**:299–303.

138. Kluge M, Schüssler P, Steiger A. Duloxetine increases stage 3 sleep and suppresses rapid eye movement (REM) sleep in patients with major depression. *Eur Neuropsychopharmacol.* 2007;**17**:527–31.

139. Nofzinger EA, Reynolds CF III, Thase ME, *et al.* REM sleep enhancement by bupropion in depressed men. *Am J Psychiatry.* 1995;**152**:274–6.

140. Ott GE, Rao U, Nuccio I, *et al.* Effect of bupropion-SR on REM sleep: relationship to antidepressant response. *Psychopharmacology.* 2002;**165**:29–36.

141. Evans L, Golshan S, Kelsoe J, *et al.* Effects of rapid tryptophan depletion on sleep electroencephalogram and mood in subjects with partially remitted depression on bupropion. *Neuropsychopharmacology.* 2002;**27**:1016–26.

142. Nicholson AN, Pascoe PA, Stone BM. Modulation of catecholamine transmission and sleep in man. *Neuropharmacology,* 1986;**25**:271–4.

143. Lelkes Z, Obál F Jr, Benedek G, *et al.* Effects of acute and chronic treatment with an atypical antidepressant drug, nomifensine, on the sleep–wake activity in rats. *Naunyn Schmiedebergs Arch Pharmacol.* 1987;**335**:149–53.

144. Scheller D, Dürmüller N, Moser P, Porsolt RD. Continuous stimulation of dopaminergic receptors by rotigotine does not interfere with the sleep–wake cycle in the rat. *Eur J Pharmacol.* 2008;**584**:111–17.

145. Stahl SM. Antidepressants. In: Stahl SM, ed. *Stahl's Essential Psychopharmacology. Neuroscientific Basis*

and Practical Applications, 3rd edn. (New York: Cambridge University Press, 2008; 511–666).

146. Montgomery I, Oswald I, Morgan K, Adam K. Trazodone enhances sleep in subjective quality but not in objective duration. Br J Clin Pharmacol. 1983;16:139–44.

147. Mouret J, Lemoine P, Minuit MP, et al. Effects of trazodone on the sleep of depressed subjects – a polygraphic study. Psychopharmacology. 1988;95:S37–S43.

148. Scharf MB, Sachais BA. Sleep laboratory evaluation of the effects and efficacy of trazodone in depressed insomniac patients. J Clin Psychiatry. 1990; 51 Suppl:13–17.

149. Van Bemmel AL, Havermans RG, van Diest R. Effects of trazodone on EEG sleep and clinical state in major depression. Psychopharmacology. 1992;107:569–74.

150. Ware JC, Rose FV, McBrayer RH. The acute effects of nefazodone, trazodone and buspirone on sleep and sleep-related penile tumescence in normal subjects. Sleep. 1994;17:544–50.

151. Saletu-Zyhlarz GM, Abu-Bakr MH, Anderer P, et al. Insomnia related to dysthymia: polysomnographic and psychometric comparison with normal controls and acute therapeutic trials with trazodone. Neuropsychobiology. 2001;44:139–49.

152. Parrino L, Spaggiari MC, Boselli M, et al. Clinical and polysomnographic effects of trazodone CR in chronic insomnia associated with dysthymia. Psychopharmacology. 1994;116:389–95.

153. Suzuki H, Yamadera H, Nakamura S, Endo S. Effects of trazodone and imipramine on the biological rhythm: an analysis of sleep EEG and body core temperature. J Nippon Med Sch. 2002;69:333–41.

154. Le Bon O, Murphy JR, Staner L, et al. Double-blind, placebo-controlled study of the efficacy of trazodone in alcohol post-withdrawal syndrome: polysomnographic and clinical evaluations. J Clin Psychopharmacol. 2003;23:377–83.

155. Saletu B, Prause W, Anderer P, et al. Insomnia in somatoform pain disorder: sleep laboratory studies on differences to controls and acute effects of trazodone, evaluated by the Somnolyzer 24 × 7 and the Siesta database. Neuropsychobiology. 2005;51:148–63.

156. Saletu-Zyhlarz GM, Abu-Bakr MH, Anderer P, et al. Insomnia in depression: differences in objective and subjective sleep and awakening quality to normal controls and acute effects of trazodone. Prog Neuropsychopharmacol Biol Psychiatry. 2002;26:249–60.

157. Sharpley AL, Walsh AE, Cowen PJ. Nefazodone – a novel antidepressant – may increase REM sleep. Biol Psychiatry. 1992;31:1070–3.

158. Rush JA, Armitage R, Gillin JC, et al. Comparative effects of nefazodone and fluoxetine on sleep in outpatients with major depression. Biol Psychiatry. 1998;44:3–14.

159. Wiegand MH, Galanakis P, Schreiner R. Nefazodone in primary insomnia: an open pilot study. Prog Neuropsychopharmacol Biol Psychiatry. 2004;28:1071–8.

160. Sharpley AL, Williamson DJ, Attenburrow ME, et al. The effects of paroxetine and nefazodone on sleep: a placebo controlled trial. Psychopharmacology. 1996;126:50–4.

161. Vogel G, Cohen J, Mullis D, et al. Nefazodone and REM sleep: how do antidepressant drugs decrease REM sleep? Sleep. 1998;21:70–7.

162. Scharf MB, McDannold M, Zaretsky N, et al. Evaluation of sleep architecture and cyclic alternating pattern rates in depressed insomniac patients treated with nefazodone hydrochloride. Am J Ther. 1999;6:77–82.

163. Gillin JC, Smith-Vaniz A, Schnierow B, et al. An open-label, 12-week clinical and sleep EEG study of nefazodone in chronic combat-related posttraumatic stress disorder. J Clin Psychiatry. 2001;62:789–96.

164. Neylan TC, Lenoci M, Maglione ML, et al. The effect of nefazodone on subjective and objective sleep quality in posttraumatic stress disorder. J Clin Psychiatry. 2003;64:445–50.

165. Shen J, Kennedy SH, Levitan RD, et al. The effects of nefazodone on women with seasonal affective disorder: clinical and polysomnographic analyses. J Psychiatry Neurosci. 2005;30:11–16.

166. Marek GJ, Carpenter LC, McDougle CJ, Price LH. Synergistic action of 5-HT2A antagonists and selective serotonin reuptake inhibitors in neuropsychiatric disorders. Neuropsychopharmacology. 2003;28:402–12.

167. Morgan K, Oswald I, Borrow S, Adam K. Effects of a single dose of mianserin on sleep. Br J Clin Pharmacol. 1980;10:525–7.

168. Tormey WP, Buckley MP, O'Kelly DA, et al. A sleep–endocrine profile of the antidepressant mianserin. Curr Med Res Opin. 1980;6:456–60.

169. Maeda Y, Hayashi T, Furuta H, et al. Effects of mianserin on human sleep. Neuropsychobiology. 1990–1991;24:198–204.

170. Mendlewicz J, Dunbar GC, Hoffman G. Changes in sleep EEG architecture during the treatment of depressed patients with mianserine. Acta Psychiatrica Scand. 1985; suppl 320:26–9.

171. Ruigt GS, Kemp B, Groenhout CM, et al. Effect of the antidepressant Org 3770 on human sleep. Eur J Clin Pharmacol. 1990;38:551–4.

172. Aslan S, Isik E, Cosar B. The effects of mirtazapine on sleep: a placebo controlled,

double-blind study in young healthy volunteers. *Sleep.* 2002;**25**:677–9.

173. Winokur A, DeMartinis NA 3rd, McNally DP, *et al.* Comparative effects of mirtazapine and fluoxetine on sleep physiology measures in patients with major depression and insomnia. *J Clin Psychiatry.* 2003;**64**:1224–9.

174. Schmid DA, Wichniak A, Uhr M, *et al.* Changes of sleep architecture, spectral composition of sleep EEG, the nocturnal secretion of cortisol, ACTH, GH, prolactin, melatonin, ghrelin, and leptin, and the DEX-CRH test in depressed patients during treatment with mirtazapine. *Neuropsychopharmacology.* 2006;**31**:832–44.

175. Shen J, Chung SA, Kayumov L, *et al.* Polysomnographic and symptomatological analyses of major depressive disorder patients treated with mirtazapine. *Can J Psychiatry.* 2006;**51**:27–34.

176. Schittecatte M, Dumont F, Machowski R, *et al.* Effects of mirtazapine on sleep polygraphic variables in major depression. *Neuropsychobiology.* 2002;**46**:197–201.

177. Cajochen C, Kräuchi K, Möri D, *et al.* Melatonin and S-20098 increase REM sleep and wake-up propensity without modifying NREM sleep homeostasis. *Am J Physiol.* 1997;**272**:R1189–96.

178. Quera Salva MA, Vanier B, Laredo J, *et al.* Major depressive disorder, sleep EEG and agomelatine: an open-label study. *Int J Neuropsychopharmacol.* 2007;**10**:691–6.

179. Macher JP, Luthringer R, Toussaint M, *et al.* Brain mapping and psychoactive drugs. In: Hindmarch I, Stonier PD, eds. *Human Psychopharmacology: Methods and Measures, Vol 3.* (New York: Wiley & Sons, 1990; 1–20).

180. Staner L, Mendlewicz J. Effect of a single dose of tianeptine in healthy volunteers on sleep electrophysiological parameters. *Eur Psychiatry.* 1994;**9** (Suppl 1):141.

181. Macher JP, Minot R, Duval F, *et al.* Neuro-electrophysiologic studies in abstinent and depressed alcoholic patients treated with tianeptine. *Presse Med.* 1991;**20**:1853–7.

182. Murck H, Nickel T, Künzel H, *et al.* State markers of depression in sleep EEG: dependency on drug and gender in patients treated with tianeptine or paroxetine. *Neuropsychopharmacology.* 2003;**28**:348–58.

183. Dzirasa K, Ribeiro S, Costa R, *et al.* Dopaminergic control of sleep-wake states. *J Neurosci.* 2006; **26**:10577–89.

184. Dahan L, Astier B, Vautrelle N, *et al.* Prominent burst firing of dopaminergic neurons in the ventral tegmental area during paradoxical sleep. *Neuropsychopharmacology.* 2007;**32**:1232–41.

185. Monti JM, Monti D. The involvement of dopamine in the modulation of sleep and waking. *Sleep Med Rev.* 2007;**11**:113–33.

186. Ehlers CL, Havstad JW, Kupfer DJ. Estimation of time course of slow-wave sleep over the night in depressed patients: effects of clomipramine and clinical response. *Br J Psychiatry.* 1996;**39**:171–81.

187. Mendlewicz J, Kempenaers C, De Martelaer V. Sleep EEG and amitriptyline treatment in depressed inpatients. *Biol Psychiatry.* 1991;**30**:691–702.

188. Reynolds CF III, Hoch CC, Buysse DJ, *et al.* Sleep in late-life recurrent depression: changes during early continuation therapy with nortriptyline. *Neuropsychopharmacology.* 1991;**5**:85–96.

189. Kupfer DJ, Ehlers CL, Franck E, *et al.* Persistent effects of antidepressants: EEG sleep studies in depressed patients during maintenance treatment. *Biol Psychiatry.* 1994;**35**:781–93.

190. Reynolds CF III, Buysse DJ, Brunner D, *et al.* Maintenance nortriptyline effects on electroencephalographic sleep in elderly patients with recurrent major depression: double-blind, placebo- and plasma-level-controlled evaluation. *Biol Psychiatry.* 1997;**42**:560–7.

191. Röschke J, Kögel P, Schlössser R, *et al.* Analysis of sleep EEG microstructure in subchronic paroxetine treatment of healthy subjects. *Psychopharmacology.* 1997;**132**:44–7.

192. Van Bemmel AL, Beersma DGM, Van Den Hoofdakker RH. Changes in EEG power density of NREM sleep in depressed patients during treatment with citalopram. *J Sleep Res.* 1993;**2**:156–62.

193. Monti JM, Hawkins M, Jantos H, *et al.* Biphasic effects of dopamine D-2 receptor agonists on sleep and wakefulness in rat. *Psychopharmacology.* 1988;**95**:395–400.

194. Monti JM, Jantos H, Ponzoni A, Monti D. Sleep and waking during acute histamine H3 agonist BP 2.94 or H3 antagonist carboperamide (MR 16155) administration in rats. *Neuropsychopharmacology.* 1996;**15**:31–5.

195. Saitou K, Kaneko Y, Sugimoto Y, Chen Z. Slow wave sleep-inducing effects of first generation H1-antagonists. *Biol Pharm Bull.* 1999;**22**:1079–82.

196. Huang ZL, Mochizuki T, Qu WM, *et al.* Altered sleep-wake characteristics and lack of arousal response to H3 receptor antagonist in histamine H1 receptor knockout mice. *Proc Natl Acad Sci USA.* 2006;**103**:4687–92.

197. Pellejero T, Monti JM, Baglietto J, *et al.* Effects of methoxamine and alpha-adrenoceptor antagonists,

prazosin and yohimbine, on the sleep-wake cycle of the rat. *Sleep.* 1984;**7**:365–72.

198. Kleinlogel H. Effects of the selective alpha 1-adrenoceptor blocker prazosin on EEG sleep and waking stages in the rat. *Neuropsychobiology.* 1989;**21**:100–3.

199. Idzikowski C, Mills FJ, Glennard R. 5-hydroxytryptamine-2 antagonist increases human slow wave sleep. *Brain Res.* 1986;**378**:164–8.

200. Sharpley AL, Solomon RA, Fernando AI, *et al.* Dose-related effects of selective 5-HT2 receptor antagonists on slow wave sleep in humans. *Psychopharmacology.* 1990;**101**:568–9.

201. Brandenberger G, Luthringer R, Muller G, *et al.* 5-HT2 receptors are partially involved in the relationship between renin release and relative delta power. *J Endocrinol Invest.* 1996;**19**:556–62.

202. Staner L, Kempenaers C, Simonnet MP, *et al.* 5-HT2 receptor antagonism and slow wave sleep in major depression, *Acta Psychiatr Scand.* 1992;**86**:133–7.

203. Teegarden BR, Shamma H, Xiong, Y. 5-HT2A inverse-agonists for the treatment of insomnia. *Curr Topics Med Chem.* 2008;**8**:969–76.

204. Adrien J. Implication of serotonin in the control of vigilance states as revealed by knockout-mouse studies. *J Soc Biol.* 2004;**198**:30–6.

205. Katsuda Y, Walch AE, Ware CJ, *et al.* Meta-chlorophenylpiperazine decreases slow wave sleep in humans. *Biol Psychiatry.* 1993;**33**:49–51.

206. Sharpley AL, Vassallo CM, Pooley EC, *et al.* Allelic variation in the 5-HT2C receptor (HT2RC) and the increase in slow wave sleep produced by olanzapine. *Psychopharmacology.* 2001;**153**:271–2.

207. Kang RH, Choi MJ, Paik JW, Hahn SW, Lee MS. Effect of serotonin receptor 2A gene polymorphism on

mirtazapine response in major depression. *Int J Psychiatry Med.* 2007;**37**:315–29.

208. Turner EH, Matthews AM, Linardatos E, *et al.* Selective publication of antidepressant trials and its influence on apparent efficacy. *N Engl J Med.* 2008;**358**:252–60.

209. Svendsen K, Christensen PG. Duration of REM sleep latency as predictor of effect of antidepressant therapy. A preliminary report. *Acta Psychiatr Scand.* 1981;**64**:238–43.

210. Rush AJ, Erman MK, Schlesser MA, *et al.* Alprazolam vs amitriptyline in depressions with reduced REM latencies. *Arch Gen Psychiatry.* 1985;**42**:1154–9.

211. Rush AJ, Giles DE, Jarrett RB, *et al.* Reduced REM latency predicts response to tricyclic medication in depressed outpatients. *Biol Psychiatry.* 1989;**26**:61–72.

212. Coble PA, Kupfer DJ, Spiker DG, *et al.* EEG sleep in primary depression. A longitudinal placebo study. *J Affect Disord.* 1979;**1**:131–8.

213. Clark C, Dupont R, Golshan S, *et al.* Preliminary evidence of an association between increased REM density and poor antidepressant response to partial sleep deprivation. *J Affect Disord.* 2000;**59**:77–83.

214. Staner L. Sleep-wake mechanism and drug discovery. Sleep EEG as a tool for the development of CNS-acting drugs. *Dialogues Clin Neurosci.* 2005;**7**:33–41.

215. Modell S, Lauer CJ. Rapid eye movement (REM) sleep: an endophenotype for depression. *Curr Psychiatry Rep.* 2007;**9**:480–5.

216. Gottesmann C, Gottesman I. The neurobiological characteristics of rapid eye movement (REM) sleep are candidate endophenotypes of depression, schizophrenia, mental retardation and dementia. *Prog Neurobiol.* 2007;**81**:237–50.

217. Antonijevic I. HPA axis and sleep: identifying subtypes of major depression. *Stress.* 2008;**11**:15–27.

Rapid eye movement sleep interruption as a therapy for major depression

M. Y. Agargun

Changes in rapid eye movement (REM) sleep and dreaming are some of the most popular issues in major depression. On the other hand, sleep deprivation studies showed that REM sleep deprivation is effective, at least partially, in treatment of mood disorders. Recent data suggest that sleep manipulations regarding REM sleep cause psychological/behavioral and neuroendocrine changes in depressed patients. In this chapter, first, I briefly present REM sleep abnormalities and dream variables in depression. Second, I review the consequences of REM sleep and dream manipulations in normal healthy subjects, in particular, in terms of diurnal rhythms. Finally, I discuss REM sleep and dream interruption as a therapy modality in depressive disorders.

Rapid eye movement sleep abnormalities and dream variables in depression

The main characteristics of REM sleep in depression are short sleep latency (<65 minutes), an increase in the number of eye movements per minute of sleep in the first REM sleep period (increased REM density), and a prolongation of the first REM episode [1]. These suggest a phase advance of the REM cycle in depression [2]. Clearly, these REM sleep signs are reported to correlate with the severity of the mood disorder [3]. On the other hand, Giles *et al.* [4] have reported concordance for shorter REM latency among family members who share the diagnosis of depression. This indicates a genetic propensity for depression indicated by the presence of this sleep sign.

With regard to dreams, recall of dreams is also typically reduced in depressed patients [5]. Reports of no recall, or of only fragmentary thoughts, are more common than are the more typical dream reports of perceptual imagery with some narrative continuity. Dream affect, too, is more often absent or blunted and, when present, is predominantly negative in nature.

In major depression, frightening and recurrent bad dreams are associated with suicidal behavior [6]. Previous studies suggested that dreams in which the dreamer is deserted, frustrated, deprived, or injured are characteristic of depression-prone people. "Masochistic" dreaming had been reported to characterize depressive patients before, during, and after episodes as a stable psychological variable [7, 8]. Using Beck's scale for dream masochism, Cartwright [9] examined whether masochistic dreaming was associated with the presence of major depression, whether women have higher masochistic dream scores than depressed men, and whether depressed women have higher masochistic dream scores than depressed men. This study found that masochistic dreaming was not significantly associated with the presence of a major depression. Women, whether depressed or not, have higher masochistic dream scores than depressed men, and depressed women have higher masochistic dream scores than depressed men. In another study, Cartwright and Wood [10] studied 25 women and 21 men undergoing divorce for three nights of sleep laboratory monitoring on two occasions one year apart. In this study, women also showed less improvement at follow-up and had more need for emotional support. These findings suggested that dream masochism might be a continuing cognitive characteristic that contributes to the vulnerability of women to major depression. A recent study (Agargun and Cartwright, unpublished data) investigated whether untreated depressed subjects with melancholic features have higher dream masochism scores than those without melancholic features,

---

Sleep and Mental Illness, eds. S. R. Pandi-Perumal and M. Kramer. Published by Cambridge University Press.

the dreams of a group of community volunteers undergoing divorce were recorded in the sleep laboratory. Subjects with melancholic features had higher dream masochism scores than those who did not meet depression criteria. Melancholic depressed individuals had higher dream masochism scores in the second half than the first half, whereas non-melancholic depressed individuals and non-depressed subjects did not differ between the halves of the night.

Rapid eye movement sleep and dream manipulations in normal healthy subjects

It is well known that long-lasting sleep interruptions normally occur preferentially out of REM sleep episodes. The proportion of episodes of wakefulness following REM sleep that were long-lasting progressively increased over the course of the night, because of the homeostatic drive for sleep [11–13]. Murphy et al. [14] have recently reported that REM episodes from which spontaneous sleep terminated were truncated relative to those that did not end the sleep period. Another study [15] suggested that REM density was higher in REM periods that ended in wakefulness than in those that did not. The authors concluded that REM sleep mechanisms appear to be the main force controlling sleep after a spontaneous sleep interruption, presumably because during the second half of the night, where more sleep interruptions occur, the pressure for NREM sleep is reduced and the circadian rhythm in REM sleep propensity reaches its peak. On the other hand, REM latency in sleep cycles that followed a period of sleep interruption was short, regardless of whether the duration of the interruption was short or long [16, 17]. Rapid eye movement sleep state is neurophysiologically close to wake. After spontaneous wakefulness, REM sleep mechanisms appear to be the main forces controlling sleep [15].

Greenberg et al. [18] examined the hypothesis that a critical intervening process in adaptation to a stressful situation is dreaming or the REM stage of sleep. They studied a group of volunteer subjects who, after adaptation to laboratory conditions, were shown a stressful movie on two consecutive days. During the night between these two viewings, some subjects were REM deprived, some awakened an equivalent number of times during NREM sleep, and some were allowed

to sleep undisturbed. They suggested that the subjects who were REM deprived showed significantly less habituation to the second viewing than the control subjects. They also hypthesized that REM sleep serves to integrate memories of similar experiences with the current stress, allowing the use of the individual's characteristic defenses. In this study, REM-deprived subjects showed a decreased ability to adapt to the specific stress. Thus, REM sleep and dreaming play an important role in adaptation to stressful events and condition in healthy subjects. A disruption in REM sleep may cause failure in psychological adaptation. However, the mechanism is clearly different in depressives than healthy subjects.

Rapid eye movement sleep and dream interruption in depressive disorders

In depressed patients, increased REM density has shown to be correlated with more intensely negative cognitions and affects [19]. Although severely depressed patients report that they have poorer dream recall and blunted dream affect [5], less severely depressed patients report higher rates of unpleasant dreams than other psychiatric patients or normal subjects [9]. Cartwright et al. [20] found that the subjects reporting more negative dreams at the beginning of the night were more likely to be in remission one year later than those reporting more negative dreams at the end of the night. In another study, Agargun and Cartwright [21] found that when end-of-night dream narratives were more negative in affect type but low in narrative quality, the affect appeared to be less integrated with older affective memory material close to the morning awaking, indicating a failure to regulate negative mood. It might be that this pattern of affect processing is pathogenic. Thus, Agargun and Cartwright note that early negative dreams reflect a within-sleep mood-regulation process taking place while those that occur later may indicate a failure in the completion of this process. There is a strong relationship between clinical features of depression and REM sleep abnormalities.

On the other hand, terminal insomnia, pervasive anhedonia, unreactive mood, and appetite loss, endogenous depressive symptoms, are reported to be related to short REM latency and increased REM density in depressed patients [22]. A negative affective state in the morning is an essential feature of melancholia. This might be related to the intervening dream

223

content and affect. Recently Besiroglu *et al.* [23] hypothesized terminal insomnia occurs adaptively in depressed patients with melancholic features having a therapeutic effect on mood regulation and improving negative dream affect and content. In this study, the authors found that terminal insomnia and nightmares were significantly more frequent in depressed patients with melancholic features. They concluded that an association between frequent nightmares and terminal insomnia exists in melancholic depression. In major depressed patients, in particular with melancholic features (MF), an adaptive function for spontaneous early morning awakening may shield mood from the effects of negative dream affect. Clearly, this reflects a within-sleep, mood-regulation process taking place. Nightmares might reflect a negative dream affect, and terminal insomnia might play a role in preventing depressed morning mood, although a failure in the completion of this process takes place during a depressive episode, in particular with melancholia.

Moreover, the masochistic dreams in melancholic depressed individuals may be regarded as a manifestation of the individual's negative bias in interpreting this experience and in his or her expectations [24]. It may be suggested that masochism in frightening dreams such as nightmares is associated with a deeper level of self-criticism and self-blaming in melancholic depressed individuals. Feeling worse in the morning than later in the day may be related to the intervening dream content and affect. Thus, REM sleep deprivation that occurs closer to morning may have a therapeutic effect on mood regulation and diminish negative dream affect and content in depressed subjects with MF or diurnal mood symptoms.

A recent report [25] indicates that remission from an untreated episode of major depression, consequent on the loss of an attachment relationship, can be accounted for in large part by the initial severity of symptoms as self-reported; the presence, direction, and intensity of diurnal variability of symptoms; the degree of the downregulation of depressed mood following REM interruptions; and the ability to report dreams when awakened from REM sleep. Those whose level of self-rated symptom severity is higher than that indicated by the clinical rating, who report few dreams, who feel at their worst in the morning hours, and who are less able to maintain the benefits during the day of sleep-related mood improvement have little chance of remission without treatment.

Finally, with melancholic features, major depression seems to be a prototype for therapeutic effect of REM/dream interruption, in particular, in terms of improvement of negative affect. Insomnia, one of the most common depressive sysmptoms, might reflect as an adaptive deprivation to deal with negative morning affect. The downregulation of depressed mood following REM interruptions allows therapeutic improvement in depressed patients.

References

1. Benca R, Obermeyer W, Thisted R, Gillin JC. Sleep and psychiatric disorders: a meta-analysis. *Arch Gen Psychiatry.* 1992;**49**:651–668.

2. Wehr T, Wirz-Justice A, Goodwin F, Duncan W, Gillin JC. Phase advance of the circadian sleep–wake cycle as an anti-depressant. *Science.* 1979;**206**:710–13.

3. Reynolds C, Kupfer D. Sleep research in affective illness: state of the art circa 1987. *Sleep.* 1987;**10**:199–215.

4. Giles DE, Kupfer DJ, Rush AJ, Roffwarg HP. Controlled comparison of electrophysiological sleep in families of probands with unipolar depression. *Am J Psychiatry.* 1998;**155**:192–9.

5. Armitage R, Rochler A, Fitch T, Trivedi M, Rush J. Dream recall and major depression: a preliminary report. *Dreaming.* 1995;**5**:189–98.

6. Agargun MY, Cilli AS, Kara H, *et al.* Repetitive and frightening dreams and suicidal behavior in patients with major depression. *Compr Psychiatry.* 1998;**39**:198–202.

7. Beck A, War C. Dreams of depressed patients. *Arch Gen Psychiatry.* 1961;**5**:66–71.

8. Hauri P. Dreams in patients remitted from reactive depression. *J Abnorm Psychology.* 1976;**85**:1–10.

9. Cartwright RD. "Masochism" in dreaming and its relation to depression. *Dreaming.* 1992;**2**:79–84.

10. Cartwright RD, Wood E. The contribution of dream masochism to the sex ratio difference in major depression. *Psychiatry Res.* 1993;**46**:165–73.

11. Feinberg I. Changes in sleep cycle patterns with age. *J Psychiatr Res* 1974;**10**:283–306.

12. Borbély A, Baumann F, Brandeis D, Strauch I, Lehmann D. Sleep deprivation: effect on sleep stages and EEG power density in man. *Electroenceph Clin Neurophysiol.* 1981;**51**:483–93.

13. Borbély AA. A two process model of sleep regulation. *Hum Neurobiol.* 1982;**1**:195–204.

14. Murphy PJ, Rogers NL, Campbell SS. Age differences in the spontaneous termination of sleep. *J Sleep Res.* 2000;**9**:27–34.

15. Barbato G, Barker C, Wehr T. Spontaneous sleep interruptions during extended nights. Relationships with NREM and REM sleep phases and effects on REM sleep regulation. *Clin Neurophysiol.* 2002; **113**:892–900.

16. Brezinova V, Beck U, Oswald I. Sleep cycle duration and timing of REM periods in interrupted night sleep. *Int J Chronobiol.* 1975;**3**:81–7.

17. Campbell SC. Evolution of sleep structure following brief intervals of wakefulness. *Electroenceph Clin Neurophysiol.* 1987;**66**:175–84.

18. Greenberg R, Pillard R, Pearlman C. The effect of dream (stage REM) deprivation on adaptation to stress. *Psychosom Med.* 1972; **34**(3):257–62.

19. Nofzinger EA, Schwartz RM, Reynolds CF III, *et al.* Affect intensity and phasic REM sleep in depressed men before and after treatment with cognitive behavioral therapy. *J Consult Clin Psychol.* 1994; **62**:83–91.

20. Cartwright R, Young MA, Mercer P, Bears M. Role of REM sleep and dream variables in the prediction of remission from depression. *Psychiatry Res.* 1998;**80**:249–55.

21. Agargun MY, Cartwright R. REM sleep, dream variables and suicidality in depressed patients. *Psychiatry Res.* 2003;**119**:33–9.

22. Giles DE, Rush AJ, Roffwarg HP. Sleep parameters in bipolar I, bipolar II, and unipolar depressions. *Biol Psychiatry.* 1986;**2**:1340–3.

23. Besiroglu L, Agargun MY, Inci R. Nightmares and terminal insomnia in depressed patients with and without melancholic features. *Psychiatry Res.* 2005;**133**:285–7.

24. Beck AT. *Depression.* (New York: Harper and Row, 1967).

25. Cartwright R, Baehr B, Kirkby J, Pandi-Perumal SR, Kabat J. REM sleep reduction, mood regulation and remission in untreated depression. *Psychiatry Res.* 2003;**121**(2):159–67.

225

Sleep in dementia

Jürgen Staedt and Stefan Rupprecht-Mrozek

Introduction

With increasing age, qualitative as well as quantitative changes in sleep occur, and approximately 38% of over 65-year-olds report sleep disturbances according to epidemiological studies. It is found that 36% suffer from sleep onset disturbances and up to 29% suffer from disturbances of sleep continuity [1]. Subjectively experienced sleep disturbances correlated negatively with cognitive performance in a three-year follow-up [2]. According to the literature, 34 to 43% of patients with Alzheimer's disease (AD) experience sleep disturbances [3, 4]. The extent to which night sleep is disturbed by the number of awakenings is said to correlate strongly with the level of severity of dementia [5–7]. On the other hand, aggressiveness and behavioral disturbances seemed to be a strong predictor for sleep disturbances in AD [8]. According to a large study in Germany, 51% of caregivers experience disruptions of sleep continuity, on average 2.4 per night [9]. In fact, many caregivers cite sleep disturbances, including night wandering and confusion, as the main reason for institutionalizing the elderly [10, 11]. Aside from somatic disorders, sleep disorders in AD are facilitated by a lack of day structure, reduced physical activity, and napping (Figure 20.1). For the therapy of sleep disorders and sleep–wake rhythm disturbances in dementia it is helpful to understand the function of the chronobiological system and pathophysiological changes of the central nervous system in the elderly.

Chronobiology and aging

The evolution of the chronobiological system is a consequence of the Earth rotating around the sun. Corresponding internal circadian clocks are found in all eukaryotic and at least in some prokaryotic organisms [12–14]. These internal clocks make sure that the rhythm of physiological processes and metabolism or even behavior occur in tune with the day/night cycle of the Earth. But internal clocks are inaccurate. In humans they are up to half an hour too fast or too slow [15]. In other words biological clocks do not run in isolation from the day/night cycle and need ongoing synchronization with the environment. In mammals this synchronization takes place in the suprachiasmatic nucleus (SCN) [16]. Here the perception of light information is ensured by three systems. In addition to the rod and cone receptors that are responsible for visual perception, melanopsin-containing retinal ganglion cells have been recently discovered in the human retina [17]. These melanopsin-expressing retinal ganglion cells are implicated in non-visual responses to light and project to numerous brain structures including hypothalamic and non-hypothalamic structures [18, 19]. Recent studies revealed that human non-visual responses are more sensitive to short wavelength light (460 nm) than to longer wavelength light (550 nm) [20]. This so-called biological, non-visual effect of short wavelength light is of tremendous importance for human melatonin levels, alertness, and thermophysiology. In this direction, data from Vandewalle et al. [21] pointed out that brain activity is highly light-wavelength dependent and that melanopsin-expressing retinal ganglion cells are of major importance in this context.

Exactly this short wavelength light spectrum of about 450 nm is filtered out with increasing age due to yellowing and opacity of the eye lenses [22]. Therefore the biological light effect is reduced by up to 50% in normal aging!

Sleep and Mental Illness, eds. S. R. Pandi-Perumal and M. Kramer. Published by Cambridge University Press.
© Cambridge University Press 2010.

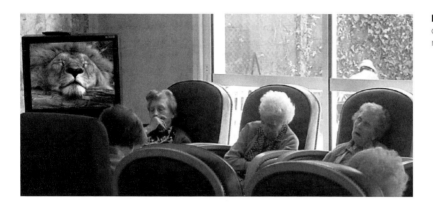

Figure 20.1 Destabilization of the circadian rhythm by excessive daytime napping in a German nursing home.

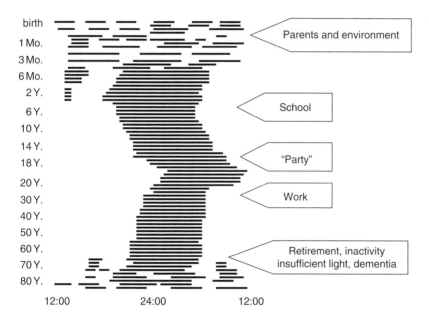

Figure 20.2 Importance of "zeitgebers" (Modified with permission from Staedt & Riemann [151]).

This biological light information is projected to the SCN via the retinohypothalamic tract and the melatonin secretion is immediately suppressed by bright light and increased at night, and therefore a very sensitive marker of circadian rhythm disturbances.

Besides light, in humans circadian rhythms are influenced mainly through "social zeitgebers". So after birth there is still an ultradian rhythm, and the circadian rhythm is slowly achieved by the synchronization of mother–infant interactions.

At the latest when starting at school or work, individuals are forced to have very stable rest–activity rhythms. This rest–activity rhythm remains stable until the children move out of the family home and/or retirement age is reached. At this point retirement-associated restrictions in social life, as well as age-related physical and psychiatric diseases, can diminish activities of daily living and favor excessive napping and early bedtimes (Figure 20.2). This point of view is supported by Fetveit and Bjorvatn [23]. They found that demented nursing home patients spent nearly thirteen hours asleep, distributed as more than nine hours of night-time sleep and more than three hours of daytime sleep.

These factors together with lens opacity-related reduced biological light effects and the well known insufficient illumination level, especially in nursing homes [24, 25], are able to promote circadian rhythm disorders in dementia.

Circadian rhythm disorders in dementia

Circadian rhythms are altered as a consequence of both normal aging and Alzheimer's disease (AD) associated brain pathologies. The elderly typically develop a phase advance, whereas in AD a phase delay of body temperature can be observed [26, 27]. In this context many studies have reported disrupted melatonin production and rhythms in AD that are taking place as early as in the very first preclinical AD stages (neuropathological Braak stage I–II) [28–30]. Since Alzheimer's pathology underlies approximately 70% of dementing diseases [31], the potential impact of the neurophysiological changes of Alzheimer's dementia on rest–activity regulation should be discussed. Neuronal degeneration in the nucleus basalis Meynert (NBM) is one of the most prominent features [32, 33]. The NBM could be defined as a cholinergic nuclear area that belongs to the ascending reticular activation system (ARAS) and innervates the neocortex. There, acetylcholine reduces the resting/voltage-dependent potassium membrane potential and thus increases neuronal excitability (reagibility). Nucleus basalis Meynert neurons show a bursting and a tonic firing pattern. Whereas the latter might be associated with NREM sleep, faster release of acetylcholine might underlie wakefulness [34]. During the wake phase, cholinergic pathways also inhibit the nuclei reticulares thalami [35]. During the sleep phase this inhibitory influence disappears and the nuclei reticulares thalami induce a GABA-modulated NREM sleep synchronization. Thus it is understandable that in AD an increasing cholinergic deficit produces EEG frequency decelerations that complicate the differentiation of the sleep–wake EEG with increasing severity of dementia. Accordingly, an extremely low cell density in the NBM and a low activity of the choline acetyltransferase in the cortex of patients with the highest delta activity is found [36]. The decreasing activity of the SCN and the synthesis of melatonin that diminishes in accordance with the progression of the AD (as determined by the Braak stages) [28, 30] facilitate rest–activity disturbances in AD along with the above-mentioned reduced "social zeitgebers" (physical activity, social isolation, insufficient illumination level in living areas). While napping may be an expression of a disrupted sleep–night structure, it has been shown to induce changes in the circadian rhythm when performed in the evening hours [37].

Sleep disturbances in dementia

There are two main types of sleep: rapid eye movement (REM) sleep and non-rapid eye movement (NREM) sleep, which has four stages. People normally cycle through the four stages of NREM sleep, usually followed by a brief interval of REM sleep, from four to five times every night.

Sleep progresses from stage 1, during which the sleeper can be awakened easily, to stage 4, during which the sleeper can be awakened only with difficulty. In stage 4, blood pressure is at its lowest, and heart and breathing rates are at their slowest.

During REM sleep, electrical activity in the brain is unusually high, somewhat resembling that during wakefulness. The eyes move rapidly, and muscles may jerk involuntarily. The rate and depth of breathing increase, but the muscles, except for the diaphragm, are greatly relaxed. The first REM period typically lasts ten minutes, with each recurring REM stage lengthening, and the final one lasting up to 40 minutes (see Figure 20.3).

Sleep architecture changes relative to age. In particular, there is a diminished consolidation of NREM sleep [38]. In dementia, the sleep consolidation is aggravated by an increase in frequency and/or duration of awakenings and a decrease in slow-wave sleep (NREM stage 3 and stage 4) [39–41]. The above-mentioned disturbed consolidation in NREM sleep in the elderly and especially in dementia can cause worsening of cognitive abilities, as NREM sleep is thought to be of importance for declarative memory [42]. This causal relationship becomes even more likely considering the fact that memory performance on a neuronal level is specifically related to gene upregulation and is reflected by the facilitation of certain connections and the sensitivity and density of receptors [43]. In this line sleep-related neurogenesis in the hippocampus is markedly suppressed by sleep deprivation [44]. Sleep disturbances therefore can alter sleep-related brain protein synthesis, synaptic consolidation/depression, and at least the consolidation of experience-dependent cortical plasticity [45, 46].

In summary, one can say that sleep and memory disturbances in dementia are partly related to each other. Treatment of sleep/wake rhythm disorders in dementia should therefore be planned with regard to both aspects.

(a)

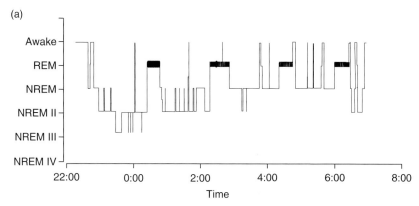

(b)

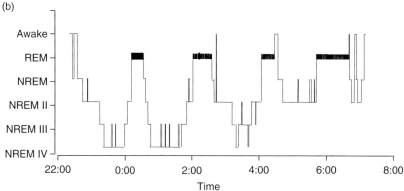

Figure 20.3 (a) Polysomnogram in dementia. REM: rapid eye movement sleep; NREM I–IV: non-rapid eye movement sleep stage 1–4.
(b) Polysomnogram in young adulthood with four sleep cycles. REM: rapid eye movement sleep; NREM I–IV: non rapid eye movement sleep stage 1–4.

Different kinds of sleep disturbances in dementia: sundowning

The synopsis of the neuropathological changes in the SCN and the NBM makes the occurrence of rest–activity disturbances more easily understandable. The most spectacular disturbance is "sundowning". This term describes a delusional and often delirious state that occurs at twilight or during early evening [47]. People with dementia may become more confused, restless, and insecure, and hallucinations may occur. It can be worse after a move or a change in the person's routine. Data on the prevalence are varying from 10 to 25% in institutionalized patients [48, 49] and even higher numbers in Alzheimer's patients living at home, reaching up to 66% [50]. A decrease in activity of the SCN, the so-called "internal zeitgeber", could play a major role for the occurrence of sundowning. In favor of this assumption is the fact that sundowning usually occurs at twilight with reduced light intensity and the fact that rays of light have a stimulating effect on the locus ceruleus via the SCN [21, 51]. The reduced light-mediated activation of the locus ceruleus could thus negatively influence cognition and executive functioning and may promote a desynchronization of the rest–activity rhythm. In line with the latter assumption, sundowning intensity increases with reduction and phase delay of the temperature amplitude [52].

In our opinion, the sundowning observed in AD is pathophysiologically based on a cortical activation (arousal reaction) with concurrently reduced indirect SCN-mediated base activation, which is additionally enhanced by the cholinergic deafferentiation of the cortex and the reduced cholinergic inhibition of the nuclei reticulares thalami.

Putting it more simply, sundowning is characterized by an arousal (e.g., fear due to impaired visual orientation, or vocalizations of other residents) whereas the neocortex is "turned off", programmed towards NREM sleep. Because of the cholinergic deafferentiation of the cortex the patient is then not able to build up the attentional capacity necessary for the processing of arousal. As a consequence, the stimulus causing the arousal cannot be processed and agitation persists or even becomes worse. In this line, disruptive vocalizations of elderly demented patients typically occur more often during the afternoon and evening hours [53].

Interestingly, patients with dementia with Lewy bodies (DLB) are especially sensitive to anticholinergic agents, indicating marked cholinergic dysfunction. Post-mortem studies of brain tissue from patients with DLB revealed a severe depletion of the NBM with 75 to 80% loss of large cholinergic neurons (in Alzheimer's disease 50 to 70% loss of cholinergic neurons) [54], and a severely reduced cholinergic activity in the reticular thalamic nucleus associated with hallucinations and fluctuating consciousness [55].

Sedative psychotropic medication applied in the treatment of sundowning and nocturnal agitation is to be considered problematic since benzodiazepines or neuroleptics further weaken the already instable sleep–wake rhythms and further decrease neuronal metabolic activity. Furthermore, antipsychotic treatment is associated with increased risk for death in patients with dementia [56–58]. Beside pre-existing cerebrovascular risk factors, affect on blood pressure, Q-T prolongation with conduction delays, thromboembolism, and extra-pyramidal symptoms causing potential swallowing problems might increase these risks [59–64].

Therefore it seems plausible that sedative psychotropic medication on the one hand increases duration of hospitalization [65] and on the other hand promotes confusion, impaired cognition, and excessive sedation with the danger of falling [66, 67]. Consequently, substances physiologically stimulating the circadian timing system in a specific way should be applied in first line. Pharmacological candidates are cholinesterase inhibitors and melatonin.

Cholinesterase inhibitors are the therapy of choice for the treatment of AD and have also shown efficacy in other forms of dementia [68–79]. Meta-analysis showed that they also influence non-cognitive symptoms and reduce psychotic symptoms, especially in Lewy body dementia [76, 80]. They should be applied at daytime in demented patients, especially when disturbances of circadian rhythms or sundowning occur.

Melatonin is believed to predominantly inhibit the activity of the SCN via $Mel_{1a,b}$ receptors [81, 82] and possesses a circadian phase-dependent hypnotic property [83]. Melatonin improves sleep only when endogenous melatonin is absent and should be given after light therapy at 20:00 to 21:00 hours.

Results of a functional MRI study demonstrate that melatonin modulates brain activity in a manner resembling actual sleep, although subjects are fully awake. Furthermore, the fatigue-inducing effect of melatonin on brain activity is essentially different from that of sleep deprivation thus revealing differences between fatigue related to the circadian sleep regulation as opposed to increased homeostatic sleep need [84]. However, placebo-controlled studies on the application of melatonin showed contradictory results. Asayama et al. [85] found a significant decrease in nocturnal activity, a prolongation of sleep, and an improvement of cognition after four weeks of administering melatonin (3 mg), whereas Serfaty et al. [86] did not find an amelioration of sleep after the administering of 6 mg of melatonin over a period of two weeks. Singer et al. [87] found after two months of administration of either 2.5 mg sustained-release melatonin, 10 mg melatonin, or placebo, there were no statistically significant differences in objective sleep measures for any of these groups, although non-significant trends for increased nocturnal total sleep time and decreased wake after sleep onset were observed in the melatonin groups relative to placebo. Trends for a greater percentage of subjects having more than a 30-minute increase in nocturnal total sleep time in the 10 mg melatonin group and for a decline in the day–night sleep ratio in the 2.5 mg sustained-release melatonin group, compared to placebo, were also seen. On subjective measures, caregiver ratings of sleep quality showed improvement in the 2.5 mg sustained-release melatonin group relative to placebo.

Thus, melatonin might need a longer time to exert an effect on sleep and other relevant symptoms of dementia. This supports the study of Riemersma-van der Lek et al. [88], who found a significant positive influence on sleep onset latency and sleep duration under the application of 2.5 mg of melatonin in a 12-month, double-blind, placebo-controlled trail.

Different kinds of sleep disturbances in dementia: REM-sleep behavior disorder

The REM-sleep behavior disorder (RBD) has to be distinguished from sundowning. REM-sleep behavior disorder exists either in an idiopathic form or it is found as an early manifestation of neurodegenerative disorders mainly of the synucleinopathies like dementia with Lewy bodies, Parkinson's disease, or multiple system atrophy [89]. REM-sleep behavior disorder is characterized by loss of usually occurring REM sleep skeletal muscle atonia, resulting in the acting out of dream mentation [90]. This occurs usually once to twice a week, sometimes up to four times per night during REM sleep episodes. Sleeping partners often report intermittent motor activity with screaming, shouting, and jumping or falling out of bed. Typical RBD-associated injuries are ecchymoses and lacerations. The behavioral manifestations can also be simple like sitting up, talking, and laughing. But an assault of bed partners is not uncommon. Up to 90% of patients with RBD are men of older age and it appears as well in the prodrome of demential diseases, so that its occurrence is not dependent on an existing dementia [91]. As a potential cause for RBD the degeneration of pedunculopontine neurons is discussed, which influences the muscle tone in sleep. In the patient's history, speaking during sleep is often found [92]. It should be mentioned that some drugs commonly prescribed in psychiatry, such as TCAs, serotonin reuptake inhibitors, or serotonin and noradrenalin reuptake inhibitors, suppress the REM-related muscle atonia and can therefore promote RBD. Treatment of choice is 0.25 mg to 1.50 mg of the well tolerated clonazepam. In the case of RBD with sleep apnea syndrome, instead of clonazepam, melatonin (3 mg to 9 mg) is preferred.

Sleep disorders with somatic conditions: sleep apnea syndrome

In addition, other factors causing sleep disturbances have to be considered in old age, such as sleep apnea syndrome (SAS), restless legs syndrome (RLS), nycturia and enuresis nocturna [93].

The age-associated increase in bodyweight, decline in muscular strength, and enhanced upper airway collapsibility are risk factors for SAS. The prevalence of SAS in the elderly is about 28% in men and 20% in women. But in patients with AD the prevalence is much higher – up to 70% [94, 95]. Sleep apnea is defined as an absence of air flow at the nose and mouth for at least ten seconds. Obstructive apnea is defined as the absence of air flow despite respiratory efforts. Central apnea, less common, is characterized by absence of respiratory efforts. Mixed apneas begin centrally, followed by obstruction.

People with SAS may experience waking with gasping, confused wandering in the night, and thrashing during sleep. One of the main risk factors for obstructive SAS is obesity, causing an increased size and fat content of the pharyngeal tissues, soft palate, and uvula. During the apneas, the oxygen level in the blood falls causing many of the daytime symptoms such as excessive drowsiness. In some cases pulmonary hypertension may develop leading to right-sided heart failure or cor pulmonale. Obstructive SAS is also associated with systemic hypertension, cardiac arrhythmia, ischemic heart disease, and stroke. Therefore sleep apnea is often associated with multi-infarct or vascular dementia [96]. Weight management and avoiding alcohol and sedatives (which can exacerbate SAS by further relaxing the pharyngeal muscles) at bedtime may relieve SAS. In mild to moderate AD short-term continuous positive airway pressure (CPAP) may be well tolerated and effective in reducing daytime sleepiness [94, 97]. But CPAP compliance in long-term use may be difficult [98]. Alternative therapy with theophylline can be considered, but because of the high anticholinergic potency of this substance delirious symptoms can be triggered. In this context it should be mentioned that the acetylcholine esterase inhibitor donepezil improved SAS in a double-blind, placebo-controlled study [99].

Sleep disorders with somatic conditions: restless legs syndrome

Another common cause for sleep disturbances is the prevalence of RLS in about 29% of the elderly [100]. It is characterized by unpleasant limb sensations, usually described as a creeping or crawling feeling, sometimes as a tingling, cramping, burning, or just plain pain, that are precipitated by rest and relieved by activity. Some patients have no definite sensation, except for the need to move. In up to 50% the arms are affected as well. There is a definite worsening of the discomfort when lying down at night or during other forms of inactivity, including just sitting. About 80% of RLS patients also experience periodic limb movements in sleep (PLMS). Periodic limb movements in sleep are characterized by sudden jerking or bending of the legs during sleep, ranging from small shudders of the ankles and toes to kicking and flailing of the arms and legs. The periodic jerking often wakes the individual and significantly disturbs their quality of sleep. Periodic limb movements in sleep can occur independently in up to 45% of the elderly [101]. Restless legs syndrome is caused by a functional disturbance in the dopaminergic system [102]. Treatments of first choice are dopamine agonists such as ropinirol (0.5 to 4 mg) or pramipexole

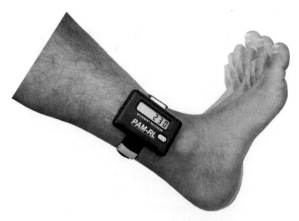

Figure 20.4 PAM-RL can record leg movements continuously for 72 hours. It can also differentiate between standing and lying using a integrated position sensor. Somnomedics®.

(0.088 to 0.540 mg) [103–105]. Because of the sometimes observed initial nausea, we recommend domperidone (30 mg/day) as an add-on during the first week of treatment. Periodic limb movements in sleep are greatly underdiagnosed, especially in people with dementia who are unable to describe their symptoms. However, if a deterioration or disruption of sleep is noticed in patients taking antidepressants or neuroleptics, PLMS should be considered, since antidepressants, in particular SSRIs and SNRIs and also neuroleptics, potentially induce or exacerbate PLMS [106–110]. Periodic limb movements in sleep can be easily diagnosed by actigraphy placed on the ankle of each leg [111–113]. Actigraphy is highly tolerated even in severely demented patients and makes home recordings more accessible, permitting the evaluation of patients in their natural sleeping environment and minimizing laboratory effects likely to alter the patient's typical sleep patterns (see Figure 20.4).

In planning therapeutic interventions one should consider that the quality of life and the sleep quality of patients with RLS is notably limited. Therefore it is important to avoid prescribing antidepressants that can worsen RLS and PLMS, such as SSRIs, SNRIs, and tricyclic antidepressants, in demented patients with RLS. For the same reason prescription of antipsychotics for sedation is not recommended. Good alternatives for the treatment of depressive symptoms in dementia are, for example, 150 mg bupropione in the morning for drive improving and 25 mg to 150 mg trazodone for sleep disturbances in the evening, as both substances lead to decreased PLMS [114, 115]. In addition, we

should mentioned that trazodone (50 mg to 300 mg) has shown benefits in AD patients with irritability in long-term treatment [116].

Non-pharmacologic treatment: sleep hygiene, light therapy

However, studies provide evidence that in some nursing-home environments a median light intensity of only 54 lux was measured, and the residents only spent approximately ten minutes in light of more than 1,000 lux [25]. In comparison with that we reach 300 to 500 lux in our illuminated workspaces. Even on cloudy days during winter the light intensity reaches 2,000 to 4,000 lux outdoors. The positive effect of daylight on sleep could be proven in a study on elderly with sleep disorders [117]. In this study an exposure to daylight for two hours in the morning and for two hours in the afternoon resulted in increased melatonin levels and sleep amelioration. In demented patients, light therapy during the evening hours reduces nocturnal motoric agitation [118, 119], but light therapy during the morning hours is also effective [120, 121] and even an amelioration of cognition in the Mini Mental State Examination can be achieved [122, 123]. Also indirect light therapy (~1,000 lux) in the living room stabilizes the sleep–wake cycle [88, 124]. Stimulation exerted by sunrise and sunset also had positive effects on sleep onset latency, nocturnal agitation states, and sleep duration in elderly patients with advanced dementia [125]. According to the available data and the routines of (nursing) homes, we recommend for demented patients a 30-minute light therapy of 10,000 lux, which in consideration of the load on the time schedule can be easily fitted into the ward routine. Alternatively, we recommend 2,500 lux indirect light therapy for two hours in the morning and in the afternoon. However, it has to be noted that severely demented patients with substantial degeneration of the SCN can only benefit to a limited extent [126]. Pharmacologic therapy should only be considered when all the above-mentioned measures have failed to achieve positive results.

Pharmacologic treatment

Before prescribing the existing medication it should be critically revised from different aspects. (1) In respect to causing sleep disturbances: several drugs produce daytime sleepiness, insomnia, or nightmares (Table 20.1),

Table 20.1 Medication with potentially adverse effects of sleep–wake rhythm[a]

Substance groups	Generic	Fatigue	Insomnia	Nightmares
Alpha-agonists[b]	e.g., clonidine, methyldopa	+	+	+
Anti-arrhythmics	Amiodarone	+	+	+
Beta-blockers[b]	Atenolole, propanolole	–	+	+
Broncholytics	Theophylline	–	+	–
Ca-antagonists	Diltiazem	+	+	+
Corticosteroids	Dexamethasone, prednisolone	–	+	–
Statins	Lovastatine, simvastatine	–	+ (Amnesia)	–
Parkinson's medication (at high dosage)	Levodopa, pergolide	–	+	–

Notes: [a] Generally data from case reports;
[b] α-receptor agonists and β$_1$-blockers can disturb circadian rhythms by suppression of melatonin secretion (adapted from Staedt & Riemann [151]).

which can partly be ameliorated if an appropriate daily intake time is selected. (2) The anticholinergic potential has to be considered: in most entities of dementia a cholinergic deficit exists as described above. Due to this deficit, delirious episodes can be provoked and it is therefore crucial to avoid anticholinergic medication as far as possible. (3) It should be taken into consideration that by specific medications the above-mentioned somatic conditions (RLS and SAS) can be worsened or if subclinically present can become clinically relevant. After changing a prescription patients should be monitored for the appearance of these disorders.

In selecting medication for the treatment of sleep disorders in demented patients hangover effects should be taken into account to avoid falls and reduced activity during the day. It is important to mention that the effectiveness of medication for the long-term treatment of sleep disorders in the elderly and demented has generally not been sufficiently investigated in double-blind, placebo-controlled trials.

Antidepressants

Sedating antidepressants are licensed for the treatment of depression, which often comes along with insomnia [127]. Nevertheless they are useful for treating sleep disturbances without accompanying depression [128]. They have no addictive potential,

but one should reflect on the anticholinergic potency of these drugs. An intake between 19:00 and 21:00 hours is advisable, because of the delayed action and to avoid hangover effects the next day.

The following drugs can be taken into consideration. Trimipramine (25–100 mg) facilitates deep sleep without REM-sleep suppression. Indeed there are no data of efficacy in the treatment of insomnia in elderly and demented patients available. The moderate anticholinergic potency should always be taken into account. For the same reason one should refrain from prescribing amitriptyline, which shows a five-fold higher anticholinergic potency than other TCAs [129].

The significantly less anticholinergic mirtazapine (15–45 mg) represents an alternative. However its potency for treatment of insomnia in elderly or demented persons has not yet been proven and it is according to clinical experience in severe cases less potent than trimipramine. In either case it should be used with caution in patients with known cardiac disease or renal impairment [130].

A treatment alternative without anticholinergic side effects is trazodone with combined properties as a 5-HT agonist and an antagonist with antihistaminergic activity. As orthostatic dysregulation and induction or aggravation of arrhythmias have been described as side effects it should be used with care and slowly titrated to the required dose from 25 mg to 300 mg [131]. In long-term follow-up in patients with AD compared to untreated patients significant reduction in irritability was observed [116]. In addition this drug does not worsen RLS like other tricyclic sedating antidepressants and mirtazapine.

Benzodiazepines and non-benzodiazepine hypnotics

All these substances can be used in principle up to a time period of four to six weeks for treatment of sleep disorder in dementia. Due to the risk of falling, their dependency potential, and the possibility of development of tolerance their use should be monitored [132, 133]. Especially in patients with sleep apnea syndrome, one should consider that benzodiazepines can increase oxygen depletion by muscle relaxation and elevation of the arousal threshold. Older benzodiazepines with long half-life time should not be prescribed to elderly patients, as they can increase the risk of falls and worsen cognition [134]. Clonazepam represents an exception, because it has proven positive effects in two large case series of patients with REM sleep behavior disorder [89]. But there are no controlled studies with regard to the use of clonazepam in sleep disorders in dementia. Therefore for short-time therapy the short-acting non-benzodiazepine hypnotics zolpidem and zopiclone are preferred, although one needs to mention that these substances can also elevate the risk of falling.

Zolpidem is the best studied drug with the best long-term effects for the treatment of sleep disorders at older ages. In a six-month trial it was well tolerated and dependency did not develop [135]. In contrast to zopiclone and lormetazepam, zolpidem showed no difference in comparison to placebo nine to eleven hours after intake with respect to driving ability in driving simulators [136]. So far zolpidem seems to be appropriate for the therapy of sleep disorders in elderly and demented patients. In this context it should be mentioned that we recommend 20 mg zolpidem per night for sleep disturbances in dementia.

At least eszopiclone's (the S-isomere of zopiclone) effectiveness in sleep disorders in the elderly has been proven in a two-week long trial [137]. During a 12-month, open-label treatment, eszopiclone 3 mg was well tolerated; tolerance was not observed [138].

Last but not least, it should be mentioned that chloraldurate had been used in the treatment of

insomnia before benzodiazepines became available as sleeping pills. Nowadays it is not used any more because of its high dependency potential, the possible liver and kidney side effects, and its arrhythmia-causing potential [139].

Melatonin

It is known that about half of elderly persons with sleep disorders produce less melatonin at night than age-matched persons without sleep disorders. Therefore it should be intended to increase melatonin levels through sufficient physical exercise in the open air (two hours each in the morning and afternoon). If sufficient activity in the fresh air is not feasible, melatonin levels may be improved through the use of synthetic melatonin. When trying to support the sleep–wake rhythm through the intake of melatonin (3 mg) one should consider the following: melatonin is secreted by the pineal gland usually between 20:00 and 06:00 hours. To stabilize the sleep–wake rhythm it is therefore essential to take the additional melatonin regularly at a fixed time point. In order to achieve a good response it is recommended to supplement it during the dark winter months at 20:00 hours and in the summer at 21:00 hours. This is because melatonin only acts on stabilizing and intensifying sleep if it is taken at the beginning of endogenous melatonin secretion. Long-term melatonin treatment is able to positively influence sleep–wake circadian rhythms, even in elderly demented persons. It is important to mention that in the above-mentioned study by Riemersma-van der Lek et al. [88] it was found that treatment with melatonin alone led to negative effects on mood, which could be compensated by additional bright light therapy of at least 1,000 lux in communal rooms. So it is crucial to guarantee sufficient illumination in melatonin treatment.

Antipsychotics

The prescription of antipsychotics in dementia should be judged critically and they are not recommended for the sole treatment of sleep disorders. With the use of antipsychotics in demented patients an elevated risk of cerebrovascular incidents and increased overall mortality has been observed. The following are discussed as possible mechanisms [57, 58]. In the FDA analysis on which its public health advisory was based, heart-related events (heart failure, sudden death) and infections (mostly pneumonia) accounted for the most deaths. Anticholinergic properties (affecting blood pressure and heart rate), Q-T-prolongation (causing conduction delays), and extrapyramidal symptoms (causing swallowing problems and compromised respiration) are at least as common and sometimes more common with conventional than with atypical antipsychotic agents, and are therefore possible candidates for the underlying causes. Furthermore it had been shown that classical antipsychotic drug use increases the risk of venous thromboembolism seven-fold [140]. In this context it has to be mentioned that the above-mentioned complications have to be seen as class effects, which seem to be stronger in classical antipsychotic drugs than in atypicals. For this reason the use of atypical antipsychotic medications should be preferred over classical antipsychotic medications [56, 141, 142]. Interestingly, in the study of Kozma [142] it became evident that benzodiazepine therapy as well was associated with an increase in cerebrovascular incidents. If there is no alternative available to the utilization of antipsychotics, it is suggested that risperidone (0.5–1 mg) is used as first-line therapy, especially in patients with concomitant dangerous behavioral disturbances. In clinical trials with demented patients it has been observed that treatment with riperidone results in stabilization of the sleep–wake rhythm and that in comparison to melperone, risperidone causes less dizziness, daytime sedation, and fewer gait disturbances without influencing sleep behavior. There are no data supporting positive effects of melperone on sleep in the long-term treatment in older patients. In patients with Parkinson's disease quetiapine can partially contribute to amelioration of sleep if they suffer from nocturnal agitation with hallucinations.

Acetylcholine esterase inhibitors

Nocturnal agitation in context of sleep–wake rhythm abnormalities is sometimes difficult to distinguish from delirious symptoms. The difficulties in differentiation are mainly caused by the fact that cholinergic tracts of the arousal system influence substantially arousal, attention, memory, and sleep–wake circadian rhythm. Therefore disorders of the cholinergic system can have an impact along a continuum and depending on vulnerability and peculiarity on different higher cortical functions (consciousness, attention) and/or the sleep–wake rhythm. With regard to these

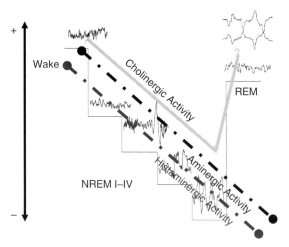

Figure 20.5 Activation of neurotransmitters throughout the sleep cycle (modified with permission from Staedt & Riemann [151]).

considerations it is comprehensible that demented patients during the course of febrile infections develop delirious symptoms. Here endogenous anticholinergic substances are produced [143]. They are able to enhance the existing cholinergic deficit by blocking of muscarinic receptors. Accordingly cholinergic neocortical activation is insufficient and a reversible delirium with restriction of higher cortical function develops.

Hence it is crucial in prescriptions of acetylcholine esterase inhibitors not only to think of cognition but also of stabilization of the sleep–wake circadian rhythm, because both areas are significantly influenced by the cholinergic system. In this context, it has to be mentioned that the effectiveness of acetylcholine esterase inhibitors in the therapy of non-cognitive symptoms is well documented [144, 145].For the above-mentioned view also indicates that under therapy with acetylcholine esterase inhibitors partial reduced prescriptions of other psychotropic drugs in demented patients were observed [146, 147]. Nevertheless acetylcholine esterase inhibitors are able to evoke in 8 to 10% of patients sleep disorders or enhanced dreams when taken in the evening [148].

As shown in Figure 20.5 the cholinergic activity drastically decreases in NREM sleep in contrast to the wake state [149, 150]. So acetylcholine esterase inhibitor induced cholinergic activation can suppress NREM sleep. For this reason in vulnerable patients the time of intake should be the morning.

References

1. Foley DJ, Monjan AA, Brown SL, *et al.* Sleep complaints among elderly persons: an epidemiologic study of three communities. *Sleep.* 1995;**18**:425–32.

2. Jelicic M, Bosma H, Ponds RW, *et al.* Subjective sleep problems in later life as predictors of cognitive decline. Report from the Maastricht Ageing Study (MAAS). *Int J Geriatr Psychiatry.* 2002;**17**:73–77.

3. Cacabelos R, Rodriguez B, Carrera C, *et al.* APOE-related frequency of cognitive and noncognitive symptoms in dementia. *Methods Find Exp Clin Pharmacol.* 1996;**18**:693–706.

4. Tractenberg RE, Singer CM, Cummings JL, *et al.* The sleep disorders inventory: an instrument for studies of sleep disturbance in persons with Alzheimer's disease. *J Sleep Res.* 2003;**12**:331–7.

5. Bliwise DL, Hughes M, McMahon PM, *et al.* Observed sleep/wakefulness and severity of dementia in an Alzheimer's disease special care unit. *J Gerontol A Biol Sci Med Sci.* 1995;**50**:303–6.

6. Prinz PN, Peskind ER, Vitaliano PP, *et al.* Changes in the sleep and waking EEGs of nondemented and demented elderly subjects. *J Am Geriatr Soc.* 1982; **30**(2):86–93.

7. Vitiello MV, Prinz PN, Williams DE, Frommlet MS, Ries RK. Sleep disturbances in patients with mild-stage Alzheimer's disease. *J Gerontol.* 1990; **45**(4):M131–8.

8. Moran M, Lynch CA, Walsh C. Sleep disturbance in mild to moderate Alzheimer's disease. *Sleep Med.* 2005;**6**(4):347–52.

9. Grassel E. Warum pflegen Angehörige? Ein Pflegemodell für die häusliche Pflege im höheren Lebensalter. *Zschr Gerontopsychol & Psychiatr.* 2000;**13**:85–94.

10. Coen RF, Swanwick GR, O'Boyle CA, *et al.* Behaviour disturbance and other predictors of carer burden Alzheimer's disease. *Int J Geriatr Psychiatry.* 1997; **12**:331–6.

11. Pollak CP, Perlick D, Linsner JP, *et al.* Sleep problem in the community elderly as predictors of death and nursing home placement. *J Commun Hlth.* 1990; **15**:123–35.

12. Kondo T, Strayer CA, Kulkarni RD, *et al.* Circadian rhythms in prokaryotes: luciferase as a reporter of circadian gene expression in cyanobacteria. *Proc Natl Acad Sci USA.* 1993;**90**(12):5672–6.

13. Sogin ML. The origin of eukaryontes and evolution into mayor kingdoms. In: Begston S, ed. *Early Life on Earth. Nobel Symposium No. 84.* (New York: Columbia University Press; 181–92).

14. Vitaterna MH, Takahashi JS, Turek FW. Overview of circadian rhythms. *Alcohol Res Health.* 2001; **25**(2):85–93.

15. Czeisler CA, Duffy JF, Shanahan TL, *et al.* Stability, precision, and near-24-hour period of the human circadian pacemaker. *Science.* 1999; **284**(5423):2177–81.

16. Edgar DM, Dement WC, Fuller CA. Effect of SCN lesions on sleep in squirrel monkeys: Evidence for opponent processes in sleep-wake regulation. *J Neurosci.* 1993;**13**(3):1065–79.

17. Provencio I, Rodriguez IR, Jiang G, *et al.* A novel human opsin in the inner retina. *J Neurosci.* 2000;**20**:600–5.

18. Hattar S, Kumar M, Park A, Tong P, Tung J, *et al.* Central projections of melanopsin-expressing retinal ganglion cells in the mouse. *J Comp Neurol.* 2006;**497**:326–49.

19. Gooley JJ, Lu J, Fischer D, Saper CB. A broad role for melanopsin in nonvisual photoreception. *J Neurosci.* 2003;**23**:7093–106.

20. Cajochen C, Münch M, Kobialka S, *et al.* High sensitivity of human melatonin, alertness, thermoregulation, and heart rate to short wavelength light. *J Clin Endocrinol Metab.* 2005;**90**(3):1311–16.

21. Vandewalle G, Schmidt C, Albouy G, *et al.* Brain responses to violet, blue, and green monochromatic light exposures in humans: prominent role of blue light and the brainstem. *PLoS One.* 2007;**2**(11):e1247.

22. Gaillard ER, Zheng L, Merriam JC, Dillon J. Age-related changes in the absorption characteristics of the primate lens. *Invest Ophthalmol Vis Sci.* 2000; **41**(6):1454–9.

23. Fetveit A, Bjorvatn B. Sleep duration during the 24-hour day is associated with the severity of dementia in nursing home patients. *J Geriatr Psychiatry.* 2006; **21**(10):945–50.

24. De Lepeleire J, Bouwen A, De Connick L, Buntinx F. Insufficient lighting in nursing homes. *J Am Med Dir Assoc.* 2007;**8**:314–17.

25. Shochat T, Martin J, Marler M, *et al.* Illumination levels in nursing home patients: effects on sleep and activity rhythms. *J Sleep Res.* 2000;**9**:373–7.

26. Harper DG, Volicer L, Stopa EG, *et al.* Disturbance of endogenous circadian rhythm in aging and Alzheimer disease. *Am J Geriatr Psychiatry.* 2005;**13**(5):359–68.

27. Tozawa T, Mishima K, Satoh K, *et al.* Stability of sleep timing against the melatonin secretion rhythm with advancing age: clinical implications. *J Clin Endocrinol Metab.* 2003;**88**(10):4689–95.

28. Wu YH, Feenstra MG, Zhou JN, *et al.* Molecular changes underlying reduced pineal melatonin levels in

Alzheimer's disease: alterations in preclinical and clinical stages. *J Clin Endocrinol Metab.* 2003;**88**:5898–906.

29. Wu YH, Swaab DF. The human pineal gland and melatonin in aging and Alzheimer's disease. *J Pineal Res.* 2005;**38**:145–52.

30. Wu YH, Fischer DF, Kalsbeek A, *et al.* Pineal clock gene oscillation is disturbed in Alzheimer's disease, due to functional disconnection from the "master clock". *FASEB J.* 2006;**20**(11):1874–6.

31. Neuropathology Group. Medical Research Council Cognitive Function and Ageing Study. Pathological correlates of late-onset dementia in a multicenter, community-based population in England and Wales. *Lancet.* 2001;**357**:169–75.

32. McGeer PL, McGeer EG, Suzuki J, *et al.* Aging, Alzheimer's disease, and the cholinergic system of the basal forebrain. *Neurology.* 1984;**34**:741–5.

33. Reinikainen KJ, Riekkinen PJ, Paljärvi L, *et al.* Cholinergic deficit in Alzheimer's disease: a study based on CSF and autopsy data. *Neurochem Res.* 1988;**13**:135–46.

34. Nunez A. Unit activity of rat basal forebrain neurons: relationship to cortical activity. *Neuroscience.* 1996;**72**:757–66.

35. Steriade M. Acetylcholine systems and rhythmic activities during the waking–sleep cycle. *Prog Brain Res.* 2004;**145**:179–96.

36. Riekkinen J Jr., Sirviö J, Riekkinen P. Relation between EEG delta power and the cortical choline acetyltransferase content. *Neurosci Res.* 1990;**8**:12–20.

37. Yoon IY, Kripke DF, Elliott JA, *et al.* Age-related changes of circadian rhythms and sleep–wake cycles. *Am Geriatr Soc.* 2003;**51**:1085–91.

38. Dijk DJ, Duffy JF, Czeisler CA. Age-related increase in awakenings: impaired consolidation of nonREM sleep at all circadian phases. *Sleep.* 2001;**24**(5):565–77.

39. Onen F, Onen SH. Sleep rhythm disturbances in Alzheimer's disease. *Rev Med Interne.* 2003;**24**:165–71.

40. Reynolds CF 3rd, Monk TH, Hoch CC, *et al.* Electroencephalographic sleep in the healthy "old old": a comparison with the "young old" in visually scored and automated measures. *J Gerontol.* 1991;**46**(2):M39–46.

41. Staedt J, Riemann D. Alzheimer-Demenz. In: J Staedt, D Riemann eds. *Diagnostik und Therapie von Schlafstörungen.* (Kohlhammer, Germany: Publisher Stuttgart, 2007; 65–7).

42. Walker MP, Stickgold R. Sleep, memory, and plasticity. *Annu Rev Psychol.* 2006;**57**:139–66.

43. Staedt J, Stoppe G. Are sleep and its disorders of interest for psychiatric and psychosomatic medicine? In: Diefenbacher A, ed. *Advances in Psychosomatic Medicine, Vol 26.* (Basel: Karger, 2004; 1–6).

44. Guzman-Marin R, Suntsova N, Methippara M, *et al.* Sleep deprivation suppresses neurogenesis in the adult hippocampus of rats. *Eur J Neurosci.* 2005; **22**(8):2111–16.

45. Cirelli C. A molecular window on sleep: changes in gene expression between sleep and wakefulness. *Neuroscientist.* 2005;**11**(1):63–74.

46. Frank MG, Jha SK, Coleman T. Blockade of postsynaptic activity in sleep inhibits developmental plasticity in visual cortex. *Neuroreport.* 2006; **17**(13):1459–63.

47. Bliwise DL. What is sundowning? *J Am Geriatr Soc.* 1994;**42**:1009–11.

48. Evans LK. Sundown syndrome in institutionalized elderly. *J Am Geriatr Soc.* 1987;**35**:101–8.

49. Martin J, Marler M, Shochat T, *et al.* Circadian rhythms of agitation in institutionalized patients with Alzheimer's disease. *Chronobiol Int.* 2000; **17**:405–18.

50. Gallagher-Thompson D, Brooks JO III, *et al.* The relations among caregiver stress, "sundowning" symptoms, and cognitive decline in Alzheimer's disease. *J Am Geriatr Soc.* 1992;**40**:807–10.

51. Aston-Jones G, Chen S, Zhu Y, Oshinsky ML. A neural circuit for circadian regulation of arousal. *Nat Neurosci.* 2001;**4**:732–8.

52. Volicer L, Harper DG, Manning BC, *et al.* Sundowning and circadian rhythms in Alzheimer's disease. *Am J Psychiatry.* 2001;**158**:704–11.

53. Burgio LD, Scilley K, Hardin M, *et al.* Temporal patterns of disruptive vocalization in elderly nursing home residents. *Int J Geriatr Psychiatry.* 2001;**16**:378–86.

54. Jellinger K. Alterations of muscarinic acetylcholine receptor subtypes in diffuse Lewy body disease: relation to Alzheimer's disease. *J Neurol Neurosurg Psychiatry.* 2000;**68**:253–4.

55. Perry R, McKeith I, Perry E. Lewy body dementia – clinical, pathological and neurochemical interconnections. *J Neural Transm Suppl.* 1997; **51**:95–109.

56. Gill SS, Bronskill SE, Normand ST, *et al.* Antipsychotic drug use and mortality in older adults with dementia. *Ann Intern Med.* 2007;**146**:775–86.

57. Setoguchi S, Wang PS, Brookhart MA, *et al.* Potential causes of higher mortality in elderly users of conventional and atypical antipsychotic medications. *JAGS.* 2008;**56**:1644–50.

237

58. Schneeweiss S, Setoguchi S, Brookhart MA, Dormuth C, Wang PS. Risk of death associated with the use of conventional versus atypical antipsychotic drugs among elderly patients. *CMAJ.* 2007;**176**(5):627–32.

59. Chan YC, Pariser SF, Neufeld G. Atypical antipsychotics in older adults. *Pharmacotherapy.* 1999;**19**:811–22.

60. Lacut K, Le Gal G, Couturaud F, *et al.* Association between antipsychotic drugs, antidepressant drugs and venous thromboembolism: results from the EDITH case-control study. *Fundam Clin Pharmacol.* 2007; **21**(6):643–50.

61. Lawlor BA. Behavioral and psychological symptoms in dementia: The role of atypical antipsychotics. *J Clin Psychiatry.* 2004;**65** (Suppl 11):5–10.

62. Liperoti R, Gambassi G, Lapane KL, *et al.* Cerebrovascular events among elderly nursing home patients treated with conventional or atypical antipsychotics. *J Clin Psychiatry.* 2005;**66**:1090–6.

63. Maixner SM, Mellow AM, Tandon R. The efficacy, safety, and tolerability of antipsychotics in the elderly. *J Clin Psychiatry.* 1999;**60** (Suppl 8):29–41.

64. Tariot PN. The older patient: the ongoing challenge of efficacy and tolerability. *J Clin Psychiatry.* 1999; **60** (Suppl 23):29–33.

65. Yuen EJ, Zisselman MH, Louis DZ, *et al.* Sedative-hypnotic use by the elderly: Effects on hospital length of stay and costs. *J Ment Hlth Administr.* 1997;**24**:90–7.

66. Ancoli-Israel S, Kripke DF. Now I lay me down to sleep: the problem of sleep fragmentation in the elderly and demented residents of nursing homes. *Bull Clin Neurosci.* 1989;**1154**:127–32.

67. Stoppe G, Brandt C, Staedt J. Behavioural problems associated with dementia: the role of newer antipsychotics. *Drugs Aging.* 1999;**14**:41–54.

68. Aarsland D, Laake K, Larsen JP, *et al.* Donepezil for cognitive impairment in Parkinson's disease: a randomised controlled study. *J Neurol Neurosurg Psychiatry.* 2002;**72**:708–12.

69. Black S, Roman GC, Geldmacher DS, *et al.* Donepezil 307 Vascular Dementia Study Group. Efficacy and tolerability of donepezil in vascular dementia: positive results of a 24-week, multicenter, international, randomized, placebo-controlled clinical trial. *Stroke.* 2003;**34**:2323–30.

70. Bullock R. Cholinesterase inhibitors and vascular dementia: another string to their bow? *CNS Drugs.* 2004;**18**:79–92.

71. Burns A, Spiegel R, Quarg P. Efficacy of rivastigmine in subjects with moderately severe Alzheimer's disease. *Int J Geriatr Psychiatry.* 2004;**19**:243–9.

72. Erkinjuntti T, Kurz A, Gauthier S, *et al.* Efficacy of galantamine in probable vascular dementia and Alzheimer's disease combined with cerebrovascular disease: a randomised trial. *Lancet.* 2002;**359**:1283–90.

73. Feldman H, Gauthier S, Hecker J, *et al.* Donepezil MSAD Study Investigators Group. A 24-week, randomized, double-blind study of donepezil in moderate to severe Alzheimer's disease. *Neurology.* 2001;**57**:613–20.

74. Kurz AF, Erkinjuntti T, Small GW, *et al.* Long-term safety and cognitive effects of galantamine in the treatment of probable vascular dementia or Alzheimer's disease with cerebrovascular disease. *Eur J Neurol.* 2003;**10**:633–40.

75. Malouf R, Birks J. Donepezil for vascular cognitive impairment. *Cochrane Database.* 2004;Syst Rev(1): CD004395.

76. McKeith IG, Grace JB, Walker Z, *et al.* Rivastigmine in the treatment of dementia with Lewy bodies: preliminary findings from an open trial. *Int J Geriatr Psychiatry.* 2000;**15**:387–92.

77. Moretti R, Torre P, Antonello RM, *et al.* Rivastigmine in subcortical vascular dementia: a randomized, controlled, open 12-month study in 208 patients. *Am J Alzheimers Dis Other Demen.* 2003;**18**:265–72.

78. Wilkinson D, Doody R, Helme R, *et al.* Donepezil in vascular dementia: a randomized, placebo-controlled study. *Neurology.* 2003;**61**:479–86.

79. Samuel W, Caligiuri M, Galasko D, *et al.* Better cognitive and psychopathologic response to donepezil in patients prospectively diagnosed as dementia with Lewy bodies: a preliminary study. *Int J Geriatr Psychiatry.* 2000;**15**:794–802.

80. Trinh NH, Hoblyn J, Mohanty S, *et al.* Efficacy of cholinesterase inhibitors in the treatment of neuropsychiatric symptoms and functional impairment in Alzheimer disease: a meta-analysis. *JAMA.* 2003;**289**:210–16.

81. Liu C, Weaver DR, Jin X, *et al.* Molecular dissection of two distinct actions of melatonin on suprachiasmatic circadian clock. *Neuron.* 1997;**19**:91–102.

82. Jin X, von Gall C, Pieschl RL, *et al.* Targeted disruption of the mouse Mel(1b) melatonin receptor. *Mol Cell Biol.* 2003;**23**:1054–60.

83. Wyatt JK, Dijk DJ, Ritz-de Cecco A, Ronda JM, vi CA. Sleep-facilitating effect of exogenous melatonin in healthy young men and women is circadian-phase dependent. *Sleep.* 2006;**29**(5):609–18.

84. Gorfine T, Assaf Y, Goshen-Gottstein Y, *et al.* Sleep-anticipating effects of melatonin in the human brain. *Neuroimage.* 2006;**31**:410–18.

85. Asayama K, Yamadera H, Ito T, *et al.* Double blind study of melatonin effects on the sleep–wake rhythm, cognitive and noncognitive functions in Alzheimer type dementia. *J Nippon Med Sch.* 2003;**70**:334–41.

86. Serfaty M, Kennell-Webb S, Warner J, *et al.* Double blind randomised placebo controlled trial of low dose melatonin for sleep disorders in dementia. *Int J Geriatr Psychiatry.* 2002;**17**:1120–7.

87. Singer C, Tractenberg RE, Kaye J, *et al.* Alzheimer's Disease Cooperative Study. A multicenter, placebo-controlled trial of melatonin for sleep disturbance in Alzheimer's disease. *Sleep.* 2003; **26**:893–901.

88. Riemersma-van der Lek RF, Swaab DF, Twisk J, *et al.* Effect of bright light and melatonin on cognitive and noncognitive function in elderly residents of group care facilities: a randomized controlled trial. *JAMA.* 2008;**299**(22):2642–55.

89. Gagnon JF, Postuma RB, Montplaisir J. Update on the pharmacology of REM sleep behavior disorder. *Neurology.* 2006;**67**(5):742–7.

90. Schenk CH, Mahowald MW. REM sleep behavior disorder: clinical, developmental, and neuroscience perspectives 16 years after its formal identification. *Sleep.* 2002;**25**:120–38.

91. Olson EJ, Boeve BF, Silber MH. Rapid eye movement sleep behaviour disorder: demographic, clinical and laboratory findings in 93 cases. *Brain.* 2000;**123**:331–9.

92. Takakusaki K, Saitoh K, Harada H, Kashiwayanagi M. Role of basal ganglia-brainstem pathways in the control of motor behaviours. *Neurosci Res.* 2004;**50**:137–51.

93. Bliwise DL, Adelman CL, Ouslander JG. Polysomnographic correlates of spontaneous nocturnal wetness episodes in incontinent geriatric patients. *Sleep.* 2004;**27**:153–7.

94. Chong MS, Ayalon L, Marler M, *et al.* Continuous positive airway pressure reduces subjective daytime sleepiness in patients with mild to moderate Alzheimer's disease with sleep disordered breathing. *J Am Geriatr Soc.* 2006;**54**(5):777–81.

95. Martin JL, Mory AK, Alessi CA. Nighttime oxygen desaturation and symptoms of sleep-disordered breathing in long-stay nursing home residents. *J Gerontol A Biol Sci Med Sci.* 2005;**60**:104–8.

96. Bassetti C, Aldrich MS, Chervin RD, *et al.* Sleep apnea in patients with transient ischemic attack and stroke. *Neurology.* 1996;**47**:1167–73.

97. Ancoli-Israel S, Palmer BW, Cooke JR, *et al.* Cognitive effects of treating obstructive sleep apnea in Alzheimer's disease: a randomized controlled study. *J Am Geriatr Soc.* 2008;**56**(11):2076–81.

98. Ayalon L, Ancoli-Israel S, Stepnowsky C, *et al.* Adherence to continuous positive airway pressure treatment in patients with Alzheimer's disease and obstructive sleep apnea. *Am J Geriatr Psychiatry.* 2006;**14**:176–80.

99. Moraes W, Poyares D, Sukys-Claudino L, Guilleminault C, Tufik S. Donepezil improves obstructive sleep apnea in Alzheimer disease: a double-blind, placebo-controlled study. *Chest.* 2008;**133**(3):677–83.

100. Obler SK. Leg symptoms in outpatient veterans. *West J Med.* 1991;**155**:256.

101. Ancoli-Israel S, Kripke DF, Klauber MR, *et al.* Periodic limb movements in sleep in community dwelling elderly. *Sleep.* 1991;**14**:496–500.

102. Staedt J, Stoppe G, Kogler A, *et al.* Nocturnal myoclonus syndrome (periodic movements in sleep) related to central dopamine D2-receptor alteration. *Eur Arch Psychiatry Clin Neurosci.* 1995;**245**:8–10.

103. Garcia-Borreguero D, Grunstein R, Sridhar G, *et al.* A 52-week open-label study of the long-term safety of ropinirole in patients with restless legs syndrome. *Sleep Med.* 2007;**8**(7–8):742–52.

104. Montplaisir J, Fantini ML, Desautels A, *et al.* Long-term treatment with pramipexol in restless legs syndrome. *Eur J Neurol.* 2006;**13**(12):1306–11.

105. Staedt J, Hünerjager H, Rüther E, *et al.* Pergolide: treatment of choice in restless legs syndrome (RLS) and nocturnal myoclonus syndrome (NMS). Longterm follow up on pergolide. *J Neural Transm.* 1998;**105**:265–8.

106. Hohl-Radke F, Dewes D, Staedt J. Schlafstörungen und periodische Beinbewegungen bei Patienten mit Schizophrenien und schizoaffektiven Psychosen. Korrelation mit dem Lebensalter und mit der Dauer der Antipsychotikaeinnahme. *NeuroGer.* 2006;**1**(2):85–92.

107. Horiguchi J, Yamashita H, Mizuno S, *et al.* Nocturnal eating/drinking syndrome and neuroleptic-induced restless legs syndrome. *Int Clin Psychopharmacol.* 1999;**14**:33–6.

108. Kraus T, Schuld A, Pollmacher T. Restless legs syndrome probably caused by olanzapine. *J Clin Psychopharmacol.* 1999;**19**:478–9.

109. Yang C, White DP, Winkelman JW. Antidepressants and periodic leg movements of sleep. *Biol Psychiatry.* 2005;**58**:510–14.

110. Wetter TC, Brunner J, Bronisch T. Restless legs syndrome probably induced by risperidone treatment. *Pharmacopsychiatry.* 2002;**35**:109–11.

111. Ancoli-Israel S, Cole R, Alessi C, *et al.* The role of actigraphy in the study of sleep and circadian rhythms. *Sleep.* 2003;**26**:342–92.

112. Sforza E, Johannes M, Claudio B. The PAM-RL ambulatory device for detection of periodic leg movements: a validation study. *Sleep Med.* 2005;**6**:407–13.

113. King MA, Jaffre MO, Morrish E, *et al.* The validation of a new actigraphy system for the measurement of periodic leg movements in sleep. *Sleep Med.* 2005;**6**:1–7.

114. Nofzinger EA, Fasiczka A, Berman S, Thase ME. Bupropion SR reduces periodic limb movements associated with arousal from sleep in depressed patients with periodic limb movements. *J Clin Psychiatry.* 2000;**61**(11):858–62.

115. Saletu-Zyhlarz GM, Abu-Bakr MH, Anderer P, *et al.* Insomnia related to dysthymia: polysomnographic and psychometric comparison with normal controls and acute therapeutic trials with trazodone. *Neuropsychobiology.* 2001;**44**(3):139–49.

116. López-Pousa S, Garre-Olmo J, Vilalta-Franch J, Turon-Estrada A, Pericot-Nierga I. Trazodone for Alzheimer's disease: a naturalistic follow-up study. *Arch Gerontol Geriatr.* 2008;**47**(2):207–15.

117. Mishima K, Okawa M, Shimizu T, *et al.* Diminished melatonin secretion in the elderly caused by insufficient environmental illumination. *J Clin Endocrinol Metabol.* 2001;**86**:129–34.

118. Haffmans PM, Sival RC, Lucius SA, *et al.* Bright light therapy and melatonin in motor restless behaviour in dementia: a placebo-controlled study. *Int J Geriatr Psychiatry.* 2001;**16**:106–10.

119. Satlin A, Volicer L, Ross V, *et al.* Bright light treatment of behavioural and sleep disturbances in patients with Alzheimer's disease. *Am J Psychiatry.* 1992;**149**:1028–32.

120. Lyketsos CG, Lindell Veiel L, Baker A, *et al.* A randomized, controlled trial of bright light therapy for agitated behaviours in dementia patients residing in long-term care. *Int J Geriatr Psychiatry.* 1999;**14**:520–5.

121. Okumoto Y, Koyama E, Matsubara H, *et al.* Sleep improvement by light in a demented aged individual. *Psychiatry Clin Neurosci.* 1998,**52**:194–6.

122. Graf A, Wallner C, Schubert V, *et al.* The effects of light therapy on mini-mental state examination scores in demented patients. *Biol Psychiatry.* 2001;**50**:725–7.

123. Yamadera H, Ito T, Suzuki H, *et al.* Effects of bright light on cognitive and sleep-wake (circadian) rhythm disturbances in Alzheimer-type dementia. *Psychiatry Clin Neurosci.* 2000;**54**:352.

124. Van Someren EJ, Kessler A, Mirmiran M, *et al.* Indirect bright light improves circadian rest-activity rhythm disturbances in demented patients. *Biol Psychiatry.* 1997;**41**:955–63.

125. Fontana Gasio PF, Krauchli K, Cajochen C, *et al.* Dawn-dusk simulation light therapy of disturbed circadian rest-activity cycles in demented elderly. *Experiment Gerontol.* 2003;**38**:207–16.

126. Ancoli-Israel S, Martin JL, Gehrman P, *et al.* Effect of light on agitation in institutionalized patients with severe Alzheimer disease. *Am J Geriatr Psychiatry.* 2003;**11**:194–203.

127. McCall WV, Fleischer AB Jr., Feldman SR. Diagnose codes associated with hypnotic medications during outpatient physician-patient encounters in the United States from 1990–1998. *Sleep.* 2002;**25**:221–3.

128. Silber MH. Clinical practice. Chronic insomnia. *N Engl J Med.* 2005;**353**(8):803–10.

129. Richelson E. The clinical relevance of antidepressant interaction with neurotransmitter transporters and receptors. *Psychopharmacol Bull.* 2002; **36**:133–50.

130. Chavez B. Pharmacotherapy in managing insomnia. Assessing patient needs and outcomes [serial online]. *Pharm.* 2005;**2**:HS23–6.

131. Benca RM. Diagnosis and treatment of chronic insomnia: a review. *Psychiatr Serv.* 2005;**56**:332–43.

132. Holbrook AM, Crowther R, Lotter A, *et al.* Metaanalysis of benzodiazepine use in the treatment of insomnia. *CMAJ.* 2000;**162**:225–33.

133. Leipzig RM, Cumming RG, Tinetti ME. Drugs and falls in older people: a systemic review and metaanalysis: I. Psychotropic drugs. *J Am Geriatr Soc.* 1999;**47**:30–9.

134. Barker MJ, Greenwood KM, Jackson M, Crowe SF. Persistence of cognitive effects after withdrawal from long-term benzodiazepine use: a meta analysis. *Arch Clin Neuropsychol.* 2004;**19**:437–54.

135. Schlich D, L'Heritier C, Coquelin JP, *et al.* Long-term treatment of insomnia with zolpidem: a multicenter general practitioner study of 107 patients. *J Int Med Res.* 1991;**19**:271–9.

136. Staner L, Ertlé S, Boeijinga P, *et al.* Next-day residual effects of hypnotics in DSM-IV primary insomnia: a driving simulator study with simultaneous electroencephalogram monitoring. *Psychopharmacology (Berl).* 2005;**181**(4):790–8.

137. Scharf M, Erman M, Rosenberg R, *et al.* A 2-week efficacy and safety study of eszopiclone in elderly patients with primary insomnia. *Sleep.* 2005; **28**:720–7.

138. Roth T, Stubbs C, Walsh JK. Ramelteon (TAK-375), a selective MT1/MT2-receptor agonist, reduces latency to persistent sleep in a model of transient insomnia related to a novel sleep environment. *Sleep.* 2005;**28**(3):303–7.

139. Simonson W. Pharmacists' role in recognizing and managing patients with insomnia. *Pharm Times.* 2004;**70** Suppl:1–8.

140. Zornberg GL, Jick H. Antipsychotic drug use and risk of first-time idiopathic venous thromboembolism: a case-control study. *Lancet.* 2000;**356**:1219–23.

141. Wang PS, Schneeweiss S, Avorn J, *et al.* Risk of death in elderly users of conventional vs. atypical antipsychotic medications. *N Engl J Med.* 2005;**353**:2335–41.

142. Kozma CM, Engelhart LM, Long S, *et al.* Absence of increased relative stroke risk in elderly dementia patients treated with risperidone versus other antipsychotics. *ICGP Program Book.* 2003.

143. Flacker JM, Wie JY. Endogenous anticholinergic substances may exist during acute illness in elderly medical patients. *J Gerontol.* 2001;**56A**:M353–5.

144. Holmes C, Wilkinson D, Dean C, *et al.* The efficacy of donepezil in the treatment of neuropsychiatric symptoms in Alzheimer's disease. *Neurology.* 2004;**63**:214–19.

145. Trinh NH, Hoblyn J, Mohanty S, Yaffe K. Efficacy of cholinesterase inhibitors in the treatment of neuropsychiatric symptoms and functional impairment in Alzheimer's disease: a meta-analysis. *JAMA.* 2003;**289**(2):210–16.

146. Robert P. Understanding and managing behavioural symptoms in Alzheimer's disease and related dementias: focus on rivastigmine. *Curr Med Res Opin.* **18**:156–71.

147. Edwards K, Koumaras B, Chen M, Gunay I, Mirski D; and the Rivastigmine Nursing Home Study Team. Long-term effects of rivastigmine treatment on the need for psychotropic medications in nursing home patients with Alzheimer's disease: results of a 52-week open-label study. *Clin Drug Investig.* 2005; **25**(8):507–15.

148. Stahl SM, Markowitz JS, Gutterman EM, Papadopoulos G. Co-use of donepezil and hypnotics among Alzheimer's disease patients living in the community. *J Clin Psychiatry.* 2003;**64**(4):466–72.

149. Hobson JA. Sleep and dreaming: induction and mediation of REM sleep by cholinergic mechanisms. *Curr Opin Neurobiol.* 1992;**2**:759–63.

150. Marrosu F, Portas C, Mascia MS, *et al.* Microdialysis measurement of cortical and hippocampal acetylcholine release during sleep-wake cycle in freely moving cats. *Brain Res.* 1995; **671**:329–32.

151. Staedt J, Riemann D. *Diagnostik und Therapie von Schlafstörungen.* (Stuttgart, Germany: Kohlhammer Publisher, 2007).

Sleep and attention-deficit/hyperactivity disorder: science and clinical practice

Reut Gruber and Paolo De Luca

Overview

Attention-deficit/hyperactivity disorder (ADHD) is characterized by impulsivity/hyperactivity and inattention [1]. Attention-deficit/hyperactivity disorder is estimated to occur in 3 to 7.5% of school-age children, making it one of the most prevalent child psychiatric conditions. A recent report demonstrated that 50% of children diagnosed with ADHD show clinically significant symptoms and impairment as young adults [2]. Onset before the age of seven years and impaired functioning in two or more settings are required for diagnosis. The DSM-IV [1] defines four types of ADHD: "predominantly inattentive," "predominantly hyperactive-impulsive," "combined," and "not otherwise specified."

The Center for Disease Control and Prevention has labeled ADHD "a serious public health problem" [2], citing the high estimated prevalence of the disorder, significant child impairment in the areas of school performance and socialization, the chronicity of the disorder, and the limited effectiveness of current interventions in the treatment of impairments associated with ADHD. If untreated, individuals with ADHD struggle with difficulties in crucial areas of life [3].

Sleep problems, particularly difficulties in initiating and maintaining sleep, are reported in clinical practice in an estimated 25 to 50% of children and adolescents with ADHD [4]. Restless and disturbed sleep was initially included in the DSM diagnostic criteria for ADHD, but was later excluded as non-specific. In general, the association between ADHD and sleep disturbance has been relatively overlooked in research conducted on ADHD populations.

Understanding the association between sleep and ADHD is important from both neurobiological and clinical perspectives. From a neurobiological viewpoint,

such understanding will offer insight into ADHD pathophysiological mechanisms. From a clinical standpoint, such work might allow better management of ADHD sleep problems, and development of intervention strategies. This chapter reviews information on research methods used in the study of sleep and ADHD, empirical findings regarding the association between sleep and ADHD, and potential explanations of the neurobiological mechanisms that underlie this association. In addition, clinical implications for treatment of sleep disorders in youths with ADHD are discussed.

Research methods used to study sleep in ADHD patients

It has been suggested that both children and adults with ADHD may be especially sensitive to perturbations in the sleep environment, and may have a heightened or altered perception of disturbances in sleep quality [3, 4]. This stresses the importance of selecting sleep-recording methods that are both objective, to minimize bias, but that also offer minimal interference with or change in the sleep environment. Both objective and subjective measures have been used to record sleep in ADHD individuals. Each approach has both advantages and limitations, as will be described below.

Objective measures used to study sleep in individuals with ADHD

The objective measures used are actigraphy and polysomnography. Actigraphy is continuous activity monitoring using a wristwatch-like device that measures body movements. Movement patterns are analyzed and used to differentiate between sleep and wake time, and to derive information on sleep onset latency, sleep duration, number of arousals, sleep schedule, and other variables. The simple, non-intrusive nature of the technique, and the fact that objective information may be obtained over long periods, makes actigraphy useful in ADHD research. This is because intrusion is minimal and several consecutive night sleep patterns may be recorded at home. Unstable sleep patterns are common in ADHD children and medium-term monitoring is important. However, the technique does not record important biophysiological parameters.

Polysomnographic (PSG) analysis, a multi-parametric test used to record biophysiological changes during sleep, has also been used to record sleep in individuals with ADHD. Given the relatively high prevalence of restless legs syndrome (RLS)/periodic leg movement disorder (PLMD) and breathing problems in ADHD children, as well as increased daytime fatigue, these measures are of scientific interest and clinical relevance. However, a disadvantage of this method is that the child is required to sleep in a laboratory, decreasing the ecological validity of the measurement. The technique can also lead to stress or sleep-adjustment difficulties causing alterations in typical sleep characteristics, such as longer sleep latency or lower sleep efficiency. Finally, the approach increases demands on participants and their families who have to change their routine and sleep away from home. Indeed, an increase in "first night" PSG effects and responsiveness to an adaptation night have been found in children and adults with ADHD [4]. In addition, there are consistent discrepancies between subjective reports and objective sleep-parameter measurements in ADHD individuals. These findings challenge the validity of the data in a population that may be relatively more sensitive and vulnerable to environmental perturbations.

Recently, portable PSG equipment has been used for in-home measurement of sleep architecture parameters in ADHD children [5]; this solves some of the problems mentioned above. The use of portable PSG equipment has been validated and successfully used in clinical populations [6, 7]. This approach offers a number of benefits for researchers: (1) ecological validity is improved; (2) laboratory stress or adjustment difficulties manifested in distinct sleep characteristics (e.g., longer sleep latency, lower sleep efficiency) [8] are eliminated; and (3) family inconvenience is minimized.

Subjective measures used to study sleep in individuals with ADHD

Parental reports are frequently used as measures of major pediatric sleep complaints. Such measures include the Pediatric Sleep Questionnaire addressing sleep-disordered breathing, snoring, and sleepiness [9], and the Children's Sleep Habits Questionnaire (CSHQ) [10]. The CSHQ is a retrospective, 45-item parent questionnaire that has been used in a number of studies to examine sleep behavior in young children. The CSHQ includes items relating to a number of key sleep domains, including sleep duration, sleep anxiety (e.g., whether the child needs a parent in the room to sleep or is afraid of sleeping in the dark), night waking, parasomnias, sleep disordered breathing, and daytime sleepiness.

In addition, sleep logs documenting bedtime, wake-up time, and night-time arousals, are frequently used either alone or to supplement actigraphic evaluation.

Empirical findings on the association between sleep and ADHD

Integration of findings from objective and subjective sources offers a comprehensive picture of sleep architecture, sleep movement, patterns, and disorders in ADHD individuals. Interestingly, whereas parental reports indicate a two- to three-fold higher prevalence of sleep problems in children with ADHD compared to controls [11–18], objective studies have yielded inconsistent findings. The next section will therefore review findings from objective and subjective measures[1].

Findings from objective measures
Sleep architecture in children with ADHD

Polysomnographic studies have failed to reveal consistent differences in objective sleep parameters between children with ADHD and controls [4]. Some studies have found no differences at all, whereas others have yielded varied and often contradictory findings, principally in relation to rapid eye movement (REM) sleep abnormalities in ADHD children [19, 20]. For example, whereas some studies have documented significant decreases in REM sleep [21, 22], others have shown significant increases [21], and also notable decreases in REM latency [21, 22], in ADHD children compared to controls. In addition, some studies have found a significantly higher number of sleep cycles in ADHD children relative to healthy controls [21], as well as shorter mean total sleep times [5].

Two recent meta-analyses reviewed data on sleep disorders in ADHD children, seeking factors that might account for the seemingly inconsistent results derived from PSG studies on ADHD children [23, 24], as well as for the differences observed in studies using objective versus subjective sleep. It was shown that age, gender, diagnostic criteria, the use of clinical samples, the need for the child to adapt to the laboratory environment, the presence of comorbid psychiatric problems, and the use of stimulant medication moderate the observed associations between sleep characteristics and ADHD.

A recent study aimed to increase ecological validity, and to limit the problems associated with laboratory recordings, by using portable PSG equipment. This approach minimized interference with normal sleep conditions. The study recruited children with ADHD without comorbid conditions, and controlled for the impact of family factors on child sleep. The findings indicated that ADHD children had less REM sleep than controls. A limitation of the study was small sample size. Future work, using the portable equipment in larger samples, and comparison of ADHD children either taking or not taking medication, will be valuable.

Findings from actigraphic studies
Sleep patterns in children with ADHD

Sleep patterning refers to timing of sleep and wake-up over a prolonged period of time. Actigraphic studies have suggested that ADHD children tend to have unstable sleep patterns [25, 26]. Increased instability in sleep onset, sleep duration, and less true sleep, were found in ADHD individuals compared to controls. Clinical and research data have suggested that delayed endogenous circadian rhythm impairs the timing of sleep and waking periods. Indication of delayed endogenous circadian rhythm has been found in ADHD individuals [27]. A possible association between circadian-related sleep parameters and daytime functioning in ADHD children requires further research that could benefit from the use of actigraphy.

Findings from subjective sleep measures regarding sleep problems in children with ADHD
Reported sleep problems in children with ADHD

The most commonly reported sleep problems include difficulty falling asleep, as reported by parents [28–30] or documented by actigraphy [31], and recorded in some PSG studies [32]. In addition, bedtime resistance, night awakening, restless sleep, and difficulties wakening in the morning have been documented in ADHD populations. Recently, a few studies have shown that ADHD symptomatology (whether the child is of the ADHD-inattentive subtype or the ADHD-hyperactive subtype) appears to be related to ADHD sleep problems.

However, the nature of this association is inconsistent, with one study showing that sleep problems are more common in the ADHD-hyperactive and ADHD-comorbid subtypes, and not in the ADHD-inattentive subtype [34]; in the ADHD-inattentive subtype [33]; or in the ADHD-comorbid subtype [35]. Hence, additional study in this area would help provide an increasingly clearer understanding about the association between sleep and ADHD. Additionally, further insight can also be gained by examining the potential mechanisms that underlie this association.

Potential mechanisms underlying the association between sleep and ADHD

The following section examines the hypothesis that sleep deprivation underlies neurobehavioral symptoms and daytime sleepiness in ADHD children.

Previous studies have shown an association between sleep disturbance and ADHD, and that the symptoms of ADHD and sleep disorders frequently overlap. Given the complexity of these relationships and the magnitude of both ADHD and sleep disorders in the pediatric population, it is vital to identify the mechanism by which these disorders interact.

Does sleep deprivation underlie neurobehavioral symptoms and daytime sleepiness in ADHD children?

Pediatric, clinical, and research data have suggested that inadequate sleep results in tiredness and daytime difficulties with focused attention, learning, and impulse modulation [36–38]. In 1991, Dahl and colleagues [39] observed that these difficulties are very similar to the core symptoms of ADHD. Subsequently, Chervin and others [40], Gozal and colleagues [41–43], and other researchers [44, 45] have studied the association between sleep and neurobehavioral functioning in ADHD children with sleep-disordered breathing (ADHD-SDB) and in children with ADHD and RLS/PLMD. These studies consistently showed that sleep disruption was associated with hyperactivity and inattention. Additional work showed that treatment of sleep problems resulted in improved behavior and a decreased need for stimulant medication in children with ADHD-SDB [46] or ADHD with RLS/PLMD [47–49]. Although these studies provide convincing evidence that sleep and neurobehavioral functioning interact in children with ADHD-SDB, it is unknown whether this holds true for the larger cohort of children with ADHD that do not suffer from sleep apnea, SDB, or RLS/PLMD.

Sleep is thought to be involved in restoring brain function after the day's activities [50], and this process is believed to be intimately linked to daily neuronal workload [51]. Beebe and Gozal [52] suggested that in children with ADHD-SDB, sleep disruption interferes with the completion of sleep-related restorative processes, which are thought to be critical for recovery of the prefrontal regions of the brain cortex (PFC) from intensive effort during wakefulness [53–55]. These findings led researchers to hypothesize that sleep disruption impairs PFC function and results in "executive dysfunctions," such as the cognitive and behavioral deficits found in children with ADHD-SDB [56]. The following sections review evidence that supports such a hypothesis in children with ADHD that do not suffer from sleep apnea, SDB, or RLS/PLM.

Relationship between insufficient sleep and ADHD

Evidence for excessive daytime sleepiness in children with ADHD

From both clinical and experimental standpoints, the most reliable observable manifestation of insufficient or poor-quality sleep is excessive daytime sleepiness. Objective studies designed to assess fatigue/alertness revealed that children with ADHD exhibited significantly more daytime sleepiness than controls [57–59]. These studies used the Multiple Sleep Latency Test (MSLT), which measures the speed of falling asleep under standard conditions, and in which a shorter sleep latency period indicates a higher level of physiological sleepiness [60, 61]. Children with ADHD had shorter sleep onset latency periods than had controls, suggesting a pathological level of sleepiness.

Electroencephalography studies have shown that children with ADHD are prone to daytime hypo-arousal characterized by increased theta activity (primarily in the frontal areas), decreased alpha and beta activity, and increased theta/alpha and theta/beta ratios [61–63], compared to normal children. Sustained wakefulness and sleep deprivation caused similarly increased theta and decreased alpha activities in normal participants [64], suggesting that children with ADHD suffer from daytime sleepiness.

The most common treatment for ADHD is methylphenidate (MPH), a central nervous system stimulant that produces increased vigilance, superior mental activity, a decreased need for sleep, and less awareness of fatigue [65]. Partial normalization of EEG patterns has been found following the administration of stimulant medication to children with ADHD [66–69], indicating that such medication acts to stimulate the underaroused cortex [70, 71] and providing support for the hypothesis that children with ADHD suffer from hypoarousal.

The findings suggesting that objective sleep parameters are comparable in all children with ADHD, combined with the fact that ADHD children are sleepier (as measured by the number of sleep onsets and their rapidity) than normal children, raise the possibility that ADHD is associated with hypo- rather than hyperarousal. This hypothesis also provides an explanation for the seemingly paradoxical effectiveness of psychostimulants in treating ADHD.

Evidence that sleep deprivation affects brain areas associated with ADHD

Neuroimaging studies have shown that activity in the cerebrum (which mediates alertness, attention, and higher-order cognitive processes) changes in response to sleep deprivation, and that these alterations are associated with differences in cognitive performance [72–74]. Decreased regional glucose activity following sleep deprivation has been observed in the thalamus [72–74], as well as in the temporal [74], prefrontal, and parietal cortices [73]. Comparisons of individuals performing a serial subtraction task and a verbal learning task under conditions of normal wakefulness and sleep deprivation revealed a sleep deprivation-associated decrease in the blood oxygen level-dependent (BOLD) activity in the prefrontal anterior cingulate gyrus, lateral posterior parietal lobules, pulvinar thalamus, temporal lobes, and visual cortices [79]. Sleep-deprived individuals showed large deactivations in the prefrontal and posterior parietal cortices, the heteromodal association areas, and Brodmann's areas in the prefrontal and posterior parietal cortices [75, 76], which are involved in higher-order analysis and integration of sensory–motor information and cognition [75].

These cortical regions are also among the major sites implicated in ADHD patients, who show abnormalities in their frontal, dorsolateral prefrontal, ventrolateral prefrontal, and dorsal anterior cingulate cortices, along with the striatum (caudate and putamen) and lateral temporal and parietal regions [73, 74, 75]. These regions together are thought to form a broadly distributed action-attentional network system [77, 78], which functions to initiate and maintain an alert state (alerting), select information from sensory input (orienting), and resolve conflict among responses (executive control). Attention-deficit/hyperactivity disorder has been associated with deficits in the alerting and executive systems. The alerting mechanism is associated with norepinephrine (NE), and the executive control network involves dopamine (DA) [78, 79]. These systems, as well as the frontal brain areas implicated in ADHD, are particularly vulnerable to sleep deprivation.

These studies showing preliminary support for the involvement of arousal-related mechanisms in ADHD deficits suggest that insufficient sleep is likely involved in ADHD pathophysiology. Empirical studies examining this hypothesis are needed to further support and specify the nature and the significance of this association.

Clinical implications

The human functions that are mostly affected by fatigue and insufficient sleep, the executive functions, self-regulation, and arousal, are also the key domains of dysfunction in children with ADHD [80]. The clearest direct health consequences of insufficient sleep are impairment in cognitive functioning, and high-risk behaviors such as substance abuse and car accidents [81, 82]. Among children predisposed to behavioral and academic difficulties, such as those with ADHD, the impact of disrupted sleep may be amplified [83–85]. Hence, ADHD may

increase both the risk of, and vulnerability to, insufficient sleep.

From a clinical perspective, diagnosing and treating sleep problems in ADHD individuals is thus of great importance. Sleep disturbances and ADHD could interact in several ways. First, sleep disturbances may worsen ADHD symptoms and/or associated mood disorders. Therefore, the treatment of comorbid sleep disorders and interventions targeted at ensuring adequate sleep may substantially improve daytime ADHD symptoms. Second, any sleep disorder that results in inadequate sleep duration, fragmented/disrupted sleep, or excessive daytime sleepiness may cause problems with mood, attention, and behavior. Therefore, sleep disturbances may mimic ADHD symptoms in children misdiagnosed with ADHD. As a consequence, symptoms of inattention, hyperactivity, and/or impulsivity may be improved or even eliminated by treatment of the primary sleep disorder. Finally, a child's sleep disruption may interrupt the sleep of his/her parents, which increases stress in the family and causes negative parent–child interactions. This cycle results in sleep deprivation and negative outcomes for both the parents and the child. Sleep deprivation has previously been related to an accumulation of stress and a deterioration of mood, which are likely to negatively affect the ability of parents to care for their children [86], and could be responsible for a negative cascade in the family.

Diagnosis and treatment

Diagnosis

The aim of assessing sleep in individuals with ADHD is to characterize the abnormal sleep pattern and to identify potential behavioral and psychological factors that might be contributing to the presence and/or exacerbation of the condition using objective and subjective sleep measures. The first step in diagnosis is to obtain symptom information. Patient and parent evaluations can be used to determine the presence of symptoms defined in the International Classification of Sleep Disorders – Revised [87]. Next, assessments over at least seven days should be made using sleep diaries. Important data to record include clock times for "lights off" and "lights on" (to estimate time in bed), sleep latency, number of awakenings, time spent awake after initial sleep onset, terminal time spent awake prior to arising from bed, and total sleep time. Concurrent objective verification can be obtained over this period using wrist actigraphy to gather data on patterns of estimated sleep and wakefulness. In addition, a detailed description of bedtime routine; caffeine, alcohol, or drug use in adolescents; exercise habits; and sleep environment should be used to determine the contribution of sleep-hygiene factors to presenting symptoms.

When assessing a child or adolescent with ADHD, it is necessary to distinguish a physiological sleep problem from an emotional problem (e.g., depression or anxiety) in which the sleep problem is but one of the symptoms. It is critical to be aware of the potential contribution of psychiatric comorbidity. A detailed history of psychiatric symptoms and psychoactive substance use should therefore be part of routine evaluation.

It is also important to assess the impact of medication on sleep onset, sleep duration, and insomnia. The best practice is to measure sleep on medication for five consecutive nights, to next have a wash-out period (with duration based on the half-life of the medication used to treat ADHD symptoms), and then to reassess sleep for another five consecutive nights. Comparing the two sleep patterns will discriminate between intrinsic and medication-related sleep alterations.

Treatment

Once a diagnosis has been made, a treatment plan should follow. Sleep problems reported by patients with ADHD are multifactorial, and may result from habit, medication, or underlying pathophysiology. Therefore, the appropriate management of sleep problems in ADHD patients is based on the correct identification of factors underlying the problem.

Sleep hygiene

Sleep hygiene issues should be addressed by development of instructions to help children develop healthy sleeping habits to diminish the likelihood that further problems may arise. Lifestyle changes may be necessary. Coping with certain sleep problems can be made easier for children by adjusting their exposure to daylight, by changing the timing of daily routines, and by strategically scheduling naps. A well organized and regular schedule of wake-up time, bedtime, meals, and activities is important.

Circadian sleep disorder

With circadian sleep disorder, therapies aim to synchronize the individual circadian clock with the environmental light–dark cycle. Various therapies target either the schedule per se (chronotherapy), or mechanisms (i.e., light, melatonin) that can reset the circadian timing system, or employ non-photic time cues [88].

The impact of ADHD medication on sleep

If the sleep disorder is related to the commencement of ADHD medication, adjusting the dose, changing the dosing schedule to avoid night interruption, a change in stimulant formulation, a trial of another stimulant, or a switch to a non-stimulant medication (clonidine), should all be considered.

Primary sleep disorders associated with periodic leg movement disorder/restless legs movement disorder or sleep apnea are discussed in Chapter 16.

Summary

In conclusion, the available data indicate an association between sleep and ADHD and an overlap between the consequences of sleep deprivation and symptoms of ADHD. Basic mechanisms within these systems are intimately connected to individual regulation of sleep and arousal; should these mechanisms be disrupted, there may be considerable ramifications for development, effective functioning, and the appearance of behavioral disorders. Sleep difficulties in children with ADHD may increase daytime ADHD symptoms, may be associated with the underlying pathophysiology of the disorder, and can pose a considerable challenge for clinicians attempting to develop effective ADHD treatment strategies. Consequently, diagnosis of sleep problems in children with ADHD should be made using subjective and objective measures. Treatment of individuals presenting with ADHD and sleep disorders must be based upon an understanding of interactions among the underlying systems, with an appreciation of the importance of such systems in the presentation and exacerbation of symptoms.

References

1. American Psychiatric Association. *Diagnostic and Statistical Manual of Mental Disorders*, 4th edn. (Washington, DC: American Psychiatric Association, 1994).

2. National Center on Birth Defects and Developmental Disabilities, Centers for Disease Control

and Prevention. Attention-deficit/hyperactivity disorder: a public health perspective. (Atlanta, GA: NCBDDD publication, 2001;01–0602).

3. Brown T, McMullen WJ. Attention Deficit Disorders and sleep arousal disturbance. *Ann NY Acad Sci.* 2001;**931**:271–86.

4. Owens J. The ADHD and sleep conundrum: a review. *J Dev Behav Pediatr.* 2005;**26**:312–22.

5. Gruber R, Xi T, Frenette S. Sleep disturbances in prepubertal children with attention deficit hyperactivity disorder: a home polysomnography study. *Sleep.* 32(3):343–50.

6. Collop NA, Anderson WM, Boehlecke B, *et al.* Clinical guidelines for the use of unattended portable monitors in the diagnosis of obstructive sleep apnea in adult patients. *J Clin Sleep Med.* 2007;**3**(7):737–47.

7. Zou D, Grote L, Peker Y, Lindblad U, Hedner J. Validation of a portable monitoring device for sleep apnea diagnosis in a population based cohort using synchronized home polysomnography. *Sleep.* 2006;**29**(3):367–74.

8. Sadeh A, Pergamin L, Bar-Haim Y. Sleep in children with attention-deficit hyperactivity disorder: a meta-analysis of polysomnographic studies. *Sleep Med Rev.* 2006;**10**(6):381–98.

9. Chervin R, Hedger K. Clinical prediction of periodic leg movements during sleep in children. *Sleep Med.* 2001;**2**:501–10.

10. Owens J, Spirito A, McGuinn M. The children's sleep habits questionnaire (CSHQ): psychometric properties of a survey instrument for school-aged children. *Sleep.* 2000;**23**:1043–51.

11. Ball J, Koloian B. Sleep patterns among ADHD children. *Clin Psychology Rev.* 1995;**15**:681–91.

12. Ball J, Tiernan M, Janusz J, Furr A. Sleep patterns among children with attention-deficit hyperactivity disorder: a re-examination of parent perceptions. *J Pediatr Psychol.* 1997;**22**:389–98.

13. Day H, Abmayr S. Parent reports of sleep disturbances in stimulant-medicated children with attention-deficit hyperactivity disorder. *J Clin Psychol.* 1998;**54**:701–16.

14. Kaplan B, McNicol J, Conte R, Moghadam H. Sleep disturbance in preschool-aged hyperactive and nonhyperactive children. *Pediatrics.* 1987;**80**:839–44.

15. Marcotte A, Thacher P, Butters M, *et al.* Parental report of sleep problems in children with attentional and learning disorders. *J Dev Behav Pediatr.* 1998;**19**:178–86.

16. Ring A, Stein D, Barak Y. Sleep disturbances in children with attention-deficit/hyperactivity: a comparative study with healthy siblings. *J Learn Disabil.* 1998;**31**:572–8.

17. Stein M. Unravelling sleep problems in treated and untreated children with ADHD. *J Child Adolesc Psychopharmacol.* 1999;**9**:157–68.

18. Trommer B, Hoeppner J, Rosenberg R, Armstrong K, Rothstein J. Sleep disturbance in children with attention deficit disorder. *Ann Neurol.* 1988;**24**:322.

19. O'Brien LM, Holbrook CR, Mervis CB, *et al.* Sleep and neurobehavioral characteristics of 5- to 7-year-old children with parentally reported symptoms of attention-deficit/hyperactivity disorder. *Pediatrics.* 2003;**111**:554–63.

20. O'Brien LM, Ivanenko A, Crabtree VM, *et al.* Sleep disturbances in children with attention deficit hyperactivity disorder. *Pediatr Res.* 2003;**54**(2):237–43.

21. Kirov R, Kinkelbur J, Heipke S, *et al.* Is there a specific polysomnographic sleep pattern in children with attention deficit/hyperactivity disorder? *J Sleep Res.* 2004;**13**(1):87–93.

22. Khan A. Sleep REM latency in hyperkinetic boys. *Am J Psychiatry.* 1982;**139**(10):1358–60.

23. Sadeh A, Pergamin L, Bar-Haim Y. Sleep in children with attention-deficit hyperactivity disorder: a meta-analysis of polysomnographic studies. *Sleep Med Rev.* 2006;**10**(6):381–98.

24. Cortese S, Konofal E, Yateman N, Mouren M, Lecendreux M. Sleep and alertness in children with attention-deficit/hyperactivity disorder: a systematic review of the literature. *Sleep.* 2006; **29**(4):504–11.

25. Gruber R, Sadeh A, Raviv A. Instability of sleep patterns in children with ADHD. *J Am Acad Child Adolesc Psychiatry.* 2000;**39**:495–501.

26. Gruber R, Sadeh A. Sleep and neurobehavioral functioning in children with ADHD. *Sleep.* 2004;**27**:267–73.

27. Van der Heijden KB, Smits MG, Van Someren EJ, Ridderinkhof KR, Gunning WB. Effect of melatonin on sleep, behavior, and cognition in ADHD and chronic sleep-onset insomnia. *J Am Acad Child Adolesc Psychiatry.* 2007;**46**(2):233–41.

28. Owens J, Sangal RB, Sutton VK, *et al.* Subjective and objective measures of sleep in children with attention-deficit/hyperactivity disorder. *Sleep Med.* 2009;**10**(4):446–56.

29. Hvolby A, Jørgensen J, Bilenberg N. Actigraphic and parental reports of sleep difficulties in children with attention-deficit/hyperactivity disorder. *Arch Pediatr Adolesc Med.* 2008;**162**(4):323–9.

30. Owens JA, Maxim R, Nobile C, McGuinn M, Msall M. Parental and self-report of sleep in children with attention-deficit/hyperactivity disorder. *Arch Pediatr Adolesc Med.* 2000;**154**(6):549–55.

31. Hvolby A, Jørgensen J, Bilenberg N. Actigraphic and parental reports of sleep difficulties in children with attention-deficit/hyperactivity disorder. *Arch Pediatr Adolesc Med.* 2008;**162**(4):323–9.

32. Corkum P, Panton R, Ironside S, Macpherson M, Williams T. Acute impact of immediate release methylphenidate administered three times a day on sleep in children with attention-deficit/hyperactivity disorder. *J Pediatr Psychol.* 2008;**33**(4):368–79.

33. LeBourgeois MK, Avis K, Mixon M, Olmi J, Harsh J. Snoring, sleep quality, and sleepiness across attention-deficit/hyperactivity disorder subtypes. *Sleep.* 2004;**27**:520–5.

34. Mayes SD, Calhoun SL, Bixler EO, *et al.* ADHD subtypes and comorbid anxiety, depression, and oppositional-defiant disorder: differences in sleep problems. *J Pediatr Psychol.* 2009;**34**(3):328–37.

35. Willoughby MT, Angold A, Egger HL. Parent-reported attention-deficit/hyperactivity disorder symptomatology and sleep problems in a preschool-age pediatric clinic sample. *J Am Acad Child Adolesc Psychiatry.* 2008;**47**(9):1086–94.

36. Bell-McGinty S, Habeck C, Hilton H, *et al.* Identification and differential vulnerability of a neural network in sleep deprivation. *Cerebral Cortex.* 2004;**14**:496–502.

37. Carskadon M, Harvey K, Dement W. Acute restriction of nocturnal sleep in children. *Perceptual Motor Skills.* 1981;**53**:103–12.

38. Archbold K, Giordani B, Ruzicka D, Chervin R. Cognitive executive dysfunction in children with mild sleep-disordered breathing. *Biol Res Nurs.* 2004;**5**:168–76.

39. Dahl R, Pelham W, Wieron M. The role of sleep disturbances in attention deficit disorder symptoms: a case study. *J Pediatr Psychol.* 1991;**16**:229–39.

40. Chervin R, Dillon J, Bassetti C, Ganoczy D, Pituch K. Symptoms of sleep disorders, inattention, and hyperparactivity in children. *Sleep.* 1997;**20**:1185–92.

41. O'Brien L, Mervis C, Holbrook C, *et al.* Neurobehavioral correlates of sleep-disordered breathing in children. *J Sleep Res.* 2004;**13**:165–72.

42. O'Brien L, Mervis C, Holbrook C, *et al.* Neurobehavioral implications of habitual snoring in children. *Pediatrics.* 2004;**114**:44–9.

43. Bass J, Corwin M, Gozal D, *et al.* The effect of chronic or intermittent hypoxia on cognition in childhood: a review of the evidence. *Pediatrics.* 2004;**114**(3):805–16.

44. Kennedy J, Blunden S, Hirte C, *et al.* Reduced neurocognition in children who snore. *Pediatr Pulmon.* 2004;**37**(4):330–7.

45. Melendres M, Lutz J, Rubin E, Marcus C. Daytime sleepiness and hyperactivity in children with suspected sleep-disordered breathing. *Pediatrics.* 2004; **114**(3):768–75.

46. Ali N, Pitson D, Stradling J. Sleep disordered breathing: effects of adenotonsillectomy on behavior and psychological functioning. *Eur J Pediatr.* 1996; **155**(1):56–62.

47. Picchietti D. Restless legs syndrome and periodic limb movement disorders in children and adolescents. *Child Adolesc Psychiatr Clin North Am.* 1996;**5**:729–40.

48. Picchietti DL, Underwood DJ, Farris WA. Further studies on periodic limb movement disorder and restless legs syndrome in children with attention-deficit hyperactivity disorder. *Mov Disord.* 1999;**14**:1000–7.

49. Pichietti DL, England SJ, Walters AS, Willis K, Verrico T. Periodic limb movement disorder and restless legs syndrome in children with attention-deficit/hyperactivity disorder. *J Child Neurol.* 1998;**13**:588–94.

50. Marquet P, Peigneux P, Laureys S, Smith C. Be caught napping: you're doing more than resting your eyes. *Nat Neurosci.* 2002;**5**:618–19.

51. Mednick S, Nakayama K, Cantero J, *et al.* The restorative effect of naps on perceptual deterioration. *Nat Neurosci.* 2002;**5**:677–81.

52. Beebe D, Gozal D. Obstructive sleep apnea and the prefrontal cortex: towards a comprehensive model linking nocturnal upper airway obstruction to daytime cognitive and behavioral deficits. *J Sleep Res.* 2002;**11**:1–16.

53. Harrison Y, Horne J. The impact of sleep deprivation on decision making: a review. *J Exper Psychol.* 2000;**6**:236–49.

54. Horne JA. Sleep loss and divergent thinking ability. *Sleep.* 1988;**11**:528–36.

55. Horne JA. *Why We Sleep.* (Oxford: Oxford University Press, 1988).

56. Montgomery-Downs H, Crabtree V, Gozal D. Cognition, sleep and respiration in at-risk children treated for obstructive sleep apnoea. *Eur Respir J.* 2005;**25**:336–42.

57. Golan N, Shahar E, Ravid S, Pillar G. Sleep disorders and daytime sleepiness in children with attention-deficit/hyperactive disorder. *Sleep.* 2004;**27**:261–6.

58. Lecendreux M, Konofal E, Bouvard M, Falissard B, Mouren-Siméoni M. Sleep and alertness in children with ADHD. *J Child Psychol Psychiatry.* 2000;**41**:803–12.

59. Palm L, Persson E, Bjerre I, Elmqvist D, Blennow G. Sleep and wakefulness in preadolescent children with deficits in attention, motor control and perception. *Acta Paediatrica.* 1992;**81**:618–24.

60. Littner M, Kushida C, Wise M, *et al.* Standards of Practice Committee of the American Academy of Sleep Medicine: Practice parameters for clinical use of the multiple sleep latency test and the maintenance of wakefulness test. *Sleep.* 2005;**28**:113–21.

61. Barry R, Clarke A, Johnstone S. A review of electrophysiology in attention-deficit/hyperactivity disorder: I. Qualitative and quantitative electroencephalography. *Clin Neurophysiol.* 2003; **114**(2)171–83.

62. Clarke A, Barry R, McCarthy R, Selikowitz M. Excess beta activity in children with attention-deficit/hyperactivity disorder: an atypical electrophysiological group. *Psychiatr Res.* 2001;**103**:205–18.

63. Crawford H, Knebel T, Vendemia J, Kaplan L, Ratcliff B. EEG activation patterns during tracking and decision-making tasks: differences between low and high sustained attention. 8th International Symposium on Aviation Psychology. (Colombus, Ohio: 1995).

64. van den Berg J, Neely G, Nilsson L, Knutsson A, Landstrom U. Electroencephalography and subjective ratings of sleep deprivation. *Sleep Med.* 2005;**6**:231–40.

65. Johnson L, Safranek S, Friemoth J. Clinical inquiries. What is the most effective treament for ADHD in children? *J Fam Pract.* 2005;**54**:166–8.

66. Clarke A, Barry A, McCarthy R, *et al.* Effects of stimulant medications on the EEG of children with attention-deficit/hyperactivity disorder predominantly inattentive subtype. *Int J Psychophysiol.* 2003;**47**:129–37.

67. Clarke A, Barry A, Bond D, McCarthy R, Selikowitz M. Effects of stimulant medications on the EEG of children with attention-deficit/hyperactivity disorder. *Psychopharmacol.* 2002;**164**:277–84.

68. Hermens D, Williams L, Clarke S, *et al.* Responses to methylphenidate in adolescent AD/HD: evidence from concurrently recorded autonomic (EDA) and central (EEG and ERP) measures. *Int J Psychophysiol.* 2005; **58**(1):21–33.

69. Lubar J, White JJ, Swartwood M, Swartwood J. Methylphedinate effects on global and complex measures of EEG. *Pediatr Neurol.* 1999;**21**:633–7.

70. Rowe D, Robinson P, Gordon E. Stimulant drug action in attention-deficit/hyperactivity disorder (ADHD): interference of neurophysiological mechanisms via quantitative modelling. *Clin Neurophysiol.* 2005;**116**:324–35.

71. Swartwood M, Swartwood J, Lubar J, *et al.* Methylphenidate effects on EEG, behavior, and performance in boys with ADHD. *Pediatr Neurol.* 1998;**18**:244–50.

72. Drummond S, Brown G, Gillin J, *et al.* Altered brain response to verbal learning following sleep deprivation. *Nature.* 2000;**403**:655–7.

73. Drummond S, Brown G, Stricker J, *et al.* Sleep deprivation-induced reduction in cortical functional response to serial subtraction. *Neuroreport.* 1999;**10**:3745–8.

74. Wu J, Gillin J, Buchsbaum M, *et al.* The effect of sleep deprivation on cerebral glucose metabolic rate in normal humans assessed with positron emission tomography. *Sleep.* 1991:155–62.

75. Mesulam M. Large-scale neurocognitive networks and distributed processing for attention, language, and memory. *Ann Neurol.* 1990;**28**:597–613.

76. Mesulam M. *Principles of Behavioral Neurology.* (Philadelphia: F.A. Davis Company, 1985).

77. Fan J, McCandliss B, Fossella J, Flombaum J, Posner M. The activation of attentional networks. *Neuroimage.* 2005;**26**:471–9.

78. Arnsten A, Li B. Neurobiology of executive functions: catecholamine influences on prefrontal cortical functions. *Biological Psychiatry.* 2005;**57**:1377–84.

79. Oades R. Attention deficit disorder with hyperactivity (ADDH): the contribution of catecholaminergic activity. *Prog Neurobiol.* 1998;**29**:365–91.

80. Connor J, Norton R, Ameratunga S, *et al.* Driver sleepiness and risk of serious injury to car occupants: population based case control study. *BMJ.* 2002;**324**:1125.

81. Bootzin RR, Stevens SJ. Adolescents, substance abuse, and the treatment of insomnia and daytime sleepiness. *Clin Psychol Rev.* 2005;**25**(5):629–44.

82. Crum RM, Storr CL, Chan YF, Ford DE. Sleep disturbance and risk for alcohol-related problems. *Am J Psychiatry.* 2004;**161**:1197–203.

83. Fried R, Aleardi M. Behavior differences in drivers with attention deficit hyperactivity disorder: the driving behavior questionnaire. *Accidents Analysis and Prevention.* 2005;**37**(6):996–1004.

84. Ercan ES, Coskunol H, Varan A, Toksöz K. Childhood attention deficit/hyperactivity disorder and alcohol dependence: a 1-year follow-up. *Alcohol Alcohol.* 2003;**38**:352–6.

85. Wilens TE. Attention-deficit/hyperactivity disorder and the substance use disorders: the nature of the relationship, subtypes at risk, and treatment issues. *Psychiatr Clin North Am.* 2004;**27**:283–301.

86. Zahn-Waxler C, Duggal S, Gruber R. The effects on parenting of parental psychopathology. In M. Bornstein, ed. *Handbook of Parenting,* 2nd edn, Vol. 4. (Hillsdale: Lawrence Erlbaum Associates, 2002).

87. Circadian rhythm sleep disorders. In: *The International Classification of Sleep Disorders: Diagnostic & Coding Manual*, 2nd edn. (Westchester, IL: American Academy of Sleep Medicine, 2005; 117–28).

88. Gruber R, Sheshko D. Circadian sleep disorders in children and adolescents. In: A Ivanenko, ed. *Sleep and Psychiatric Disorders in Children and Adolescents.*

(Informa Healthcare USA, Inc., 2007; 61–77).

Endnote

1. We focus on individuals who do not suffer from medical or neurological conditions that interfere with sleep [19].

Chapter

22

Interaction between primary sleep disorders and attention-deficit/ hyperactivity disorder

Anna Ivanenko and Sricharan Moturi

Sleep regulation and ADHD: conceptual framework

Attention-deficit/hyperactivity disorder (ADHD) is a neurobehavioral syndrome characterized by impulsivity, hyperactivity, inattention, distractibility, and symptoms of executive dysfunction. Similar symptoms of behavioral disinhibition, poor concentration, emotional dysregulation, and performance deficits have been described in children and adolescents subjected to sleep loss or resulting from sleep fragmentation.

Several theoretical models have been proposed to explain the interface between sleep disruption and symptoms of ADHD based on the common neuropathophysiological pathways involved in the regulation of attention, behavior, and the sleep–wakefulness cycle.

For example, neurotransmitters like norepinephrine (NE) and serotonin (5-HT) have been implicated in the regulation of attentional processes and sleep–wakefulness cycle with NE being hypothesized to cause hyperarousal in subjects with ADHD resulting in delayed sleep onset [1]. Structural and functional abnormalities in the prefrontal cortex seen in patients with ADHD and primary sleep disorders support the hypothesis of executive function abnormalities as one of the underlying mechanisms of neurocognitive and behavioral deficits seen in ADHD and primary sleep disorders [2, 3].

Possible association of hypoarousal and ADHD has been proposed based on the clinical findings, thereby raising the question of whether the hyperactivity is an adaptive behavior against the underlying daytime sleepiness (resulting from hypoarousal) [4]. Inter-subject variability in sleep patterns observed in subjects with ADHD appears to be related to disturbances in arousal regulation associated with ADHD [5].

Finally, several research studies indicated circadian mechanisms of sleep disruption with melatonin mediated sleep phase delay and intrinsic homeostatic regulatory dysfunction being part of pathophysiological pathways of increased sleep onset latency in patients with ADHD [6].

Sleep related breathing disorders (SRBD) and ADHD
Clinical characteristics and prevalence of SRBD in children

Sleep related breathing disorders (SRBD) are best understood as occurring across a spectrum that includes habitual snoring at its least severe, lowermost end, and obstructive sleep apnea (OSA) at its most severe, uppermost end. Sleep related breathing disorders include upper airway resistance syndrome (UARS) and obstructive hypoventilation syndrome as part of the spectrum. Obstructive sleep apnea appears to be related to upper airway collapse during inspiration either due to anatomical factors (obstruction related to lymphoid tissue proliferation) and/or functional factors such as increased pharyngeal muscle collapsibility. Obesity related fatty infiltration of the upper airway structures and/or subcutaneous fat deposits in anterior neck region along with increased adipose tissue in the abdominal wall causes reduced intrathoracic volume and diaphragmatic excursion in the supine position leading to obstructive hypoventilation during sleep. Although obesity appears to be one of the leading causes of SRBD in adults, adenotonsillar hypertrophy is the predominant cause of SRBD in children, other than craniofacial and soft tissue abnormalities.

Sleep and Mental Illness, eds. S. R. Pandi-Perumal and M. Kramer. Published by Cambridge University Press. © Cambridge University Press 2010.

Recently, Gozal and colleagues proposed a new classification of OSA in children to elucidate the relationship between the anatomical and functional risk factors [7]. Type I OSA is characterized by the presence of marked adenotonsillar hypertrophy in the absence of obesity, and Type II is OSA associated with obesity in the presence of only minimal adenotonsillar hypertrophy. Independent risk factors for development of adenotonsillar hypertrophy include cigarette smoke, recurrent viral infections, asthma, and allergic rhinitis. Genetic factors have also been implicated in the pathophysiology of OSA. Overnight polysomnography (PSG) has been recommended as a "gold standard" for the diagnosis of OSA in children and adolescents [8].

Pathophysiology of SRBD and ADHD

Pathophysiology of SRBD and ADHD has been investigated using animal models of SRBD. Studies in rodents revealed that intermittent hypoxia was associated with increased oxidative stress [9], induction of excessive nitric oxide (NO) levels and upregulation of pro-inflammatory cytokines [10]. These pathophysiologic changes were proposed to cause neuronal cell death in the cortex and hippocampus [11], thereby causing perturbations in higher cognitive functions like vigilance, task switching, and working memory consistent with a distinct ADHD phenotype.

Although animal research cannot be exactly replicated in the pediatric population, some of the animal studies' findings could be extrapolated to children. For example, Larkin et al. showed increased levels of inflammatory markers such as C-reactive proteins in adolescents with SRBD and disrupted sleep, which could confer additional risk for cardiovascular disease independent of obesity [12], while Gozal and colleagues showed elevated C-reactive proteins in children with OSA who later develop neurocognitive deficits [13]. A study by Halbower et al. of children with OSA demonstrated possible neuronal injury in the hippocampus and frontal cortex as evidenced by reduced N-acetyl aspartate/choline ratio compared to age- and gender-matched controls, leading to deficits of IQ and executive functions [14].

Neurocognitive impact of SRBD has been explored in numerous studies. One study, which focused on the cognitive impact of SRBD in children, found that subjects with oxygen desaturations of 3 to 4% with or without upper airway obstruction or respiratory arousals tended to have lower IQ, impaired attentional capacity and memory compared to controls [15]. Another study of children with symptoms of snoring but less prevalent oxygen desaturations as documented by the polysomnogram showed improved daytime vigilance and decreased hyperactive behavior after adenotonsillectomy [16]. There also appears to be a dose-dependent relationship between nocturnal hypoxia and neurocognitive impairment as evidenced in an early study by Lewin et al. [17]. In this study, 28 healthy children with OSA and a healthy, age-matched comparison group of ten children were assessed using standard measures of sleep, behavior, and cognitive function. Children with OSA had significantly more behavior problems than the healthy comparison group based on parents' reports. Children diagnosed with moderate to severe OSA had significantly lower scores on tasks that assessed sustained attention. A significant association was also found between OSA severity and verbal ability. Recent systematic review of literature suggested that ADHD might be involved in the development of comorbid obesity through abnormal eating behaviors like impulsive binge eating [18]. Excessive sleepiness was also shown to be associated with obesity in children possibly contributing to symptoms of ADHD [19].

To summarize and explain a complex relationship between sleep disorders and neurobehavioral/emotional development in children, a multisystem heuristic model of bidirectional relationship between SRBD and daytime functions has been proposed by Gozal and Beebe [20]. This model implies that sleep disruption can produce prefrontal cortical dysfunction leading to impaired executive functions that appear to translate into daytime cognitive and behavioral difficulties in children [21, 22]. The putative mechanisms behind the prefrontal cortical dysfunction are speculated to be related to disruption in cellular and neurochemical processes, inflammatory responses to hypoxia, and oxidative stress marked by increased production of free radicals, adhesion molecules, and decreased levels of NO, thereby leading to potential neuronal loss during a vulnerable period of brain development that includes processes such as myelination and synaptic pruning [14, 20].

Prevalence of SRBD and ADHD

A recent systematic review of epidemiological studies of SRBD in children provided estimates of

253

parent-reported symptoms of SRBD at 4 to 11% including parentally reported snoring at 7.45%, whereas prevalence of SRBD diagnosed using polysomnography ranged between 1 and 4%. Greater rates of prevalence were suggested in boys, in overweight children, and among African-American children [23]. In a recent systematic review, worldwide pooled prevalence rates of pediatric ADHD were found to be 5.9% with no significant differences between North America and Europe [24]. Prevalence of ADHD in North America alone was estimated to be 8.7% among US children aged 8 to 15, of whom fewer than half receive treatment [25].

Studies on the prevalence of ADHD in children with SRBD have been largely inconsistent. Cohen-Zion and Anconi-Israel reviewed 47 studies on sleep in children with ADHD and concluded that the data were inconclusive as to the relative prevalence of primary sleep disorders in children with ADHD when compared to controls. For example, parental reports in children without ADHD have found symptoms of SRBD and periodic limb movement disorder (PLMD) as being associated with symptoms of hyperactivity and inattention. Subjective symptoms of sleep disordered breathing have also been more frequently reported in children with ADHD than controls. However, PSG studies have so far not confirmed whether the actual prevalence of SRBD is higher in ADHD and a clear relationship could not be ascertained [26]. A more recent systematic review of literature did, however, conclude that children with ADHD were more likely to have mild SRBD [27].

Association of SRBD and ADHD

Behavioral morbidities and neurocognitive deficits in children with SRBD have been widely reported in the literature. Psychiatric symptoms associated with SRBD include hyperactivity, inattention, disruptive behaviors like aggression, and symptoms consistent with mood disorders. Association of SRBD with hyperactivity in children has been well supported by parental reports [28–30], and polysomnographic studies [17, 31, 32].

Neuropsychological assessments including auditory continuous performance tests showed impairment in selective and sustained attention in children with SRBD [21]. Other behavioral correlates of SRBD include disruptive behaviors and aggression [33, 34]. Depressive symptoms were more likely to be reported by children who snore than non-snoring children, and

appear to be independent of comorbid obesity [35]. Deficits in cognitive domains such as memory, intelligence [22], and learning problems [36] have been well documented in children with SRBD. However, some studies have failed to replicate similar deficits in memory [37] and intelligence [38] possibly due to different aspects of memory being measured (variable vs. declarative vs. working memory), use of different neuropsychological tests, as well as other confounding variables like premorbid academic functioning and socioeconomic status. Most of the studies examining behavioral and cognitive deficits in children with SRBD have been methodologically limited, and lack comprehensive diagnostic evaluations of ADHD. There is certainly a wide range of assessment tools used to measure cognitive functions across different studies that makes it difficult to conduct meta-analysis and to generalize findings to a general pediatric population.

Treatment outcome studies have provided additional insights into the causal relationship between SRBD, cognitive deficits, and behavioral problems in children. A vast majority of studies indicated significant improvement in neurocognitive and behavioral measures following the treatment of SRBD [16, 39–41]. Huang and colleagues showed that children with mild SRBD and coexistent ADHD improved across most subjectively measured behavioral and cognitive domains after adenotonsillectomy (AT) compared to children who had treatment with stimulant medications alone [42]. Another recent study examined differences in sleep and behavioral outcomes in children with SRBD using the pediatric sleep questionnaire (PSQ) and Conners' Parent Rating Scale – Revised Short form (CPRS-RS) before and after AT. Although there was no randomized control group that did not undergo AT, children with severe baseline T-scores in CPRS-RS showed greater improvements post-AT in inattention, hyperactivity, oppositional behaviors, and ADHD index [43]. A recent literature review that focused on the treatment outcomes in children with SRBD concluded that AT is associated with improvements in the quality of life, behavior, and cognitive function, although larger randomized controlled trials are needed for definitive evidence of such benefits [44].

ADHD and SRBD in adults

Prevalence of ADHD in adults has been estimated to be 4.4% [45], whereas prevalence studies of ADHD in adults with SRBD are largely lacking. However, few reports suggest the presence of SRBD in some adults with ADHD who report significant sleep problems [46, 47]. Significant deficits in alertness and attention have been shown in adults with diagnosed OSA [48]. Recent meta-analysis of 40 studies in adults with SRBD (predominantly OSA) found that executive functions were the most impaired cognitive domain of which the most often affected were working memory, phonological fluency, cognitive flexibility, and planning, with some deficits persisting even after treatment of OSA [49]. Age did not appear to interact with the effects of SRBD on the cognitive deficits [50].

Recently, a $3'$-UTR polymorphism of the circadian locomotor output cycles protein kaput (*CLOCK*) gene, rs1801260, showed a strong, significant association ($p < 0.001$) between adult ADHD and sleep patterns with at least one T-mutation being the risk allele further providing insight into the pathophysiologic overlap between ADHD and sleep disturbances [51]. Impaired executive functions related to underlying sleep disorders seem to explain daytime cognitive and behavioral difficulties in adults, and are speculated to be due to prefrontal cortical dysfunction [52]. A recent study that utilized sleep questionnaires and a symptoms checklist in adults with ADHD demonstrated that the severity of ADHD symptoms was closely related to the feeling of being refreshed in the morning, problems with the sleep–wake pattern, sleep quality, and sleep onset latency [53]. A relatively small study that evaluated the presence of attentional deficits in 41 adults with OSA before and after treatment with continuous positive airway pressure (CPAP) showed improvements in ADHD symptoms among 58% of treated subjects with elevated baseline scores of ADHD. Yet, 42% of the patients demonstrated persistent attentional deficits, raising the question of whether the duration of untreated sleep apnea is a major factor in the treatment [54].

Periodic limb movement disorder (PLMD), restless legs syndrome (RLS), and ADHD

Clinical characteristics and prevalence of RLS/PLMD in pediatric patients

Restless legs syndrome (RLS) is a neurological movement disorder that is predominantly characterized by sensorimotor symptoms affecting the limbs. It is typically characterized by unpleasant and distressing sensations in the legs accompanied by an urge to move. Most of these symptoms appear to be aggravated by inactivity and relieved by movement, and also appear to worsen at night. Although well reported and characterized in adults, diagnosis of RLS in children and adolescents can be challenging due to a variance in descriptors of sensory symptoms. Periodic limb movements in sleep (PLMS) are brief, rhythmic, stereotyped movements of legs that last between 0.5 and 5 seconds in duration occurring sequentially as four or more movements within an interval of 5 to 90 seconds [55]. Periodic limb movement disorder (PLMD) is diagnosed when periodic limb movement index (PLMI) exceeds five per hour in most cases, and is associated with clinical sleep disturbance or a complaint of daytime fatigue. Also, the PLMS cannot be explained by another sleep disorder (e.g., a sleep related breathing disorder such as obstructive sleep apnea), medical or neurological disorder, mental disorder, medication use, or substance use disorder.

A recent epidemiological study of the general population with regards to the prevalence of RLS in adults reported that symptoms of RLS are present in approximately 7% of the general population, and that 2.7% reported experiencing moderately or severely distressing symptoms at least two to three times per week [56]. Although more than one-third of adults with RLS report onset of symptoms between the ages of 10 and 20 years [57], the prevalence of RLS symptoms was only recently studied in children [58]. Picchietti and colleagues reported 1.9% of 8- to 11-year-old children meeting criteria for definite RLS and 2.0% of 12- to 17-year-old adolescents. Moderately or severely distressing restless legs syndrome symptoms were reported to occur greater than or equal to two times per week in 0.5% and 1.0% of children respectively. Prevalence rates of PLMD in children are largely unknown, but have been reported to be 11.9% in a community survey and 8.4% in a sleep center referral population [59].

The exact etiology of RLS is largely unknown, yet the pathophysiologic mechanisms appear to be much better understood. Although genetic factors have long been implicated in the pathogenesis of RLS, this appears to be true only for primary and/or idiopathic cases of RLS. Restless legs syndrome is also associated with various neurological and psychiatric disorders, and the final common pathway appears to involve dopaminergic mechanisms. Thus far, five gene loci have been mapped in primary RLS to chromosomes 12q, 14q, 9p, 2q, and 20p, also known as RLS 1–5. Recently, the neuronal nitric oxide synthase (*NOS1*) gene was found to have associations with RLS and was mapped on chromosome 12 (RLS-1) [60]. In a recent study of 23 children with RLS, it was shown that family history was positive in 87% of the children and was compatible with an autosomal dominant inheritance pattern [61]. The dopaminergic hypothesis appears to be supported by treatment response of RLS to dopaminergic agonists (or worsening on dopamine antagonists like antipsychotics) as well as the recent validation of the L-DOPA test [62]. Reduced dopamine receptor (D2) binding along with hypodopaminergia in basal ganglia as shown on SPECT tends to support the dopaminergic hypothesis [63]. Pathophysiology of RLS also appears to involve iron metabolism and is associated with conditions that precipitate iron deficiency (like anemia). It is being proposed that low peripheral iron stores can mediate the levels of dopamine in the brain by affecting the cofactor for tyrosine hydroxylase, the rate-limiting enzyme in the production of dopamine [64].

The consensus criteria for pediatric RLS developed at the National Institutes of Health (NIH) workshop modified diagnostic criteria for pediatric RLS into "definite RLS," "probable RLS," and "possible RLS" [65]. The diagnosis of RLS in children should accompany age-dependent descriptors of sensations by the child, along with presence of a sleep disturbance. The diagnosis of PLMD requires an overnight polysomnogram to assess the amount of leg movements (PLMI) and disturbed sleep associated with them. Children complaining of "growing pains" have been shown to meet criteria for RLS, and therefore asking parents about leg aches in children that occur during the night can further aid in diagnosing RLS [66].

Non-pharmacological treatment options for RLS and associated sleep disturbances include incorporation of a regular sleep schedule coupled with routine bedtime and wake-up time, reducing environmental influences (like TV, music, video games, etc. prior to/at bedtime), and daily physical exercise can help children and adolescents with sleep problems associated with RLS. It can be helpful to ascertain the child's current nutritional status and need for dietary supplements of iron in cases associated with low serum ferritin level. Iron supplementation has been shown to be effective in reducing symptoms of RLS [67] and

PLMD, as well as daytime symptoms consistent with ADHD [68]. Although dopaminergic agonists like pramipexole and ropinirole are approved by the Food and Drug Administration (FDA) for treatment of RLS in adults, they are not approved for use in children. A few case reports have illustrated improvements in RLS along with improvement in associated depressive and ADHD symptoms in children on these medications [69, 70].

Association of ADHD with RLS and PLMD

Children with ADHD have been shown to consistently exhibit significant sleep difficulties. A meta-analysis of polysomnographic studies in children with ADHD revealed only one significant combined effect indicating that children with ADHD are more likely than controls to suffer from PLMS [71]. One study reported that a higher hyperactivity index on the Conners' Parent Rating Scale (CPRS) predicted symptoms of PLMD, RLS, and growing pains [72]. Conversely, a retrospective chart review by Walters and colleagues showed that 91% of children with PLMI (>5 per hour) had an associated diagnosis of ADHD. Also, 94% of a subset of this patient sample with PLMI (>25 per hour) had a 94% prevalence rate of ADHD [73]. Another study showed that at least 50% of children with ADHD have PLMI (>5 per hour), and one third of these children have a positive family history of RLS [74]. In a prospective study of 62 adults with RLS by Wagner and colleagues, 26% of adults met DSM-IV criteria for ADHD compared to 6% of patients who had insomnia and 5% of controls. The RLS symptom severity score was greater for patients who had ADHD compared with those who did not have ADHD [75]. It has been suggested that comorbidity of RLS with ADHD can be associated with increased bedtime refusal, since children with RLS associate the distressing sensations of RLS with bedtime. This can often be perceived as oppositional behavior or symptoms of ADHD [76]. The relationship, therefore, appears to be bidirectional and clinicians should thoroughly assess for symptoms of ADHD in patients with RLS and vice versa.

Potential mechanisms of association between ADHD and RLS have been explored in more recently published literature. A review by Cortese and colleagues examined the evidence of ADHD and RLS association and reported that up to 44% of subjects with ADHD have been found to have RLS or RLS symptoms, and up to 26% of subjects with RLS have been found to have ADHD or ADHD-like symptoms. The authors proposed that sleep disruption associated with RLS might lead to inattentiveness, moodiness, and paradoxical overactivity and can manifest as restlessness and inattention during daytime that mimic symptoms of ADHD. Alternatively, RLS has been shown to be comorbid with idiopathic ADHD [77].

The dopaminergic pathway has also been suggested as the "final common pathway" implicated in the pathophysiology of RLS, PLMD, and ADHD in both children and adults. In an early study by Walters and colleagues, seven children with comorbid ADHD and RLS/PLMD were successfully treated with dopaminergic therapies with reduction in RLS symptoms, PLMI, and improvement in ADHD symptoms as measured by CPRS and the Child Behavior Check List (CBCL). It was concluded that improvement could be due to enhanced dopamine levels or due to improved sleep quality [78].

Disruption in iron status has been proposed as a potential implicating factor in the association between RLS/PLMD and ADHD. Low levels of iron stores as reflected by serum ferritin less than 50 ng/ml were associated with increased prevalence and severity of RLS in adults [79] and were shown to be associated with ADHD and RLS/PLMD in children [80, 81]. Beneficial effects of increasing ferritin levels through iron supplementation in children have been demonstrated by Konofal and colleagues. In this study, 23 non-anemic children with ferritin levels less than 30 ng/ml were randomized to either receive iron supplementation (80 mg/day) or placebo for 12 weeks. Improvements on the ADHD rating scale were observed in the group receiving iron compared to placebo. However, improvements on CPRS and Conner's teacher rating scale did not reach significance [82]. These findings provide further insight into the pathophysiologic links between ADHD and RLS/PLMD.

Conclusion

Children with primary sleep disorders frequently exhibit symptoms of ADHD, and youngsters with ADHD consistently present with sleep disturbances. Sleep disorders like delayed sleep phase syndrome, sleep disordered breathing, and RLS/PLMD are shown to have a strong association with ADHD

with common pathophysiological pathways regulating sleep, arousal, and attention being proposed as neurobiological mechanisms of this association.

Clinical research indicates significant improvement in daytime behavioral and neurocognitive functions in children and adolescents treated for primary sleep disorders and emphasizes the importance of assessing children with symptoms of ADHD for the presence of sleep disturbances. Further studies are needed to delineate symptoms of primary sleep disorders and ADHD in children, and to develop treatment algorithms for sleep disturbances associated with ADHD.

References

1. Dahl RE. Regulation of sleep and arousal. *Dev Pathophysiol.* 1996;**8**:3–27.
2. Zang YF, Jin Z, Weng XC, et al. Functional MRI in attention-deficit hyperactivity disorder: evidence for hypofrontality. *Brain Dev.* 2005;**27**(8):544–50.
3. Zimmerman ME, Aloia MS. A review of neuroimaging in obstructive sleep apnea. *J Clin Sleep Med.* 2006;**2**(4):461–71.
4. Lecendreux M, Konofal E, Bouvard M, Falissard B, Mouren-Siméoni MC. Sleep and alertness in children with ADHD. *J Child Psychol Psychiatry.* 2000;**41**:803–12.
5. Gruber R, Sadeh A. Sleep and neurobehavioral functioning in boys with attention-deficit/hyperactivity disorder and no reported breathing problems. *Sleep.* 2004;**27**:267–73.
6. Owens JA. The ADHD and sleep conundrum: a review. *Dev Behav Pediatr.* 2005;**26**(4):312–22.
7. Dayyat E, Kheirandish-Gozal L, Gozal D. Childhood obstructive sleep apnea: one or two distinct disease entities? *Sleep Med Clin.* 2007;**2**:433–44.
8. Section on Pediatric Pulmonology, Subcommittee on Obstructive Sleep Apnea Syndrome. Clinical practice guideline: diagnosis and management of childhood obstructive sleep apnea syndrome. *Pediatrics.* 2002;**109**(4):704–12.
9. Row BW, Liu R, Xu W, Kheirandish L, Gozal D. Intermittent hypoxia is associated with oxidative stress and spatial learning deficits in the rat. *Am J Respir Crit Care Med.* 2003;**167**:1548–53.
10. Li RC, Row BW, Kheirandish L, et al. Nitric oxide synthase and intermittent hypoxia induced spatial learning deficits in the rat. *Neurobiol Dis.* 2004;**17**:44–53.
11. Xu W, Chi L, Row BW, et al. Increased oxidative stress is associated with chronic intermittent hypoxia-mediated brain cortical neuronal cell

apoptosis in a mouse model of sleep apnea. *Neuroscience.* 2004;**126**:313–23.

12. Larkin EK, Rosen CL, Kirchner HL, *et al.* Variation of C-reactive protein levels in adolescents: association with sleep disordered breathing and sleep duration. *Circulation.* 2005;**111**:1978–84.

13. Gozal D, Crabtree VM, Sans Capdevila O, Witcher LA, Kheirandish-Gozal L. C-Reactive protein, obstructive sleep apnea, and cognitive dysfunction in school-aged children. *Am J Respir Crit Care Med.* 2007; **176**(2):188–93.

14. Halbower AC, Degaonkar M, Barker PB, *et al.* Childhood obstructive sleep apnea associates with neuropsychological deficits and neuronal brain injury. *PLoS Med.* 2006;**3**(8):e301.

15. Rhodes SK, Shimoda KC, Waid LR, *et al.* Neurocognitive deficits in morbidly obese children with obstructive sleep apnea. *J Pediatr.* 1995;**127**:741–4.

16. Ali NJ, Pitson D, Stradling JR. Sleep disordered breathing: effects of adenotonsillectomy on behaviour and psychological functioning. *Eur J Pediatr.* 1996;**155**:56–62.

17. Lewin DS, Rosen RC, England SJ, Dahl RE. Preliminary evidence of behavioral and cognitive sequelae of obstructive sleep apnea in children. *Sleep Med.* 2002;**3**(1):5–13.

18. Cortese S, Angriman M, Maffeis C, *et al.* Attention-deficit/hyperactivity disorder (ADHD) and obesity: a systematic review of the literature. *Crit Rev Food Sci Nutr.* 2008;**48**(6):524–37.

19. Cortese S, Konofal E, Dalla Bernardina B, Mouren MC, Lecendreux M. Does excessive daytime sleepiness contribute to explaining the association between obesity and ADHD symptoms? *Med Hypotheses.* 2008;**70**(1):12–16.

20. Beebe DW, Gozal D. Obstructive sleep apnea and the prefrontal cortex: towards a comprehensive model linking nocturnal upper airway obstruction to daytime cognitive and behavioral deficits. *J Sleep Res.* 2002;**11**:1–16.

21. Blunden S, Lushington K, Kennedy D, Martin J, Dawson D. Behavior and neurocognitive performance in children aged 5–10 years who snore compared to controls. *J Clin Exper Neuropsychol.* 2000;**22**(5):554–68.

22. Kennedy JD, Blunden S, Hirte C, *et al.* Reduced neurocognition in children who snore. *Pediatric Pulmonol.* 2004;**37**(4):330–37.

23. Lumeng JC, Chervin RD. Epidemiology of pediatric obstructive sleep apnea. *Proc Am Thorac Soc.* 2008;**5**:242–52.

24. Polanczyk G, de Lima MS, Horta BL, Biederman J, Rohde LA. The worldwide prevalence of ADHD:

a systematic review and metaregression analysis. *Am J Psychiatry.* 2007;**164**:942–8.

25. Froehlich TE, Lanphear BP, Epstein JN, *et al.* Prevalence, recognition, and treatment of attention-deficit/hyperactivity disorder in a national sample of US children. *Arch Pediatr Adolesc Med.* 2007;**161**:857–64.

26. Cohen-Zion M, Ancoli-Israel S. Sleep in children with attention-deficit hyperactivity disorder (ADHD): a review of naturalistic and stimulant intervention studies. *Sleep Med Rev.* 2004;**8**:379–402.

27. Cortese S, Konofal E, Yateman N, Mouren MC, Lecendreux M. Sleep and alertness in children with attention-deficit/hyperactivity disorder: A systematic review of literature. *Sleep.* 2006;**29**(4):504–11.

28. Gottlieb DJ, Vezina RM, Chase C, *et al.* Symptoms of sleep-disordered breathing in 5-year-old children are associated with sleepiness and problem behaviors. *Pediatrics.* 2003;**112**:870–7.

29. Melendres MC, Lutz JM, Rubin ED, Marcus CL. Daytime sleepiness and hyperactivity in children with suspected sleep-disordered breathing. *Pediatrics.* 2004;**114**:768–75.

30. Chervin RD, Archbold KH, Dillon JE. Inattention, hyperactivity, and symptoms of sleep-disordered breathing. *Pediatrics.* 2002;**109**:449–56.

31. O'Brien LM, Holbrook CR, Mervis CB, *et al.* Sleep and neurobehavioral characteristics of 5- to 7-year-old children with parentally reported symptoms of attention-deficit/hyperactivity disorder. *Pediatrics.* 2003;**111**:554–63.

32. O'Brien LM, Mervis CB, Holbrook CR, *et al.* Neurobehavioral implications of habitual snoring in children. *Pediatrics.* 2004;**114**:44–9.

33. Mulvaney SA, Goodwin JL, Morgan WJ, *et al.* Behavior problems associated with sleep disordered breathing in school-aged children: the Tucson Children's Assessment of Sleep Apnea Study. *J Pediatr Psychol.* 2006;**31**:322–30.

34. Chervin R, Dillon J, Archbold K, Ruzicka D. Conduct problems and symptoms of sleep disorders in children. *J Am Acad Child Adolesc Psychiatry.* 2003;**42**(2):201–8.

35. Crabtree VM, Varni JW, Gozal D. Health-related quality of life and depressive symptoms in children with suspected sleep-disordered breathing. *Sleep.* 2004;**27**(6):1131–8.

36. Gozal D. Sleep-disordered breathing and school performance in children. *Pediatrics.* 1998;**102**:616–20.

37. Gottlieb DJ, Chase C, Vezina RM, *et al.* Sleep-disordered breathing symptoms are associated with poorer cognitive function in 5-year-old children. *J Pediatrics.* 2004;**145**(4):458–64.

38. Kaemingk KL, Pasvogel AE, Goodwin JL, *et al.*
Learning in children and sleep disordered breathing:
findings of the Tucson Children's Assessment of Sleep
Apnea (TuCASA) Prospective Cohort Study.
J Int Neuropsychol Soc. 2003;**9**:1016–26.

39. Chervin RD, Ruzicka DL, Giordani BJ, *et al.*
Sleep-disordered breathing, behavior, and cognition in
children before and after adenotonsillectomy.
Pediatrics. 2006;**117**:e769–e778.

40. Li HY, Huang YS, Chen NH, Fang TJ, Lee LA.
Impact of adenotonsillectomy on behavior in children
with sleep-disordered breathing, *Laryngoscope.*
2006;**116**:1142–7.

41. Avior G, Fishman G, Leor A, *et al.* The effect of
tonsillectomy and adenoidectomy on inattention and
impulsivity as measured by the Test of Variables of
Attention (TOVA) in children with obstructive sleep
apnea syndrome. *Otolaryngol Head Neck Surg.*
2004;**131**:367–71.

42. Huang YS, Guilleminault C, Li HY, *et al.*
Attention-deficit/hyperactivity disorder with
obstructive sleep apnea: a treatment outcome study.
Sleep Med. 2007;**8**(1):18–30.

43. Wei JL, Mayo MS, Smith HJ, Reese M, Weatherly RA.
Improved behavior and sleep after adenotonsillectomy
in children with sleep-disordered breathing. *Arch
Otolaryngol Head Neck Surg.* 2007;**133**:974–9.

44. Garetz SL. Behavior, cognition, and quality of life after
adenotonsillectomy for pediatric sleep-disordered
breathing: summary of the literature. *Otolaryngol Head
Neck Surg.* 2008;**138**(1):S19–S26.

45. Kessler RC, Adler L, Barkley R, *et al.* The prevalence
and correlates of adult ADHD in the United States:
results from the National Comorbidity Survey
Replication. *Am J Psychiatry.* 2006;**163**:716–23.

46. Surman CB, Thomas RJ, Aleardi M, Pagano C,
Biederman J. Adults With ADHD and sleep
complaints: a pilot study identifying sleep-disordered
breathing using polysomnography and sleep quality
assessment. *J Atten Disord.* 2006;**9**:550–5.

47. Naseem S, Chaudhary B, Collop N. Attention deficit
hyperactivity disorder in adults and obstructive sleep
apnea. *Chest.* 2001;**119**:294–6.

48. Mazza S, Pépin JL, Naëgelé B, *et al.* Most obstructive
sleep apnoea patients exhibit vigilance and attention
deficits on an extended battery of tests. *Eur Respir J.*
2005;**25**:75–80.

49. Saunamäki T, Jehkonen M. A review of executive
functions in obstructive sleep apnea syndrome.
Acta Neurol Scand. 2007;**115**(1):1–11.

50. Mathieu A, Mazza S, Décary A, *et al.* Effects of
obstructive sleep apnea on cognitive function:

a comparison between younger and older OSAS
patients. *Sleep Med.* 2008;**9**(2):112–20.

51. Kissling C, Retz W, Wiemann S, *et al.*
A polymorphism at the 3′-untranslated region of the
CLOCK gene is associated with adult attention-deficit
hyperactivity disorder. *Am J Med Genet
B Neuropsychiatr Genet.* 2008;**147B**(3):333–8.

52. Adams N, Strauss M, Schluchter M, Redline S.
Relation of measures of sleep-disordered breathing to
neuropsychological functioning. *Am J Respir Crit Care
Med.* 200;**163**(7):1626–31.

53. Schredl M, Alm B, Sobanski E. Sleep quality in adult
patients with attention deficit hyperactivity disorder
(ADHD). *Eur Arch Psychiatry Clin Neurosci.* 2007;
257(3):164–8.

54. Risk CG. The impact of sleep disorders on the
attention deficit disorder in the adult.
Part I: The patient with obstructive sleep apnea. *Chest.*
2005;**128**:231S.

55. American Academy of Sleep Medicine.
The International Classification of Sleep Disorders,
2nd edn. (Westchester: American Academy of Sleep
Medicine, 2005).

56. Allen RP, Walters AS, Montplaisir J, *et al.* Restless legs
syndrome prevalence and impact: REST general
population study. *Arch Intern Med.* 2005;**165**:1286–92.

57. Walters AS, Hickey K, Maltzman J, *et al.*
A questionnaire study of 138 patients with restless legs
syndrome: the 'Night-Walkers' survey. *Neurology.*
1996;**46**(1):92–5.

58. Picchietti D, Allen RP, Walters AS, *et al.* Restless legs
syndrome: prevalence and impact in children and
adolescents: Peds REST study. *Pediatrics.* 2007;
120(2):253–66.

59. Crabtree VM, Ivanenko A, O'Brien LM, Gozal D.
Periodic limb movement disorder of sleep in children.
J Sleep Res. 2003;**12**(1):73–81.

60. Winkelmann J, Lichtner P, Schormair B, *et al.* Variants
in the neuronal nitric oxide synthase (Nnos, NOS1)
gene are associated with restless legs syndrome.
Mov Disord. 2007;**23**:350–8.

61. Muhle H, Neumann A, Lohmann-Hedrich K, *et al.*
Childhood-onset restless legs syndrome: clinical and
genetic features of 22 families. *Mov Disord.* 2008;
23(8):1113–21.

62. Stiasny-Kolster K, Kohnen R, Carsten Moller J, *et al.*
Validation of the "L-DOPA Test" for diagnosis of
restless legs syndrome. *Mov Disord.* 2006;**21**:1233–9.

63. Michaud M, Soucy JP, Chabli A, *et al.* SPECT imaging
of striatal pre- and postsynaptic dopaminergic status in
restless legs syndrome with periodic leg movements in
sleep. *J Neurol.* 2002;**249**:164–70.

64. Allen RP. Race, iron status and restless legs syndrome. *Sleep Med.* 2002;**3**:467–8.

65. Allen RP, Picchietti D, Hening WA, *et al.* Restless legs syndrome: diagnostic criteria, special considerations, and epidemiology. A report from the restless legs syndrome diagnosis and epidemiology workshop at the National Institutes of Health. *Sleep Med.* 2003;**4**:101–19.

66. Rajaram SS, Walters AS, England SJ, Mehta D, Nizam F. Some children with growing pains may actually have restless legs syndrome. *Sleep.* 2004;**27**(4):767–73.

67. Kryger MH, Otake K, Foerster J. Low body stores of iron and restless legs syndrome: a correctable cause of insomnia in adolescents and teenagers. *Sleep Med.* 2002;**3**(2):127–32.

68. Simakajornboon N, Gozal D, Vlasic V, *et al.* Periodic limb movements in sleep and iron status in children. *Sleep.* 2003;**26**(6):735–8.

69. Cortese S, Konofal E, Lecendreux M. Effectiveness of ropinirole for RLS and depressive symptoms in an 11-year-old girl. *Sleep Med.* 2009;**10**(2):259–61.

70. Konofal E, Arnulf I, Lecendreux M, Mouren MC. Ropinirole in a child with attention-deficit hyperactivity disorder and restless legs syndrome. *Pediatr Neurol.* 2005;**32**(5):350–1.

71. Sadeh A, Pergamin L, Bar-Haim Y. Sleep in children with attention-deficit hyperactivity disorder: a meta-analysis of polysomnographic studies. *Sleep Med Rev.* 2006;**10**(6):381–98.

72. Chervin RD, Archbold KH, Dillon JE, *et al.* Associations between symptoms of inattention, hyperactivity, restless legs, and periodic leg movements. *Sleep.* 2002;**25**(2):213–18.

73. Picchietti DL, Walters AS. Moderate to severe periodic limb movement disorder in childhood and adolescence. *Sleep.* 1999;**22**(3):297–300.

74. Picchietti DL, Underwood DJ, Farris WA, *et al.* Further studies on periodic limb movement disorder and restless legs syndrome in children with attention-deficit hyperactivity disorder. *Mov Disord.* 1999;**14**(6):1000–7.

75. Wagner ML, Walters AS, Fisher BC. Symptoms of attention-deficit/hyperactivity disorder in adults with restless legs syndrome. *Sleep.* 2004;**27**(8):1499–504.

76. Cortese S, Lecendreux M, Mouren MC, Konofal E. ADHD and insomnia. *J Am Acad Child Adolesc Psychiatry.* 2006;**45**(4):384–5.

77. Cortese S, Konofal E, Lecendreux M, *et al.* Restless legs syndrome and attention-deficit/hyperactivity disorder: a review of the literature. *Sleep.* 2005;**28**(8):1007–13.

78. Walters AS, Mandelbaum DE, Lewin DS, *et al.* Dopaminergic therapy in children with restless legs/periodic limb movements in sleep and ADHD-Dopaminergic Therapy Study Group. *Pediatr Neurol.* 2000;**22**(3):182–6.

79. Sun ER, Chen CA, Ho G, Earley CJ, Allen RP. Iron and the restless legs syndrome. *Sleep.* 1998;**21**(4):371–7.

80. Oner P, Dirik EB, Taner Y, Caykoylu A, Anlar O. Association between low serum ferritin and restless legs syndrome in patients with attention deficit hyperactivity disorder. *Tohoku J Exp Med* 2007; **213**(3):269–76.

81. Konofal E, Cortese S, Marchand M, *et al.* Impact of restless legs syndrome and iron deficiency on attention-deficit/hyperactivity disorder in children. *Sleep Med.* 2007;**8**(7–8):711–15.

82. Konofal E, Lecendreux M, Deron J, *et al.* Effects of iron supplementation on attention deficit hyperactivity disorder in children. *Pediatr Neurol.* 2008;**38**(1):20–6.

Chapter 23

Sleep in autism spectrum disorders

Roger Godbout

Introduction

Autism is a pervasive developmental disorder with neurological origins [1], defined by a triad of symptoms in the social, communicative, and restricted interest and repetitive behaviors areas [2]. Asperger's syndrome is characterized by clinical manifestations that are very similar to autism except for the fact that the former do not suffer from a delay in the development of language. In the present chapter, autism and Asperger's syndrome will be grouped together under the term of autism spectrum disorders (ASD).

The prevalence of ASD is estimated to be 13 per 10,000 with a male:female ratio of approximately 4.5:1 [3]. The first signs of ASD appear before 36 months of age and the syndrome lasts an entire life, with the clinical picture improving throughout lifespan particularly regarding the social and communicative areas [4, 5, but see 6]. There are currently two sets of arguments suggesting an atypical brain organization in autism: impaired transfer of information between brain regions, i.e., a *connectivity disorder*, and ectopic localization of brain regions associated with some cognitive functions, i.e., *cortical reallocation*. In terms of event-related electroencephalography (EEG), the former refers to a diminished synchrony of activation, relative size, or coherence of EEG signals among pairs of functional regions normally involved in a given task. The latter refers to the activation of a brain region different from that used by typical control individuals, for example during performance on a specific cognitive task; cross-modal plasticity is an example of this phenomenon. A growing body of literature shows that sleep disorders constitute an indicator of abnormal neural functioning in autism and, therefore, a characteristic of the autism phenotype [7] and the following sections will review this literature.

Questionnaire studies

The prevalence of sleep disorders in typically developing children is approximately 30% [8] and this figure increases dramatically in children with ASD, up to 83% for an average of 65% [9–11]. These numbers that are higher than what has been described for other developmental disorders with various etiologies, although the severity itself might not be different across diagnoses [10].

Findings from questionnaire studies suggest that the sleep of persons with ASD is characterized by long sleep onset latencies, interrupted by nocturnal and early morning awakenings, and submitted to irregular circadian schedules [12–17]. Reports by parents suggest that sleep disorders may appear as early as two to three years old [12, 18] and Richdale and Prior [16] have observed that sleep disorders reported by parents of ASD children younger than eight years appeared to be more severe than in the older children. These authors proposed that sleep behavior may significantly improve with maturation in ASD, and clinical experience also shows that parental expertise and tolerance may also contribute to this prognosis. At the opposite extreme, Honomichl *et al.* [19] observed that parents of ASD children reported sleep disorders as being more severe in the six- to eleven-year-old group than in the two- to five-year-old group. Even though methodological issues can be raised to account for contradicting results in the ASD children literature [20], there is also evidence for sleep disorders in the adult ASD population from questionnaire studies [7, 21–23], suggesting that sleep disorders in ASD are not merely a question of developmental delay. The question of IQ is often rightly raised when discussing sleep disorders in autism and one study [24] has subdivided its ASD cohort using an IQ of 70 as the

Sleep and Mental Illness, eds. S. R. Pandi-Perumal and M. Kramer. Published by Cambridge University Press.
© Cambridge University Press 2010.

cut-off score; the two groups of ASD children were found to be comparable except for more nocturnal awakenings in the mentally retarded group. This contrasts with another study in which the IQ cut-off score was 55 and where the authors found a longer sleep latency in the group with the higher IQ. Besides the fact that IQ is associated to a myriad of comorbid conditions including epilepsy [25], and besides the fact that the quantification of IQ in ASD is presently a matter of debate [26], it has disputably been suggested that parents of ASD children may unreliably score the sleep of their children [27], a question that needs to be thoroughly investigated given the major clinical significance it carries. Although it is beyond the scope of this chapter, one must not forget that the parents of children with ASD also suffer from poor sleep [28], whether it is due to the burden of caregiving or to genetic factors.

One striking observation from our own study on subjective reports of sleep in adults with ASD and normal IQ [7] is that despite the fact that subjective measures of sleep in the ASD group were compatible with insomnia, and even though this was also documented with polysomnography, morning restfulness and sleep satisfaction were not different from the control group. This raises the question as to whether or not sleep disorders should be treated in ASD, keeping in mind that non-pharmacological, behavioral procedures for better sleep habits are available [29].

Objective measures

Actigraphy is a technique by which body movements are recorded with a wrist-worn meter and data are then translated into rest–activity cycles so that the main rest period can be analyzed to yield quantified sleep characteristics. A recent study for example used a one-week period to record actigraphic and sleep diary data in 32 school-age children with Asperger's syndrome and high-functioning autism [30]: compared to controls, ASD children showed sleep onset difficulties on the sleep diaries and actigraphy, while Asperger's syndrome and high-functioning autism groups were not different from one another. Subjective data on sleep in ASD may not always be supported by objective evidence, however, since another study only supported the presence of early morning awakenings in eight children with ASD, while all other actigraphy data were equivalent to those of control participants [31].

Actigraphy cannot quantify variables accessible to polysomnography such as sleep stage duration and transitions, REM sleep parameters, and the quantification of phasic sleep events (sleep spindles, K-complexes, rapid eye movements). In fact, there are very few reports on laboratory sleep recordings in autism. Early studies have revealed REM sleep abnormalities in autistic children, including dissociated REM sleep (i.e., intrusion of sleep spindle activity in the EEG tracing) [32] and fewer rapid eye movements [33]. The next study involved polysomnography in four children with ASD and revealed an increased number of stage shifts along with a decreased proportion of stage 2 sleep relative to five controls, together with increased rapid eye movements [34]. None of the aforementioned studies controlled for diagnostic tools, associated conditions, and/or IQ. One more recent study implemented such controls and recorded the sleep of 21 children aged four to ten years old and diagnosed with ASD. Interestingly enough, no significant differences were found between the ASD group and controls on any of the polysomnographic parameters recorded on night #2, following a night of adaptation to laboratory conditions [35]. This contrasts with polysomnography results obtained in adults adapted to laboratory conditions, controlled for comorbidity, and without actual complaints about their sleep. In one study [36], a group of eight adults with Asperger's syndrome showed difficulty in maintaining sleep in early parts of the night, displayed a pathological number of periodic leg movements during sleep and had unstable REM sleep despite a normal amount of rapid eye movements. It was suggested that anomalies in voluntary ocular saccades in autism were due to an impairment in neocortical areas [37, 38], some of which are also involved in the control of REM sleep ocular saccades, including the frontal cortex [39] as well as the loop made of the midpontine region, the frontal eye field, and the limbic system [40]. This paper [36] also confirmed a previous case study [41] in which low EEG spindle activity was reported. These findings were later confirmed again and extended, both in Asperger's syndrome and high-functining autism in a larger group of patients [7], including a longer sleep latency, more frequent nocturnal awakenings, lower sleep efficiency, increased duration of shallow (stage 1) sleep, decreased SWS, fewer stage 2 EEG sleep spindles, and a lower number of rapid eye movements during REM sleep.

The host of these findings indicate that micro- and macrostructure of sleep in ASD depart from what is found in comparison groups and that sleep instability may constitute a salient feature of the ASD phenotype.

References

1. London E, Haroutunian V, eds. Symposium: Neurobiology of Autism. *Brain Pathology.* 2007;**17**(4):407–59.

2. Volkmar FR, Lord C, Bailey A, Schultz RT, Klin A. Autism and pervasive developmental disorders. *J Child Psychol Psychiatry Allied Discipl.* 2004;**45**:135–70.

3. Fombonne E. Epidemiology of autistic disorder and other pervasive developmental disorders. *J Clin Psychiatry.* 2005;**66**:3–8.

4. Fecteau S, Mottron L, Burack J, Berthiaume C. Developmental changes of autistic symptoms. *Autism.* 2003;**6**:67–81.

5. Piven J, Harper J, Palmer P, Arndt S. Course of behavioral change in autism: a retrospective study of high-IQ adolescents and adults. *J Am Acad Child Adol Psychiatry.* 1996;**35**:523–9.

6. Howlin P, Goode S, Hutton J, Rutter M. Adult outcome for children with autism. *J Child Psychol Psychiatry.* 2004;**45**:212–29.

7. Limoges E, Mottron L, Bolduc C, Berthiaume C, Godbout R. Atypical sleep architecture and the autism phenotype. *Brain.* 2005;**128**:1049–61.

8. Mindell JA. Sleep disorders in children. *Health Psychology.* 1993;**12**:151–62.

9. Johnson CR. Sleep problems in children with mental retardation and autism. *Child Adol Psychiatr Clin North Am.* 1996;**5**:673–83.

10. Polimeni MA, Richdale AL, Francis JP. A survey of sleep problems in autism, Asperger's disorder and typically developing children. *J Intell Disab Res.* 2005;**49**:260–8.

11. Richdale AL. Sleep in children with autism and Asperger syndrome. In: Stores G, Wiggs L, eds. *Sleep Disturbances in Children and Adolescents with Disorders of Development: Its Significance and Management.* (London: MacKeith Press, 2001; 181–91).

12. Hoshino Y, Watanabe H, Yashima Y, Kaneko M, Kumashiro H. An investigation on sleep disturbance of autistic children. *Folia Psychiatrica et Neurologica Japonica.* 1984;**38**:45–51.

13. Lainhart JE. Psychiatric problems in individuals with autism, their parents and siblings. *Int Rev Psychiatry.* 1999;**11**:278–98.

14. Patzold LM, Richdale AL, Tonge BJ. An investigation into sleep characteristics of children with autism and Asperger's disorder. *J Paediatric Child Health.* 1998;**34**:528–33.

15. Richdale AL. Sleep problems in autism: prevalence, cause, and intervention. *Dev Med Child Neurol.* 1999;**41**:60–6.

16. Richdale AL, Prior MR. The sleep/wake rhythm in children with autism. *Eur Child Adol Psychiatry.* 1995;**4**:175–86.

17. Stores G, Wiggs L. Abnormal sleep patterns associated with autism: a brief review of research findings, assessment methods and treatment strategies. *Autism.* 1998;**2**:157–69.

18. Taira M, Takase M, Sasaki H. Sleep disorder in children with autism. *Psychiatry Clin Neurosci.* 1998;**52**:182–3.

19. Honomichl RD, Goodlin-Jones BL, Burnham M, Gaylor E, Anders TF. Sleep patterns of children with pervasive developmental disorders. *J Autism Dev Dis.* 2002;**32**:553–61.

20. Richdale AL. A comment on Honomichl RD. *et al.* (2002). *J Autism Dev Dis.* 2004;**34**:553–61.

21. Oyane NMF, Bjorvatn B. Sleep disturbances in adolescents and young adults with autism or Asperger syndrome. *Autism.* 2005;**9**:83–94.

22. Tani P, Lindberg N, Niemen-von Wendt T, *et al.* Insomnia is a frequent finding in adults with Asperger syndrome. *BMC Psychiatry.* 2003;**3**:12.

23. Tani P, Lindberg N, Joukamaa M, *et al.* Asperger syndrome, alexithymia and perception of sleep. *Neuropsychobiology.* 2004;**49**:64–70.

24. Gail Williams P, Sears LL, Allard A. Sleep problems in children with autism. *J Sleep Res.* 2004;**13**:265–8.

25. Amiet C, Gourfinkel-An I, Bouzamondo A, *et al.* Epilepsy in autism is associated with intellectual disability and gender: evidence from a meta-analysis. *Biol Psychiatry.* 2008;**64**:577–82.

26. Dawson M, Soulières I, Gernsbacher MA, Mottron L. The level and nature of autistic intelligence. *Psychol Sci.* 2007;**18**:657–62.

27. Schreck KA, Mulick JA. Parental report of sleep problems in children with autism. *J Autism Dev Dis.* 2000;**30**:127–35.

28. Meltzer LJ. Sleep in parents of children with autism spectrum disorders. *J Pediatr Psychol.* 2008;**33**:380–6.

29. Jan JE, Owens JA, Weiss MD, *et al.* Sleep hygiene for children with neurodevelopmental disabilities. *Pediatrics.* 2008;**122**:1343–50.

30. Allik H, Larsson JO, Smedje H. Sleep patterns of school-age children with Asperger syndrome or high-functioning autism. *J Autism Dev Dis.* 2006;**36**:585–95.

31. Hering E, Epstein R, Elroy S, Iancu DR, Zelnik N. Sleep patterns in autistic children. *J Autism Dev Dis.* 1999;**29**:143–7.

32. Ornitz EM, Ritvo ER, Brown MB, *et al.* The EEG and rapid eye movements during REM sleep in normal and autistic children. *Electroencephalogr Clin Neurophysiol.* 1969;**26**:167–75.

33. Tanguay PE, Ornitz EM, Forsythe AB, Ritvo ER. Rapid eye movement (REM) activity in normal and autistic children during REM sleep. *J Autism Child Schizophr.* 1976;**6**:275–88.

34. Elia M, Ferri R, Musumeci SA, Bergonzi P. Rapid eye movement modulation during night sleep in autistic subjects. *Brain Dysfunction.* 1991;**4**:348–54.

35. Malow BA, Marzec ML, McGrew SG, *et al.* Characterizing sleep in children with autism spectrum disorders: a multidimensional approach. *Sleep.* 2006;**29**:1563–71.

36. Godbout R, Bergeron C, Limoges E, Stip E, Mottron L. A laboratory study of sleep in Asperger's syndrome. *NeuroReport.* 2000;**11**:127–30.

37. Kemner C, Verbaten MN, Cuperus JM, Camfferman G, van Engeland H. Abnormal saccadic eye movements in autistic children. *J Autism Dev Disord.* 1998;**28**:61–7.

38. Minshew NJ, Luna B, Sweeney JA. Oculomotor evidence for neocortical systems but not cerebellar dysfunction in autism. *Neurology.* 1999;**52**:917–22.

39. Hong CC, Gillin JC, Dow BM, Wu J, Buchsbaum MS. Localized and lateralized cerebral glucose metabolism associated with eye movements during REM sleep and wakefulness: a positron emission tomography (PET) study. *Sleep.* 1995;**18**:570–80.

40. Ioannides AA, Corsi-Cabrera M, Fenwick PBC, *et al.* MEG tomography of human cortex and brainstem activity in waking and REM sleep saccades. *Cerebral Cortex.* 2004;**14**:56–72.

41. Godbout R, Bergeron C, Stip E, Mottron L. A laboratory study of sleep and dreaming in a case of Asperger's syndrome. *Dreaming.* 1998;**8**:75–88.

Chapter 24

Sleep in schizophrenia

Roger Godbout

Introduction

The relationship between sleep and schizophrenia has been fascinating scientists, clinicians, philosophers, and the patients themselves for immemorial times. Most probably because of the perceived similarity between the positive symptoms of schizophrenia and dreaming, psychosis has been considered as a state of waking dreams [1]. More recently, this idea has been revived both by "neuro-psychoanalysts" such as Carhart-Harris [2] and neuroscientists such as Gottesmann [3] who find not only a psychological resemblance but also strong neurobiological similarities between the dreaming state and schizophrenia. If this were true, one should expect to find fewer differences on selected appropriate dependent variables between sleep and wake cognitions in persons with schizophrenia than in healthy individuals or, alternatively, no difference between daytime cognitions of persons with schizophrenia and dreams of healthy individuals. Such a finding has not yet been reported in the scientific literature, although self-report questionnaires and laboratory-based dream narratives of patients with schizophrenia appear to be qualitatively and quantitatively different from comparison groups [4, 5]. Contrary to dreaming, the literature on sleep and schizophrenia is well documented; sleep plays a significant role in the clinical picture of this disease and it may also point to some of its pathophysiological mechanisms. This chapter is divided into three parts: the first part will discuss the clinical aspects of sleep disorders in persons with schizophrenia, the second part will review subjective reports of sleep, and the last part will cover objective findings.

Schizophrenia in the sleep disorders clinic

The International Classification of Sleep Disorders (ICSD) lists the sleep disorders in schizophrenia in the section on "Sleep Disorders Associated with Mental Disorders", under the heading of "Psychosis" [6] (it is noteworthy that the bibliography refers only to studies in schizophrenia). Sleep disorders are described as varying together with the waxing and waning phases of chronic schizophrenia, whereas insomnia may alternate with excessive sleepiness. For example, the acute exacerbation of psychotic symptoms is usually accompanied by a severe disturbance of sleep continuity while chronic stable patients may appear as having long periods of uninterrupted sleep. Below are some of the essential features of ICSD indications [6].

Diagnostic criteria

The ICSD diagnostic criteria for "Psychoses associated with sleep disturbance" are:

a. The patient has a complaint of insomnia or excessive sleepiness.

b. The patient has a clinical diagnosis of schizophrenia, schizophreniform disorder, or other functional psychosis.

c. Polysomnographic monitoring demonstrates an increased sleep latency, reduced sleep efficiency, an increased number and duration of awakenings, and often a reversed first-night effect.

d. The sleep disturbance is not associated with other medical or mental disorders (e.g., dementia).

e. The complaint does not meet diagnostic criteria for other sleep disorders.

Sleep and Mental Illness, eds. S. R. Pandi-Perumal and M. Kramer. Published by Cambridge University Press.

The ICSD minimal criteria are (a) plus (b); it is thus noteworthy that the diagnosis of a sleep disorder in a person with schizophrenia can be solely based on subjective complaints and that polysomnography, i.e., the simultaneous recording of many physiological parameters during sleep, is not required.

Possible associated features

The clinical evaluation of sleep in patients with schizophrenia should include a monitoring of the following features:

- odd bedtimes and rise times, together with a disruption of other daily activities such as mealtimes
- time course: sleep disorders may precede decompensation, acute exacerbation, and relapses
- predisposing factors: medical illness and increased stress may trigger sleep disturbance
- most psychotic patients experience some degree of sleep disruption during exacerbations of their illness, regardless of gender
- severe sleep disruption may exacerbate symptoms of schizophrenia, induce impulsivity and aggressivity, to the degree that patients can become suicidal.

Differential diagnosis

Conditions that should be ruled out include other sleep disorders such as periodic leg movement or sleep apneas, side effects of antipsychotic medication (sedation or akathisia), drug-induced psychosis, drug and alcohol withdrawal, mood disorders, and post-traumatic stress disorders.

Duration and severity criteria

The possible duration of sleep disorders is broken down into three levels: acute = four weeks or less; subacute = more than four weeks but less than two years; chronic = two years or longer.

Severity criteria have three levels that can be summarized as follows [6]: mild = an almost nightly complaint, with little or no impact on daytime functioning; moderate = nightly complaint, with mild or moderate impact on daytime functioning; severe = nightly complaint, with severe impact on daytime functioning.

Subjective reports of sleep in schizophrenia

Subjective reports of sleep disorders often precede psychotic relapse, as reported by the patients or relatives [7], and the same applies to acutely ill and chronic patients, including increased sleep latency, increased nocturnal awakenings, and disturbing dreams [8, 9]. During the prodromal phase, patients and clinicians also report a delay in the sleep–wake schedule possibly associated with insomnia and daytime somnolence. Accordingly, chronotype characterization through questionnaires has revealed a greater proportion of types in middle-aged chronic outpatients with schizophrenia compared to controls [10]. The same study showed that evening chronotype was associated with a lower quality of sleep as estimated by a standard questionnaire, i.e., the Pittsburgh Sleep Quality Index [11]. The issue of chronotype and circadian rhythms in schizophrenia is not so simple as there is also evidence for the possibility of a phase advance in this disease, with comparable consequences on sleep latency and sleep continuity [12]. The question of sleep disorders and aging is a significant one in schizophrenia and older patients are particularly concerned with the need to improve their sleep [13] and, as a matter of fact, aging is possibly associated with a phase advance of biological rhythms [14]. Although the improvement of sleep quality following treatment with atypical antipsychotics is appealing to older patients based on questionnaire studies [15], one must not forget that treatment may have to be interrupted at one point and that withdrawal may then induce serious sleep difficulties [16].

The presence of daytime somnolence/sleepiness often reported in schizophrenia can be interpreted as a consequence of poor sleep or impaired circadian rhythms, even though actual evidence in favor of one or the other is not so abundant. Sedation is also a well known secondary effect of many neuroleptics, including those of the second generation (i.e., atypical antipsychotics). A thorough evaluation of nocturnal sleep as well as daytime alertness is thus a prerequisite that has to be based on the most recent data and sound clinical tools available. The recent review of Kane and Sharif [17] includes a good discussion on antipsychotic-induced sedation and it presents clinical tools to measure the risk–benefit balance when using this last class of molecules. In this regard, on one hand, caution must be taken not to interpret sedation or daytime "somnolence" as if it were daytime "sleepiness", i.e., true sleep. Indeed, psychomotor slowing or severe negative symptoms may lead a patient to seek social isolation by retiring and resting in bed. On the other hand, true sleepiness can be induced by the sleep apnea syndrome, the incidence of which increases with age, including in persons with schizophrenia [18], often together with a sudden gain of weight following a medication change [19]. The next paragraphs will review some of the literature on objective measures of sleep in schizophrenia.

Objective findings on sleep in schizophrenia

Laboratory recordings of sleep for research purposes in patients with schizophrenia can be challenging in terms of recruitment capacity, sampling bias, and uncontrolled independent variables, and it is thus not surprising to find that published results have been equivocal [20]. Protocols are more easily achieved in strictly clinical circumstances, like testing the presence of pathological sleep apneas with or without EEG awakenings. In that context, the growth of a clinical data base may soon permit the generation of coherent results based on homogenous samples. Meanwhile, the use of statistical meta-analysis techniques has permitted us to draw general conclusions on the sleep of patients with schizophrenia [21, 22] to which other studies can be compared. In both settings, experimental and clinical, recordings should be monitored by a qualified polysomnographic technologist in order to assure quality control, management of unexpected technical events, and proper contact with patients.

It is useful to divide sleep findings into two categories. The first category of variables is related to sleep initiation and maintenance; these are useful to test the presence of insomnia and can be used to quantify sleep quality and efficiency. The second category corresponds to variables related to the NREM–REM sleep cycle; the values of these variables cannot be estimated by subjective measures and point towards neurobiological control of sleep cycles. Both sets of data can be used to identify sleep–wake mechanisms [23, 24] that can possibly share pathophysiological substrates with those underlying schizophrenia [25, 26].

Polysomnographically monitored sleep of neuroleptic-free patients with schizophrenia

There are two published statistical meta-analysis studies on sleep in drug-free patients. The first one

[21] analyzed only three published data sets and found increased sleep latency, decreased total sleep time, and decreased slow-wave sleep (SWS: stage 3 and stage 4) in groups of patients with schizophrenia compared to controls. Our own [22] meta-analysis included 20 studies, with 321 patients with schizophrenia and 331 control participants. Results indicated that neuroleptic-free patients with schizophrenia had an increased sleep latency, a decreased total sleep time, and a decreased sleep efficiency, all consistent with a difficulty of initiating and maintaining sleep, but we found no differences in SWS or REM sleep. We also found that patients withdrawn from neuroleptics had more sleep disorders than neuroleptic-naive patients. On one hand, we can conclude from these results that insomnia in schizophrenia is an intrinsic feature of the disease rather than a consequence of neuroleptic use. On the other hand, the results on SWS and REM sleep need more discussion. In the 20 studies we reviewed [22], 13 compared patients with schizophrenia to controls on SWS and only two (15%) found a significant difference between the groups. If only stage 4 were analyzed, four of the 12 available studies (33%) showed a significant difference. Since one of the main characteristics of stage 4 is to display EEG activity with high voltage and slow frequencies in the delta range (0.5–4.0 Hz), quantified analysis of EEG slow-wave activity may be the technique of choice to compare patients with schizophrenia to controls with regards to SWS. Concerning REM sleep latency, a comparable situation prevailed: 10 out of 20 studies (50%) found a significantly shorter REM sleep latency in the schizophrenia group. In this case, the duration of the neuroleptic-free period may have played a role. For example, one study [26] found that previously treated patients withdrawn for two to four weeks had a shorter REM sleep latency (and greater REM sleep duration) compared to patients withdrawn for more than four weeks. Gender differences may also play a role in REM sleep latency in schizophrenia since another study [27] found a statistically significant relationship between reduced REM sleep latency and poor outcome in female patients, but not in male patients. This also suggests that the pathophysiological mechanisms underlying REM sleep latency in schizophrenia are different in male and female patients. More generally, unconfirmed expected results may be due to the fact that studies have not always controlled for variables such as daytime napping on the day of recording, or

the inclusion of participants with comorbid sleep disorders such as sleep apnea or sleep-related periodic limb movements.

Despite its powerful capacity to generate new interpretations from scattered data sets, statistical meta-analysis has its limits. For example, meaningful dependent variables may not be entered as moderator variables in the calculations because they have not been used by a sufficient number of studies, including duration of the illness, chronicity, diagnosis subtype, scale symptoms (e.g., positive and negative symptoms), and subtypes of antipsychotic molecules.

Based on the results described above it is reasonable to conclude that sleep disorders are an intrinsic feature of schizophrenia. Since these results were extracted from the sleep of acutely ill, drug-naive, and neuroleptic-withdrawn patients, it can also be concluded that these sleep disorders are not a consequence of neuroleptic treatments, even though it must be remembered that sleep in neuroleptic-withdrawn schizophrenia patients is not comparable to that of drug-naive patients [28].

Effects of neuroleptics on polysomnographic measures in schizophrenia

Despite the large variability in methodology, data generally point toward a positive effect of neuroleptics on sleep continuity [29, 30]. The effects of neuroleptics on subjective measures of sleep have been described to be generally positive except for sedative side effects (see above). Objective measures of sleep architecture using polysomnography may vary, due to heterogeneous methodologies, but recent comprehensive literature reviews [29, 30] show the following: (a) typical neuroleptics including haloperidol, thiothixene, and flupenthixol improve sleep initiation and maintenance while they may inhibit REM sleep; (b) atypical neuroleptics such as olanzapine, risperidone, quetiapine, clozapine, and ziprazidone also generally facilitate sleep consolidation and REM sleep duration and increase SWS with the exception of quetiapine and risperidone, which may inhibit it under certain conditions [31].

In addition to current neuroleptic treatment, patients with schizophrenia are occasionally given melatonin to improve their sleep further, but published accounts are rare. Two of these studies have shown an improvement of sleep [32, 33] and a third one found that melatonin increased sleep disorders upon a first night in the laboratory (i.e., the so-called "first night effect") [34]. Whether the effects of melatonin on sleep of schizophrenia patients under neuroleptic treatment relates to basal rate of melatonin activity needs to be determined [35].

Conclusion

Although sleep disorders are not part of the required diagnostic criteria for schizophrenia, they constitute an intimate dimension of the clinical picture of this disease. There is also evidence that sleep, clinical status, and daytime performance covary in schizophrenia. Effort should be devoted to find whether this relationship is multidirectional or not, in order to adapt optimal treatment strategies.

References

1. Freud S. *The Interpretation of Dreams* (1900), translated by AA. Brill. (New York: Gramercy Books, 1996).

2. Carhart-Harris R. Waves of the unconscious: the neurophysiology of dreamlike phenomena and its implications for the psychodynamic model of the mind. *Neuro-Psychoanalysis.* 2007;**9**:183–211.

3. Gottesmann C. The dreaming sleep stage: a new neurobiological model of schizophrenia? *Neuroscience.* 2006;**140**:1105–15.

4. Kramer M. Dreams and psychopathology. In: Kryger MH, Roth T, Dement WC, eds. *Principles and Practice of Sleep Medicine*, 3rd edition. (Philadelphia: Saunders, 2000; 511–19).

5. Lusignan FA, Zadra A, Dubuc MJ, et al. Dream content in chronically-treated persons with schizophrenia. *Schizophr Res.* 2009;**112**(1–3):164–73.

6. American Academy of Sleep Medicine. *International Classification of Sleep Disorders, Revised: Diagnostic and Coding Manual.* (Chicago: American Academy of Sleep Medicine, 2001).

7. Herz M. Prodromal symptoms and prevention of relapse in schizophrenia. *J Clin Psychiatry.* 1985;**46**:22–5.

8. Royuela A, Macias JA, Gil-Verona JA, et al. Sleep in schizophrenia: a preliminary study using the Pittsburgh Sleep Quality Index. *Neurobiol Sleep Wakefulness Cycle.* 2002;**2**:37–9.

9. Ritsner M, Kurs R, Ponizovsky A, Hadjez J. Perceived quality of life in schizophrenia: relationships to sleep quality. *Qual Life Res.* 2004;**13**:783–91.

10. Hofstetter JR, Mayeda AR, Happel CG, Lysaker PH. Sleep and daily activity preferences in schizophrenia: associations with neurocognition and symptoms. *J Nerv Ment Dis.* 2003;**191**:408–10.

11. Buysse DJ, Reynolds CF III, Monk TH, Berman SR, Kupfer DJ. The Pittsburgh Sleep Quality Index: a new instrument for psychiatric practice and research. *Psych Res.* 1989;**28**:193–213.

12. Boivin DB. Influence of sleep–wake and circadian rhythm disturbances in psychiatric disorders. *J Psychiatry Neurosci.* 2000;**25**:446–58.

13. Auslander LA, Jeste DV. Perceptions of problems and needs for service among middle-aged and elderly outpatients with schizophrenia and related psychotic disorders. *Community Ment Health J.* 2002;**38**:391–402.

14. Czeisler CA, Dumont M, Duffy JF, *et al.* Association of sleep–wake habits in older people with changes in output of circadian pacemaker. *Lancet.* 1992;**340**:933–6.

15. Yamashita H, Mori K, Nagao M, *et al.* Influence of aging on the improvement of subjective sleep quality by atypical antipsychotic drugs in patients with schizophrenia: comparison of middle-aged and older adults. *Am J Geriatr Psychiatry.* 2005;**13**:377–84.

16. Chemerinski E, Ho BC, Flaum M, *et al.* Insomnia as a predictor for symptom worsening following antipsychotic withdrawal in schizophrenia. *Compr Psychiatry.* 2002;**43**:393–6.

17. Kane JM, Sharif ZA. Atypical antipsychotics: sedation versus efficacy. *J Clin Psychiatry.* 2008; **69** (Suppl 1):18–31.

18. Ancoli-Israel S, Martin J, Jones DW, *et al.* Sleep-disordered breathing and periodic limb movements in sleep in older patients with schizophrenia. *Biol Psychiatry.* 1999;**45**:1426–32.

19. Winkelman JW. Schizophrenia, obesity, and obstructive sleep apnea. *J Clin Psychiatry.* 2001;**62**:8–11.

20. Monti JM, Monti D. Sleep disturbance in schizophrenia. *Int J Psychiatry.* 2005;**17**:247–53.

21. Benca RM, Obermeyer WH, Thisted RA, Gillin JC. Sleep and psychiatric disorders. A meta-analysis. *Arch Gen Psychiatry.* 1992;**49**:651–68; discussion 669–70.

22. Chouinard S, Poulin J, Stip E, Godbout R. Sleep in untreated patients with schizophrenia: a meta-analysis. *Schizophr Bull.* 2004;**30**:957–67.

23. Fuller PM, Gooley JJ, Saper CB. Neurobiology of the sleep–wake cycle: sleep architecture, circadian regulation, and regulatory feedback. *J Biol Rhythms.* 2006;**21**:482–93.

24. Fuller PM, Saper CB, Lu J. The pontine REM switch: past and present. *J Physiol.* 2007;**584**:735–41.

25. Poulin J, Daoust AM, Forest G, Stip I, Godbout R. Sleep architecture and its clinical correlates in first episode and neuroleptic-naive patients with schizophrenia. *Schizophr Res.* 2003;**62**:147–53.

26. Forest G, Poulin J, Lussier I, Stip E, Godbout R. Attention and non-REM sleep in neuroleptic-naive persons with schizophrenia and control participants. *Psychiatry Res.* 2007;**149**:33–40.

27. Tandon R, Shipley JE, Taylor S, *et al.* Electroencephalographic sleep abnormalities in schizophrenia: relationship to positive/negative symptoms and prior neuroleptic treatment. *Arch Gen Psychiatry.* 1992;**49**:185–94.

28. Goldman M, Tandon R, DeQuard JR, *et al.* Biological predictors of 1-year outcome in schizophrenia in males and females. *Schizophr Res.* 1996;**21**:65–73.

29. Monti JM, Monti D. Sleep in schizophrenia patients and the effects of antipsychotic drugs. *Sleep Med Rev.* 2004;**8**:133–48.

30. Krystal AD, Goforth HW, Roth T. Effects of antipsychotic medications on sleep in schizophrenia. *Int Clin Psychopharmacol.* 2008;**23**:150–60.

31. Keshavan MS, Prasad KM, Montrose DM, Miewald JM, Kupfer DJ. Sleep quality and architecture in quetiapine, risperidone, or never-treated schizophrenia patients. *J Clin Psychopharmacol.* 2007;**27**:703–5.

32. Kumar PNS, Andrade C, Bhakta SG, Singh NM. Melatonin in schizophrenic outpatients with insomnia: a double-blind, placebo-controlled study. *J Clin Psychiatry.* 2007;**68**:237–41.

33. Shamir E, Laudon M, Barak Y, *et al.* Melatonin improves sleep quality of patients with chronic schizophrenia. *J Clin Psychiatry.* 2000; **61**:373–7.

34. Shamir E, Rotenberg VS, Laudon M, Zisapel N, Elizur A. First-night effect of melatonin treatment in patients with chronic schizophrenia. *J Clin Psychopharmacol.* 2000;**20**:691–4.

35. Rotenberg VS. Sleep of patients with schizophrenia on and off melatonin treatment: contradictions and hypothesis. In: Bosch P, van den Noort M, eds. *Schizophrenia, Sleep, and Acupuncture.* (Goettingen: Hogrefe & Huber Publishers, 2008; 104–21).

Chapter 25

Fatigue and sleepiness in affective illness

Jonathan Adrian Ewing Fleming

Introduction

Disrupted sleep is a core symptom of most acute psychiatric illnesses, and is a prominent feature of the mood disorders both during an acute episode and during periods of remission between episodes [1]. If disrupted sleep continues as a residual symptom of depression, after an otherwise successful treatment of a major depressive disorder (MDD), there is a significant risk for relapse. For example, two-thirds of patients with persistent insomnia following treatment with nortriptyline and interpersonal psychotherapy relapsed within one year after discontinuation of active medication (placebo washout) whereas 90% of patients with good sleep, at the end of the acute treatment period, remained well [2].

When sleep is disrupted in normal sleepers it causes a number of symptoms, including fatigue and, if sleep loss is marked or protracted, daytime sleepiness [3]. However, the symptoms of fatigue and sleepiness in patients with both primary and secondary mood disorders appear to have a more complicated etiology than simply sleep disruption or sleep loss. Indeed, improving sleep performance may not impact fatigue as the core feature of pathological fatigue is that it persists after adequate rest [4]. This chapter outlines the presentation of fatigue and sleepiness in affective illness, reviews non-evidence-based strategies that may be helpful in management, and defines the limited, evidence-based treatments known to alleviate these impairing symptoms.

The mood disorders

The DSM-IV-TR diagnostic system [1] identifies four types of mood episodes (major depressive episode, manic episode, mixed episode, and hypomanic episode)

that have their own diagnostic criteria but are not diagnosed as separate entities; they are the building blocks for the ten mood disorder diagnoses (e.g., major depressive disorder, dysthymic disorder, and bipolar I disorder) that once made must be further specified by applying one of three specifiers: (1) the clinical status of the current (or most recent) mood episode; (2) the features of the current episode; and (3) the course of recurrent episodes. See Table 25.1.

A core feature of the DSM-IV-TR system is that the clinician is required to exclude medical and substance-use disorders before making a primary mood disorder diagnosis. Of course, mood disorders are common comorbidities of medical and substance-use disorders but they are diagnosed separately as either a mood disorder due to a general medical condition (characterized by a prominent and persistent disturbance in mood associated with that medical condition) or a substance-induced mood disorder (characterized by a prominent and persistent disturbance in mood associated with medication use or substance abuse). Obviously these two conditions – mood disorder due to a general medical condition and substance-induced mood disorder – are complex and, in both the acute and chronic phases of these disorders, disturbed sleep with daytime fatigue and sleepiness are common disturbances. The discussion of fatigue and sleepiness in this chapter will address the primary mood disorders where these symptoms are known to be prominent and problematic. See Table 25.2.

Because fatigue is a common symptom and disturbed sleep a frequent accompaniment to acute and chronic psychiatric illness, it is not surprising that these two symptoms are seen in a variety of psychiatric conditions (see Tables 25.3 and 25.4) requiring the clinician to complete a full medical and

Sleep and Mental Illness, eds. S. R. Pandi-Perumal and M. Kramer. Published by Cambridge University Press.
© Cambridge University Press 2010.

Table 25.1 The DSM-IV-TR mood disorders

The mood episodes

Major depressive episode (major depressive episode)

Manic episode (manic episode)

Mixed episode (mixed episode)

Hypomanic episode (hypomanic episode)

The depressive disorders

Major depressive disorder

Dysthymic disorder

Depressive disorder not otherwise specified

The bipolar disorders

Bipolar I disorder

Bipolar II disorder (recurrent major depressive episodes with hypomanic episodes)

Cyclothymic disorder

Bipolar disorder not otherwise specified

The other mood disorders

Mood disorder due to a general medical condition

Substance-induced mood disorder

Mood disorder not otherwise specified

Table 25.2 DSM-IV-TR mood disorders known to present with prominent symptoms of fatigue and/or hypersomnia

Major depressive episodes

During an episode

As a residual symptom (partial remission of mood episode)

With atypical or melancholic features

With seasonal pattern

Bipolar I and II [5]

Table 25.3 The DSM-IV-TR differential diagnosis of decreased energy or fatigue

1. Sleep disorders

Breathing-related sleep disorder

Narcolepsy

Primary hypersomnia

Primary insomnia

Parasomnias

2. Mood and anxiety disorders

Major depressive episode

(Depressive episodes further specified as atypical, melancholic or with a seasonal pattern may present with prominent fatigue and/or hypersomnia)

Dysthymic disorder

Generalized anxiety disorder

3. Other major psychiatric disorders

Dementia

Schizoaffective disorder

Schizophrenia

Schizophreniform disorder

Undifferentiated somatoform disorder

4. Psychiatric disorders associated with medical disorders or substance use

Personality change due to a general medical condition

Substance intoxication

Substance withdrawal

psychiatric assessment to ensure that the correct diagnosis of a primary mood disorder is made.

Fatigue

Neurasthenia, defined in the 1870s, was the medical term first used to describe the states of fatigue, fatigability, muscular weakness, and mental hypersensitivity [5] but as a diagnostic entity in psychiatry, it has had a chequered history. Although the ICD-10 includes research diagnostic criteria for this disorder [6] the neurasthenic syndrome is significant but uncommon with only one in nine people complaining of fatigue meeting the current, ICD-10, research criteria for this disorder [7].

Fatigue, on the other hand, is a common symptom; the prevalence for prolonged (more than one month) fatigue ranges from 18 to 37% [7] yet a generally accepted definition for this common, subjective, non-specific symptom has remained elusive. It has been defined as an extreme and persistent tiredness, weakness, or exhaustion – mental, physical, or both [8] but no simple definition successfully captures its complexity as it can be considered a single

Table 25.4 The DSM-IV-TR differential diagnosis of hypersomnia

1. Sleep disorders

   Breathing-related sleep disorder

   Narcolepsy

   Circadian rhythm sleep disorder

   Primary hypersomnia

   Hypersomnia related to another mental disorder

   Sleep disorder due to a general medical condition

   Substance-induced sleep disorder

   Primary insomnia

   Parasomnias

2. Mood disorders

   Major depressive episode

   Dysthymic disorder

3. Other major psychiatric disorders

   Delirium

   Schizophrenia

   Schizophreniform disorder

   Schizoaffective disorder

4. Psychiatric disorders associated with medical disorders or substance use

   Adverse effects of medication not otherwise specified

   Substance intoxication

   Substance withdrawal

symptom, a cluster of symptoms, or a specific syndrome (e.g., chronic fatigue syndrome [CFS] or cancer-related fatigue) [9].

Fatigue usually lacks a clear somatic cause [10], its etiology is poorly understood, and often it is a functional symptom [11, 12]. When viewed as a multidimensional symptom, fatigue affects three domains of functioning: (1) physical (e.g., reduced activity, general weakness, decreased physical endurance, etc.); (2) cognitive (e.g., decreased concentration, attention, mental endurance, etc.); and (3) emotional (e.g., decreased motivation, enthusiasm, and initiative; feeling overwhelmed, bored, or low) [9]. When utilizing a multidimensional (physical, cognitive, and emotional) approach in evaluating fatigue it is clear that this symptom shares some commonalities with

the criterion symptoms for a major depressive episode with, for example, difficulty concentrating (mental fatigue) and anhedonia (emotional fatigue) being seen in both [9].

Fatigue, as a single symptom, is a DSM-IV-TR criterion symptom for a mood episode (major depressive episode – A6: "*fatigue or loss of energy nearly every day*") and for a disorder (dysthymic disorder – B3: "*low energy or fatigue*"). The criterion for A6 is elaborated ("*Decreased energy, tiredness, and fatigue are common. A person may report sustained fatigue without physical exertion. Even the smallest tasks seem to require substantial effort. The efficiency with which tasks are accomplished may be reduced. For example, an individual may complain that washing and dressing in the morning are exhausting and take twice as long as usual.*") whereas B3 (*low energy or fatigue*) is not.

In the DSM-III-R [13] – the manual that preceded DSM-IV – a useful glossary of technical terms was provide in an appendix that defined symptoms such as distractibility and insomnia but not fatigue, despite it being mentioned 28 times as either a criterion symptom or an epiphenomenon. The elaboration for criterion A6 in this edition states, "*A decrease in energy level is almost invariably present, and is experienced as sustained fatigue even in the absence of physical exertion. The smallest task may seem difficult or impossible to accomplish.*"

The DSM-IV-TR and the ICD-10 revision [14] use loss of energy and fatigue as apparently interchangeable terms and concepts, a view supported by a factor analysis of several depression rating scales where a lack of energy was shown to be a primary, self-rated measure of fatigue [15]. Interestingly, in a study of 57 patients with MDD, Christensen and Duncan [16] confirmed that energy level could be used to distinguish depressed from non-depressed individuals. A discriminant analysis of a self-report questionnaire, containing measures of energy level and psychosocial variables, showed that energy level correctly classified 93% as depressed or non-depressed compared with psychosocial variables that correctly classified 87%. Combining psychosocial and energy variables did not increase classification accuracy over that achieved by using the energy measures alone and the exhaustion measure provided the greatest relative contribution to the overall discriminant function.

Interesting as these findings are, the absence of an accepted definition for fatigue in mood disorders or other conditions is an impediment to research and makes it difficult to interpret studies. In multiple sclerosis (MS) research – where fatigue has been variously defined as an overwhelming sense of tiredness, lack of energy, or feelings of exhaustion [17], difficulty initiating or sustaining voluntary effort [18], or feelings of physical tiredness and lack of energy distinct from sadness or weakness [19] – the absence of a standard definition has been noted to be a significant obstacle [20].

Within psychiatry, different studies have used different definitions and a variety of assessment scales have been utilized [21]. In the ground-breaking, epidemiological catchment area studies [22–24] the presence of fatigue was assessed by asking the question, *"Has there ever been a period lasting two weeks or more when you felt tired out all the time?"* Although this assumed that the respondent was able to distinguish between the different clinical states of sleepiness and tiredness, which is not always an easy task, a positive response was only recorded if the respondent (a) told a professional about it, and/or (b) took medication for it, and/or (c) indicated that it interfered with daytime functioning. This is a clinically useful question as it ensures that significant and durable fatigue is being assessed and that it causes impairment. These studies support the findings of many other studies that, in the general population, fatigue has a high current (6.7%) and lifetime (24.4%) prevalence rate, and medically unexplained fatigue shares similarly high prevalence rates (6% current; 15.5% lifetime) [23].

A relatively new self-assessment scale – the 30-item Motivation and Energy Inventory scale [25] – was developed to detect change in three domains (mental energy, social motivation, and physical energy) in patients with MDD. Unlike other scales that have been developed and validated in different patient populations – commonly cancer patients – this new scale specifically addresses fatigue and energy in depressed patients and, with further study, may prove useful as both a measure of change over time and as a tool to compare the activation levels of a variety of patient and healthy samples.

The interrelationship between fatigue and depression is bidirectional with fatigue symptoms being associated with the development of MDD and persistent fatigue being a consequence of MDD. Addington and colleagues [22] in a prospective population-based study, showed that individuals who reported a history of unexplained fatigue at baseline and at follow-up 13 years later, were at markedly increased risk for new onset major depression as compared to those who never reported such fatigue. Similarly, those who developed new fatigue or had remitted fatigue after the baseline measurement were at increased risk for developing major depression.

Full remission of the symptoms of a major depression occurs in only 25 to 50% of patients receiving antidepressant monotherapy [26] and one of the most resistant symptoms to treatment with antidepressants is fatigue [27]. About one fifth of patients considered to have had a good treatment response to fluoxetine (final HAM-D score ≤ 7) continued to have some symptoms associated with depression, the most common being insomnia and the second most common being fatigue [28]. Interestingly, 91.7% (44/48) of those with post-treatment threshold or subthreshold insomnia had pretreatment insomnia and 92.7% (38/41) of those with post-treatment threshold or subthreshold fatigue had pretreatment fatigue.

Residual symptoms of MDD, which include but are not limited to fatigue, are clinically very important as they are associated with an earlier and higher relapse rate of depression, an increased suicide rate, increased use of healthcare services, and marked social impairment [29].

Etiology of fatigue

Understanding the etiology and pathophysiology of fatigue is critical to developing successful treatments, yet our understanding of the causes of both medically unexplained fatigue and the fatigue associated with psychiatric syndromes remains rudimentary. Although advances in neuroimaging and neuropharmacology are helping improve this understanding, currently fatigue is thought to involve different neuronal circuits than those causing changes in mood. Stahl and colleagues [30] suggest that physical fatigue and a lack of physical energy may be associated with brain areas regulating motor functioning. They note diffuse cortical projections of several key neurotransmitter systems – especially noradrenalin, dopamine, acetylcholine, and histamine – and propose that they regulate the symptom of mental fatigue at the cortical level with reduced neuronal activities in the prefrontal cortex, especially the dorsolateral prefrontal cortex, helping explain the symptom of mental fatigue. Although further work is ongoing in this area it is noteworthy that the major treatments for depression, fatigue, and hypersomnia predominantly involve noradrenergic, dopaminergic, and serotonergic mechanisms.

Converging functional neuroimaging evidence from patients with chronic fatigue syndrome and multiple sclerosis [31] supports the hypothesis that neural circuitry involved in the development of both fatigue and depression involves several regions of the prefrontal cortex and anterior cingulate cortex. Future fMRI studies may allow identification of specific subregions within these structures that are important in mediating fatigue in different clinical conditions including the mood disorders.

The assessment of fatigue

Because of the absence of a clear definition for fatigue, it is clinically important to clarify with the patient what they mean by the terms they use. Fatigue states are highly subjective and can be confused with other dysphoric states such as boredom and depression so clarity is important. How the patient responds to appropriate rest distinguishes between normal and pathological fatigue; the former being relieved by rest, the latter not. Additionally it is important to note what worsens and what alleviates fatigue and how it fluctuates throughout the day.

When fatigue is a prominent feature of depression it requires careful evaluation and particular care is required if the depression is resolving and fatigue remains a prominent, impairing residual symptom. Prior to any intervention, it is useful to quantify the degree of current fatigue both through the use of validated instruments [21] and through unvalidated strategies such as using a mild, moderate, or severe designation. Alternatively, a 0–10 rating scale can be used to record the subjective intensity of fatigue (1–3 being considered as mild, 4–6 moderate, and 7–10 severe). Although such a strategy has not been studied in depressed patients, in cancer patients, moderate and severe subjective ratings of fatigue have been associated, respectively, with distress and decreased physical functioning [32].

The assessment of the fatigued patient must include the usual domains of assessment for the psychiatrist including personal, adaptive, and maladaptive coping strategies for dysphoric states (depression, anxiety, frustration, guilt, etc.) as well as stress and should evaluate adaptive and maladaptive coping strategies the patient utilizes in handling loss of function. Understanding the assets and liabilities of a patient's family, social, and spiritual life is also important.

Patients reporting moderate or severe levels of fatigue, either at the initial assessment or following a partial reduction of other depressive symptoms, require a refocused history and consideration of undiagnosed or unmanaged comorbidities such as cardiac, pulmonary, renal, hepatic, neurologic, or endocrine dysfunction or the emergence of an infectious process or sleep disorder such as apnea. Noting the pattern of fatigue as well as factors that precipitate, relieve, or worsen it may help exclude other conditions from the differential. This reassessment must include a careful review of systems, the ordering of relevant blood tests, and a review of current recreational drug use, over-the-counter medication use – particularly long-acting antihistamines such as diphenhydramine [33] that may be used to self-manage sleep complaints – and prescribed medication use, particularly attending to drug interactions. Medications that commonly contribute to fatigue are narcotics, sedatives, hypnotics, antihistamines, antiemetics, antihypertensives, and antianxiety agents [34]. The growing, off-label use of the atypical antipsychotics exposes patients to sedation and daytime somnolence associated with the H_1 antagonist activity of these drugs [35].

Antidepressants – the core biological intervention for clinical depression – vary in their capacity to cause insomnia through direct, activating effects or through the induction of iatrogenic disorders such as periodic limb movement disorder [36]. Additionally, and probably unrelated to sleep disruptive effects, they can through their effects on cholinergic and histaminic circuits be sedating. See Table 25.5.

The nutritional status of "at risk" patients (prolonged anorexia, chronic debilitation from any cause, and the elderly) needs to be carefully evaluated with the regularity of meals, the quantity and quality of nutritional calories, and the preponderance of low-glycemic index foods also being assessed.

Inactivity associated with social avoidance, anergy, or frank depression can lead to a deconditioned physical state with a reduced tolerance for normal activities of daily living, including exercise, similar to that seen in cancer patients [37] and those with CFS [38]. Inactivity, high-calorie diets and medications that cause weight gain [39] may cause significant obesity resulting in the later emergence of a respiratory sleep disorder such as upper airway resistance syndrome [40] or frank sleep apnea [41].

Table 25.5 Relative sedation of antidepressants and mood stabilizers

First-generation antidepressants	
Amitriptyline	+++
Clomipramine	+++
Doxepin	+++
Trimipramine	+++
Trazodone	+++
Desipramine	+
Nortriptyline	+
Amoxapine	+
Second-generation antidepressants	
Mirtazapine	+++
Fluvoxamine	++
Sertraline	+
Paroxetine	+
Duloxetine	+
Venlafaxine	+
Bupropion	+
Reversible and non-reversible monoamine oxidase inhibitors	
Phenelzine	+
Tranylcypromine	+
Moclobemide	+
Mood stabilizers	
Quetiapine	++++
Carbamezepine	+++
Lithium	++
Valproic acid	++
Topiramate	+
Lamotrigine	+

Although self-administered stress management training has been shown to increase vitality in cancer patients [42], specific studies of stress management strategies – sometimes incorporated into cognitive behavioral therapy (CBT), a general form of psychotherapy directed at changing disorder-specific cognitions and behaviors that helps patients gain control over their unique symptoms – in fatigued, depressed patients have not been completed. Nonetheless any intervention that decreases stress, or improves maladaptive responses to it, is likely to be beneficial.

Although energy conservation strategies, including brief scheduled rest periods [43], are important in combating fatigue in chronically ill patients, their role in fatigued depressed patients has not been assessed, although it is likely that structuring a daytime routine in which priorities are set and activities are scheduled at times of anticipated peak energy will be helpful. Protracted sleeping can induce or worsen dysphoria in some instances; generally naps, if taken, should be brief and less than 20 minutes in duration [44].

Psychosocial treatment of fatigue

There are over 35 self-help interventions for depression ranging from using St John's Wort to singing and prayer [45]. Few of these have been systematically studied but may be helpful in an individualized program for a patient with depression and fatigue. Clinically it can be useful to have the fatigued patient catalog their activities into energizing or enervating events and to help them alternate activities to maximize energy utilization.

There are no evidence-based guidelines for managing fatigue associated with mood disorders or their treatments. However, strategies that have been proven effective in managing fatigue states associated with other medical disorders – for example cancer [34], MS [46], and CFS [47] – can inform us. Distraction techniques such as playing board or video games, listening to music, reading, and socializing can be helpful. Practicing good sleep hygiene [48], although lacking strong evidence to support it as a therapeutic intervention for all cases of disturbed sleep, is widely considered as being important in both normal and ill populations and reinforcing the circadian rhythm of sleep is especially important in bipolar disorder [49]. Other non-specific interventions such as relaxation training [46] may be helpful, especially in patients with high levels of somatized tension, and this is a useful self-management strategy that can help minimize the effects of stress.

Cognitive behavioral therapy enjoys about a 70% response rate in CFS [50]. Core components of CBT for CFS include (a) explanation of the etiological model; (b) assessing and encouraging motivation for CBT; (c) challenging and changing fatigue-associated cognitions (e.g., "I can't do anything if I feel this way");

(d) achievement and maintenance of a basic amount of physical activity; (e) a gradual increase in physical activity; (f) rehabilitation strategies for activities of daily living or the workplace. Cognitive behavioral therapists may not be widely available so it is encouraging to note that alternative delivery systems for CBT – such as telephone or self-instruction – can be helpful [51].

Cognitive behavioral therapy for depression [52] – that does not specifically target fatigue – can significantly improve residual depressive symptoms, improvements that are maintained for up to four years. Fava and colleagues [53] showed that patients who received CBT emphasizing management of cognitive distortions and maladaptive beliefs were 40% less likely to relapse during a four-year follow-up than those who were treated according to standard clinical management.

Similarly CBT-I, a specific cognitive behavioral therapy focusing on the treatment of insomnia can improve the overall outcome of patients treated with antidepressant monotherapy. In a randomized, controlled pilot study [54], patients with MDD successfully treated with escitalopram yet suffering continued insomnia obtained a higher rate of remission of depression (61.5%) than in the control group (33.3%), and the combination of antidepressant and CBT-I was associated with a greater remission from insomnia (50.0%) than in the controls (7.7%).

Another form of behavioral treatment for CFS is graded exercise therapy (GET) that may address cognitions or beliefs that discourage graded exercise [55] but is significantly different from CBT and has a less robust response rate of around 55% for the amelioration of fatigue. Because GET is based on a physiological model of deconditioning and utilizes activity as the main intervention for fatigue, and as exercise has been shown to improve sub-syndromal and mild to moderate depression [56], exercise may play a role in the management of fatigue associated with mood disorders although no studies have directly addressed this possibility. Patients with CFS note that pacing – management of daily activities through the use of strategic resting – is helpful but there are no published studies comparing pacing with CBT or GET [50].

The pharmacotherapy of fatigue

Antidepressants and stimulants have been the predominant pharmacological treatments for fatigue and within these two distinct classes of medications there are individual differences both in efficacy and side effects. With mixed results, antidepressants have been utilized to treat fatigue in patients with a variety of heterogeneous medical conditions, with and without depressive symptoms, but the nature of the studies and the number of subjects included raise significant concerns about their validity and generalizability. There are no controlled trials supporting superiority of one antidepressant over another in the treatment of fatigue associated with mood disorders but of the monotherapies, antidepressants that increase norepinephrine or dopamine are considered preferable for patients with prominent fatigue or energy complaints. Venlafaxine [57], bupropion [58], fluoxetine [59], and sertraline [59] share pharmacological profiles that are likely to benefit the fatigued or anergic depressed patient but this has never been adequately tested through formal, comparative studies.

All antidepressants affect sleep and cause sedation to varying degrees (Table 25.5) in variable populations and for different reasons [36]. If an activating antidepressant is utilized, sleep disruption may occur and therapy with a sleep-promoting agent may be required. Interestingly combined therapy of this type may result in the earlier expression of an antidepressant response with no significant withdrawal or rebound phenomena on discontinuing the sedative-hypnotic [60]. Obviously, using the least sedating sleep-promoting agent is always preferred and short acting benzodiazepines and benzodiazepine agonists are much less sedating than trazodone, which is commonly used for its sedative rather than its antidepressant properties [61].

Additionally, antidepressants can induce sleep disorders that can further disrupt sleep [62, 63]. Some evidence supports bupropion as being a relatively "sleep friendly" antidepressant that may also target fatigue [64] and it has been used effectively as an augmenting agent in open-label trials with treatment-resistant depression [65].

Psychostimulants have been used both as antidepressants since their introduction, and continue to be used as augmenting agents in treatment-resistant depression [66], and as a stand alone treatment for depression in vulnerable populations [67]. However, the evidence for efficacy is not substantial as the number of subjects treated is small and the duration of treatment limited. Methylphenidate and atomoxetine have been used to manage fatigue and as augmenting agents in treatment-resistant depression [15] but, again, this is not supported by large, randomized controlled trials. With a small number of patients in open-label trials, varying doses of methylphenidate have been shown to accelerate the response to an antidepressant and to specifically benefit fatigue and anergic symptoms. A recent controlled study of osmotic release methylphenidate failed to show an augmenting, antidepressant effect although it significantly improved energy and fatigue [68]. Studies on atomoxetine are limited currently to a chart review and an open-label study for a total of 29 patients so a specific recommendation for its use cannot be made.

The novel wake-promoting agent modafinil – a piperidine derivative pharmacologically different from other stimulants – has no useful antidepressant effect but has been shown to improve fatigue in both depression and other illnesses although this effect is not consistent across all studies [69]. In a randomized, controlled study of 200 mg of modafinil in 311 patients with a partial response to SSRI monotherapy, Fava and colleagues showed a statistically significant improvement in their overall clinical condition (based on CGI-I scores) but with no significant differences between modafinil and placebo in fatigue or depression scales [70].

Hypersomnia

Hypersomnia is defined as sleep in excess of nine to ten hours, within a 24-hour period, and affects 3 to 8% of the population [71]. Commonly excessive daytime sleepiness (EDS) reflects acute and/or chronic sleep loss and is not considered pathological if the nocturnal sleep period is inadequate for an individual's needs. Indeed, the most common cause of daytime sleepiness in the general population is inadequate nocturnal sleep. Hypersomnia and EDS are core features of the primary sleep disorders obstructive sleep apnea and narcolepsy but are commonly reported in four of the subtypes of MDD (see Table 25.2): MDD with atypical features, also known as atypical depression (AD); MDD with melancholic features; major depressive episode with seasonal pattern, also known as seasonal affective disorder (SAD); and bipolar disorders, during the depressed, euthymic, or mixed phases.

Although there is some overlap in symptoms, the patient with EDS usually struggles to maintain wakefulness in dull, unstimulating situations whereas the fatigued patient struggles with lethargy and listlessness. Like fatigue, hypersomnia can be a residual symptom of treated MDD and be resistant to treatment – Nierenberg and colleagues [28] showed that 70% of patients who had otherwise responded to fluoxetine continued to complain of excessive daytime sleepiness; a rate almost twice as high as complaints of fatigue (35.8%). Although hypersomnia is not as common as fatigue in MDD it is prevalent, occurring in 10 to 20% of patients with MDD and 36.2% of patients with AD [72].

Unlike fatigue, sleepiness can be evaluated by objective testing with the Multiple Sleep Latency Test (MSLT), measuring propensity for sleep or physiological sleep pressure, and the Maintenance of Wakefulness Test (MWT), measuring the ability to resist sleep, although these objective measures correlate poorly with subjective reports of sleepiness. Additionally, neither test correlates well with standard subjective measures of sleepiness such as the Epworth Sleepiness and Stanford Sleepiness Scales [73]. In one of the few MSLT studies in depressed patients, Nofzinger and colleagues [74] studied 25 bipolar depressed patients utilizing the MSLT and found that none demonstrated pathological sleepiness with the mean Sleepiness Index (100 – the sum of sleep latencies for five naps) being within the normal range at 31.59 ± 19.1. Only 20% of the subjectively sleepy depressed group fell asleep in all nap opportunities and, unlike the comparative group of narcoleptics, objective sleepiness decreased as the day progressed. They concluded that either hypersomnia complaints may reflect the subjective state of an anergic depression rather than a truly greater propensity for sleep, or that the MSLT may be an inappropriate test for this subgroup. As the MSLT is designed as a marker of sleep initiation, patients with hypersomnia may have difficulty initiating sleep yet, once asleep, may spend a larger portion of the day asleep. Additional factors such as the nature of an individual's stressors, their personality, and coping pattern may also be important variables in depressed patients with hypersomnia.

According to DSM-IV-TR rules an affective episode can be classified as atypical when mood reactivity (for example, the brightening of mood in response to positive experiences) occurs within the context of two of the following four symptoms: (1) significant weight gain or increase in appetite; (2) hypersomnia; (3) leaden paralysis (i.e., heavy, leaden feelings in arms or legs); and/or (4) a long-standing pattern of interpersonal rejection sensitivity (not limited to episodes of mood disturbance) that results in significant social or occupational impairment. Atypical features are diagnosed when they predominate within the most recent two weeks of a current major depressive episode – in major depressive disorder – or in bipolar I or bipolar II disorder when a current major depressive episode is the most recent type of mood episode, or when these features predominate during the most recent two years of dysthymic disorder.

The predictive validity of atypical features is unclear [75] although these features are two to three times more common in women and are associated with an earlier age of onset of depressive episodes. Frequently patients with atypical features have a more chronic, less episodic course, with only partial inter-episode recovery [1]. Mood episodes with atypical features are more common in bipolar I disorder, bipolar II disorder, and the seasonal pattern of major depressive disorder, recurrent.

The "melancholic features" specification is applied to a major depressive episode either as part of a major depressive disorder or when the depressive episode is the most recent mood episode associated with a bipolar I or bipolar II disorder. It is characterized by a loss of pleasure in all, or almost all, activities and an absence of reactivity to pleasurable stimuli (i.e., the patient does not feel much better, even for a moment, when something good happens). Additionally there are unique features to the depressed mood; it is regularly worse in the morning (diurnal variation) and is associated with early morning awakening (at least two hours before usual time of awakening), psychomotor retardation or agitation, significant anorexia and/or weight loss, and excessive or inappropriate guilt. Although often viewed as an anergic depression with an associated maintenance insomnia there are no data indicating that this subset is more sleepy than patients with MDD [76].

The specification "with seasonal pattern" can be applied to major depressive episodes occurring in bipolar I disorder, bipolar II disorder, or major depressive disorder, recurrent. The core feature is a regular temporal relationship between the onset of major depressive episodes and a particular time of the year (e.g., regular appearance of the major depressive episode in the fall or winter). The prevalence of winter-type, seasonal pattern appears to vary with latitude, age, and sex; increasing with higher latitudes, younger age, and the female gender (women comprise

60 to 90% of patients). Seasonal hypersomnia and sleep difficulties are common symptoms of this type of depression and although circadian factors have been implicated it is probably best viewed as a multi-faceted disorder in which behavioral, emotional, environmental, cognitive, and physiological changes are important in its onset and maintenance [77].

Hypersomnia is a common complaint of patients during major depressive episodes that follow mania or hypomania and EDS – although not confirmed objectively by Multiple Sleep Latency Tests [74] – is a known accompaniment of these disorders [78].

Assessment

The same assessment issues – previously discussed for the fatigued patient – are germane to the assessment of the sleepy, depressed patient. Because of the clear interrelationship between sleep disorders manifesting prominent sleepiness (e.g., obstructive sleep apnea, narcolepsy) [71] and comorbid depression it is important to pay particular attention to the sleep history and rule in or out these disorders and other causes of disrupted sleep.

As treating the hypersomnia associated with atypical or seasonal features and depressive episodes following mania or hypomania with stimulants or antidepressants may risk precipitating hypomania or mania, it is important to take a careful history – utilizing collateral information when possible – of previous past episodes of hypomania or mania. Similarly the family history, particularly of first-degree blood relatives, of mood and sleep disorders should be taken and recorded.

Patients with chronic mood disorders may disattend to their health so a full work-up, if not completed recently, is appropriate particularly in the elderly, who may require a current evaluation of their cardiovascular, renal, and hepatic functioning before undertaking pharmacotherapy. Additionally these patients often seek relief from their dysphoric states by abusing or misusing recreational drugs or prescribed medications, requiring a detailed history of substance and medication use and attending particularly to drug–drug interactions.

Assessing the patient's safety is an ongoing requirement in patients with hypersomnia associated with mood disorders because of the correlation between disrupted sleep and suicidality and because the overlay of sleepiness, with or without the sedative effects of medications, is likely to affect performance of complex tasks such as driving.

Psychosocial treatments of sleepiness

There are limited psychosocial interventions of proven efficacy for this patient population. Attending to sleep hygiene is always important and facilitating entrainment of circadian rhythms by regulating activity (e.g., arising time, meal times, light exposure, etc.) is known to be important in the management of patients with bipolar disorder. A midday walk outdoors has remitted symptoms of SAD in 50% of participating patients [79]; exercise, dawn stimulation, and negative air ions are all being investigated as potential treatments for this disorder. Cognitive behavioral therapy studies in patients with depression have shown that behavioral disengagement is an important variable both as a manifestation of the disorder and as an obstacle to its relief. Early work suggests that incorporating a personalized behavioral activation program may be helpful [77] and, by inference, this may help sleep performance and possibly daytime alertness.

Pharmacological interventions

Unsupported by large-scale RCTs the traditional intervention for AD has been the irreversible monoamine oxidase inhibitors (e.g., phenylzine and selegiline) and the reversible monoamine oxidase inhibitor, moclobemide. A variety of other medications and CBT have been shown to be effective. Although the SSRI drugs are effective and have a more favorable side-effect and safety profile, sufficiently powered studies are required before they can be recommended as first-line treatments [80]. A recent, non-controlled study comparing electroconvulsive therapy (ECT) in MDD and MDD with atypical features showed that ECT caused a remission in 80.6% of the atypical group, which was 2.6 times the rate in patients with MDD [81].

Melancholic depressions are usually considered to be a more severe form of mood disorder and tend to occur later in life when other comorbidities may complicate the clinical picture [82]. Refractoriness of symptoms may require complex pharmacological interventions that have never been formally studied for their direct effects on sleep–wake processes and,

not infrequently, ECT becomes the treatment of either first choice or last resort.

Light therapy

Although seasonal mood disorders respond to antidepressants, the traditional treatment is with timed bright light [83]. In a recent RCT of group CBT adapted for seasonal affective disorder, Rohan and colleagues [77] showed that CBT, light therapy, and CBT combined with light therapy improved depression but the combined treatment had the highest remission rates (73%). Modafinil (100–200 mg) in an open-label trial was effective in reducing hypersomnia and depression in a small group of patients with SAD [84].

There is no clear consensus of the management of the depressed pole of bipolar disorder; the absence of large, adequately powered RCTs in this patient group is part of the problem but utilizing antidepressants risks "switching" patients into hypomania or mania or inducing rapid mood cycling. Guidance from studies is also confusing; conventional clinical wisdom is that antidepressants and stimulants should not be used yet a recent meta-analysis of heterogeneous trials involving conventional antidepressants in bipolar disorder suggests a more favorable therapeutic index [85] although not supported by other trials [86]. A recent review of this complicated area has been carried out [87].

Conclusion

Although fatigue is poorly defined, as an acute symptom it is a core feature of clinical depression that interferes with functioning and the affected patient's quality of life. Fatigue can be resistant to treatment with standard, antidepressant monotherapy and when it persists as a residual symptom causes significant impairment in all domains of functioning and is a risk factor for recurrence, self-destructive behavior, and increased utilization of health services. Similarly, EDS is seen in specific subtypes of depression as an acute symptom and, like fatigue, can be a residual symptom resistant to conventional treatment. Additionally, fatigue and EDS are shared symptoms with significant sleep disorders requiring the clinician to complete a comprehensive assessment, including a sleep history, of all patients with mood disorders but particularly in those whose mood syndrome may not have responded as expected to standard treatments.

References

1. American Psychiatric Association. *Diagnostic and Statistical Manual of Mental Disorders* (*DSM-IV-TR*), 4th edn. (Washington: DC: American Psychiatric Press, Inc., 2000).

2. Reynolds CF III, Frank E, Houck PR, *et al.* Which elderly patients with remitted depression remain well with continued interpersonal psychotherapy after discontinuation of antidepressant medication? *Am J Psychiatry.* 1997;**154**:958–62.

3. Caldwell JA, Caldwell JL, Schmidt RM. Alertness management strategies for operational contexts. *Sleep Med Rev.* 2008;**12**:257–73.

4. Radbruch L, Strasser F, Elsner F, *et al.* Fatigue in palliative care patients: an EAPC approach. *Palliative Medicine.* 2008;**22**:13–22.

5. Beard G. Neurasthenia, or nervous exhaustion. *Boston Med Surg J.* 1869;**3**:217–21.

6. World Health Organization. *The ICD-10 classification of Mental and Behavioural Disorders: Diagnostic Criteria for Research.* (Geneva: World Health Organization, 1993).

7. Hickie I, Davenport T, Issakidis C, *et al.* Neurasthenia: prevalence, disability and health care characteristics in the Australian community. *Br J Psychiatry.* 2002;**181**:56–61.

8. Dittnera AJ, Wessely SC, Brown RG. The assessment of fatigue: a practical guide for clinicians and researchers. *J Psychosom Res.* 2004;**56**(2):157–70.

9. Arnold L. Understanding fatigue in major depressive disorder and other medical disorders. *Psychosomatics.* 2008;**49**:185–90.

10. Sharpe M, Wilks D. ABC of psychological medicine: fatigue. *BMJ.* 2002;**325**:480–3.

11. Wessely S, Nimnuan C, Sharpe M. Functional somatic syndromes: one or many? *Lancet.* 1999;**354**:936–9.

12. Mayou R, Farmer A. ABC of psychological medicine: functional somatic symptoms and syndromes. *BMJ.* 2002;**325**:265–8.

13. American Psychiatric Association. *Diagnostic and Statistical Manual of Mental Disorders* (*DSM-III-R*), 3th edn, revised. (Washington, DC: American Psychiatric Press, Inc., 1987).

14. World Health Organization. *The International Statistical Classification of Disease and Related Health Problems* (*ICD-10*), 10th revision. (VA, USA: American Psychiatric Publishing, Inc., 1992).

15. Demyttenaere K, De Fruyt J, Stahl SM. The many faces of fatigue in major depressive disorder. *Int J Neuropsychopharmacol.* 2005;**8**:93–105.

16. Christensen L, Duncan K. Distinguishing depressed from nondepressed individuals using energy and psychosocial variables. *J Consult Clin Psychol.* 1995;**63**:495–8.

17. Comi G, Leocani L, Rossi P, *et al.* Physiopathology and treatment of fatigue in multiple sclerosis. *J Neurol.* 2001;**248**:174–9.

18. Chaudhuri A, Behan PO. Fatigue in neurological disorders. *Lancet.* 2004;**363**:978–88.

19. Krupp LB, Alvarez LA, LaRocca NG, *et al.* Fatigue in multiple sclerosis. *Arch Neurol.* 1988;**45**:435–7.

20. Krupp LB. Fatigue in multiple sclerosis: definition, pathophysiology and treatment. *CNS Drugs.* 2003;**17**:225–34.

21. Dittner AJ, Wessely SC, Brown RG. The assessment of fatigue: a practical guide for clinicians and researchers. *J Psychosom Res.* 2004;**56**:157–70.

22. Addington AM, Gallo JJ, Ford DE, *et al.* Epidemiology of unexplained fatigue and major depression in the community: the Baltimore ECA followup, 1981–1994. *Psychol Med.* 2001;**31**:1037–44.

23. Walker EA, Katon WJ, Jemelka RP. Psychiatric disorders and medical care utilization among people in the general population who report fatigue. *J Gen Intern Med.* 1993;**8**:436–40.

24. Kroenke K, Price RK. Symptoms in the community. Prevalence, classification, and psychiatric comorbidity. *Arch Intern Med.* 1993;**153**:2474–80.

25. Fehnel SE, Bann CM, Hogue SL, *et al.* The development and psychometric evaluation of the Motivation and Energy Inventory (MEI). *Qual Life Res.* 2004;**13**:1321–36.

26. Nierenberg AA, DeCecco LM. Definitions of antidepressant treatment response, remission, non-response, partial response and other relevant outcomes: a focus on treatment resistant depression. *J Clin Psychiatry.* 2002;**62** (Suppl 16):5–9.

27. Paykel ES. Remission and residual symptomatology in major depression. *Psychopathology.* 1998;**31**:5–14.

28. Nierenberg AA, Keefe BR, Leslie VC, *et al.* Residual symptoms in depressed patients who respond acutely to fluoxetine. *J Clin Psychiatry.* 1999;**60**:221–5.

29. Mouchabac S, Ferreri M, Cabanac F, *et al.* Residual symptoms after a treated major depressive disorder: in practice ambulatory observatory carried out of city. *Encephale.* 2003;**29**:438–44.

30. Stahl SM, Zhang L, Damatarca C, *et al.* Brain circuits determine destiny in depression: a novel approach to the psychopharmacology of wakefulness, fatigue, and executive dysfunction in major depressive disorder. *J Clin Psychiatry.* 2003;**64** (Suppl 14):6–17.

31. Matthews SC, Paulus MP, Dimsdale JE. Contribution of functional neuroimaging to understanding neuropsychiatric side effects of interferon in hepatitis C. *Psychosomatics.* 2004;**45**:281–6.

32. Cleeland CS, Wang XS. NCCN proceeding: measuring and understanding fatigue. *Oncology.* 1999;**13**:91–7.

33. Witek TJ Jr., Canestrari DA, Miller RD, *et al.* Characterization of daytime sleepiness and psychomotor performance following H1 receptor antagonists. *Ann Allergy Asthma Immunol.* 1995;**74**:419–26.

34. Mock V. Fatigue management: evidence and guidelines for practice. *Cancer.* 2001;**92** (Suppl 6):1699–707.

35. Kane JM, Sharif ZA. Atypical antipsychotics: sedation versus efficacy. *J Clin Psychiatry.* 2008;**69** (Suppl 1):18–31.

36. Mayers AG, Baldwin DS. Antidepressants and their effect on sleep. *Hum Psychopharmacol.* 2005;**20**:533–59.

37. Marciniak CM, Sliwa JA, Spill G, *et al.* Functional outcome following rehabilitation of the cancer patient. *Arch Phys Med Rehabil.* 1996;**77**:54–7.

38. De Lorenzo F, Xiao H, Mukherjee M, *et al.* Chronic fatigue syndrome: physical and cardiovascular deconditioning. *QJM.* 1998;**91**:475–81.

39. Fava M. Weight gain and antidepressants. *J Clin Psychiatry.* 2000;**61** (Suppl 11):37–41.

40. Guilleminault C, Kirisoglu C, Poyares D, *et al.* Upper airway resistance syndrome: a long-term outcome study. *J Psychiatr Res.* 2006;**40**:273–9.

41. Bardwell WA, Moore P, Ancoli-Israel S, *et al.* Fatigue in obstructive sleep apnea: driven by depressive symptoms instead of apnea severity? *Am J Psychiatry.* 2003;**160**:350–5.

42. Jacobsen PB, Meade CD, Stein KD, *et al.* Efficacy and costs of two forms of stress management training for cancer patients undergoing chemotherapy. *J Clin Oncol.* 2002;**20**:2851–62.

43. Franklin DJ, Packel L. Cancer-related fatigue. *Arch Phys Med Rehabil.* 2006;**87** (Suppl 1):S91–S93.

44. Hayashi M, Watanabe M, Hori T. The effects of a 20 min nap in the mid-afternoon on mood, performance and EEG activity. *Clin Neurophysiol.* 1999;**110**:272–9.

45. Morgan AJ, Jorm AF. Self-help interventions for depressive disorders and depressive symptoms: a systematic review. *Ann Gen Psychiatry.* 2008;**7**:13.

46. van Kessel K, Moss-Morris R, Willoughby E, *et al.* A randomized controlled trial of cognitive behavior therapy for multiple sclerosis fatigue. *Psychosom Med.* 2008;**70**:205–13.

47. Price JR, Mitchell E, Tidy E, *et al.* Cognitive behaviour therapy for chronic fatigue syndrome in adults. *Cochrane Database Syst Rev.* 2008;**16**(3):CD001027.

48. Martínez-Manzano C, Levario-Carrillo M. The efficacy of sleep hygiene measures in the treatment of insomnia. *Gac Med Mex.* 1997;**133**:3–6.

49. Harvey AG. Sleep and circadian rhythms in bipolar disorder: seeking synchrony, harmony, and regulation. *Am J Psychiatry.* 2008;**165**:820–9.

50. Prins JB, van der Meer JW, Bleijenberg G. Chronic fatigue syndrome. *Lancet.* 2006;**367**(9507):346–55.

51. Knoop H, van der Meer JW, Bleijenberg G. Guided self-instructions for people with chronic fatigue syndrome: randomised controlled trial. *Br J Psychiatry.* 2008;**193**:340–1.

52. Beck AT, Rush AJ, Shaw BF, Emery G. *Cognitive Therapy of Depression.* (New York: Guilfond Press, 1979).

53. Fava GA, Grandi S, Zielezny M, *et al.* Four-year outcome for cognitive behavioral treatment of residual symptoms in major depression. *Am J Psychiatry.* 1996;**153**:945–7.

54. Manber R, Edinger JD, Gress JL, *et al.* Cognitive behavioral therapy for insomnia enhances depression outcome in patients with comorbid major depressive disorder and insomnia. *Sleep.* 2008;**31**:489–95.

55. Powell P, Bentall RP, Nye FJ, *et al.* Randomised controlled trial of patient education to encourage graded exercise in chronic fatigue syndrome. *BMJ.* 2001;**322**:1–5.

56. Otto MW, Church TS, Craft LL, *et al.* Exercise for mood and anxiety disorders. *J Clin Psychiatry.* 2007;**68**:669–76.

57. Stahl SM. Neurotransmission of cognition, part 1. Dopamine is a hitchhiker in frontal cortex: norepinephrine transporters regulate dopamine. *J Clin Psychiatry.* 2003;**64**:4–5.

58. Stahl SM. *Essential Psychopharmacology,* 2nd edn. (New York: Cambridge University Press, 2000).

59. Stahl SM. Not so selective serotonin reuptake inhibitors. *J Clin Psychiatry.* 1998;**59**:343–4.

60. Krystal A, Fava M, Rubens R, *et al.* Evaluation of eszopiclone discontinuation after cotherapy with fluoxetine for insomnia with coexisting depression. *J Clin Sleep Med.* 2007;**3**:48–55.

61. James SP, Mendelson WB. The use of trazodone as a hypnotic: a critical review. *J Clin Psychiatry.* 2004;**65**:752–5.

62. Rottach KG, Schaner BM, Kirch MH, *et al.* Restless legs syndrome as side effect of second generation antidepressants. *J Psychiatr Res.* 2008;**43**:70–5.

63. Yang C, White DP, Winkelman JW. Antidepressants and periodic leg movements of sleep. *Biol Psychiatry.* 2005;**58**:510–14.

64. Pae CU, Lim HK, Han C, Patkar AA, *et al.* Fatigue as a core symptom in major depressive disorder: overview and the role of bupropion. *Expert Rev Neurother.* 2007;**7**:1251–63.

65. DeBattista C, Solvason HB, Poirier J. A prospective trial of bupropion SR augmentation of partial and non-responders to serotonergic antidepressants. *J Clin Psychopharmacol.* 2003;**23**:27–30.

66. Patkar AA, Massand PS, Pae CU, *et al.* A randomized, double-blind, placebo-controlled trial of augmentation with an extended release formulation of methylphenidate in outpatients with treatment resistant depression. *J Clin Psychopharmacol.* 2006;**26**:653–6.

67. Wagner GJ, Rabkin R. Effects of dextroamphetamine on depression and fatigue in men with HIV: a double-blind, placebo-controlled trial. *J Clin Psychiatry.* 2000;**61**:436–40.

68. Ravindran AV, Kennedy SH, O'Donovan MC, *et al.* Osmotic-release oral system methylphenidate augmentation of antidepressant monotherapy in major depressive disorder: results of a double-blind, randomized, placebo-controlled trial. *J Clin Psychiatry.* 2008;**69**:87–94.

69. Kumar R. Approved and investigational uses of modafinil: an evidence-based review. *Drugs.* 2008;**68**:1803–39.

70. Fava M, Thase ME, DeBattista C. A multicenter, placebo-controlled study of modafinil augmentation in partial responders to selective serotonin reuptake inhibitors with persistent fatigue and sleepiness. *J Clin Psychiatry.* 2005;**66**:85–93.

71. Peterson MJ, Benca RM. Sleep in mood disorders. *Sleep Med Clin.* 2008;**3**:231–49.

72. Baldwin DS, Papakostas GI. Symptoms of fatigue and sleepiness in major depressive disorder. *J Clin Psychiatry.* 2006;**67** (Suppl 6):9–15.

73. Sullivan SS, Kushida CA. Multiple sleep latency test and maintenance of wakefulness test. *Chest.* 2008;**134**:854–61.

74. Nofzinger EA, Thase ME, Reynolds CF 3rd, *et al.* Hypersomnia in bipolar depression: a comparison with narcolepsy using the multiple sleep latency test. *Am J Psychiatry.* 1991;**148**:1177–81.

75. Seemüller F, Riedel M, Wickelmaier F, *et al.* Atypical symptoms in hospitalised patients with major

76. depressive episode: frequency, clinical characteristics, and internal validity. *J Affect Disord.* 2008;**108**:271–8.

76. Blazer D, Bachar JR, Hughes DC. Major depression with melancholia: a comparison of middle-aged and elderly adults. *J Am Geriatr Soc.* 1987;**35**:927–32.

77. Rohan KJ, Roecklein KA, Tierney Lindsey K, *et al.* A randomized controlled trial of cognitive-behavioral therapy, light therapy, and their combination for seasonal affective disorder. *J Consult Clin Psychol.* 2007;**75**:489–500.

78. Tsuno N, Jaussent I, Dauvilliers Y, *et al.* Determinants of excessive daytime sleepiness in a French community-dwelling elderly population. *J Sleep Res.* 2007;**16**:364–71.

79. Wirz-Justice A, Graw P, Kräuchi K, *et al.* 'Natural' light treatment of seasonal affective disorder. *J Affect Disord.* 1996;**37**:109–20.

80. Stewart JW. Treating depression with atypical features. *J Clin Psychiatry.* 2007;**68** (Suppl 3):25–9.

81. Husain MM, McClintock SM, Rush AJ, *et al.* The efficacy of acute electroconvulsive therapy in atypical depression. *J Clin Psychiatry.* 2008;**69**:406–11.

82. Koukopoulos A, Sani G, Koukopoulos AE, *et al.* Melancholia agitata and mixed depression. *Acta Psychiatr Scand Suppl.* 2007;**433**:50–7.

83. Westrin A, Lam RW. Seasonal affective disorder: a clinical update. *Ann Clin Psychiatry.* 2007;**19**:239–46.

84. Lundt L. Modafinil treatment in patients with seasonal affective disorder/winter depression: an open-label pilot study. *J Affect Disord.* 2004;**81**:173–8.

85. Gijsman HJ, Geddes JR, Rendell JM, *et al.* Antidepressants for bipolar depression: a systematic review of randomized, controlled trials. *Am J Psychiatry.* 2004;**161**:1537–47.

86. Sachs GS, Nierenberg AA, Calabrese JR, *et al.* Effectiveness of adjunctive antidepressant treatment for bipolar depression. *N Engl J Med.* 2007;**356**(17)1711–22.

87. Salvi V, Fagiolini A, Swartz HA, Maina G, Frank E. The use of antidepressants in bipolar disorder. *J Clin Psychiatry.* 2008;**69**:1307–18.

Chapter 26

Sleep in seasonal affective disorder

Timo Partonen, D. Warren Spence, and S. R. Pandi-Perumal

Introduction

There is considerable evidence that a number of sleep-related problems are influenced by seasonal changes throughout the year. Difficulty in falling asleep is the most common form of insomnia, but tends to increase in winter and summer, and shows only a weak relationship with age. Difficulties with sleep maintenance and terminal insomnia are two problems that increase considerably with advancing age, but these problems are also influenced by the time of year. To every thing there is a season, and this literally applies to sleep as well. In the absence of time cues, sleep tends to become longer in autumn and shorter in spring [1]. Changes in sleep patterns in response to seasonal changes are seen throughout the animal kingdom. Wehr *et al.* [2] have shown for instance that the duration of melatonin secretion in healthy humans responds to changes in photoperiod in ways that resemble the responses seen in other animals.

Winter challenge

The timing of sleep, the sleep phase, is delayed by about 90 minutes in winter compared with summer [3]. Under these conditions, healthy individuals go to bed earlier in summer, at an intermediate time in spring and autumn, and later in winter. There is a similar, but more robust, change in the wake-up time, which is earlier in summer compared with winter [4].

In winter, the length of sleep episodes generally increases, but can be divided into two symmetrical bouts of several hours each, with a waking interval of one to three hours in between [5]. There are coincident changes in sleep structure as well, because the duration of slow-wave sleep (SWS) usually decreases

and rapid eye movement (REM) sleep increases in winter [3]. These increases in sleep duration are in turn associated with alterations in melatonin secretion. The duration of melatonin secretion might be shortened or lengthened by sleep curtailment or extension, respectively.

The colder temperatures of winter can also have adverse effects, with evidence showing that sleeping in the cold under poor sleep-hygiene conditions reduces REM sleep. On average, a cold night will decrease REM sleep by 25%, but a greater degree of deprivation can occur during very cold nights [6]. Although core body temperature guides sleep induction and follows the length of day across the year, it has a much smaller range of seasonal variation than sleep. The circadian rhythm of core body temperature is phase delayed by about 45 minutes and the onset of SWS by about 40 minutes in winter compared with summer [7].

Latitude and the seasonal effect on sleep

The prevalence of insomnia has been assessed at population level in two Nordic countries recently. In both of these countries, Norway and Finland, a similar proportion of the population was living at the equal northerly latitudes. In one study, the one-month point prevalence of insomnia, as defined by DSM-IV criteria, was 12% in a representative sample of the adult Norwegian population [8]. In this study, which was conducted over 12 months, sleep onset problems and daytime impairment were generally found to be more common in winter than summer. Interestingly, the prevalence of sleep onset problems increased in southern Norway from summer to winter, while the opposite pattern was found in the

---

northerly regions. Physical and mental health appeared to be the strongest predictors of insomnia in this study.

The second study, which used a representative sample of the adult Finnish population, similarly showed a 12% prevalence rate for insomnia as assessed by DSM-IV and the Sleep-EVAL system [9]. An equal number of individuals reported global dissatisfaction with sleep. In general, sleep deterioration in summer or winter was linked to more complaints of poor-quality sleep. The prevalence of insomnia symptoms occurring at least three nights per week was 38%. Difficulty in initiating sleep was reported by 12%, difficulty in maintaining sleep by 32%, early morning awakenings by 11%, and non-restorative sleep by 8%. Compared to studies that used similar measurement techniques, the investigators found that insomnia is twice as prevalent in Finland as in other European countries, which are located closer to the equator.

Since mood is influenced by a complex interaction of circadian phase and the duration of prior wakefulness, even moderate changes in the timing of the sleep–wake cycle may have profound effects on mood [10]. Studies of workers in expedition stations located at the extreme southerly latitudes of Antarctica have shown that exposure to total darkness affects total sleep time, time of sleep onset, and quality of sleep [11]. Anxiety and depression seem to be preceded by changes in the sleep characteristics, and mood, in turn, appears to affect sleep quality.

Spring challenge

The onset of spring is a particularly challenging period with regard to sleep. During the winter months, and in particular when compared to the summer, the duration of melatonin secretion at night increases [5], while the peak phase of melatonin rhythm is typically delayed by one to two hours [12]. At the end of the winter season when the hours of sunlight increase very rapidly, there is a decrease in melatonin levels and a phase advance in the secretion of melatonin begins [13]. At this point, individuals with sleeping problems tend to need a longer time to adapt, and serum levels of melatonin, which are typically elevated in affected patients, together with morning tiredness, are symptoms that may last late into spring. The occurrence of melatonin peaks coincides with spontaneous waking at night, whereas melatonin nadirs are

associated with REM sleep [14]. Selective deprivation of SWS results in reduced levels of melatonin for the rest of the night [15].

In addition to the actions of melatonin, mechanisms related to REM sleep specifically appear to control sleep after a spontaneous sleep interruption. This occurs presumably because the propensity for circadian rhythm in REM sleep reaches its peak during the second half of the night [16]. Rapid eye movement sleep increases the frequency of electrical activity in the suprachiasmatic nuclei [17], thereby transmitting information about the phase of a circadian rhythm to the circadian pacemaker.

Genetic influences may influence how the circadian pacemaker processes information about the passage of time that takes place during REM sleep. This conclusion is based on the finding that the theta frequency, which occurs during REM sleep, slows down notably only in individuals who have a deficiency in the enzyme encoded by the *Acads* (acyl-coenzyme A dehydrogenase, C-2 to C-3 short chain) gene [18]. Mutation in this gene leads to activation of a gene involved in the detoxification of metabolic byproducts. Thus, theta activity may be an informative measure not only of the length of sleep [19], but also of the function of the circadian pacemaker.

Summer challenge

The next challenge after spring is summer. Whereas sleep phase, or the daily rest–activity cycle, is primarily reset by the work schedule, the circadian clockwork is substantially influenced by natural daylight. First, there is a seasonal pattern in the phases of circadian temperature and melatonin rhythms, peaking at an earlier time of day in summer compared with winter. Second, there is also a seasonal pattern in the phase relation, or angle, between temperature rhythm and sleep, with a relatively low core body temperature preceding sleep in spring and summer [4]. The mismatch therefore emerges most often during summer [1]. In six weeks, for example, most individuals may develop a free-running sleep–wake cycle longer than 24 hours and exhibit no harmony in rhythms under isolated conditions [20]. It is of note that the temporal relationship between the circadian phase of core body temperature and the timing of SWS is usually well preserved throughout the year [7].

It seems that not only the external (circadian pacemaker in relation to the local time) but also the internal (circadian rhythm in relation to another) phase relations of the circadian rhythms are dependent on the season. These experimental results can be simulated with dual oscillators that are reset separately to dawn and dusk, or with a model of the circadian and sleep processes that have a lowered threshold for the onset of sleep in the dark period.

Seasonal affective disorder

Seasonal affective disorder (SAD) was originally defined as a syndrome in which depression developed during the autumn or winter and remitted the following spring or summer for two successive years or more [21]. In addition, the SAD patient had to show a history of major depressive or bipolar disorder. Approximately 10% of affective disorders have seasonally dependent characteristics [22]. Two subtypes of SAD have been described in the literature: winter SAD (winter depression) and summer SAD, of which the former is far more frequent.

Epidemiological studies have shown that there is a greater incidence of SAD or atypical symptoms of depression at higher latitudes. For example, over 10% of the Siberian population has clear seasonal variations in mood and behavior, whereas the prevalence of these variations to the extent of a problem is about 40% in Finland. One model that has been proposed for SAD is that it is a multifactorial illness in which the genetic influence interacts with seasonal changes, including light exposure or ambient temperature. The genetic effect seems to contribute 29% to the seasonal variations in mood and behavior (sleep duration, social activity, mood, appetite, weight, and energy level), which can be summarized as the global seasonality score.

These original, operational conceptualizations of SAD were eventually transformed into diagnostic criteria based on the *Diagnostic and Statistical Manual of Mental Disorders*, in the latest version (DSM-IV) of which SAD is regarded as a specifier of either bipolar or recurrent major depressive disorder with a seasonal pattern of major depressive episodes [23]. The latest version of the *Classification of Mental and Behavioural Disorders* (ICD-10) provides provisional diagnostic criteria for SAD only on the grounds that its status is best regarded as uncertain [24]. Subject to these reservations, SAD is recognized as a form of bipolar affective or recurrent depressive disorder, with episodes varying in degrees of severity.

Clinical features associated with winter SAD are rather consistent across patients from diverse, industrialized cultures. So-called atypical depressive symptoms such as prolonged sleep duration (hypersomnia), increased appetite, weight gain, and carbohydrate craving frequently precede impaired functioning [25]. Atypical depressive symptoms, rather than the overall severity of a depressive episode, are the best predictors of a favorable response to treatment [26, 27]. Somatic symptoms are often the presenting complaint at visits to general practice. Mixed disorders often compromise the search for winter SAD, and each may require specific intervention.

Interestingly, whereas healthy subjects report sedation after ingestion of carbohydrates, depressed winter SAD patients experience activation and are less sensitive to the sweet taste [28, 29]. Resting metabolic rates may also be increased in depressed winter SAD patients secondary to changes in appetite and caloric intake [30].

Sleep abnormalities in seasonal affective disorder

Among patients with winter SAD, complaints of hypersomnia greatly exceed those of insomnia or reports of no sleeping problems. Although the extent of prolonged sleep observed in depressed patients with winter SAD does not differ markedly from that reported by the general population, their sleep-related complaints are accompanied by abnormal findings in the structure of sleep, including decreased SWS, increased REM density, and impaired sleep efficiency [31–33]. In patients with winter SAD, the band-specific electroencephalogram of non-REM (NREM) sleep resembles those of individuals who have been sleep deprived [34]. Night-time sleep polygraphic findings in patients with winter SAD are summarized in Table 26.1.

Studies of the pathophysiology of SAD have demonstrated the multilevel nature of its biological dysfunction. Alterations in sleep-related events, such as the regulation of core body temperature, may influence the occurrence of disordered sleep often seen in winter SAD. Although there is no evidence of abnormal homeostatic regulation of sleep as assessed by constant routine protocols, alterations in sleep-related events, such as in the regulation of core body temperature at night, may influence the emergence of disturbances often seen in winter SAD [35, 36].

285

Table 26.1 Sleep characteristics in patients with seasonal affective disorder

	Reference [29] Mean (SD)	Reference [30] Mean (SD)	Reference [31] Mean (SEM)	Reference [34] Mean (SD)
Baseline				
Total sleep time, minutes	386.1 (37.9)	399.2 (73.3)	427.3 (13.5)	430.8 (46.3)
REM sleep latency, minutes	92.7 (40.1)	77.4 (31.0)	112.4 (13.8)	112.2 (81.0)
Sleep efficiency, index	0.88 (0.07)	0.80 (0.15)	0.84 (0.02)	0.94 (0.06)
After light therapy				
Total sleep time, minutes	390.3 (64.7)	408.9 (55.6)	444.5 (11.4)	–
REM sleep latency, minutes	85.7 (58.6)	70.1 (40.0)	105.1 (15.3)	–
Sleep efficiency, index	0.89 (0.13)	0.87 (0.08)	0.88 (0.03)	–

Notes: SD = standard deviation; SEM = standard error of the mean.

Avery *et al.* [27] speculated that a phase delay of circadian rhythms relative to sleep might explain why SAD subjects experience hypersomnia. When, under conditions of internal desynchronization, the temperature minimum is phase delayed relative to the sleep onset, the subsequent sleep duration is relatively long [37, 38]. The circadian pacemaker also drives seasonal changes in functions and behavior by transmitting a signal of day length in the form of the duration of melatonin production to its receptors. Patients with winter SAD do generate a biological signal of change of season that is absent in healthy volunteers, a phenomenon similar to the signaling used by other mammals for regulating seasonal changes in their behavior [39].

In addition, winter SAD patients also show characteristic changes in overall levels of melatonin secretion. In related studies the discrepancies between day- and night-time urinary melatonin levels that are typically seen in healthy subjects have been found to be reduced in SAD patients who were living in Siberia. The excretion pattern normalized, however, following remission of SAD symptoms as a result of interventions or environmental changes such as bright light therapy, changes in season, or flight to a more southerly region. Consistent with other research, additional studies have demonstrated that, in winter, the daytime serum melatonin levels of SAD patients were increased compared to controls. These differences disappeared during the summer months or after bright light therapy.

In this context, the possibility that evolutionary selection for or against the unique response to cold exposure needs to be considered, and that this capability may confer some adaptive advantage. On the one hand, reaction time measures tend to show incomplete recovery, whereas detection performance gradually improves [6]. On the other hand, selection for or against the unique response to light exposure may have resulted in a difference in the circadian clockwork function. It may have affected the temporal organization of circadian rhythms and made the circadian clock more or less flexible to stimuli respectively.

From the circadian process to the sleep process

In winter, the amplitude of the circadian rhythm in core body temperature is smaller in depressed SAD patients, as well as in those in remission, than in healthy controls [40]. This finding strengthens the view that low circadian amplitudes characterize patients with SAD [41]. Compared to healthy controls, the circadian cycle in patients with winter SAD symptoms appears to be more elastic, having greater deviations from the 24-hour cycle and peaking at less regular times [42]. The circadian disturbances evident among children with winter SAD differ from those in adults by having rhythms that are well timed but attenuated in amplitude [43].

The decreasing daylight period as winter approaches is thought to trigger a depressive episode in individuals predisposed to winter SAD in particular. However, no causal relationship can be drawn between the incidence of winter SAD and the relative shortage of light exposure, or cooler temperatures. Winter SAD may also be sensitive to factors that are common to a range of recurrent affective disorders and produce sleep abnormalities seen in these patients [44].

Recent evidence provides some support for the hypothesis that there is abnormal photosensitivity in SAD, possibly secondary to pineal dysfunction. This may lead to the circadian abnormalities discovered in patients with SAD that can be normalized by scheduled exposures to light. For example, the decrease in plasma melatonin levels that normally occurs in the early morning is delayed by two hours, and the rest–activity rhythm is delayed by up to 70 minutes with respect to healthy controls [42]. The importance of the circadian rhythm of melatonin in the pathogenesis of SAD is underscored by the finding that morning light therapy, which acts by inducing a phase advance of the circadian rhythms, is generally effective, and is a treatment of choice.

Despite a considerable amount of experimental work, the pathophysiological basis of winter depression and its response to bright light remain unknown. While differences exist in emphases, the majority of the proposed explanations link them to the circadian clockwork, the regulation of the daily sleep–wake cycles, and subsequent mood variation on a seasonal basis. It has been observed that most of the extant hypotheses are not mutually exclusive.

References

1. Wirz-Justice A, Wever RA, Aschoff J. Seasonality in freerunning circadian rhythms in man. *Naturwissenschaften.* 1984;**71**:316–9.

2. Wehr TA, Moul DE, Barbato G, *et al.* Conservation of photoperiod-responsive mechanisms in humans. *Am J Physiol.* 1993;**265**:R846–57.

3. Kohsaka M, Fukuda N, Honma K, Honma S, Morita N. Seasonality in human sleep. *Experientia.* 1992;**48**:231–3.

4. Honma K, Honma S, Kohsaka M, Fukuda N. Seasonal variation in the human circadian rhythm: dissociation between sleep and temperature rhythm. *Am J Physiol.* 1992;**262**:R885–91.

5. Wehr TA. In short photoperiods, human sleep is biphasic. *J Sleep Res.* 1992;**1**:103–7.

6. Angus RG, Pearce DG, Buguet AG, Olsen L. Vigilance performance of men sleeping under arctic conditions. *Aviat Space Environ Med.* 1979;**50**:692–6.

7. Van Dongen HP, Kerkhof GA, Kloppel HB. Seasonal covariation of the circadian phases of rectal temperature and slow wave sleep onset. *J Sleep Res.* 1997;**6**:19–25.

8. Pallesen S, Nordhus IH, Nielsen GH, *et al.* Prevalence of insomnia in the adult Norwegian population. *Sleep.* 2001;**24**:771–9.

9. Ohayon MM, Partinen M. Insomnia and global sleep dissatisfaction in Finland. *J Sleep Res.* 2002;**11**:339–46.

10. Boivin DB, Czeisler CA, Dijk DJ, *et al.* Complex interaction of the sleep-wake cycle and circadian phase modulates mood in healthy subjects. *Arch Gen Psychiatry.* 1997;**54**:145–52.

11. Palinkas LA, Houseal M, Miller C. Sleep and mood during a winter in Antarctica. *Int J Circumpolar Health.* 2000;**59**:63–73.

12. Yoneyama S, Hashimoto S, Honma K. Seasonal changes of human circadian rhythms in Antarctica. *Am J Physiol.* 1999;**277**:R1091–7.

13. Bratlid T, Wahlund B. Alterations in serum melatonin and sleep in individuals in a sub-Arctic region from winter to spring. *Int J Circumpolar Health.* 2003;**62**:242–54.

14. Birkeland AJ. Plasma melatonin levels and nocturnal transitions between sleep and wakefulness. *Neuroendocrinology.* 1982;**34**:126–31.

15. Rao ML, Pelzer E, Papassotiropoulos A, *et al.* Selective slow-wave sleep deprivation influences blood serotonin profiles and serum melatonin concentrations in healthy subjects. *Biol Psychiatry.* 1996;**40**:664–7.

16. Barbato G, Barker C, Bender C, Wehr TA. Spontaneous sleep interruptions during extended nights: relationships with NREM and REM sleep phases and effects on REM sleep regulation. *Clin Neurophysiol.* 2002;**113**:892–900.

17. Deboer T, Vansteensel MJ, Detari L, Meijer JH. Sleep states alter activity of suprachiasmatic nucleus neurons. *Nat Neurosci.* 2003;**6**:1086–90.

18. Tafti M, Petit B, Chollet D, *et al.* Deficiency in short-chain fatty acid beta-oxidation affects theta oscillations during sleep. *Nat Genet.* 2003;**34**:320–5.

19. Hasan J, Toivonen S, Mikola H, *et al.* A study of sleep patterns on two Finnish icebreakers, ambulatory recording and automatic analysis. *Bull Inst Marit Trop Med Gdynia.* 1987;**38**:17–24.

20. Steel GD, Callaway M, Suedfeld P, Palinkas L. Human sleep–wake cycles in the high Arctic: effects of unusual photoperiodicity in a natural setting. *Biol Rhythm Res.* 1995;**26**:582–92.

21. Rosenthal NE, Sack DA, Gillin JC, *et al.* Seasonal affective disorder: a description of the syndrome and preliminary findings with light therapy. *Arch Gen Psychiatry.* 1984;**41**:72–80.

22. Faedda GL, Tondo L, Teicher MH, *et al.* Seasonal mood disoders: patterns of seasonal recurrence in

mania and depression. *Arch Gen Psychiatry.* 1993;**50**:17–23.

23. American Psychiatric Association. *Diagnostic and Statistical Manual of Mental Disorders (DSM-IV)*, 4th edn. (Washington, DC: American Psychiatric Press, 1994).

24. World Health Organization. *The ICD-10 Classification of Mental and Behavioural Disorders: Diagnostic Criteria for Research.* (Geneva: World Health Organization, 1993).

25. Tam EM, Lam RW, Robertson HA, *et al.* Atypical depressive symptoms in seasonal and non-seasonal mood disorders. *J Affect Disord.* 1997;**44**:39–44.

26. Terman M, Amira L, Terman JS, Ross DC. Predictors of response and nonresponse to light treatment for winter depression. *Am J Psychiatry.* 1996;**153**:1423–9.

27. Avery DH, Dahl K, Savage MV, *et al.* Circadian temperature and cortisol rhythms during a constant routine are phase-delayed in hypersomnic winter depression. *Biol Psychiatry.* 1997;**41**:1109–23.

28. Rosenthal NE, Genhart MJ, Caballero B, *et al.* Psychobiological effects of carbohydrate- and protein-rich meals in patients with seasonal affective disorder and normal controls. *Biol Psychiatry.* 1989;**25**:1029–40.

29. Arbisi PA, Levine AS, Nerenberg J, Wolf J. Seasonal alteration in taste detection and recognition threshold in seasonal affective disorder: the proximate source of carbohydrate craving. *Psychiatry Res.* 1996;**59**:171–82.

30. Gaist PA, Obarzanek E, Skwerer RG, *et al.* Effects of bright light on resting metabolic rate in patients with seasonal affective disorder and control subjects. *Biol Psychiatry.* 1990;**28**:989–96.

31. Partonen T, Appelberg B, Partinen M. Effects of light treatment on sleep structure in seasonal affective disorder. *Eur Arch Psychiatry Clin Neurosci.* 1993;**242**:310–13.

32. Anderson JL, Rosen LN, Mendelson WB, *et al.* Sleep in fall/winter seasonal affective disorder: effects of light and changing seasons. *J Psychosom Res.* 1994;**38**:323–37.

33. Brunner DP, Kräuchi K, Dijk D-J, *et al.* Sleep electroencephalogram in seasonal affective disorder and in control women: effects of midday light treatment and sleep deprivation. *Biol Psychiatry.* 1996;**40**:485–96.

34. Schwartz PJ, Rosenthal NE, Wehr TA. Band-specific electroencephalogram and brain cooling abnormalities during NREM sleep in patients with winter depression. *Biol Psychiatry.* 2001;**50**:627–32.

35. Schwartz PJ, Rosenthal NE, Turner EH, *et al.* Seasonal variation in core temperature regulation during sleep in patients with winter seasonal affective disorder. *Biol Psychiatry.* 1997;**42**:122–31.

36. Schwartz PJ, Rosenthal NE, Kajimura N, *et al.* Ultradian oscillations in cranial thermoregulation and electroencephalographic slow-wave activity during sleep are abnormal in humans with annual winter depression. *Brain Res.* 2000;**866**:152–67.

37. Czeisler CA, Weitzman ED, Moore-Ede MC, Zimmerman JC, Knauer RS. Human sleep: its duration and organization depend on its circadian phase. *Science.* 1980;**210**:1264–7.

38. Zulley J, Wever R, Aschoff J. The dependence of onset and duration of sleep on the circadian rhythm of rectal temperature. *Pflugers Arch.* 1981;**391**:314–18.

39. Wehr TA, Duncan WC Jr., Sher L, *et al.* A circadian signal of change of season in patients with seasonal affective disorder. *Arch Gen Psychiatry.* 2001;**58**:1108–14.

40. Koorengevel KM, Beersma DG, den Boer JA, van den Hoofdakker RH. A forced desynchrony study of circadian pacemaker characteristics in seasonal affective disorder. *J Biol Rhythms.* 2002;**17**:463–75.

41. Czeisler CA, Kronauer RE, Mooney JJ, Anderson JL, Allan JS. Biologic rhythm disorders, depression, and phototherapy: a new hypothesis. *Psychiatr Clin North Am.* 1987;**10**:687–709.

42. Teicher MH, Glod CA, Magnus E, *et al.* Circadian rest-activity disturbances in seasonal affective disorder. *Arch Gen Psychiatry.* 1997;**54**:124–30.

43. Glod CA, Teicher MH, Polcari A, McGreenery CE, Ito Y. Circadian rest-activity disturbances in children with seasonal affective disorder. *J Am Acad Child Adolesc Psychiatry.* 1997;**36**:188–95.

44. Partonen T, Lönnqvist J. Seasonal affective disorder. *Lancet.* 1998;**352**:1369–74.

Sleep during antipsychotic treatment

Andreas Schuld, Christoph J. Lauer, and Thomas Pollmächer

Summary

Like all other major psychiatric disorders, schizophrenia is associated with sleep disturbances, but the changes in sleep parameters are less specific than, for example, in major depression. Antipsychotics used to treat schizophrenia do relevantly influence sleep parameters. As a potent tool of behavioural characterization of drug effects, polysomnographic studies were performed in healthy volunteers as well as in patients with schizophrenia. A series of such studies focusing on classical substances and modern second-generation antipsychotics will be reviewed. Moreover, sleep-specific side effects like induction of parasomnic behavior also are frequent during antipsychotic treatment and will be mentioned in the present review.

Introduction

In patients suffering from psychiatric disorders, sleep is often changed. There are many studies recording sleep in acute or chronic phases of the disorders, and even in remission there seem to be some changes in sleep representing scars of the earlier manifestations and/or reflecting pre-existing vulnerability. The most popular findings in the field of psychiatric sleep medicine are related to major depression: sleep in depression is characterized by reduced REM latency, increased REM density, early morning awakening, and a possibly secondary shift of slow-wave sleep to the second sleep cycle [1]. Many studies replicated these findings. Pathophysiologically, certain aminergic–cholinergic imbalances were thought to cause these changes. In contrast, sleep changes in other major psychiatric disorders are much less specific: there are studies in patients suffering from dementia, anxiety disorders, obsessive–compulsive disorders,

eating disorders, and personality disorders [2]. Also patients suffering from schizophrenia were intensively studied in sleep laboratories, but studying those patients is confounded by a variety of problems: frequently the acute phase of the disease is characterized by very severe psychopathologic symptomatology that does not permit sleep recording. Additionally, some signs and symptoms like, for example, acoustic hallucinations or delusions of persecution keep the patients awake. Thus, early studies usually were performed in patients already treated for the disease and on more or less stable antipsychotic medication [3].

From a psychiatric research point of view this bears certain problems because psychotropic medication of various classes has influences on sleep structure (like, for example, the REM suppression during treatment with anticholinergic substances) or even on the EEG itself (see, for example, the induction of beta-spindles during treatment with GABAergic drugs). Thus, the above-mentioned early studies on sleep in schizophrenia raised the question of the influences that antipsychotic drugs exert on sleep by themselves. Therefore, as a first research strategy, some studies tried to examine schizophrenia patients twice, first under stable medication and later after withdrawal of the drugs.

For behavioral pharmacologists, additional sleep recordings in healthy subjects during or following experimental intake of psychotropic drugs are powerful tools for the neurobiological in-vivo characterization of psychotropic drugs.

The precise knowledge about the pharmacology of the drugs alone is of scientific interest, but also from a clinical perspective the influences of the drugs on sleep are important: during acute phases of the disease, sedative properties may be a positive aspect of

Sleep and Mental Illness, eds. S. R. Pandi-Perumal and M. Kramer. Published by Cambridge University Press.
© Cambridge University Press 2010.

the pharmacology of such drugs, whereas for relapse prevention most patients and their physicians prefer drugs that are less sedating.

The present article will summarize studies on sleep influenced by antipsychotic treatment. Therefore, first we will review the most important findings on sleep changes in schizophrenia. Later, findings on changes in sleep following acute or during chronic treatment with certain drugs will be reported. This includes experimental studies in healthy humans and clinical studies in patients with schizophrenia. A focus is set on some modern second-generation antipsychotics and on some older paradigmatic substances like haloperidol, chlorpromazine, and clozapine. Finally, some sleep-related side effects of antipsychotics will be discussed like the induction of parasomnic behavior or movement disorders and possibly indirect side effects on bodyweight and sleep-related breathing.

Sleep in schizophrenia

Whereas early studies on sleep in schizophrenia often did not properly control for antipsychotic treatment, later there were a series of studies on patients with stable treatment or off-treatment during remission. But even those studies were flawed by possible long-lasting changes in sleep persisting even after drug withdrawal [3]. Thus, in the 1990s, studies were performed that examined drug-naïve patients.

These studies taken together suggest that sleep in schizophrenia is characterized by disturbed sleep continuity, prolonged sleep onset, and, as a consequence, reduced sleep efficacy [2–5]. There also were some studies reporting findings on reduced REM-latency and a slow-wave sleep deficit [6, 7]. In recent years, combined studies linked certain neuropsychological abnormalities in schizophrenia to changes in sleep architecture [8–10].

Although sleep studies are of high value for the understanding of the disorder, they nevertheless have certain shortcomings: because sleep recording is a quite invasive manoeuvre for psychiatric patients, a selection bias preferring certain subtypes of patients is very likely. Moreover, disturbed sleep in schizophrenia is not alone a consequence of the neurobiology of the disorder and therefore only reflects changes in dopaminergic or serotonergic circuits in the CNS. Schizophrenia also is characterized by a variety of other signs and symptoms, which secondarily might influence sleep: first, so-called positive symptoms

of the psychosis, like delusions or hallucinations, by themselves may disturb sleep. Additionally, the patients also show changes in other fields of behavior, which indirectly influence sleep: even in the pre-neuroleptic era schizophrenia was associated with abnormal high bodyweight and some unhealthy behaviors like increased smoking or reduced physical activity. Possibly as a consequence of this, obesity is more frequent in those patients and their sleep thus is also disturbed, for example, by disordered breathing [11].

Hence, sleep abnormalities in schizophrenia are of multifactorial origin. Additionally, antipsychotic treatment of the disorder changes sleep and wakefulness. Thus, studies on sleep changes during or following intake of antipsychotic drugs are of particular interest for the understanding of the pharmacological features of the drugs and for the understanding of the pathophysiology of schizophrenia.

Sleep following antipsychotic treatment

For the understanding of sleep changes during or following intake of antipsychotic drugs, the basic principles of pharmacological treatment of schizophrenia must be summarized: the most specific pharmacological feature of antipsychotics is a substantial antagonism at CNS dopaminergic D_2-receptors. Moreover, most of the remaining dopaminergic receptor subtypes also are antagonized by these drugs, but also some drugs are partial agonists on these receptors. Dopamine receptors are widely spread in the CNS in cortical and basal brain regions. They are responsible for many brain functions including movement regulation and endocrine systems [12]. Antipsychotics also often antagonize serotonergic receptors to a variable extent; primarily clozapine and second-generation antipsychotics like risperidone or olanzapine have this pharmacologic feature. Moreover, these drugs exert effects on other neurotransmitter systems relevant for sleep–wake behavior, such as the histaminergic and the cholinergic system [13]. Finally, antipsychotic drugs not only change classical neurotransmitter systems but also may indirectly exert their effects via changing immunological and/or neuroendocrine systems, which also are involved in sleep regulation [14].

Studies in healthy subjects and in patients suffering from schizophrenia

Even a very precise knowledge of the molecular pharmacology of every single drug does not allow the prediction of sleep changes during the use of the drugs. Experimental designs using healthy subjects are a powerful tool for the behavioral characterization of those substances. Usually, the polysomnographic characterization of sleep changes in healthy volunteers only allows showing acute, single-dose effects. Studies on long-lasting stable treatment only were performed in patients. For the present review a focus was set on studies in patients with schizophrenia, whereas the use of antipsychotics in patients with other psychiatric disorders is just mentioned briefly below.

Phenothiazines (e.g., chlorpromazine)

Chlorpromazine is a classical tricyclic phenothiazine, which was very popular in earlier times of antipsychotic treatment. The substance is characterized by antidopaminergic, but also antiserotonergic and antihistaminergic, properties and has strong sedative properties. In healthy subjects, chlorpromazine induced an increased sleep amount with only little influence on sleep architecture [15, 16].

In patients with schizophrenia, treatment with chlorpromazine also increased total sleep amount [17]. In a study on long-term administration it was shown that this was mainly due to increasing non-REM sleep [18].

Butyrophenones (e.g., haloperidol)

Butyrophenones, especially *haloperidol*, were the most important drugs for the treatment of schizophrenia for many years. Besides the very robust anti-D_2 properties, haloperidol exerts just very weak anticholinergic, antiadrenergic, and antiserotonergic effects. Even in quite recent experimental studies, sleep in healthy volunteers was examined following haloperidol intake: in one study, sleep architecture was just very slightly altered, only slight increases in total sleep amount were found [19]. Another group reported changes in sleep microstructure: REM sleep following haloperidol seemed to have more saw-tooth waves [20]. In general, very similar results were reported in patients suffering from schizophrenia [21].

Clozapine

Clozapine is a very important antipsychotic substance with certain unique pharmacological features: the major difference to most of the other antipsychotics is a very complex pharmacology, which is characterized

by an antidopaminergic property not only at D_1 and D_2 receptors but also at D_3 and D_4 receptors. Moreover, the antidopaminergic effect on D_2 receptors is even smaller than the antiserotonergic features. Additionally, it is antihistaminergic and anticholinergic [18]. Because the drug already robustly changes awake EEG [22], results from sleep studies are confounded in a very complex manner. Possibly due to the complex side effects of clozapine, no polysomnographic studies in healthy subjects have been published to date. Clozapine treatment in schizophrenia results in increases in sleep efficacy by increasing stage 2, but decreasing slow-wave, sleep [21, 23].

Second-generation antipsychotics

Second-generation antipsychotics are a highly variable group of substances known to be effective in schizophrenia, but inducing fewer motor side effects, mainly due to less robust anti-D_2 properties in combination with antiserotonergic features [24]. Some of these drugs were tested in polysomnographic studies, the respective results are shown below in detail.

Risperidone is a robust blocker of D_2, 5-HT, and α_1 and α_2 adrenergic receptors. It is slightly antihistaminergic, but has almost no anticholinergic properties. In healthy subjects, risperidone reduced wakefulness and REM sleep and increased stage 2 [19]. In patients suffering from schizophrenia, risperidone reduced wakefulness and increased stage 2 sleep and non-significantly also slow-wave sleep [25]. The closely related substance *paliperone* also increased stage 2 and additionally REM sleep [26].

Olanzapine is an antagonist at muscarinergic receptors, 5-HT, D_{1-5}, α_1, α_2, and histamine receptors. It is possibly the second-generation antipsychotic that has been most widely studied using sleep laboratory techniques. In healthy volunteers, olanzapine increased sleep efficacy by increasing slow-wave sleep [27, 28]. Comparable findings were observed also in patients with schizophrenia: even in awake EEG, increased slowing and signs of sleepiness were observed [22, 29]. In nocturnal polysomnography in patients slow-wave sleep was also increased [30, 31]. Moreover, small amounts of slow-wave sleep before treatment seemed to be a good predictor for a sufficient antipsychotic response to olanzapin later on [32].

Ziprasidone is a complex drug with antagonistic effects on 5-HT$_{2A}$ and 5-HT$_{2C}$, D_2 and very slight effects on α_1 and histamine receptors. So far it has only been studied in healthy volunteers [33]. In this study, non-REM sleep amount increased, but the amount of REM sleep was reduced.

Quetiapine, a 5-HT$_1$ and 5-HT$_2$, D$_{1-3}$, α_1, α_2 and histamine blocker without affinity for D$_4$ and cholinergic receptors was also examined by the same research group. In healthy subjects it resulted in increases in total sleep time mainly due to increases in stage 2 sleep [34].

Studies in patients suffering from other major psychiatric disorders and/or insomnia

During very recent years there has been a growing interest in the development of new pharmacological strategies for the treatment of insomnia or insomnia related to affective disorders. Earlier treatment strategies often used benzodiazepines or non-benzodiazepine agonists at the BZD-binding site of the GABA receptor. Unfortunately, GABAergic treatment is typically associated with a considerable risk for tolerance or dependency. Thus, other classes of CNS drugs were screened for their sleep-inducing properties. A series of studies used antidepressants, but also second-generation antipsychotics, which bear a reduced risk of inducing extrapyramidal side effects, were tested. Unfortunately, only some of the studies used sleep laboratory techniques: in patients with major depression, Sharpley and coworkers [27] reported increases in slow-wave sleep during olanzapine treatment comparable to those in patients suffering from schizophrenia. Quetiapine was tested in a pilot study on patients with primary insomnia and showed subjective and objective improvements of sleep continuity and length [35].

Sleep-related side effects during/following antipsychotic treatment

Basically, for psychopharmacological interventions in acutely ill psychiatric patients, especially in those with schizophrenia or mania, sedation is a well accepted feature of antipsychotic drugs. Nevertheless, during chronic treatment after remission of acute stages of the disorder sedation might be scored as a negative side effect. Because this is true for most of the substances mentioned before, sedation as a side effect is not separately described in the present review.

Interestingly, some specific sleep-related side effects were observed in single cases during treatment with antipsychotics. Episodes of somnambulism for

example were reported during treatment with chlorpromazine in combination with benzodiazepines and lithium [36], quetiapine [37], and olanzapine [38].

Clinically relevant complaints of restless legs symptomatology were observed in case reports during treatment with olanzapine [39] and with risperidone [40]. In a first systematic study, also an increased prevalence and incidence of restless legs was reported during treatment with antidepressants [41]; comparable systematic studies in antipsychotics have not been published to date. Not only can the induction of restless legs syndrome be observed, but even in healthy subjects following intake of quetiapine increased amounts of periodic limb movements in sleep were found [34].

As mentioned above, other side effects of antipsychotic drugs may indirectly also alter sleep in the patients treated: for example, excessive salivation or sleep-related breathing disorders as a result of drug-induced weight gain may disturb sleep continuity [11, 42].

Conclusions

Treatment with antipsychotic drugs is associated with a variety of changes in sleep–wake behavior. Some of the clinical properties of these drugs fit very well their pharmacological properties; antihistaminergic and anticholinergic features especially often correlate very well to sleep changes. But as for all psychotropic medication, the molecular pharmacology alone does not always sufficiently explain drug effects. First, the disturbed sleep continuity often reported in schizophrenia might be also related to disease-specific symptomatology like delusions or hallucinations, thus successful treatment of these so called "positive symptoms" might have an indirect effect on sleep. Second, side effects such as the induction of movement disorders during sleep or severe weight gain and sleep apnea may cause sleep disruption. Thus behavioral characterization of antipsychotic drugs should regularly include systematic observation of sleep in the patients and, if possible, also sleep laboratory examination in small groups of healthy subjects and patients to increase our knowledge and understanding of the mechanisms of drug action. Moreover, this still could increase our knowledge about sleep in general and the clinical features and pathophysiology of schizophrenia.

If all these aspects are kept in mind, one can conclude that, in general, antipsychotic substances have sleep-enhancing properties in healthy subjects and in patients with schizophrenia. This is due mainly to increasing non-REM sleep to a variable extent, whereas only minor or conflicing findings were published regarding REM sleep. This is different from antidepressant drugs: sedative antidepressants often robustly alter sleep architecture by suppressing REM sleep and/or slow-wave sleep, whereas other antidepressants disturb sleep continuity. Also GABAergic drugs such as benzodiazepines do significantly change sleep architecture by suppressing REM sleep and decreasing slow-wave sleep. Thus, substances like certain second-generation antipsychotics, which increase sleep continuity and increase slow-wave sleep with more or less no suppression of REM sleep, could be very interesting substances for the treatment of disturbed sleep in patients with psychiatric disorders and possibly also in insomia patients.

References

1. Lauer CJ, Schreiber W, Holsboer F, Krieg JC. In quest of identifying vulnerability markers for psychiatric disorders by all-night polysomnography. *Arch Gen Psychiatry.* 1995;**52**:145–53.

2. Benca RM, Obermeyer WH, Thisted RA, Gillin JC. Sleep and psychiatric disorders. A meta-analysis. *Arch Gen Psychiatry.* 1992;**49**:651–68.

3. Lauer CJ, Schreiber W, Pollmächer T, *et al.* Sleep in schizophrenia: A polysomnographic study on drug-naïve patients. *Neuropsychopharmacology.* 1997;**16**:51–60.

4. Taylor SF, Tandon R, Shipley JE, Eiser AS. Effect of neuroleptic treatment on polysomnographic measures in schizophrenia. *Biol Psychiatry.* 1991;**30**:904–12.

5. Tandon R, Shipley JE, Taylor S, *et al.* Electroencephalographic sleep abnormalities in schizophrenia. Relationship to positive/negative symptoms and prior neuroleptic treatment. *Arch Gen Psychiatry.* 1992;**49**:185–94.

6. Keshavan MS, Reynolds CF 3rd, Miewald JM, Montrose DM. A longitudinal study of EEG sleep in schizophrenia. *Psychiatry Res.* 1996;**59**:203–11.

7. Keshavan MS, Prasad KM, Montrose DM, *et al.* Sleep quality and architecture in quetiapine, risperidone, or never-treated schizophrenia patients. *J Clin Psychopharmacol.* 2007;**27**:703–5.

8. Göder R, Aldenhoff JB, Boigs M, *et al.* Delta power in sleep in relation to neuropsychological performance in healthy subjects and schizophrenia patients. *J Neuropsychiatry Clin Neurosci.* 2006;**18**:529–35.

9. Göder R, Boigs M, Braun S, *et al.* Impairment of visuospatial memory is associated with decreased slow wave sleep in schizophrenia. *J Psychiatr Res.* 2004;**38**:591–9.

10. Forest G, Poulin J, Daoust AM, *et al.* Attention and non-REM sleep in neuroleptic-naive persons with schizophrenia and control participants. *Psychiatry Res.* 2007;**149**:33–40.

11. Ancoli-Israel S, Martin J, Jones DW, *et al.* Sleep-disordered breathing and periodic limb movements in sleep in older patients with schizophrenia. *Biol Psychiatry.* 1999;**45**:1426–32.

12. Freedman R. Schizophrenia. *N Engl J Med.* 2003;**349**:1738–49.

13. Kinon BJ, Lieberman JA. Mechanisms of action of atypical antipsychotic drugs: a critical analysis. *Psychopharmacology (Berl).* 1996;**124**:2–34.

14. Pollmächer T, Haack M, Schuld A, *et al.* Effects of antipsychotic drugs on cytokine networks. *J Psychiatr Res.* 1999;**35**:369–82.

15. Lewis SA, Evans JI. Dose effects of chlorpromazine on human sleep. *Psychopharmacologia.* 1969;**14**:342–8.

16. Lester BK, Coulter JD, Cowden LC, Williams HL. Chlorpromazine and human sleep. *Psychopharmacologia.* 1971;**20**:280–7.

17. Kupfer DJ, Wyatt RJ, Synder F, Davis JM. Chlorpromazine and sleep in psychiatric patients. *Arch Gen Psychiatry.* 1971;**24**:185–9.

18. Kaplan J, Dawson S, Vaughan T, *et al.* Effect of prolonged chlorpromazine administration on the sleep of chronic schizophrenics. *Arch Gen Psychiatry.* 1974;**31**:62–6.

19. Giménez S, Clos S, Romero S, *et al.* Effects of olanzapine, risperidone and haloperidol on sleep after a single oral morning dose in healthy volunteers. *Psychopharmacology (Berl).* 2007;**190**:507–16.

20. Pinto LR Jr., Peres CA, Russo RH, *et al.* Sawtooth waves during REM sleep after administration of haloperidol combined with total sleep deprivation in healthy young subjects. *Braz J Med Biol Res.* 2002;**35**:599–604.

21. Wetter TC, Lauer CJ, Gillich G, Pollmächer T. The electroencephalographic sleep pattern in schizophrenic patients treated with clozapine or classical antipsychotic drugs. *J Psychiatr Res.* 1996;**30**:411–19.

22. Schuld A, Kühn M, Haack M, *et al.* A comparison of the effects of clozapine and olanzapine on the EEG in patients with schizophrenia. *Pharmacopsychiatry.* 2000;**33**:109–11.

23. Hinze-Selch D, Mullington J, Orth A, *et al.* Effects of clozapine on sleep: a longitudinal study. *Biol Psychiatry.* 1997;**42**:260–6.

293

24. Cutler A, Ball S, Stahl SM. Dosing atypical antipsychotics. *CNS Spectr.* 2008;**5** (Suppl 9):1–16.

25. Yamashita H, Morinobu S, Yamawaki S, *et al.* Effect of risperidone on sleep in schizophrenia: a comparison with haloperidol. *Psychiatry Res.* 2002;**109**:137–42.

26. Luthringer R, Staner L, Noel N, *et al.* A double-blind, placebo-controlled, randomized study evaluating the effect of paliperidone extended-release tablets on sleep architecture in patients with schizophrenia. *Int Clin Psychopharmacol.* 2007;**22**:299–308.

27. Sharpley AL, Vassallo CM, Cowen PJ. Olanzapine increases slow-wave sleep: evidence for blockade of central 5-HT(2C) receptors in vivo. *Biol Psychiatry.* 2000;**47**:468–70.

28. Lindberg N, Virkkunen M, Tani P, *et al.* Effect of a single-dose of olanzapine on sleep in healthy females and males. *Int Clin Psychopharmacol.* 2002;**17**:177–84.

29. Wichniak A, Szafranski T, Wierzbicka A, *et al.* Electroencephalogram slowing, sleepiness and treatment response in patients with schizophrenia during olanzapine treatment. *J Psychopharmacol.* 2006;**20**:80–5.

30. Salín-Pascual RJ, Herrera-Estrella M, Galicia-Polo L, *et al.* Low delta sleep predicted a good clinical response to olanzapine administration in schizophrenic patients. *Rev Invest Clin.* 2004;**56**:345–50.

31. Müller MJ, Rossbach W, Mann K, *et al.* Subchronic effects of olanzapine on sleep EEG in schizophrenic patients with predominantly negative symptoms. *Pharmacopsychiatry.* 2004;**37**:157–62.

32. Salin-Pascual RJ, Herrera-Estrella M, Galicia-Polo L, Laurrabaquio MR. Olanzapine acute administration in schizophrenic patients increases delta sleep and sleep efficiency. *Biol Psychiatry.* 1999;**46**:141–3.

33. Cohrs S, Meier A, Neumann AC, *et al.* Improved sleep continuity and increased slow wave sleep and REM latency during ziprasidone treatment: a randomized, controlled, crossover trial of 12 healthy male subjects. *J Clin Psychiatry.* 2005;**66**:989–96.

34. Cohrs S, Rodenbeck A, Guan Z, *et al.* Sleep-promoting properties of quetiapine in healthy subjects. *Psychopharmacology (Berl).* 2004;**174**:421–9.

35. Wiegand MH, Landry F, Brückner T, *et al. Psychopharmacology (Berl).* 2008;**196**:337–8.

36. Glassman JN, Darko D, Gillin JC. Medication-induced somnambulism in a patient with schizoaffective disorder. *J Clin Psychiatry.* 1986;**47**:523–4.

37. Hafeez ZH, Kalinowski CM. Somnambulism induced by quetiapine: two case reports and a review of the literature CNS. *Spectr.* 2007;**12**:910–12.

38. Chiu YH, Chen CH, Shen WW. Somnambulism secondary to olanzapine treatment in one patient with bipolar disorder. *Prog Neuropsychopharmacol Biol Psychiatry.* 2008;**32**:581–2.

39. Kraus T, Schuld A, Pollmächer T. Periodic leg movements in sleep and restless legs syndrome probably caused by olanzapine. *J Clin Psychopharmacol.* 1999;**19**:478–9.

40. Wetter TC, Brunner J, Bronisch T. Restless legs syndrome probably induced by risperidone treatment. *Pharmacopsychiatry.* 2002;**35**:109–11.

41. Rottach KG, Schaner BM, Kirch AH, *et al.* Restless legs syndrome as side effect of second generation antidepressants. *J Psychiatr Res.* 2008;**43**:70–5.

42. Zimmermann U, Kraus T, Himmerich H, *et al.* Epidemiology, implications and mechanisms underlying drug-induced weigh gain in psychiatric patients. *J Psychiatr Res.* 2003;**37**:193–220.

Chapter 28

Sleep-related memory consolidation in mental illnesses

Nathalie Pross and Luc Staner

Introduction

The medial temporal lobe and more especially the hippocampal formation are crucial for memory learning and storage activities. This was outlined in the famous case study of H. M. [1], a patient with an anterograde amnesia following bilateral damage to the medial temporal lobe and hippocampus. This neurological patient was severely impaired in declarative memory activities but his perceptual and motor skill learning as well as his working memory were preserved. In other words, H. M. had an intact short-term memory and an intact long-term memory, but was unable to transfer new verbal information to long-term memory. During the last four decades, a lot of experimental and functional imaging studies brought further support to the role of the hippocampus in memory transferring activities, also known as memory consolidation activities [2, 3].

Memory consolidation is also a major field in the sleep research domain. At this stage, it is well demonstrated that the different sleep stages are implicated in the consolidation of different kinds of information (i.e., verbal, visuo-spatial, declarative, procedural, explicit, and implicit) [4, 5]. However, there is no consensus about the precise role of each sleep stage in memory consolidation, and more generally there is no real consensus about the exact role of sleep in memory. Nevertheless, the existence of strong functional relationships between the hippocampus, sleep, and memory consolidation are well recognized in the literature [6, 7].

More recently, a growing body of literature converges in identifying the prefrontal cortex as a major player in sleep-dependent memory consolidation processes. The prefrontal cortex is not directly implicated in the long-term storage processes, but it plays a crucial role in memory processing and retrieval activities [8]. Indeed sleep-deprivation studies indicate that the efficiency of the prefrontal cortex during a memory task is particularly vulnerable to sleep loss [9]. Thus, even if the hippocampus seems to play the most important role, evidence is mounting that the functioning of the frontal areas should also be examined in studies investigating sleep-dependent memory consolidation processes.

Of particular note is the fact that the prefrontal cortex is strongly connected to a variety of brain networks including the hippocampal and amygdala network. The amygdala plays an important role in the processing of emotional information, and there is some clinical evidence suggesting a relationship between the regulation of sleep and the regulation of emotional processes [10]. Consequently, a growing number of studies examine whether the emotional valence of the learned material (i.e., neutral items vs. positive or negative items) influence sleep-related memory consolidation.

Several neuropsychiatric disorders, such as schizophrenia, depression, Alzheimer's disease, and post-traumatic stress disorder (PTSD) are associated with alterations of both sleep as well as memory. Recent anatomical and functional imaging studies demonstrated that the hippocampal formation is affected in Alzheimer's disease and in schizophrenia [11]. It is also well recognized that schizophrenic and depressive patients present wide frontal-lobe related functional impairments [12, 13]. And finally, depression and PTSD are commonly associated with an amygdala-dependent emotional processing disorder [14, 15]. However, at this stage, few studies have investigated the field of sleep-related memory consolidation in these neuropsychiatric disorders.

The aim of this chapter is to examine the links between memory-consolidation impairment and sleep alterations in different mental illnesses. However,

---

Sleep and Mental Illness, eds. S. R. Pandi-Perumal and M. Kramer. Published by Cambridge University Press.
© Cambridge University Press 2010.

before getting to the heart of the matter, the different memory systems will be detailed. Indeed, as the different memory concepts are often confused with terms describing materials, tasks, or procedures, it seems important to define the different kinds of memory and to explain their underlying mechanisms. Then, the possible roles of sleep in these different memory systems in healthy subjects will be presented. Finally, memory-consolidation disorders occurring in schizophrenia, depression, Alzheimer's disease, and PTSD will be discussed according to the specific sleep, cognitive, and mood disorders that characterize each of these mental illnesses.

Memory systems, memory processes, memory tasks, and to-be-remembered material

The theoretical domain of *memory* is a very complex research field for the non-initiated as well as for initiated people! Researchers have agreed for 50 years, with the fact that memory is not a unitary entity. As a result, numerous classifications have been proposed to distinguish different forms of memory. Some of them refer to structural distinctions (e.g., short-term vs. long-term memory; declarative vs. procedural memory; episodic vs. semantic memory...), others refer to the material differences (e.g., verbal vs. visuo-spatial vs. olfactory items; neutral vs. positive or negative items...) or the cognitive processes implicated in the task (e.g., immediate vs. delayed recall task, recognition task, span task, executive task...) and others directly relate to the memory process itself (e.g., encoding, recoding, rehearsal, consolidation, storage, or retrieval).

Historically, the first distinction was based on the short-term vs. long-term dichotomy [16]. At the present time, there are many experimental and neuro-psychological data supporting the existence of a short-term memory system and a long-term memory system [17, 18]. However, several concurrent distinctions progressively appeared in the literature and authors in this field currently refer to other kinds of classification schemes. The most current distinctions are the dichotomy explicit/implicit memory proposed by Graf and Schacter [19] and the dichotomy declarative/non-declarative memory proposed by Squire [20]. However, references to other distinctions like semantic/episodic [21] (Tulving), declarative/procedural [22]

(Cohen and Eichenbaum), or memory with/without consciousness [23] (Jacoby and Witherspoon) are also found in the literature. It has to be noted that certain distinctions such as explicit/implicit and with/without consciousness refer more or less to the same concept, as well as the distinctions declarative/non-declarative and declarative/procedural. More precisely, the latter concern different memory systems and the former concern different kinds (or forms, or expressions) of memory.

Different memory systems and memory models

In their chapter "What are the memory systems of 1994?" Schacter and Tulving [24] indicated that "a memory system is defined in terms of its brain mechanisms, the kind of information it processes, and the principles of its operation" (p. 13). In the same volume, Nadel [25] indicated that the length of time that information is stored in the system is also an important feature in the definition of a memory system. According to these conceptual issues, and to a review of evidence coming from cognitive and neuropsychological data, the most achieved and consensual memory model appears to be the SPI (serial–parallel–independent) model proposed by Tulving [26] (see Figure 28.1).

This model encompasses five memory systems: the episodic memory, the working memory, the semantic memory, the perceptual representation systems, and the procedural memory. These five major memory systems can be classified in two categories according to both a classical structural point of view (i.e., a short-term memory system – the working memory – and four systems of long-term memory), and a functional point of view (i.e., an action system – the procedural memory – and four cognitive representation systems). *Procedural memory* is defined by Schacter and Tulving [24] as a system "involved in learning various kinds of behavioral and cognitive skills and algorithms". Broadly speaking, the information stored in the procedural system is characterized by its difficulty to verbalize and by the fact that this system operates at an automatic level (i.e., without a controlled retrieval). Conversely, the four cognitive representation systems are highly dependent on cognition and/or thought, and can be classified as declarative knowledge (i.e., knowledge that can be verbalized). *Episodic memory* refers to the "memory of personally experienced events" [27].

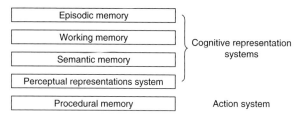

Figure 28.1 Tulving's SPI (serial–parallel–independent) model.

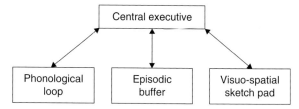

Figure 28.2 The working memory model according to the last update proposed by Baddeley [33].

The episodic information is directly related to the temporal–spatial context in which it was acquired. *Semantic memory* is defined as the general knowledge about the world, objects, and facts (i.e., unrelated to a personal experience). The *perceptual representations system* stores the information about the perceptual features of physical objects. And finally, the last cognitive representation system (i.e., *working memory*) differs from the three others in that it is concerned about the temporary features of its storage and processing activities. The working memory is the less well defined system in the SPI model. Indeed in one of his key publications, Tulving [26] refers to a primary memory that "registers and retains incoming information in a highly accessible form for a short period of time after the input". However, in his subsequent publication [27] no specifications between working memory and the other memory systems defined in the SPI model are mentioned. This lack of interest accorded to the working memory represents probably one of the major weaknesses in Tulving's model. Indeed, working memory is an important memory system due to its role in encoding and retrieval activities. Moreover, working memory is highly dependent on sleep efficiency, and is known to be impaired in several mental illnesses such as schizophrenia or depression.

The *working memory model* was proposed by Baddeley and Hitch in 1974 [28] (see Figure 28.2). Working memory was then defined as a memory system involved in temporary information storage and manipulation during ongoing cognitive tasks like comprehension, reasoning, and learning. In 1974, working memory was conceived as a multicomponent system composed by a specific storage unit and by an executive system. During more than ten years, most of the studies were focused on the storage system functioning. In 1986, Baddeley published the first update of his model [29], which he then described as being composed of three subunits: the executive system called the central executive and two slave systems, one dedicated to verbal storage (i.e., the phonological loop) and the other

dedicated to visuo-spatial storage (i.e., the visuo-spatial sketchpad). The distinction between the storage of verbal material and the storage of visuo-spatial material proposed by Baddeley highlights the importance of the nature of the to-be-memorized materials in memory tasks. This is illustrated for instance in the distinction between dyslexia, where verbal storage deficits are observed [30], and schizophrenia, where visuo-spatial storage deficits are found [31]. In 1996, Baddeley published the first detailed review about the major subunit of the working memory: the central executive [32]. With regard to functional neuroanatomy, the central executive is assumed to be linked to the frontal lobes. It is postulated to be responsible for planning, cognitive flexibility, abstract thinking, rule acquisition, initiating appropriate actions and inhibiting inappropriate actions, selecting relevant sensory information, selective attention, long-term memory activation, and so on. According to this description, the central executive is related to attentional control and processing activities more than to storage activities. In the last update of the multicomponent model of working memory, Baddeley added a new component, the episodic buffer [33, 34]. This component is expected to be responsible for the "temporary storage of information held in a multimodal code, and is capable of binding information from the subsidiary systems, and from long-term memory, into a unitary episodic representation" [33]. According to the author, the episodic buffer has a crucial role in encoding but also retrieving information from episodic memory.

Even if memory consolidation is an important research field in sleep studies, very few memory models account for this phenomenon. Tulving's model is the most commonly cited in the literature; however, the recent MNESIS model [35] (see Figure 28.3) is probably a more appropriate theoretical conception to explain the sleep-related memory consolidation phenomenon.

MNESIS is a new memory model based on experimental and neuropsychological data, which encompasses Baddeley's last updated working memory model and

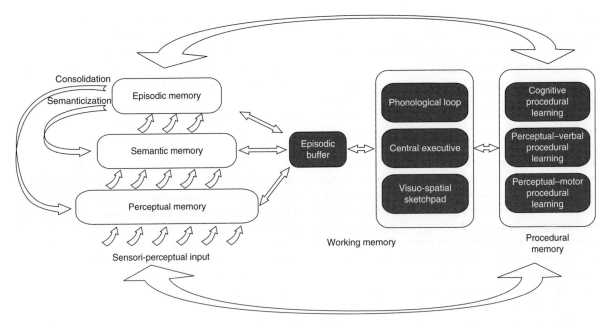

Figure 28.3 MNESIS (Memory NEoStructural Inter-Systemic model) proposed by Eustache and Desgranges [35]. (Reproduced with the authors' permission).

Tulving's classical SPI model. From a structural point of view, the model is interesting because it takes into account the memory systems supposed to be influenced by sleep. From a functional point of view, the MNESIS model tries to theorize the memory consolidation process. Further, as discussed in the following sections, it permits also the explanation of discrepancies in memory sleep-related studies by considering the working memory system as an interface between several memory systems.

In studies investigating the role of sleep in memory consolidation, the concept of memory system plays a crucial role. Indeed, as shown in the following sections, an REM sleep deprivation will not have the same effects on episodic memory as on procedural memory. However, at the same time, the way task-related memory is processed plays a determinant role in the memory-consolidation mechanisms.

Different memory processes

The classical memory tasks are characterized by a succession of different memory processes. The major and the most studied memory processes are the encoding, the storage, and the retrieval processes. However, other kinds of processes like recoding, consolidation, rehearsal, or forgetting, take place between the encoding phase and the retrieving phase. The process of *consolidation* can be studied at different levels (i.e., molecular, electrophysiological, or behavioral [5]). For the behaviorists, memory consolidation refers to a time-dependent process that allows the transformation of a new memory from a fragile to a more stable state that is resistant to interference without further practice [36, 37]. Recently, Walker [38] (see also Stickgold and Walker [39]) extended the definition of the consolidation process. According to this author, consolidation can be subdivided into two phases: stabilization and enhancement. Stabilization will be independent of sleep whereas enhancement will occur primarily but not exclusively during sleep. In terms of brain region, one may say that, broadly speaking, the principal player in memory consolidation is the hippocampus [40]. More precisely, it is assumed that the memory-consolidation process requires an interaction between the neocortex and the hippocampus [7]. In this dialog between the neocortex and hippocampus, the concept of "episodic buffer" appears to have a particular interest. Marshall and Born [7] indicated for example that "to prevent interference with pre-existing long-term memories during incorporation of new memories, information is encoded temporarily into an intermediate buffer from where, in an offline process, it is gradually transferred to the long-term store." Interestingly, we know that patients with schizophrenia or Alzheimer's disease are impaired both in tasks measuring the efficiency of the episodic buffer [11] and in sleep-related memory consolidation [41, 42].

Although mounting evidence supports the idea that sleep plays a key role in memory consolidation, it has to be kept in mind that memory consolidation is also highly dependent on encoding and/or retrieval processes. Indeed, since memory consolidation is appreciated through the retrieval of pre-encoded material, disturbances in the encoding and/or in the retrieval processes will affect performance on a task supposed to assess memory consolidation processes. In this regard, Craik and Lockart [43] postulated that memory performance is a function of the depth of initial processing (i.e., the level of processing theory). Even if memory researchers agree today that this postulate is a little simplistic, it remains a useful proposal. Consequently, the strength of the encoding process should be considered systematically in studies investigating the effects of sleep on memory consolidation. This is illustrated for instance by the studies of Drummond et al. [44] showing the deleterious effect of sleep deprivation on immediate verbal learning and of Walker and Stickgold [45] showing that, in an immediate recall task of emotionally valenced words, the sleep-deprived group recalled significantly fewer positive words than the group that was allowed to sleep. Accordingly, sleep disturbances observed in mental illnesses, as well as their daytime consequence on vigilance, will probably influence memory performance through their effects on several intercorrelated memory processes.

In a same way, the relationships between consolidation and retrieval should also be considered. During the last ten years, a lot of research has been focused on sleep-deprivation effects on memory and, more especially, on frontal lobe-dependent tasks [46]. As previously explained frontal lobe-dependent tasks are related to Baddeley's central executive unit and encompass different kinds of activities, like planning, selective attention, long-term memory activation, and so on. The retrieval process is highly dependent on frontal-lobe functions. Thus, when the memory recall task involves a conscious strategic retrieval process, memory performance is a function of memory consolidation but also of central executive efficiency. This could affect the results of sleep-related memory studies in schizophrenic patients who present simultaneously with sleep impairments and executive dysfunctions.

Relationships between memory and sleep are complex since they are linked to both the memory system and the memory process involved. In the next section, two other determinants will be discussed: the memory task and the to-be-remembered material.

Different kinds of memory tasks and different to-be-remembered materials

Sleep-related memory consolidation is highly dependent on the kind of memory task. In fact, each memory task is different because a given task will tap one memory system more than another, and tasks that tap the same memory system will not necessary assess exactly the same aspect of memory. For instance, there are short-term memory vs. long-term memory tasks; simple vs. complex tasks; explicit vs. implicit tasks. The methodology used to assess the strength of the memory-consolidation process is also a crucial point. As an example, the amount of attentional demands required by a free recall task is higher than that required by a cued recall task or by a recognition task. As we saw previously, it is well demonstrated that attentional/executive demands are dependent on frontal lobe functioning, and there is also increasing evidence that sleep deprivation impairs frontal lobe functions. The literature indicates that in order to study the consolidation process, most of the studies use partial or selective sleep-deprivation paradigms. Therefore, the choice of the memory task should be a crucial point for the assessment of memory consolidation following sleep deprivation. For instance, the memory task should not require a large amount of executive resources like a free recall memory task. It has to be underlined that this kind of consideration is not systematically taken into account in studies investigating the effects of sleep on memory consolidation. As stressed in the introduction section, there is a lack of consensus in the methodology of sleep-dependent memory studies. The discrepancies between studies in this research field could relate to the confusion of concepts as memory systems, tasks or processes, or in a misunderstanding of some interactions in memory systems. Moreover, contradictory results can also be explained by differences in the to-be-remembered materials used in the study protocols. For instance, Sterpenich et al. [47] demonstrated that the emotional significance of the encoded information plays an important role in a sleep-related recollection memory task. In this study, by using a classical remember/known paradigm [27], the authors showed that young healthy subjects recognized significantly fewer neutral and positive pictures after a 72-hour total sleep-deprivation period in comparison to the subjects who had a regular sleep night. But interestingly, no difference in the recognition of negative pictures between both groups was noticed in this study. This result shows that the material plays an important role in sleep-related memory tasks. This study tells us that the emotional valence of the material in studies dealing with sleep paradigms has to be taken into account. More generally, the role of the nature of the to-be-remembered material in the memory consolidation processes has been stressed by Rauchs *et al.* [4] who expect that the different sleep stages are probably also differently related to verbal or visuo-spatial memorization processes.

Sleep-related memory consolidation in healthy subjects and in mental illnesses

Like memory, *sleep* is a very complex research field for the non-initiated as well as for initiated people! At this stage the main role of sleep is not clearly identified. In a general way, researchers agree that the functions of sleep are most probably multiple [48], and according to the manifold literature, memory consolidation is indisputably one of these sleep functions.

The involvement of sleep in information reprocessing was suggested for the first time in 1900 by Müller and Pilzecker [49]. However, more than one hundred years later, there is still no consensus regarding the relationships between sleep and memory, or more exactly between sleep stages and memory systems. Indeed, although a growing body of evidence suggests a strong relationship between sleep and memory consolidation, it still remains unclear which memory system depends on which sleep-related consolidation process.

In the sleep-related memory research field, two key theories try to explain the links between sleep and memory. On the one hand, the sequential hypothesis [50] postulates that memory processing during sleep depends on the initial involvement of slow-wave sleep (SWS) in addition to the subsequent contribution of paradoxical sleep (i.e., rapid eye movement – REM – sleep). On the other hand, the dual process theory [51] postulates that memory processing during sleep differs regarding the sleep stages. In other words, according to the sequential hypothesis, the processing of newly acquired memories would be highly dependent on the succession of the sleep stages during the night, whereas the dual process theory postulates that SWS and REM sleep contribute differently to the processing of new information, or, in other words that the sleep-dependent memory processes differ according to sleep stages and memory systems. As indicated by Rauchs and colleagues [4] these theories are probably not antinomic and could be viewed as complementary.

Many studies have been conducted in order to determine which kind of information is related to SWS or to REM sleep. This question has been examined at different description levels (i.e., molecular, neuronal, brain structural, and behavioral [5]). These studies were mostly conducted in samples of healthy volunteers. Nevertheless, some recent data examined sleep-related memory consolidation processes in mental illnesses.

Sleep-related memory consolidation in healthy volunteers

It is well demonstrated that early night sleep is characterized by a dominance of SWS, whereas late night sleep is characterized by a greater proportion of REM sleep. In 1997, Plihal and Born [51] published a key paper that evidenced differential effects of early and late nocturnal sleep on two main memory systems (i.e., declarative and procedural memory). This study showed that early nocturnal sleep was beneficial for declarative memory consolidation, which was assessed with a paired-associate word list task, and that late nocturnal sleep improved mirror-tracing skills (i.e., a procedural memory task). In a same vein, Smith [52] published a review paper in which the strong relationship between procedural learning and REM sleep was demonstrated. According to this author, REM sleep is not involved in declarative information processing. In fact, declarative memory is presented as depending on stage 3/4 or non-REM sleep.

Nevertheless, less than ten years later, this sleep-dependent dissociation in memory consolidation (i.e., declarative memory/SWS vs. procedural memory/REM sleep) seems to be less evident. Indeed, a recent publication [53] concluded that REM sleep is probably not required for procedural memory consolidation. To date, the REM sleep–memory consolidation hypothesis is an active topic of debate in the literature. According to some authors [54, 55], REM sleep would not be involved in memory consolidation. The main argument in favor of this hypothesis is that the pharmacological or brain lesion-induced suppression of REM sleep has no deleterious effect on memory. In this sense, the results presented by Rasch et al. [53] are largely consistent with this hypothesis. Indeed, this study showed that a pharmacological REM sleep suppression enhances rather than impairs a procedural memory task (i.e., finger tapping). However, the defenders of the REM sleep–memory consolidation hypothesis argue that REM sleep is not definitively suppressed in cases of chronic drug treatment [5] and that many methodological aspects can also explain the discrepancies in these study results [52]. According to some recent publications, REM sleep could also be associated with declarative memory consolidation. Indeed, Nishida and colleagues [56] demonstrated that REM sleep was correlated with memory recognition performance. In this study, the authors made the hypothesis that REM sleep has a beneficial effect on emotional but not on neutral memories. The hypothesis was tested with a nap paradigm (i.e., half of the participants were allowed to nap, whereas the other half were not). The experimental task consisted of watching two sets of 120 pictures (60 neutral and 60 negative) 4 hours and 15 minutes before the recognition test, respectively. The nap group had the opportunity to sleep for 90 minutes after the first session. The recognition test was composed of 360 pictures (i.e., 120 old neutral + 60 new, and 120 old negative + 60 new pictures). The results indicated that memory recognition performances were selectively better for negative pictures than for neutral pictures and that the recognition performances were better for the pictures presented 4 hours prior to the test in comparison to the pictures presented 15 minutes prior to the recognition test in the nap group. Within the nap group, the offline emotional memory benefit was significantly correlated with the amount of REM sleep observed during the nap as well as with the extent of right-lateralized prefrontal theta power during REM. As indicated by the authors, these results have some interesting implications in memory consolidation dysfunctions in psychiatric and mood disorders like depression or PTSD (i.e., pathologies characterized by REM sleep dysfunctions). In a same way, Nishida and Walker [57] showed that procedural memory consolidation is not exclusively dependent on REM sleep. Indeed, the authors showed in a nap paradigm, that motor memory performance (assessed by a finger

tapping task) was improved only in subjects who nap. Interestingly, these improvements were correlated with stage 2 non-REM sleep. This study underscores that consolidation of procedural memories is not only related to REM sleep as expected by several authors. Thus, even if many studies tend to demonstrate the strong relationship between REM sleep and procedural memory consolidation, some discrepancies remain.

In the same vein, there is currently less clear evidence in favor of a specific relationship between SWS and declarative memories than ten years ago. In fact, as indicated previously, Plihal and Born [51] as well as Gais and Born [58] demonstrated that the consolidation of declarative information assessed with a paired associate word list task was correlated with SWS-rich early sleep. However, several data indicate that this relationship is probably more complex and that sleep-related memory consolidation of declarative information is probably mediated by and/or dependent on other factors than only SWS, such as task difficulty and spindle activity. Indeed, a growing body of literature shows that sleep spindles occurring during phase 2 sleep also play an important role in declarative memory consolidation [48, 59, 60]. Schmidt and colleagues [61] demonstrated a strong relationship between sleep spindle activity and memory consolidation during daytime napping. In their study, the material was composed of associate word pairs containing concrete nouns (i.e., low task difficulty) and by word pairs characterized by a more abstract relationship (i.e., high task difficulty). The results indicated that the sleep-related consolidation was dependent on the nature of the learned material. Indeed, EEG power density and sleep spindle activity were differently affected after the learning of difficult versus easy word pairs. This study underlines that memory consolidation of declarative memories is not only related to SWS but depends more generally on non-REM sleep. It also indicates that the role of sleep in declarative memory consolidation might also depend on the kind of to-be-remembered materials. As described previously, the latter is particularly evidenced in studies that contain emotional material [56, 62].

To sum up, these different data demonstrate that even if declarative (i.e., facts and events) memory consolidation seems preferentially related to SWS and procedural (i.e., skills) memory consolidation to REM sleep, the reality is probably more complicated. Indeed, studies in healthy volunteers showed that several other aspects underlie memory consolidation. Some of them are directly related to sleep characteristics, whereas others depend on the to-be-remembered material.

Sleep-related consolidation in mental illnesses

Because previous research has focused on healthy young adults, only very few studies on sleep-related memory consolidation have been conducted in patients with neuropsychiatric disorders so far. However, many neuropsychiatric illnesses such as Alzheimer's disease, schizophrenia, post-traumatic stress disorder (PTSD), and depression are characterized by sleep disorders and by memory impairments. For instance, patients with schizophrenia suffer from several sleep disturbances [63, 64], some of them being probably due to their medication [65, 66]. Alterations of stage 2 sleep, SWS, and deficiency of delta activity can be outlined among these sleep disturbances. Conjointly, schizophrenic patients present also several cognitive impairments like executive dysfunctions [67] or long-term memory deficiencies [68]. In the same way, Alzheimer's disease is characterized by massive memory impairments [69] and by different sleep disturbances [41]. Another similarity between these illnesses is the existence of hippocampal abnormalities. In fact, recent studies indicated a reduced hippocampal volume in schizophrenic patients [70, 71] while there is a growing body of literature showing a positive correlation between Alzheimer's disease severity and hippocampal atrophy [72–74].

As previously discussed, the hippocampus is an important brain structure for memory. Recent research has demonstrated the role of the hippocampus in declarative memory [75]; relationships between this brain structure and memory deficits in schizophrenia [76] and Alzheimer's disease [77] were also evidenced. In studies investigating sleep-related memory consolidation, the recently demonstrated role of the hippocampus in the integration or binding function of memory traces is of particular interest [78, 79]. According to Eustache and Desgranges' [35] cognitive point of view, the binding function is assumed by the episodic buffer [33, 80]. From a functional neuroanatomical point of view, the integration or binding function is known to be dependent on the hippocampal areas [81, 82].

As discussed earlier, there is now much evidence coming from sleep studies that the hippocampus is a key structure for memory consolidation since it is supposed to be a time-dependent process involving a dialog between the hippocampal areas and the neocortex [40]. In their model of declarative memory consolidation, Wagner and Born [83] explain that the hippocampus is responsible for the encoding of different features concerning the new information. The model posits that, during wakefulness, both the hippocampus and neocortical circuits are implicated in the treatment of new materials, with the hippocampus being described as an intermediate buffer (i.e., episodic buffer) responsible for the temporary storage of the newly encoded information. During sleep, or more precisely during SWS, this new information is simultaneously replayed (or reactivated) in both the hippocampus and neocortex, and then progressively transferred from the hippocampus to the neocortex, described as the long-term store. At an electrophysiological level, it has been suggested that the hippocampal to neocortical information transfer during sleep is linked to coordinate hippocampal high-frequency ripple activities and thalamo-cortical spindle activities, with both activities being synchronized to cortical slow oscillations [84, 85].

In a healthy matched controlled study, Göder et al. [86] showed that, in patients with schizophrenia, the reduction in the amount of SWS and sleep efficiency were correlated to next-day visuo-spatial declarative memory impairments assessed with the Rey–Osterrieth Complex Figure Test and a spatial location recall test. The authors concluded that schizophrenic patients presented a deficient sleep-related memory consolidation. However, Bódizs and Lázár [87] proposed an alternative interpretation based on the structural brain abnormalities observed in schizophrenic patients that relate to the encoding impairments observed in schizophrenic patients [88]. As discussed above, memory consolidation is a process highly dependent on encoding and retrieval processes. Consequently, the next-day memory impairments observed by Göder et al. [86] in schizophrenic patients could be explained by a binding deficit (i.e., integration) of the different features of new information in a coherent representation during the encoding process. Indeed, several recent researchers have demonstrated a binding deficit in schizophrenic patients [89, 90]. The spatial deficit observed in schizophrenia [91] is another possible explanation of the finding of Göder et al. [86]. Indeed, Luck et al. [92] assessed working memory-binding efficiency in schizophrenic patients

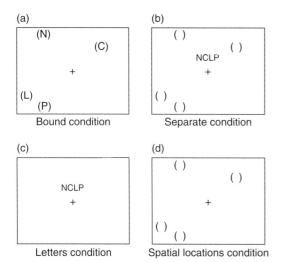

Figure 28.4 Luck and colleagues [92] used two kind of tasks: a binding task and a single-feature task. The aim of the binding task was to retain letters within locations (bound condition) or letters separated from locations (separate condition). In the single-feature task, the subjects had to retain letters (letters condition) or spatial locations (spatial locations condition).

and healthy subjects. The binding task consisted of retaining four letters and four locations, and was declined in two conditions. The bound condition (A) was characterized by the fact that letters were included within locations. In separate condition (B), the letters were presented centrally and separated from the locations. In order to assess the maintenance abilities, a single-feature task declined in two conditions was also administered: the letters condition (C) where only four letters were centrally presented and the spatial locations condition (D) where four locations were presented instead of the letters (see Figure 28.4). The results showed that both groups performed better in the bound condition (A) in comparison to the separate condition (B); nevertheless the patients' performances were lower in comparison to healthy subjects. In single-feature conditions, the patients presented a significant impairment in maintenance of spatial locations (D) but not in letter maintenance (C). The authors concluded that the lower working memory-binding performances in patients were probably due to their spatial maintenance memory deficit, and that consequently not all forms of binding would be disturbed in schizophrenia. On basis of the observations of structural brain abnormalities [70, 71] and of a binding deficit [89, 90], one may advocate the existence of a disturbed functioning of the

episodic buffer, to explain the next-day memory impairments observed by Göder et al. [86] in schizophrenic patients. Other factors that may have contributed to a lower memory consolidation effect of sleep in schizophrenic patients are a deficit in the working memory's visuo-spatial subunit (i.e., the visuo-spatial sketch pad) during encoding and a central executive deficit. Indeed there is evidence for a deficit of spatial working memory [92] and of the central executive [93] in schizophrenia. The latter deficit, which encompasses frontal or executive function, is particularly implicated in memory retrieval processes. Indeed it has been shown that patients with schizophrenia are impaired in all activities requiring high control abilities such as planning, selective attention, or long-term memory activation [67]. Thus, discrepancies observed in two sleep-related procedural memory consolidation studies in patients with schizophrenia [42, 94] could be explained by a deficit in the control abilities involved in the retrieval process. Indeed, Manoach and colleagues [94] showed that chronically medicated patients with schizophrenia failed to improve their performances in a procedural memory learning task after one night of sleep (i.e., finger tapping motor sequence task). On the other side, Göder and colleagues [42] demonstrated an improvement in a sleep-related procedural memory task (i.e., mirror-tracing task) in medicated patients with schizophrenia. The discrepancies observed in these studies could be explained by examining cognitive processes involved in both procedural tasks. Indeed, the mirror-tracing task, which is considered an implicit memory task, does not involve a great amount of control ability during the retrieval process. On the contrary, the finger tapping is an explicit memory task, and in this way its retrieval performance is dependent on control (or executive) abilities. Thus, these studies in patients with schizophrenia demonstrate that in sleep-related memory consolidation studies it is important to examine the encoding and retrieval processes. In this way, it could also be postulated that even if Alzheimer's patients experience sleep disturbances and long-term memory deficits, the lack of memory consolidation in these patients is probably not only due to sleep disturbances but could be related to the encoding deficits and the retrieval impairments observed in Alzheimer's patients.

To the best of our knowledge, very few sleep-related memory consolidation studies have been conducted in patients with mood disorders to date [95]. Nevertheless, the existence of a deficiency in sleep-related memory consolidation in patients presenting mood disorders is frequently hypothesized in the literature [56, 96]. This hypothesis is conceivable, as several facts speak in favor of a relationship between sleep disturbances and the memory dysfunctions observed in these illnesses. For instance, on the one side, REM sleep disturbances as well as amygdala and frontal dysfunctions coexist in mood disorders such as PTSD [97–99] or depression [100]. On the other side, a growing body of evidence suggests that the consolidation of emotional memories is enhanced after a period of sleep [101, 102]. More precisely, Wagner and colleagues [62] demonstrated that REM sleep is involved in the formation of emotional memory in humans [62]. Since the amygdala is activated during REM sleep [103], and since this brain structure is well known to be involved in the processing of emotional information [104], some authors postulated that the amygdala mediates hippocampal memory consolidation of emotional valenced information [83, 105]. Recent studies using total sleep deprivation paradigms demonstrated that the prefrontal cortex exerts an inhibitory top–down control of amygdala [47], and thereby plays a role in sleep-related emotional memory consolidation. Thus, according to the sleep disturbances and to the limbic and frontal dysfunctions observed in mood disorders, several authors postulated that these patients present disturbances in sleep-related memory consolidation of emotional information [96, 106]. Taken together, these dysfunctions should lead to a "maladaptative consolidation process" [56] or an "overconsolidation" [106] of negative affective memories. According to this hypothesis, this overconsolidation of negative memories should reinforce the mood disorder. Moreover, this hypothesis also allows us to explain the antidepressant effect of sleep deprivation observed in depressive patients [107].

Additionally, attentional bias could influence sleep-related memory consolidation in depressive and PTSD patients. This attentional bias is characterized by a deficit of inhibition toward mood congruent information [108]. In other words, during the encoding process, mood congruent information is more deeply processed and therefore better retained because the working memory's central executive subunit allows a greater amount of attention toward this mood congruent information. Thus, depressive patients exhibit biased attention toward negative information [109–111],

while PTSD patients present a deficit of inhibition in trauma-relevant stimuli [112]. Accordingly, the over-consolidation of negative memories in mood disorders is certainly also underlain by an abnormal encoding process. As a consequence, studies in patients having mood disorders that assess sleep-related memory consolidation need to be carefully designed in order to take into account this emotional bias and designs used in healthy subjects are probably not suitable.

Conclusion

Even if some studies dealing with sleep-related memory consolidation impairments in mental illnesses were published, very few data supporting such a specific deficit in neuropsychiatric disorders could be evidenced. Indeed, on the one hand some of these studies concluded in favor of the existence of a sleep-related memory consolidation deficit in mental illness, but several methodological pitfalls have led us to cast doubt on their results. On the other hand, some interesting hypotheses are defended in the literature but were unfortunately at this stage not tested in patient studies. However, data issued both from empirical healthy subject studies and from academic cognitive theories permitted us to cast light on several important points that should more often be considered in sleep-related memory consolidation research. Among these points we can retain the importance of the to-be-remembered material and of the task difficulty. Indeed, as memory processing is highly dependent on material features, the choice of the memory task material is crucial in sleep-related memory consolidation studies. Task difficulty can affect performance on a task supposed to assess memory consolidation processes, because it has a direct incidence on the depth of encoding and/or can lead to more or less memory retrieving facilitation. The relationship between the consolidation process and the other memory processes appears also of particular interest. Indeed, memory consolidation is strongly linked to encoding and retrieving processes. However, studies investigating the effect of sleep on memory consolidation often do not consider the relationships between these processes. Finally, it can be concluded that, according to specific deficits in the particular memory processes, systems, to-be-remembered material, or memory-related brain areas in mental illnesses, sleep-related memory consolidation study designs in patient studies should be constructed very cautiously!

References

1. Scoville WB, Milner B. Loss of recent memory after bilateral hippocampal lesions. *J Neurol Neurosurg Psychiatry.* 1957;**20**:11–12.

2. Eichenbaum H. Hippocampus: cognitive processes and neural representations that underlie declarative memory. *Neuron.* 2004;**44**:109–20.

3. Zola SM, Squire L. The medial temporal lobe and the hippocampus. In: Tulving E, Craik FIM, eds. *The Oxford Handbook of Memory.* (New York: Oxford University Press, 2000; 485–500).

4. Rauchs G, Desgranges B, Foret J, Eustache F. The relationships between memory systems and sleep stages. *J Sleep Res.* 2005;**14**:123–40.

5. Walker MP, Stickgold R. Sleep-dependent learning and memory consolidation. *Neuron.* 2004;**44**(1):121–33.

6. Morini F, Nobili L, Curcio G, De Carli F. Sleep in the human hippocampus: a stereo-EEG study. *PloS ONE.* 2007;**2**(9):e867.

7. Marshall L, Born J. The contribution of sleep to hippocampus-dependent memory consolidation. *Trends Cogn Sci.* 2007;**11**(10):442–50.

8. Baddeley A, Della Sala S. Working memory and executive control. *Philos Trans R Soc Lond B Biol Sci.* 1996;**351**(1346):1397–403; discussion 1403–4.

9. Chuah YML, Venkatraman V, Dinges DF, Chee MWL. The neural basis of interindividual variability in inhibitory efficiency after sleep deprivation. *J Neurosci.* 2006;**26**(27):7156–62.

10. Benca RM, Obermeyer WH, Thisted RA, Gillin JC. Sleep and psychiatric disorders. A meta-analysis. *Arch Gen Psychiatry.* 1992;**49**(8):651–68; discussion 669–70.

11. Lange N, Lake S, Sperling R, *et al.* Two macroscopic and microscopic brain imaging studies of human hippocampus in early Alzheimer's disease and schizophrenia research. *Stat Med.* 2004;**23**(2):327–50.

12. Martino DJ, Bucay D, Butman JT, Allegri RF. Neuropsychological frontal impairments and negative symptoms in schizophrenia. *Psychiatry Res.* 2007;**152**(2–3):121–8.

13. Drevets WC, Price JL, Furey ML. Brain structural and functional abnormalities in mood disorders: implications for neurocircuitry models of depression. *Brain Struct Funct.* 2008;**213**(1–2):93–118.

14. Siegle GJ, Thompson W, Carter CS, Steinhauer SR, Thase ME. Increased amygdala and decreased dorsolateral prefrontal BOLD responses in unipolar depression: related and independent features. *Biol Psychiatry.* 2007;**61**(2):198–209.

15. Etkin A, Wager TD. Functional neuroimaging of anxiety: a meta-analysis of emotional processing in PTSD, social anxiety disorder, and specific phobia. *Am J Psychiatry.* 2007;**164**(10):1476–88.

16. Atkinson RC, Shiffrin RM. Human memory: a proposed system and its control processes. In: Spence KW, ed. *The Psychology of Learning and Motivation. Advances in Research and Theory*, Vol. 2. (New York: Academic Press, 1968; 89–195).

17. Bower GH. A brief history of memory research. In: Tulving E, Craik FIM, eds. *The Oxford Handbook of Memory.* (New York: Oxford University Press, 2000; 3–32).

18. Cowan N. What are the differences between long-term, short-term, and working memory? *Prog Brain Res.* 2008;**169**:323–38.

19. Graf P, Schacter D. Implicit and explicit memory for new associations in normal subjects and amnesic patients. *J Exper Psychol Learn Mem Cogn.* 1985;**11**:501–18.

20. Squire L. Memory and the hippocampus: a synthesis of findings with rats, monkeys, and humans. *Psychol Rev.* 1992;**99**:195–231.

21. Tulving E. Episodic and semantic memory. In: Tulving E, Donaldson W, eds. *Organization of Memory.* (New York: Academic Press, 1972; 381–403).

22. Cohen NJ, Eichenbaum H. *Memory, Amnesia, and the Hippocampal System.* (MA: MIT Press, 1993).

23. Jacoby LL, Witherspoon D. Remembering without awareness. *Can J Psychol.* 1982;**36**:300–24.

24. Schacter DL, Tulving E. What are the memory systems of 1994? In: Schacter DL, Tulving E, eds. *Memory Systems.* (Cambridge: MIT Press, 1994; 1–38).

25. Nadel L. Multiple memory systems: what and why. An update. In: Schacter D, Tulving E, eds. *Memory Systems.* (Cambridge: MIT Press, 1994; 39–63).

26. Tulving E. Organization of memory: quo vadis? In: Gazzaniga MS, ed. *The Cognitive Neuroscience.* (Cambridge, MA: MIT Press, 1995; 839–47).

27. Tulving E. Episodic memory and common sense: how far apart? *Philos Trans R Soc Lond B Biol Sci.* 2001;**356**(1413):1505–15.

28. Baddeley A, Hitch G. Working memory. In: Bower GA, ed. *Recent Advances in Learning and Motivation*, Vol. 8. (New York: Academic Press, 1974; 47–89).

29. Baddeley A. *Working Memory.* (Oxford: Clarendon Press, 1986).

30. Kibby MY, Marks W, Morgan S, Long CJ. Specific impairment in developmental reading disabilities: a working memory approach. *J Learn Disabil.* 2004;**37**(4):349–63.

31. Cocchi L, Schenk F, Volken H, *et al.* Visuo-spatial processing in a dynamic and a static working memory

paradigm in schizophrenia. *Psychiatry Res.* 2007;**152**(2–3):129–42.

32. Baddeley AD. Exploring the central executive. *Q J Exper Psychol.* 1996;**49A**:5–28.

33. Baddeley A. The episodic buffer: a new component of working memory? *Trends Cogn Sci.* 2000;**4**(11):417–23.

34. Repovs G, Baddeley A. The multi-component model of working memory: explorations in experimental cognitive psychology. *Neuroscience.* 2006;**139**(1):5–21.

35. Eustache F, Desgranges B. MNESIS: Towards the integration of current multisystem models of memory. *Neuropsychol Rev.* 2008;**18**: 53–69.

36. McGaugh JL. Memory: a century of consolidation. *Science.* 2000;**287**:248–57.

37. Squire L. Rapid consolidation. *Science.* 2007;**316**:57–8.

38. Walker MP. Sleep-dependent memory processing. *Harv Rev Psychiatry.* 2008;**16**(5):287–98.

39. Stickgold R, Walker MP. Sleep-dependent memory consolidation and reconsolidation. *Sleep Med.* 2007;**8**(4):331–43.

40. Murray EA, Bussey TJ. Consolidation and the medial temporal lobe revisited: methodological considerations. *Hippocampus.* 2001;**11**(1):1–7.

41. Rauchs G, Schabus M, Parapatics S, *et al.* Is there a link between sleep changes and memory in Alzheimer's disease? *Neuroreport.* 2008;**19**(11):1159–62.

42. Göder R, Fritzer G, Gottwald B, *et al.* Effects of olanzapine on slow wave sleep, sleep spindles and sleep-related memory consolidation in schizophrenia. *Pharmacopsychiatry.* 2008;**41**(3):92–9.

43. Craik F, Lockhart R. Levels of processing: a framework for memory research. *J Verb Learn Verb Behav,* 1972;**11**:671–84.

44. Drummond SPA, Brown GG, Gillin JC, *et al.* Altered brain response to verbal learning following sleep deprivation. *Nature.* 2000;**403**(6770):655–7.

45. Walker MP, Stickgold R. Sleep, memory, and plasticity. *Annu Rev Psychol.* 2006;**57**:139–66.

46. Jones K, Harrison Y. Frontal lobe function, sleep loss and fragmented sleep. *Sleep Med Rev.* 2001;**5**(6):463–75.

47. Sterpenich V, Albouy G, Boly M, *et al.* Sleep-related hippocampo-cortical interplay during emotional memory recollection. *PLoS Biol.* 2007;**5**(11):e282.

48. Schabus M, Gruber G, Parapatics S, *et al.* Sleep spindles and their significance for declarative memory consolidation. *Sleep.* 2004;**27**(8):1479–85.

49. Müller GE, Pilzecker A. Experimentalle Beiträge zur Lehre vom Gedächtnis. *Z. Psychol. Ergänzungsband.* 1900;**1**:1–300.

50. Ambrosini MV, Giuditta A. Learning and sleep: the sequential hypothesis. *Sleep Med Rev.* 2001;**5**(6):477–90.

51. Plihal W, Born J. Effects of early and late nocturnal sleep on declarative and procedural memory. *J Cogn Neurosci.* 1997;**9**(4):534–47.

52. Smith C. Sleep states and memory processes in humans: procedural versus declarative memory systems. *Sleep Med Rev.* 2001;**5**(6):491–506.

53. Rasch B, Pommer J, Diekelmann S, Born J. Pharmacological REM sleep suppression paradoxically improves rather than impairs skill memory. *Nat Neurosci.* 2009;**12**(4):396–7.

54. Siegel JM. The REM sleep-memory consolidation hypothesis. *Science.* 2001;**294**(5544):1058–63.

55. Vertes RP. Memory consolidation in sleep; dream or reality. *Neuron.* 2004;**44**(1):135–48.

56. Nishida M, Pearsall J, Buckner RL, Walker MP. REM sleep, prefrontal theta, and the consolidation of human emotional memory. *Cerebral Cortex.* 2009;**19**(5):1158–66.

57. Nishida M, Walker MP. Daytime naps, motor memory consolidation and regionally specific sleep spindles. *PLoS ONE,* 2007;**2**(4):e341.

58. Gais S, Born J. Declarative memory consolidation: mechanisms acting during human sleep. *Learn Mem.* 2004;**11**(6):679–85.

59. Buzsaki G. Memory consolidation during sleep: a neurophysiological perspective. *J Sleep Res.* 1998;**7**(1):17–23.

60. Sirota A, Csicsvari J, Buhl D, Buzsaki G. Communication between neocortex and hippocampus during sleep in rodents. *PNAS.* 2003;**100**(4):2065–9.

61. Schmidt C, Peigneux P, Muto V, *et al.* Encoding difficulty promotes postlearning changes in sleep spindle activity during napping. *J Neurosci.* 2006;**26**(35):8976–82.

62. Wagner U, Gais S, Born J. Emotional memory formation is enhanced across sleep intervals with high amounts of rapid eye movement sleep. *Learn Mem.* 2001;**8**:112–19.

63. Staner L, Noël N, Luthringer R. Schizophrenia, sleep, and antipsychotic drugs. In: Pandi-Perumal SR, Verster J, Monti J, Langer S, eds. *Sleep Disorders: Diagnosis and Therapeutics.* (Informa Healthcare, 2008; 417–26).

64. Chouinard S, Poulin J, Stip E, Godbout R. Sleep in untreated patients with schizophrenia: a meta-analysis. *Schizophr Bull.* 2004;**30**(4):957–67.

65. Cohrs S. Sleep disturbances in patients with schizophrenia: impact and effect of antipsychotics. *CNS Drugs.* 2008;**22**(11):939–62.

66. Krystal AD, Goforth HW, Roth T. Effects of antipsychotic medications on sleep in schizophrenia. *Int Clin Psychopharmacol.* 2008;**23**(3):150–60.

67. Kerns JG, Nuechterlein KH, Braver TS, Barch DM. Executive functioning component mechanisms and schizophrenia. *Biol Psychiatry.* 2008;**64**(1):26–33.

68. Danion JM, Huron C, Vidailhet P, Berna F. Functional mechanisms of episodic memory impairment in schizophrenia. *Can J Psychiatry.* 2007;**52**(11):693–701.

69. Eustache F, Giffard B, Rauchs G, et al. La maladie d'Alzheimer et la mémore humaine. *Rev Neurol.* 2006;**162**(10):929–39.

70. Vita A, De Peri L, Silenzi C, Dieci M. Brain morphology in first-episode schizophrenia: a meta-analysis of quantitative magnetic resonance imaging studies. *Schizophr Res.* 2006;**82**(1):75–88.

71. Velakoulis D, Wood SJ, Wong MT, et al. Hippocampal and amygdala volumes according to psychosis stage and diagnosis: a magnetic resonance imaging study of chronic schizophrenia, first-episode psychosis, and ultra-high-risk individuals. *Arch Gen Psychiatry.* 2006;**63**(2):139–49.

72. deToledo-Morrell L, Stoub TR, Wang C. Hippocampal atrophy and disconnection in incipient and mild Alzheimer's disease. *Prog Brain Res.* 2007;**163**:741–53.

73. Sperling R. Functional MRI studies of associative encoding in normal aging, mild cognitive impairment, and Alzheimer's disease. *Ann N Y Acad Sci.* 2007;**1097**:146–55.

74. Di Paola M, Macaluso E, Carlesimo GA, et al. Episodic memory impairment in patients with Alzheimer's disease is correlated with entorhinal cortex atrophy. A voxel-based morphometry study. *J Neurol.* 2007;**254**(6):774–81.

75. Stoub TR, Rogalski EJ, Leurgans S, Bennett DA, Detoledo-Morrell L. Rate of entorhinal and hippocampal atrophy in incipient and mild AD: Relation to memory function. *Neurobiol Aging.* 2008 Sep 20. [Epub ahead of print].

76. Boyer P, Phillips JL, Rousseau FL, Ilivitsky S. Hippocampal abnormalities and memory deficits: new evidences of a strong pathophysiological link in schizophrenia. *Brain Res Rev.* 2007;**54**(1):92–112.

77. Elgh E, Lindqvist Astot A, Fagerlund M, et al. Cognitive dysfunction, hippocampal atrophy and glucocorticoid feedback in Alzheimer's disease. *Biol Psychiatry.* 2006;**59**(2):155–61.

78. Chua EF, Schacter DL, Rand-Giovannetti E, Sperling RA. Evidence for a specific role of the anterior hippocampal region in successful associative encoding. *Hippocampus.* 2007;**17**(11):1071–80.

79. Suzuki WA. Integrating associative learning signals across the brain. *Hippocampus.* 2007;**17**(9):842–50.

80. Rudner M, Fransson P, Ingvar M, Nyberg L, Rönnberg J. Neural representation of binding lexical signs and words in the episodic buffer of working memory. *Neuropsychologia.* 2007;**45**(10):2258–76.

81. Piekema C, Fernández G, Postma A, et al. Spatial and non-spatial contextual working memory in patients with diencephalic or hippocampal dysfunction. *Brain Res.* 2007;**1172**:103–9.

82. Staresina BP, Davachi L. Selective and shared contributions of the hippocampus and perirhinal cortex to episodic item and associative encoding. *J Cogn Neurosci.* 2008;**20**(8):1478–89.

83. Wagner U, Born J. Memory consolidation during sleep: interactive effects of sleep stages and HPA regulation. *Stress.* 2008;**11**(1):28–41.

84. Born J, Rasch B, Gais S. Sleep to remember. *Neuroscientist.* 2006;**12**(5):410–24.

85. Clemens Z, Mölle M, Erros L, et al. Temporal coupling of parahippocampal ripples, sleep spindles and slow oscillations in humans. *Brain.* 2007;**130**:2868–78.

86. Göder R, Boigs M, Braun S, et al. Impairment of visuospatial memory is associated with decreased slow wave sleep in schizophrenia. *J Psychiatr Res.* 2004;**38**(6):591–9.

87. Bódizs R, Lázár AS. Schizophrenia, slow wave sleep and visuospatial memory: sleep-dependent consolidation or trait-like correlation? *J Psychiatr Res.* 2006;**40**(1):89–90.

88. Forbes NF, Carrick LA, McIntosh AM, Lawrie SM. Working memory in schizophrenia: a meta-analysis. *Psychol Med.* 2008;**23**:1–17.

89. Doré MC, Caza N, Gingras N, Rouleau N. Deficient relational binding processes in adolescents with psychosis: evidence from impaired memory for source and temporal context. *Cogn Neuropsychiatry.* 2007;**12**(6):511–36.

90. Diaz-Asper C, Malley J, Genderson M, Apud J, Elvevåg B. Context binding in schizophrenia: effects of clinical symptomatology and item content. *Psychiatry Res.* 2008;**159**(3):259–70.

91. Glahn DC, Therman S, Manninen M, et al. Spatial working memory as an endophenotype for schizophrenia. *Biol Psychiatry.* 2003;**53**(7):624–6.

92. Luck D, Foucher JR, Offerlin-Meyer I, Lepage M, Danion JM. Assessment of single and bound features in a working memory task in schizophrenia. *Schizophr Res.* 2008;**100**(1–3):153–60.

93. Kim J, Glahn DC, Nuechterlein KH, Cannon TD. Maintenance and manipulation of information in

schizophrenia: further evidence for impairment in the central executive component of working memory. *Schizophr Res.* 2004;**68**(2–3):173–87.

94. Manoach DS, Cain MS, Vangel MG, *et al.* A failure of sleep-dependent procedural learning in chronic, medicated schizophrenia. *Biol Psychiatry.* 2004;**56**(12):951–6.

95. Göder R, Fritzer G, Hinze-Selch D, *et al.* Sleep in major depression: relation to memory performance and outcome after interpersonal psychotherapy. *Neuropsychobiology.* 2007;**55**(1):36–42.

96. Hornung OP, Regen F, Danker-Hopfe H, Heuser I, Anghelescu I. Sleep-related memory consolidation in depression: an emerging field of research. *Depress Anxiety.* 2008;**25**(12):E163–5.

97. Spoormaker VI, Montgomery P. Disturbed sleep in post-traumatic stress disorder: secondary symptom or core feature? *Sleep Med Rev.* 2008;**12**(3):169–84.

98. Singareddy RK, Balon R. Sleep in posttraumatic stress disorder. *Ann Clin Psychiatry.* 2002;**14**(3):183–90.

99. Liberzon I, Sripada CS. The functional neuroanatomy of PTSD: a critical review. *Prog Brain Res.* 2008;**167**:151–69.

100. Drevets WC. Prefrontal cortical-amygdalar metabolism in major depression. *Ann N Y Acad Sci.* 1999;**877**:614–37.

101. Wagner U, Hallschmid M, Rasch B, Born J. Brief sleep after learning keeps emotional memories alive for years. *Biol Psychiatry.* 2006;**60**(7):788–90.

102. Hu P, Stylos-Allan M, Walker MP. Sleep facilitates consolidation of emotional declarative memory. *Psychol Sci.* 2006;**17**(10):891–8.

103. Maquet P, Péters J, Aerts J, *et al.* Functional neuroanatomy of human rapid-eye-movement sleep and dreaming. *Nature.* 1996;**383**(6596): 163–6.

104. Seymour B, Dolan R. Emotion, decision making, and the amygdala. *Neuron.* 2008;**58**(5):662–71.

105. McGaugh JL. The amygdala modulates the consolidation of memories of emotionally arousing experiences. *Annu Rev Neurosci.* 2004;**27**:1–28.

106. Holland P, Lewis PA. Emotional memory: selective enhancement by sleep. *Curr Biol.* 2007;**17**(5):R179–81.

107. Voderholzer U, Hohagen F, Klein T, *et al.* Impact of sleep deprivation and subsequent recovery sleep on cortisol in unmedicated depressed patients. *Am J Psychiatry.* 2004;**161**(8):1404–10.

108. Watkins PC, Mathews A, Williamson DA, Fuller RD. Mood-congruent memory in depression: emotional priming or elaboration? *J Abnorm Psychol.* 1992;**101**:581–6.

109. Goeleven E, De Raedt R, Baert S, Koster EH. Deficient inhibition of emotional information in depression. *J Affect Disord.* 2006;**93**(1–3):149–57.

110. Joormann J, Gotlib IH. Selective attention to emotional faces following recovery from depression. *J Abnorm Psychol.* 2007;**116**(1):80–5.

111. Joormann J, Yoon KL, Zetsche U. Cognitive inhibition in depression. *Applied Preventive Psychology.* 2007;**12**:128–39.

112. Moore SA. Cognitive abnormalities in posttraumatic stress disorder. *Curr Opin Psychiatry.* 2008;**22**:19–24.

Chapter 29

Sleep-associated cognitive side effects of psychoactive medications

James F. Pagel

Introduction: psychoactive effects of medications

The cognitive effects of psychoactive medications on sleep have historically been considered as global and non-specific, with electrophysiological effects defined by the alteration of sleep stages. However, in the last 25 years the selective neurotransmitter effects of many psychoactive drugs have been clarified. As a result of this work, it is currently questionable as to whether the theoretical postulates of global and electrophysiological sleep stage effects have an actual contribution to known psychoactive drug effects and side effects.

Our understanding of the neurotransmitter effects of psychoactive agents has been derived from two divergent yet contributory data bases of neurochemical knowledge. The specific neurochemical effects of many of these agents have been studied in animal models and analyzed to determine the specific neurosynaptic effects for each pharmacologically active compound. Although such data serve as the basis of most textbook presentations that note pharmacologic drug effects, this approach has known limitations when applied to the study of central nervous system (CNS) medication effects and side effects.

a. The human CNS is extraordinarily complex and only a few cells and neuroanatomic interactions have been studied (there are over a hundred billon neurons in the human CNS with each utilizing multiple neurotransmitters and signaling systems) [1–3].

b. This approach is almost exclusively limited to animal models, from which data must be extrapolated as applying to humans.

c. This approach is limited by the theoretical postulates for neurochemical interactions in a research mileu where new neurochemicals, cellular transponders, and neuro-hormones are constantly being discovered.

d. Neuroreceptor effects are likely to differ at different sites throughout the CNS. Specific neural site effects can induce changes at the microscopic level that directly contrast with net changes and effects on behavioral states and cortical arousal [2–4].

e. This approach is expensive requiring the complex infrastructure of a neuroanatomically oriented neurochemistry laboratory.

Because of these limitations, much of classic basic-science neurochemistry is based on data derived from a different data base – the clinical reports of effects and side effects of clinically utilized pharmaceutical agents. Clinical trials required for the use and release of new agents provide an extensive base of drug effect and side-effect information. Most such studies are large, specific, and well designed. Physicians in medical practice can also submit case reports of drug side effects for drugs in clinical use. These case reports often address the psychoactive side of particular agents. This information is less specific than that derived from animal studies; however, it has the advantages of large group study size, being human based, and not being limited to known or theoretical effects of particular types of medication. Limitations of this approach include its reliance on human subject reports, limitations in the studies of older agents that are sometimes used in the assessment and approval of current drugs, the lack of such assessments in some clinical trials of agents presumed not to have

Sleep and Mental Illness, eds. S. R. Pandi-Perumal and M. Kramer. Published by Cambridge University Press.
© Cambridge University Press 2010.

cognitive side effects, and the fact that such studies are not done on agents not approved for clinical use in the practice of medicine [5, 6]. Our current knowledge of the psychoactive effects of medications is based on a coupling of this clinical knowledge with specific neurochemical effects that can be studied in animal models.

The cognitive state of sleep

Sleep is defined both behaviorally and cognitively as a reversible behavioral state of perceptual disengagement from, and unresponsiveness to, the environment. This is a very complex amalgam of physiological and behavioral processes, a process that, unlike coma, is physiologic, recurrent, and reversible. Sleep is generally described, not defined, by polysomnographic correlates that can be recorded and analyzed in the sleep laboratory. The sleep state and its spectrum of electrophysiologic correlates are affected by almost all medications with behavioral or cognitive effects and/or side effects. Medications affect sleep in at least three general ways: (1) altering cognitive levels of sleepiness/alertness; (2) altering cognitive activity during sleep – generally reported as dreaming; and (3) affecting the symptoms of medical and psychiatric diagnoses known to affect sleep.

Drug-induced sleepiness is perhaps the most commonly reported side effect of CNS active pharmacological agents [7] (the 1990 Drug Interactions and Side Effect Index of the *Physicians' Desk Reference* lists drowsiness as a side effect of 584 prescription or over-the-counter preparations). The terminology describing daytime sleepiness, generally considered to be "the subjective state of sleep need," is poorly defined, interchangeably including such contextual terminology as sleepiness, drowsiness, languor, inertness, fatigue, and sluggishness [8, 9]. Psychological tests utilized in assessing daytime sleepiness include validated questionnaires, spontaneously occurring psychological variations, and performance measures. The most widely used questionnaires for sleepiness include the Stanford Sleepiness Scale (SSS) and the Epworth Sleepiness Scale assessing patient reports of sleepiness-induced limitations on waking behavior. Subjective behavioral complaints may not accurately reflect the results of tests for physiological sleepiness [10]. The most prominent tests developed to utilize spontaneously occurring psychological variations are the Multiple Sleep Latency Test (MSLT) and the Maintenance of Wakefulness Test (MWT). Both of these tests use modified polysomnography to assess sleep onset latency during a series of waking nap periods. The effects of sleepiness on daytime performance can be assessed by tests of complex reaction and coordination, or by tests that assess complex behavioral tasks likely to be affected by sleepiness (e.g., tests of driving performance) [11]. Many of these tests have been shown in general and controlled (i.e., clinical trial) populations to have sensitivity to low-level sedation, highly reproducible results, and correlations. However, the results of questionnaire, cognitive, and performance tests for daytime sleepiness correlate only loosely with the actual effects of sleepiness on complex performance tasks such as the operation of a motor vehicle [11]. These effects are often inferred based on the actual real-life analog of driving performance and accident data [12]. These data have been shown to correlate with epidemiological studies suggesting that several groups of drugs known to induce daytime sleepiness are associated with increased rates of automobile accidents (e.g., sedating antihistamines, long-acting benzodiazepines, and sedating antidepressants [12, 13]). Few of these tests have, however, been generally applied to the vast majority of drugs noted to induce sleepiness as a side effect. Since performance measures are susceptible to non-task related influences of motivation, distraction, and comprehension of instructions, the results of performance and questionnaire rating tests do not always correlate with the results obtained from the MSLT and MWT [8].

Medication effects on sleep and wakefulness

The neuronal systems modulating waking and sleep are contained within the isodendritic core of the brain extending from the medulla though the brainstem and hypothalamus up to the basal forebrain. Multiple factors and systems are involved, with no single chemical neurotransmitter identified as necessary or sufficient for modulating sleep and wakefulness. Almost all drugs with sleep and dreaming effects or sedative side effects can be shown to affect one or more of the widely dispersed central neurotransmitters important in the neuromodulation of sleep and wakefulness. These primary neurotransmitters include dopamine, epinephrine, norepinephrine, acetylcholine, serotonin, histamine, glutamate, gamma-aminobutyrate (GABA), orexin, and adenosine. The effects and/or side effects of these agents can directly affect the synapse or have effects on neurotransmitters active at those sites.

There are other neurochemical mechanisms through which drugs can affect neuronal function; however, these systems and these compounds are generally not as well described as the neurotransmitter systems. Some agents exert their effect at the cell membrane, affecting cellular membrane transduction, ATP production, or ionic flux. Among these agents known to affect sleep and wakefulness are substance P, G-proteins, corticotropin-releasing factor, thyrotropin-releasing factor, nitric oxide, vasoactive intestinal peptide, melatonin, and neurotensin [4, 14]. Neuroendocrine agents such as melatonin can also affect sleep and wakefulness exerting effects outside the neural-transmission network. Most of the medications approved for the treatment of insomnia are benzodiazepine or benzodiazepine-like agents that affect GABA receptor activity. These agents, for which sleep induction is the primary therapeutic effect, will not be addressed in this chapter, which concentrates on medication side effects. However, the sedative side effects of many psychoactive medications are clinically utilized in the effort to induce sleepiness for patients with insomnia. Antidepressants are often used to treat disturbances in sleep. Antidepressant medications can induce both sleepiness and insomnia based on specific neurotransmitter effects (Table 29.1). Drug-induced sleepiness is a commonly reported side effect of a wide variety of other medications that can limit their usefulness (Table 29.2). Such sedative effects have sometimes been clinically utilized as off-label approaches to inducing sleepiness. Drug-induced insomnia is reported somewhat less commonly as a side effect of medications; however, multiple groups of medications can cause insomnia in some patients (Table 29.3). Chronic and long-term sedative/hypnotic use to induce sleep may cause tolerance to the sedative effect, and can contribute to chronic insomnia [15]. Many of the drugs reported to induce sleepiness and/or insomnia as effects or side effects are the same agents reported to induce nightmares and disordered dreaming (Table 29.4).

Medications affecting dreaming

Dreaming is defined by most of the sleep medicine community as mental activity reported from sleep [16]. However, this definition is not generally accepted and contradicts accepted psychoanalytic and neuroscientific definitions of dreaming. The psychoanalytic definition (dreaming as bizarre, hallucinatory mentation occurring in wake or sleep) has been incorporated into psychiatry [17]. The neuroscientific and theoretical definition (dreaming as REM sleep) is often used for studies of dreaming in animal models and human CNS scanning studies despite the large number of studies indicating that dreaming can occur without REM sleep and REM sleep without reported dreaming [18, 19]. Few studies have looked at the effects of medications on dreaming in human beings: the only species that can currently report both the content and an experience of whether a dream has occurred. General population groups such as those included in clinical trials define dreaming in multiple ways [17].

Neurochemists interested in dreaming have concentrated on the effects of neurochemicals on REM sleep, generally assuming that medications affecting REM sleep also affect dreaming. The medications proposed to affect dreaming are the same ones known to affect REM sleep. Agents that suppress REM sleep such as ethanol and benzodiazepines such as valium induce episodes of REM sleep rebound on withdrawal. These REM sleep rebound episodes have been associated with reports of nightmares and disturbed dreaming, and have generally been considered the primary mechanism resulting in drug-induced disordered dreaming and nightmares.

The original and quite simple model of REM sleep neurochemistry is called the reciprocal interaction model [20]. This theoretical model describes the interplay between two major neurotransmitter systems (aminergic and cholinergic) involved in REM sleep generation in the brainstem. Subsequent work by the original authors and others has led to revised versions that incorporate the effects of other neurotransmitter systems that have been shown to affect the generation of REM sleep in the brainstem. These authors' most recent version of this once simple system has become increasingly complex as other neurotransmitters and neuromodulators have been shown to affect REM sleep generation. The systems known to affect the generation of REM sleep include GABA, nitric oxide, glutamate, glycine, histamine, adenosine, dopamine, and other less well described neuropeptides [21].

Table 29.1 Antidepressants [sedating agents in bold, insomnia-inducing agents in italics]

Class	Drug	Sleep stage effects	Indications
Tricyclic	**Trimipramine**	Increased – REMS latency	Depression with insomnia, REMS & SWS supression, chronic pain, fibromyalgia, enuresis [etc.]
	Nortriptyline	Decreased – REMS(++), SWS latency	
	Doxepin	Deep sleep, sleep latency	
	Amoxapine		
	Amitriptyline		
	Imipramine		
	Amoxapine		
	Protriptyline*		
Non-tricyclic sedating	**Desimiprinine**	Increased – REMS latency	Depression, depression with insomnia, REMS supression
	Maprotiline	Decreased – SWS latency, REMS(++)	
	Mirtazapine	Sleep latency	
MAOI	**Phenelzine**	Increased – stage 4	Depression, REMS supression
	Tranylcypromine	Decreased – REMS latency, REMS(+++)	
SSRI	*Fluoxetine**	Increased – REMS latency, sleep latency, stage 1	Depression, PTSD, obsessive–compulsive disorder, phobias, cataplexy [etc.]
	Paroxetine	Decreased – REMS	
	Sertraline		
	Fluvoxamine		
	Citalopram HBr.		
Serotonin + norepinephrine reuptake inhibitor	*Venlafaxine*	Increased – REMS	Depression, nicotine withdrawal, neuropathic pain, generalized anxiety
	Duloxetine	Latency	
		Decreased – sleep latency, REMS	
Dopamine + norepinephrine reuptake inhibitor	*Bupropion*	Increased – REMS latency, sleep latency	Depression, nicotine withdrawal
Non-tricyclic non-SSRI	**Nefazodone**	Increased – REMS	Depression, depression with insomnia and anxiety
		Decreased – sleep latency	
Serotonin 1a agonist	Buspirone	Increased – REMS latency	Anxiety
		Decreased – REMS	

Keys: (++) higher levels of effect; REMS: REM sleep; *: documented as respiratory stimulant.

Table 29.2 Medication types reported in clinical trials and case reports to have sleepiness as a side effect

Medication class	Neurochemical basis for sleepiness
Antihistamines	Histaminine receptor blockade
Antiparkinsonian agents	Dopamine receptor agonists
Antimuscarinic/ antispasmodic	Varied effects
Skeletal muscle relaxants	Varied effects
Alpha-adrenergic blocking agents	Alpha-1 adrenergic antagonists
Beta-adrenergic blocking agents	Beta-adrenergic antagonists
Opiate agonists	Opioid receptor agonists (general CNS depression)
Opiate partial agonists	Opioid receptor agonists (general CNS depression)
Anticonvulsants	
– barbituates	GABA receptor agonists
– benzodiazepines	GABA receptor agonists
– hydantoins	General effects?
– succinimides	General effects?
– other	Varied effects including GABA potentiation
Antidepressants	
– MAOI	Norepinephrine, 5-HT and dopamine effects
– tricyclic	Acetylcholine blockade, norepinephrine and 5-HT uptake inhibition
– SSRI	5-HT uptake inhibition
– others	5-HT, dopamine, and norepinephrine effects
Antipsychotics	Dopamine receptor blockade, varied effects on histaminic, cholenergic, and alpha-adrenergic receptors
Barbiturates	GABA agonists
Benzodiazepines	GABA agonists
Anxiolytics, misc. sedatives and hypnotics	GABA agonists, varied effects
Antitussives	General?
Antidiarrhea agents	Opioid, general?
Antiemetics	Antihistamine and varied effects
Genitourinary smooth muscle relaxants	General?

Table 29.3 Medication types known to cause insomnia

Adrenocorticotropin (ACTH) and cortisone

Antibiotics (quinolones)

Anticonvulsants

Antihypertensives (alpha-agonists, beta-blockers, central acting agents)

Antidepressants (SSRIs)

Antineoplastic agents

Appetite supressants

Beta agonists

Caffeine

Decongestants

Diuretics

Dopamine agonists

Ephedrine and pseudoephedrine

Ethanol

Ginsing

Lipid and cholesterol lowering agents

Niacin

Nicotine agonists

Oral contraceptives

Psycho-stimulants and amphetamines

Sedative/hypnotics

Theophylline

Thyroid preparations

Data based on clinical trials and case reports of effects and side effects of clinically utilized pharmaceutical agents indicate that a very different pattern of medication classes contributes to the induction of disordered dreaming and nightmares (Table 29.4). These data suggest that the medications associated with clinical reports of disordered dreaming differ from those postulated to induce nightmares based on the association of dreaming with REM sleep rebound [5, 6]. Medications such as the acetylcholinesterase inhibitors that affect cholinergic receptors are rarely associated with clinical trial and case reports of nightmares and disordered dreaming. Medications known to suppress REM sleep such as the various antidepressants and benzodiazepines are often reported to induce disordered dreaming and nightmares. Almost all of the medications reported to induce daytime sleepiness (Tables 29.1 and 29.2) are also reported to induce nightmares and disordered dreaming. The neurochemistry of dreaming appears to be far more complex than even the modified reciprocal interaction model of REM sleep. Nightmares are classified as a REM sleep parasomnia, and are more closely associated with REM sleep than dreaming except in the case of post-traumatic stress disorder where they often occur at sleep onset [22].

Disordered dreaming and nightmares are also commonly reported during the withdrawal from addictive medications and drugs of abuse. This finding has been postulated to be secondary to the occurrence of REM sleep rebound during withdrawal from REM sleep suppressant medication. In the case of withdrawal from REM sleep depressant addictive medications such as ethanol and benzodiazepines this explanation may be correct at least in part. However, nightmares and disordered dreaming are often reported as part of the withdrawal syndrome from non-REM sleep suppressant addictive medications such as cannabis, cocaine, and opiates [23, 24]. This finding suggests that disturbed dreaming and nightmares are potentially an intrinsic part of the process of withdrawal from addictive agents rather than a symptom of REM sleep rebound.

Medication effects on sleep-associated diagnoses

A wide spectrum of physiological processes are altered during sleep. There are more than 60 recognized sleep diagnoses each with clear diagnostic criteria, and many are treated with specific pharmacological therapies. Most medical and psychiatric diseases produce mental or physical discomfort that can adversely affect sleep. Medications utilized in the treatment of sleep disorders can adversely affect the disease process for some patients, while medications for other diagnoses can alter sleep cognitive levels of alertness/sleepiness, dreaming, and sometimes inducing unwanted behaviors during sleep (i.e., parasomnias).

Diagnostic groups with abnormalities of alertness/sleepiness respiratory effects

Obstructive sleep apnea (OSA) with its well described effect of daytime somnolence may affect up to 25% of the population. Medications that lead to weight gain may precipitate the development of OSA. Some patients with OSA also have chronic insomnia, yet treatment of these patients with sedative/hypnotic medications can cause respiratory depression, increased apnea, and worsened sleep in these patients. Most sedative medications depress respiratory drive with increasing dosage. Benzodiazepines, barbiturates, and opiates can exacerbate respiratory failure in patients with chronic obstructive pulmonary disease (COPD), central sleep apnea, and restrictive lung disease. These medications can also negatively affect OSA and may increase the potential for symptomatic sleep apnea in some population groups such as patients being treated for chronic pain. Treatment of chronic pain with opiates can induce central sleep apnea as well as worsen the severity of sleep apnea [25]. The newer non-benzodiazepine hypnotics have demonstrated lower potential for respiratory depression. Methylprogesterone (Provera), protriptyline (Vivactyl), and fluoxetine (Prozac) have been documented to have respiratory stimulant effects that may be clinically useful in some patients [26].

Other sleep diagnoses

Periodic limb movement disorder (PLMD) and restless leg syndrome (RLS) may positively respond to treatment with benzodiazepines and opiates yet increase in intensity with the use of some antidepressants particularly the selective serotonin reuptake

Table 29.4 Medications reported to induce nightmares (medications included in each class are considered most likely to induce nightmares based on a quantitative meta-analysis of clinical trials, clinical studies, and case reports)

Affected neuroreceptor	Patient reports of nightmares: evidence base = clinical trials (CT); case reports (CR); clinical study (CS)	Probability assesment of drug effect
Drug		
Acetylcholine – cholinergic agonists		
Donepezil	CT [3/747 report disordered dreaming]	Possible
Rivastigmine	CT [abnormal dreaming in 1/100–1/1,000 of patients]	Possible
Norepinephine – beta-blockers		
Atenolol	CT [3/20 patients]	Probable
Bisopropol	CT [3/68 patients]: CR [1] – de-challenge	Probable
Labetalol	CT [5/175 patients]	Probable
Oxprenolol	CT [11/130 patients]	Probable
Propranolol	CT [8/107 patients]	Probable
Norepinephine affecting agents		
Guanethidine	CT [4/48 patients]	Probable
Serotonin – SSRI		
Fluoxetine	CT [1–5% – greater frequency in OCD and bulimic trials]: CR [4] – de & re-challenge	Probable
Escitalopram oxylate	CT [abnormal dreaming – 1% of 999 patients]	Probable
Nefazodone	CT [3% (372) versus 2% control]	Probable
Paroxetine	CT [4% (392) versus 1% control]	Significant
Agents affecting serotonin and norepinephrine		
Duloxetine	CT [>1% report of nightmare/abnormal dreaming – 23,983 patients]	Probable
Risperidone	CT [1% increased dream activity – 2,607 patients]	Probable
Venlafaxine	CT [4% (1,033) versus 3% control]	Probable
Agents affecting norepinephrine and dopamine		
Buproprion	CT [13/244 – dream abnormality]	Probable
Norepinephrine, serotonin, and dopamine reuptake inhibitor		
Sibutramine	Post-marketing case report	Possible
Dopamine – agonists		
Amantadine	CT [5% report abnormal dreams]: CR [1]	Probable
Levodopa	CT [2/9 patients]	Probable
Ropinirole	CT [3% (208) report abnormal dreaming versus 2% placebo]	Probable
Selegiline	CT [2/49 reporting vivid dreams]	Probable
Amphetamine-like agents		
Bethanidine	CT [2/44 patients]	Probable
Fenfluramine	CT [7/28 patients]: CR [1] de & re-challenge	Probable
Phenmetrazine	CT [3/81 patients]	Probable

315

Table 29.4 (cont.)

GABA		
GABA hydroxyl buterate	CT [nightmares >1% 473 patients]	Probable
Triazolam	CT [7/21 patients]	Probable
Zopiclone	CT [3–5/83 patients]	Probable
Nicotine agonists		
Varenicline	CT [abnormal dreams 14/821 patients]	Probable
Nicotine patches	CS [disturbed dreaming in up to 12%, affects tendency to use threatment]	Probable
Anti-infectives and immunosuppressants		
Amantadine	CT [5% reporting abnormal dreams]: CR [1]	Probable
Fleroxacin	CT [7/84 patients]	Probable
Ganciclovir	CR [1] – de & re-challenge	Probable
Gusperimus	CT [13/36 patient]	Probable
Antipsychotics		
Clozapine	CT [4%]	Probable
Antihistamine		
Chlorpheniramine	CT [4/80 patients]	Probable
ACE inhibitors		
Enalapril	CT [0.5–1% abnormal dreaming – 2,987 patients]	Probable
Losartin potassium	CT [>1% dream abnormality – 858 patients]	Probable
Quinapril	CT	Probable
Other agents		
Digoxin	CR [1] – de & re-challenge	Probable
Naproxen	CR [1] – de & re-challenge	Probable
Verapamil	CR [1] – de & re-challenge	Probable

inhibitors (SSRIs) [27]. L-dopa, while initially being useful in the treatment of RLS/PLMD, will eventually induce tachyphylaxsis and a worsening of symptoms [28]. Increased daytime alertness typifies a spectrum of common diagnoses including chronic insomnia, anxiety disorder, and post-traumatic stress disorder. Such patients may demonstrate altered responses to medications inducing alertness and/or sleepiness with unexpected results. Patients with narcolepsy often report improved sleep with daytime amphetamine use. Stimulants may induce sleepiness in some patients while hypnotics may induce agitation and

insomnia even when used in anesthetic settings and dosages [29].

Parasomnia-precipitating medications
Medication effects on sleep stages and EEG

Medication-induced changes in sleep stages can lead to an increase in symptoms occurring during those specific sleep/dream states. For example, insomnia and nightmares are associated with the REM sleep rebound that occurs after discontinuation of REM-suppressive drugs (i.e., ethanol, barbiturates, benzodiazepines). Medications such as lithium, opiates, and GABA-hydroxy-butyrate (sodium oxybate) that can cause an increase in deep sleep can induce the occurrence of arousal disorders such as somnambulism [30]. Nicotine, caffeine, and alcohol have been implicated, as well, in somnambulism, possibly due to their tendencies to increase nocturnal arousals [31].

REM behavior disorder (RBD) can be triggered by a variety of antidepressant medications as well as dopamine agonists and anticholinergics used to treat Alzheimer's disease. Acute RBD has been noted to occur during the withdrawal from cocaine, amphetamines, benzodiazepines, ethanol, barbiturates, and meprobamate [32]. Caffeine may unmask RBD.

Sleep-related eating disorder (SRED) is often associated with the use of zolpidem, triazolam, and other psychotrophic agents including lithium carbonate, amitriptyline, olanzapine, and risperidone [33]. Sleep-related eating disorder can also develop in individuals withdrawing from ethanol or other substance abuse.

The influence of psychoactive medications on sleep states has a positive side as well. For example, REM sleep suppressive medications can be useful adjuncts in the treatment of REM sleep parasomnias and other REM sleep stage specific symptoms. Both benzodiazepines and antidepressants can be used to decrease REM sleep. Similarly, the arousal disorders can be treated with medications affecting deep sleep (benzodiazepines and others). Clonazepam (Klonopin) is the medication most commonly utilized in the treatment of parasomnias, particularly in REM behavior disorder.

Medication types documented to affect sleep and dreaming

The pharmacodynamics of psychoactive medications are affected by half-life of activity, which varies based on gastrointestinal uptake, competition with other agents, and efficacy of hepatic or urinary elimination systems. The ability of an agent to cross the blood–brain barrier into the CNS affects the ability of that agent to induce CNS effects and side effects. Once these variables have been addressed, the potential CNS effects of any agent remain complex. It is the rare drug that is a pure agonist for a single neuron type, with most, if not all, medications affecting the binding of multiple CNS neuroreceptors.

Neuroreceptors vary locally in concentration and response throughout the CNS. Subtypes exist for each neuroreceptor that vary genetically between individuals as well as locally depending on CNS location. Neurons are likely to respond to multiple neurotransmitters [2, 3, 34]. Despite these limitations and the complexity of the applicable neuropharmacology, the primary neuroreceptor effects for many CNS active agents have been identified.

Primary neurotransmitter and neuromodulator effects
Acetylcholine

The electrical nature of the action potential conveying nerve impulses from neuron to neuron was first described by Ramon y Cajal and Charles Sheridan at the turn of the nineteenth century. The chemical medication of that spike potential between neurons was not clarified until the 1930s. The Austrian pharmacologist Otto Loewi had postulated the possibility that the effects of the vagal nerve on heart rate were chemically mediated. He could not, however, determine how to experimentally prove his postulate. One night he awakened after a dream in which he was sure that he had discovered the experimental solution to the problem. But, try as he might, he was unable to remember his dream. The next night he went to bed intent on redreaming the solution. He awoke and rushed to the lab where he electrically stimulated the vagus nerve of a frog to induce a slowing of the heart rate. He took the blood from that frog and injected it into another, inducing in that frog a slowing of the heart rate as well. This demonstrated that the slowing of the heart rate caused by stimulation of the vagus nerve was mediated by a chemical in the blood. That chemical, acetylcholine, became the first neurotransmitter to be isolated.

It has been proposed that the drive to sleep is determined by activity in basal forebrain cholinergic neurons [35]. However, such site-specific cholinergic neural effect is evidently not necessary for sleep [36]. Clinical use of medications such as the anticholinesterase inhibitors has been reported only rarely to induce somnolence and insomnia (in donepizil clinical trials, insomnia was reported in 9 and somnolence in 2 of 747 patients) [37].

Rapid eye movement sleep is affected by pharmacological alteration of acetylcholine activity in the

317

CNS. There are several lines of evidence supporting the conclusion that brainstem cholinergic neurons can be excited to induce REM sleep [1, 38]. Cholinergic agents are most likely to increase percentages of REM sleep, with cholinergic antagonists tending to decrease REM sleep. Anticholinergics are among the neurochemical agents that suppress REM sleep in the human. A wide variety of pharmaceutical agents have anticholinergic activity. The reported side effects of some of these agents include nightmares, disordered dreaming, and hallucinations. This has led some authors to postulate that it is the cholinergic effects of medications that induce hallucinations or psychosis as a side effect in some patients [39]. Recently anticholinesterase agents have come into widespread use for the treatment of the cognitive effects from early Alzheimer's disease. These agents increase acetylcholine in the CNS by blocking anticholinesterase, the primary system utilized in the breakdown of acetylcholine. Despite the known role of acetylcholine in the initiation of REM sleep, medications affecting acetylcholine are rarely reported to affect dreaming. The side effect of disturbed dreaming or nightmares was reported by only 3 of 747 patients taking the commonly used anticholinesterase drug donepezil (Aricept) in clinical trials and was rarely reported in clinical trials from other agents in this class (Table 29.4).

Norepinephrine

Many of the drugs in general use for treating high blood pressure (hypertension) affect norepinephrine receptors. Some of these agents, particularly the alpha and beta adrenergic antagonists, are commonly reported to induce sedation as a side effect [Table 29.2]. Sedation is the most common side effect reported for the alpha-2 agonists clonidine and methyldopa (30–75%). Sleep disturbance appears to be more common with the lipophilic beta-blockers, but is been reported at rates of 3 to 11% in association with the newer beta-blockers with vasodilating properties (carvedilol and labetalol). These agents and central-acting agents such as aldomet and reserpine may also induce the complaint of insomnia (Table 29.3).

Both beta and alpha-1 adrenergic antagonists have been shown to affect both REM sleep and reports of dreaming. Because these agents suppress REM sleep, they are sometimes used clinically in the treatment of recurrent nightmares in patients with post-traumatic

stress disorder (PTSD). Yet the norepinephrine affecting antihypertensive agents classified as beta-blockers and alpha-agonists are responsible for 34% of clinical trials in which nightmares are reported as an adverse effect [40]. The reported effects of these agents on both dreams and nightmares is often opposite to the drug's known pharmacological effects on REM sleep. Decreases in dream recall occur with use of both alpha-agonists (e.g., minoxidil) that are REM suppressant and beta-blockers (e.g., propranolol, atenolol) that do not suppress REM sleep. The use of beta-blockers depresses REM sleep percentages yet can result in reports of increased dreaming, nightmares, and hallucinations [41, 42]. The effects of these agents demonstrate that a drug's effect on REM sleep may or may not be associated with an associated change in reported dreaming.

Serotonin

Most antidepressants exert primary effects at serotonin receptors; however, these agents also affect a variety of other neurotransmitters (Table 29.1). Some of these agents induce significant sedation, particularly the tricyclic and quatracyclic antidepressants, and are sometimes used clinically to induce sleep. These agents are known to induce next-day sedation and diminished driving performance the day after use [13]. Other antidepressants, especially sergiline and fluoxetine, can be arousing and can induce insomnia in some patients.

Both serotonin and norepinephrine are proposed to have functional roles in the production of REM sleep. Most antidepressants suppress REM sleep. This effect is greatest for the older types of antidepressants including the monamine oxidase inhibitors (MAOIs) and the tricyclic antidepressants (TCAs, e.g., amitryptiline and imipramine). However, even the SSRIs (e.g., paroxetine and sergeline) are potent supressors of REM sleep. Rapid eye movement sleep suppression is not generally seen with buspiron [43]. Most antidepressants are reported in clinical trials to induce nightmares in some patients. Case reports of nightmares are associated with fluoxetine [44]. Intense visual dreaming and nightmares are associated with the acute withdrawal from some antidepressants [45]. This effect could be due to REM sleep rebound occurring after the withdrawal of these REM sleep suppressant agents; however, studies of reported dream recall with antidepressant use show that recall may vary independently of REM sleep suppression [46]. Studies of chronic steady state use and antidepressant withdrawal have shown inconsistent effects: increased dream recall with SSRIs and TCAs, no effect, and decreased recall [47].

Dopamine

Dopamine agonists are commonly reported to induce daytime sleepiness as a side effect (Table 29.2). The amphetamines exert primary effects at dopamine receptors and clinically induce increased alertness in most patient populations. Such agents are utilized for their contrary effect of quieting and increased focus in patients with the diagnosis of attention-deficit/hyperactivity disorder.

Dopamine receptor stimulation commonly results in the reported side effect of drug-induced nightmares. Dopamine, bromocriptine, pergoline, pergoline, pramipexole, and other dopamine agonists can lead to vivid dreaming, nightmares, and night terrors, which can be the first signs of the development of drug-induced psychosis [48]. Amphetamine use has been linked to nightmares (16% of nightmare reports from clinical trials). This effect has been postulated to occur secondary to dopamine receptor stimulation [40].

Gamma-aminobutyric acid (GABA)

Gamma-aminobutyric acid is the primary negative feedback neurotransmitter in the CNS. Most hypnotics (sleep-inducing) agents affect this receptor. Some neurochemists refer to the GABA receptor as the benzodiazepine (e.g., diazepam) receptor since this is the site where these agents exert their primary neurochemical effects resulting in diminished alertness and increased sleep propensity. It is the case that 24% of reports of nightmares come from benzodiazepine clinical trials [40]. The non-benzodiazepine hypnotic (eszopiclone), which is not associated at clinical dosages with REM sleep suppression or REM sleep rebound on withdrawal, has been associated with the occurrence of nightmares in several clinical trials as have other agents affecting GABA reuptake inhibition [49, 50]. The finding that different types of drugs known to affect the GABA receptor (agonists, modulators, and reuptake inhibitors) can result in patient complaints of nightmares and abnormal dreaming is suggestive that GABA may be a modulator of neuronal populations involved in dreaming [4, 50].

Histamine

Drugs with antihistaminergic effects induce significant sedation. This is particularly true of the type 1 antihistamines and the traditional antipsychotics (Table 29.2). Chlorpromazine and thioridazine are the most sedating of these antipsychotic agents, with sedation also reported at high frequency (46%) with the newer atypical antipsychotic clozepine. Haldol, risperidone, olanzepine, sertindole, and quetiapine induce significant sedation somewhat less frequently. Sedating antihistamines are associated with decreased performance on next-day driving tests and an increase in automobile accidents [12]. Because of side effects of daytime sedation and cognitive impairment these agents are not recommended for use in the elderly [51].

Case reports indicate that the commonly used antihistamine chlorpheniramine induces nightmares in some patients suggesting a potential role for histamine as a modulator of dreaming. Because of the high frequency of use of over-the-counter preparations containing this medication for sleep induction and the treatment of allergies, this may be the medication most likely to be responsible for drug-induced disordered dreaming and nightmares.

Neurotransmitter/neuromodulating systems

Cholinergic and aminergic neuronal populations are proposed to have prominent roles in the control of the REM–NREM sleep cycle [1]. These neurotransmitters may function in a reciprocal interaction that also involves a wide spectrum of neurotransmitters that interact in an intricate modulation of the cardinal sleep stages [4]. Proposed neurotransmitter modulators affecting this system include GABA, dopamine, orexin, adenosine, histamine, glycine, glutamate, nitric oxide, and neuropeptides [52]. Both nicotine and adenosine have multiple neurotransmitter effects and can be considered neuromodulators.

Nicotine

Nicotine affects muscarinic cholinergic receptors. However, specific nicotine receptors acting as neuromodulators have been demonstrated to be present throughout the CNS with demonstrated regional variance and with a diversity of effects on receptor systems [53]. Nicotine is proposed to exert primary effects including neurotoxicity on interpeduncular cholinergic neurons [54].

Clinically, nicotine contributes to hyperarousal and can induce insomnia (Table 29.3). Transdermal nicotine patches are reported to induce abnormal dreaming [55]. In some clinical trials this effect of inducing "bad dreams" has been serious enough to contribute to treatment failure [56]. Varenicline, a selective alpha-4 beta-2 nicotinic acetylcholine receptor partial agonist approved for smoking cessation induced abnormal dreaming in 13% and insomnia in 18% of clinical trial participants [57].

Adenosine

A primary effect of caffeine is to block adenosine receptors in the CNS, an effect shared by theophylline and nitrous oxide. The alerting effects of these agents led to the hypothesis that a primary effect of adenosine was to inhibit sleep active neurons in the basal forebrain leading to increased wakefulness [35]. Further studies have demonstrated that neither cholinergic activity nor adenosine accumulation in the basal forebrain is necessary for sleep induction [36]. Adenosine has been shown to have multiple CNS effects including inhibitory neuromodulary effects on various populations of neurons in the CNS responsive to glutamate, GABA, glycogen, and acetylcholine [58].

Other medication types reported to induce sleep-associated CNS side effects

Agents affecting host defense

Aristotle and Hippocrates pointed out that an association exists between infection and sleepiness. Both viral and bacterial infections can be associated with severe somnolence and large increases in NREM sleep [59]. Such microbial-induced changes in sleep are considered part of the acute phase response to infection. Both muramyl peptides and endotoxins are chemical mediators of infection that have been shown to induce sleepiness [59, 60]. Some of the antibiotics (i.e., fluoroquinolones [floxacin and cipro]) that are known to induce insomnia have also been reported to induce both insomnia and nightmares [40]. Other chemical mediators involved in the inflammatory response to infection (the cytokines IL-1B and TNF-α, and prostaglandin E2) are known to be involved in NREM sleep regulation [61]. Infectious diseases are sometimes associated with the complaint of nightmares. Sleep loss affects host defense and cellular immune function [59, 60, 61]. A diverse group of antibiotics, antivirals, and immunosuppressant drugs can induce the complaint of sedation, insomnia, and nightmares for some patients. An interaction exists between host defense and infectious disease, as well as between the cognitive effects on sleep and dreaming for these agents. A clear, but currently poorly defined, relationship exists between host defense and infectious disease, and sleep/dreaming.

Anesthestics

Older sedative/hypnotics were anesthetic agents given at low dosage to induce sleep. Some of these agents (i.e., benzodiazepines) are still utilized both in anesthetic and sleep induction. While the sleep-inducing effects of benzodiazepines are GABA related, the basis for effects on sleep that can persist post-anesthesia are unclear. The state induced by these agents is not clearly sleep, with significant alterations in EEG induced not corresponding to classic electrophysiologic sleep staging.

Agents that alter an individual's conscious relationship to the external environment are known to alter dream and nightmare occurrence. Many of the agents reported to cause altered dreaming are induction anesthestics utilized in surgery. An increased incidence of "pleasant" dreams are reported with propofol use [62]. The barbiturate thiopental, ketamine, and the opiate tramadol have produced disordered dreaming and nightmares [62–64]. Some of the agents associated with the complaint of nightmares also can induce waking hallucinations and confusion (fleroxacin, triazolam, ethanol withdrawal, and amphetamines). This association has, in part, led to proposals that dreams and nightmares are hallucinatory experiences occurring during sleep [65].

Anti-epileptic agents

Sedation is the most common reported side effect for many of the anti-epileptic agents, reported at levels of 70% with phenobarbitol, 42% with carbamazepine and valproate, and in 33% of patients using phenytoin and primidone [40]. Both phenobarbitol and carbamazepine have been shown to induce sleepiness as documented by multiple sleep latency testing (MSLT). Sedation is reported as a side effect in 15 to 27% of patients taking topramate, and in 5 to 10% of those taking gabapentin, lamotrigine, vigabatrin, and zonisamide. For the agents affecting GABA receptors, the side effect of sleepiness is most likely modulated through that neurotransmitter. For other agents, the neurotransmitter basis for sedation remains unidentified. None of these agents is reported to induce nightmares or disordered dreaming at frequencies higher than 1/100 to 1/1,000 in clinical trial reports [66].

Other medications inducing sleep-associated CNS side effects

Other neurotransmitter modulators proposed to affect sleep and dreaming include orexin, adenosine, histamine, glycine, glutamate, nitric acid, and neuropeptides [4]. The neurochemical and pharmacological basis for sleep-associated cognitive side effects for the remaining agents included in Tables 29.2, 29.3, and 29.4 without noted neurotransmitter basis remains poorly defined. It is possible that the induction of sedation, insomnia, nightmares, and altered dreaming by some of these agents is secondary to neurotransmitter effects that have yet to be described.

Other non-prescription agents inducing sleep-associated CNS side effects

Ethanol is probably the most widely used hypnotic agent. Twenty-two percent of patients with chronic insomnia are reported to use ethanol as a hypnotic [67, 68]. Ethanol, while inducing sleep, contributes to an overall diminishment in sleep efficiency and quality. When used in excess with other sedative/hypnotic agents, overdose can be fatal in part due to respiratory depressant effects. The H1 antihistamines, including diphenhydramine, hydroxyzine, and triprolidine, induce next-day sleepiness after use [12]. Sedation occurs as well for some individuals taking the H2 agents, but is much less common. Sedation is a potential but unexamined side effect for a wide spectrum of nutritional supplements beyond the preparations marketed for sleep induction including melatonin, tryptophan, chamomile, passion flower, valerian root, kava, and skull cap. Most of these agents have been noted to induce serious toxicity for some patients. Among drugs of abuse, marijuana, benzodiazepines, opiates, and barbiturates have significant sedating effects. Amphetamine and cocaine abuse can induce insomnia and paradoxical sleepiness after long periods of drug-induced wakefulness. Over-the-counter medications may induce insomnia, including decongestants (including nasal sprays), weight loss agents, Ginseng preparations and high dose vitamin B1 (niacin) [29].

Summary: the neurochemistry of cognitive sleep-associated medication side effects

The group of pharmacological preparations, both psychotropic and otherwise, reported to alter sleep and dreaming is extensive and quite diverse (Table 29.5). Almost all of the agents exerting their neurochemical effects on dopamine, histamine, GABA, serotonin, and norepinephrine will induce altered sleep and dreaming for some patients. Most agents affecting dopaminergic neuroreceptors induce nightmares in some patients. The neuromodulator adenosine clearly affects sleep and wakefulness, while nicotine alters both sleep and dreaming. The effects of these agents on dreaming are either unassociated with or opposite to the known effects of these agents on REM sleep. Based on medication effects and side-effect profiles, the association of the neurotransmitter acetylcholine with dreaming and sleep appears limited.

Other medications appear to affect sleep and dreaming by affecting an individual's conscious relationship to the environment (anesthetics) or by affecting chemical mediators involved in the inflammatory response. Most of the agents reported to alter dreaming also induce CNS side effects of daytime somnolence and/or insomnia. The tendency of drugs to induce such cognitive side effects may be an indicator for drugs likely to induce disordered dreaming and nightmares. When queried in clinical trials as to alterations in sleep-associated cognition, many patients will report such side effects. Currently there is limited assessment routinely utilized in the assessment of drugs without a clear theoretic history of the potential for sleep-associated cognitive side effects such as diabetic, antibiotic, host-defense and dietary suppressant medications. With our increasing understanding of the complexity of the sleep state and its effects on multiple physiological systems it would seem appropriate to incorporate such assessments into studies for most if not all medications subjected to clinical trials.

The fact that a wide spectrum of pharmacological agents is reported to induce disturbed dreaming and nightmares suggests that the biochemical basis for dreaming is more complex and less understood than

Table 29.5 Cognitive effects and side effects of medications: basis for CNS effects

Basis for CNS activity	Sleepiness	Insomnia	Alterations in dreaming
Neurotransmitter-mediated effects			
Serotonin	+++	++	+++
Norepinephrine	++	++	+++
Dopamine	+++	+++	+++
Histamine	+++	+	++
GABA	+++	+	++
Acetylcholine	–	++	–
Neuromodulator-mediated effects			
Adenosine	+	+++	–
Nicotine	–	+++	+++
Other medication effects			
Effects on inflammation	++	++	++
Addictive drug withdrawal	+	+++	+++
Altered conscious interaction with environment	+++	+	++
Alterations in sleep-associated disease	+++	+++	+

Keys: (+++) a majority of drugs with this activity cause this effect in >10% of patients;
(++) some drugs with this activity induce this effect in 1 to 10% of patients;
(+) an idiosyncratic effect for some agents in this group or a withdrawal effect;
(–) reported in less than 1% of patients using agents with this effect.

is generally suggested. Among prescription medications in clinical use, beta-blockers affecting norepinephrine neuroreceptors are the agents most likely to result in patient complaints of disturbed dreaming. The strongest clinical evidence for a drug to induce disordered dreaming or nightmares is for the SSRI paroxetine – a medication known to suppress REM sleep. Acetylcholinesterase inhibitors affecting the acetylcholine neuroreceptor system rarely result in patient complaints of drug-induced nightmares. Such studies of drug effects and side effects do not support theoretical postulates that cholinergic neurons (the triggers for REM sleep) serve as the primary neuroreceptor system involved in dreaming and nightmares. There are few data based on medication effects or side effects to support the reciprocal [REM sleep-on]–[REM sleep-off] system of AIM theory based on cholinergic triggers as a basis for dream neurochemistry [69]. Disturbed dreaming and nightmares are reported during withdrawal from addictive medications. This complaint occurs with drugs without known REM sleep suppression or REM sleep rebound during withdrawal, suggesting that disturbance in dreaming in this situation may characterize withdrawal from addictive agents rather than being secondary to REM sleep rebound as previously postulated.

These findings are more evidence that dreaming is not a simple or derivative state of REM sleep. Dreaming is a complex state that is poorly described by our current models of neuroanatomy and neurochemistry. Dreaming is a state of consciousness with an inherent neurochemical complexity similar to waking. Based on its neurochemistry, dreaming appears to be another state of consciousness, variably assessable in waking, and affected by the medications that can alter our cognitive interaction with the world.

Conclusion

Those agents known to induce CNS effects and those having CNS side effects affect the sleep-associated cognitive states. The sleep-associated cognitive states are neurochemically complex with almost all drugs reported to affect cognitive aspects of sleep and waking consciousness also affecting dreaming (Table 29.5). Medications that have the clinical effects of arousal (insomnia) and/or sedation are those that alter reports of dreaming and nightmares.

References

1. Hobson JA, Steriade M. The neuronal basis of behavioral state control: internal regulatory systems of the brain. In: Bloom F, ed. Mountcastle V, series ed. *Handbook of Psychology*. (Washington, DC: American Physiological Society, 1986; IV(14):701–823).

2. Kandle ER. The brain and behavior. In: Kandel ER, Schwartz JH, Jessell TM, eds. *Principles of Neural Science*, 4th edn. (New York: McGraw Hill, 2000; 5–18).

3. Schwartz JH. Neurotransmitters. In: Kandel ER, Schwartz JH, Jessell TM, eds. *Principles of Neural Science*, 4th edn. (New York: McGraw Hill, 2000; 280–297).

4. Pace-Schott EF. Postscript: Recent findings on the neurobiology of sleep and dreaming. In: Pace-Schott EF, Solms M, Blagrove M, Harnard S, eds. *Sleep and Dreaming: Scientific Advances and Reconsiderations*. (Cambridge: Cambridge University Press, 2003; 335–50).

5. Pagel JF, Helfer P. Drug-induced nightmares: an etiology based review. *Hum Psychopharmacol Clin Exp.* 2003;**18**:59–67.

6. Pagel JF. The neuropharmacology of nightmares. In: Pandi-Perumal SR, Cardinali DP, Lander M, eds. *Sleep and Sleep Disorders: Neuropsychopharmacologic Approach*. (Georgetown, TX: Landes Bioscience, 2006; 225–40).

7. *Physicians Desk Reference*, 44th edn. (Monfield, NJ: Thompson PDR, 1990).

8. Buysse DJ. Drugs affecting sleep, sleepiness and performance. In: TM Monk, ed. *Sleep, Sleepiness and Performance*. (West Sussex, England: John Wiley & Sons, 1991; 4–31).

9. Chervin RD. Sleepiness, fatigue, tiredness, and lack of energy in obstructive sleep apnea. *Chest.* 2000;**118**:372–9.

10. Roehrs T, Carskadon MA, Dement WC, Roth T. Daytime sleepiness and alertness. In: Kryger M, Roth T, Dement B, eds. *Principles and Practice of Sleep Medicine*, 3rd edn. (Philadelphia: W. B. Saunders Company, 2002; 43–53).

11. Pivik RT. The several qualities of sleepiness: psychophysiological considerations. In: Monk TM, ed. *Sleep, Sleepiness and Performance*. (West Sussex, England: John Wiley & Sons, 1991; 3–38).

12. O'Hanlon JF, Ramaekers JG. Antihistamine effects on actual driving performance in a standard driving test: a summary of Dutch experience, 1989–94. *Allergy.* 1995;**50**:234–42.

13. Volz HP, Sturm Y. Antidepressant drugs and psychomotor performance. *Neuropsychobiology.* 1995;**31**:146–55.

14. Jones BE. Basic mechanisms of the sleep wake states. In: Kryger MH, Roth T, Dement WC, eds. *Principles and Practice of Sleep Medicine*, 3rd edn. (Philadelphia, PA: W. B. Saunders Co., 2000; 134–54).

15. Ashton H. The effects of drugs on sleep. In: Cooper R, ed. *Sleep*. (London: Chapman & Hall Medical, 1994; 174–207).

16. Pagel JF, Myers P. Definitions of dreaming: a comparison of definitions of dreaming utilized by different study populations (college psychology students, sleep lab patients, and medical professionals). *Sleep.* 2002;**25**:A299–A300.

17. Pagel JF, Blagrove M, Levin R, *et al.* Defining dreaming: a paradigm for comparing disciplinary specific definitions of dream. *Dreaming.* 2001;**11**(4):195–202.

18. Foulkes D. *Dreaming: A Cognitive-Psychological Analysis*. (Hillsdale, NJ: Lawrence Erlbaum Associates, 1985).

19. Solms M. *The Neurophysiology of Dreams: A Clinico-anatomical Study*. (Mahwah, NJ: Lawrence Erlbaum, 1997).

20. McCarley R, Hobson J. Neuronal excitability modulation over the sleep cycle: a structural and mathematical model. *Science.* 1975;**189**:58–60.

21. Hobson J, Pace-Schott E, Stickgold R. Dreaming and the brain: toward a cognitive neuroscience of conscious states. In: Pace-Schott E, Solms M, Blagtove M, Harnad S, eds. *Sleep and Dreaming: Scientific Advances and Reconsiderations*. (Cambridge: Cambridge University Press, 2003; 1–50).

22. Pagel JF, Nielsen T. Parasomnias: nightmare disorder. In: Hauri P, ed. *The International Classification of Sleep Disorders. Diagnostic and Coding Manual (ICD-11)*. (Westchester, IL: American Academy of Sleep Medicine, 2005; 155–8).

23. Bundley AJ, Hughes JR, Moore BA, Novy PL. Marijuana abstinence effects in marijuana smokers maintained in their home environment. *Arch Gen Psychiatry.* 2001;**58**(10):917–24.

24. Wade DT, Makela PM, House H, Bateman C, Robson P. Long term use of a cannabis-based medicine in the treatment of spasticity and other symptoms in multiple sclerosis. *Mult Scler.* 2006;**12**(5):639–45.

25. Mogri M, Desai H, Webster L, Grant BJ, Mador MJ. Hypoxemia in patients on chronic opiate therapy with

and without sleep apnea. *Sleep Breath.* 2009; **13**(1):49–57.

26. Hudgel D. Pharmacological treatment of sleep disordered breathing. In: Lee-Chiong T, ed. *Sleep: A Comprehensive Handbook.* (Hoboken, NJ: J. Wiley and Sons, 2006; 347–54).

27. Stiasny K, Oertel W, Trenkwalder C. Clinical symptomatology and treatment of restless legs syndrome and periodic limb movement disorder. *Sleep Med Rev.* 2002;**6**(4):253–65.

28. Allen RP. Earley CJ. Augmentation of the restless legs syndrome with carbidopa/levodopa. *Sleep.* 1996;**19**:205–13.

29. Pagel JF. Medications that induce sleepiness. In: Lee-Chiong T, ed. *Sleep: A Comprehensive Handbook.* (Hoboken, NJ: J. Wiley and Sons, 2006; 175–82).

30. Pagel JF. Pharmacologic alterations of sleep and dream: a clinical framework for utilizing the electrophysiological and sleep stage effects of psychoactive medications. *Hum Psychopharmacol.* 1996;**11**:217–23.

31. Pagel JF. The treatment of parasomnias. In: Kushida C, ed. *Handbook of Sleep Disorders.* (Informa Publishing, 2008; 524–32).

32. Tippman-Peikert M, Morgenthaler T, Boeve B, Silber M. REM sleep behavior disorder and REM-related parasomnias. In: Lee-Chiong T, ed. *Sleep: A Comprehensive Handbook.* (Hoboken, NJ: J. Wiley and Sons, 2006; 435–42).

33. Schenck CH, Mahowald MW. Parasomnias. Managing bizarre sleep-related behavior disorders. *Postgrad Med.* 2000;**107**(3):145–56.

34. Rye DB. Contributions of the pedunculopontine region to normal and altered REM sleep. *Sleep.* 1997;**20**(9):757–88.

35. Rannie DG, Grunze HC, McCarley RW, Green RW. Adenosine inhibition of mesopontine cholinergic neurons: implications for EEG arousal. *Science.* 1996;**263**:689–92.

36. Blanco-Centurion C, Xu M, Murillo-Rodriguez E, *et al.* Adenosine and sleep homeostasis in the basal forebrain. *J Neurosci.* 2006;**26**:8092–100.

37. *Physicians Desk Reference*, 62nd edn. (Monfield, NJ: Thompson PDR; 2008).

38. Steriade M. Brain electrical activity and sensory processing during waking and sleeping states. In: Kryger MH, Roth T, Dement WC, eds. *Principles and Practice of Sleep Medicine*, 3rd edn. (Philadelphia, PA: W. B. Saunders Co., 2000; 93–111).

39. Perry E, Perry R. Acetylcholine and hallucinations: disease related compared to drug induced alterations in human consciousness. *Brain Cogn.* 1995;**28**:240–58.

40. Thompson D, Pierce D. Drug-induced nightmares. *Ann Pharmacother.* 1999;**33**:93–6.

41. Dimsdale J, Newton R. Cognitive effects of beta-blockers. *J Psychosom Res.* 1991;**36**(3):229–36.

42. Brismar K, Motgensen L, Wetterberg L. Depressed melatonin secretion in patients with nightmares due to beta-adrenoceptor blocking drugs. *Acta Med Scand.* 1987;**221**(2):155–8.

43. Gursky J, Krahn L. The effects of antidepressants on sleep: a review. *Harv Rev Psychiatry.* 2000;**8**(6):298–306.

44. Coupland NJ, Bell CJ, Potokar JP. Serotonin reuptake inhibitor withdrawal. *J Clin Psychopharmacol.* 1996;**16**(5):356–62.

45. Pace-Schott EE, Gersh T, Silvestri R, *et al.* Effects of serotonin reuptake inhibitors (SSRI) on dreaming in normal subjects. *Sleep.* 1999;**22** (Supp 1):H278D.

46. Lepkifker E, Dannon PN, Iancu I, Ziv R, Kotler M. Nightmares related to fluoxetine treatment. *Clin Neuropharmacol.* 1995;**18**(1):90–4.

47. Pace-Schott E, *et al.* Enhancement of subjective intensity of dream features in normal subjects by the SSRIs paroxetine and fluvoxamine. *Sleep.* 2000;**23** (Supp 2):A173.

48. Stacy M. Managing late complications of Parkinson's disease. *Med Clin North Am.* 1999;**83**(2):469–81.

49. Xi MC, Morales FR, Chase MH. Evidence that wakefulness and REM sleep are controlled by a GABAergic pontine mechanism. *J Neurophysiol.* 1999;**82**:2015–19.

50. Mallick BN, Kaur S, Saxena RN. Interactions between cholinergic and GABAnergic neurotransmitters in and around the locus coeruleus for the induction and maintainence of rapid eye movement sleep *Neuroscience.* 2001;**104**:467–85.

51. Ashton H. The effects of drugs on sleep. In: Cooper R, ed. *Sleep.* (London: Chapman & Hall Medical, 1994; 174–207).

52. Pace-Schott EF. Postscript: Recent findings on the neurobiology of sleep and dreaming. In: Pace-Schott EF, Solms M, Blagrove M, Harnard S, eds. *Sleep and Dreaming: Scientific Advances and Reconsiderations.* (Cambridge: Cambridge University Press, 2003; 335–50).

53. Collis S, Wade D, Londen J, Izanwassar S. Neurochemical alterations produced by daily nicotine exposure in peri-adolescent versus adult rats. *Eu J Pharmacol.* 2004;**502**:75–85.

54. Ciani E, Severi S, Bartosqui R, Constestabile A. Neurochemical correlates of nicotine neurotoxicity on rat habenulo-interpedicular cholinergic neurons. *Neurotoxicity.* 2005;**26**(3):467–74.

55. Smith TM, Winters FD. Smoking cessation: a clinical study of the transdermal nicotine patch. *J Am Osteopath Assoc.* 1995;**95**(11):655–6; 661–2.

56. Ivers RG, Farrington M, Burns CB, *et al.* A study of the use of free nicotine patches by indigenous people. *Aust NZ J Public Health.* 2003;**27**(5):486–90.

57. Lam S, Patel PN. Varenicline: a selective alpha4beta2 nicotinic acetylcholine receptor partial agonist approved for smoking cessation. *Cardiol Rev.* 2007;**15**(3):154–61.

58. Arrigoni E, Rannie D, McCarley R, Green R. Adenosine mediated presynaptic modulation of glutmagenic transmission in the laterodorsal tegmentum. *J Neurosci.* 2001;**3**:1076–85.

59. Krueger JM, Fang J. Host defense. In: Kryger M, Roth T, Dement W, eds. *Principles and Practice of Sleep Medicine*, Vol. 3. (Philadelphia: W. B. Saunders Co., 2000; 255–65).

60. Krueger JM, Kubillis S, Shoham S, *et al.* Enhancement of slow wave sleep by endotoxin and libid A. *Am J Physiol.* 1986;**251**:R591–597.

61. Jaffe SE. Sleep and infectious disease. In: Kryger M, Roth T, Dement W, eds. *Principles and Practice of Sleep Medicine*, Vol. 3. (Philadelphia: W. B. Saunders Co., 2000; 1093–102).

62. Marsh S, Schaefer HG, Tschan C, Meier B. Dreaming and anaesthesia: total i.v. anaesthesia with propofol versus balanced volatile anaesthesia with enflurane. *Eur J Anaesthesiol.* 1992;**9**:331–3.

63. Krissel J, Dick WF, Leyser KH, *et al.* Thiopentone, thiopentone/ketamine, and ketamine for induction of anesthesia in caesarean section. *Eur J Anaesthesiol.* 1994;**11**:115–22.

64. Oxorn DC, Ferris LE, Harrington E, Orser BA. The effects of midazolam on propofol-induced anesthesia: propofol dose requirements, mood profiles, and perioperative dreams, *Anesth Analg.* 1997;**85**:553–9.

65. Hobson JA. *Dreaming as Delerium.* (MIT Press, 1999).

66. AHFS drug information. (Bethesda MD: American Society of Health-System Pharmacists, 2003).

67. Breslau N, Roth T, Rosenthal L, *et al.* Sleep disturbance and psychiatric disorders: a longitudinal epidemiological study of young adults. *Biol Psychiatry.* 1996;**39**:411–18.

68. Sateia MJ, Doghramji K, Hauri PJ, *et al.* Evaluation of chronic insomnia. *Sleep.* 2000;**23**:243–314.

69. Pagel J F. *The Limits of Dream: A Scientific Exploration of the Mind/Brain Interface.* (Oxford: Academic Press/ Elsiever, 2008).

Chapter 30

Sleep and post-traumatic stress disorder

Andrea Iaboni and Harvey Moldofsky

Introduction to post-traumatic stress disorder

Post-traumatic stress disorder (PTSD) is a psychiatric disorder arising out of exposure to life- or bodily-threatening traumatic events, witnessing such an event, or learning about such an event from a relative or friend. Such occurrences are met with considerable psychological distress including fear, helplessness, and horror. According to the *Diagnostic and Statistical Manual* (DSM-IV) of the American Psychiatric Association [1] five criteria define PTSD. These include re-experiencing of the trauma, hyperarousal, avoidance behaviors, persistence of the symptoms for more than one month after the traumatic event, and the disturbance being sufficiently distressing to result in social or occupational impairment. The hyperarousal symptoms are similar to those of panic and generalized anxiety disorders, while the avoidant symptoms and numbing have a phobic and depressive quality. The intrusive symptoms, which include flashbacks, recurrent nightmares of the event, obsessive memories of trauma, and unpleasant reactions with trauma reminders, are the symptoms of PTSD that distinguish it from other anxiety and mood disorders. These intrusive symptoms are often quite disabling. Post-traumatic stress disorder is considered to be acute when present for less than three months, and chronic when more than three months.

Traumatic experiences are common, with one study finding nearly 90% of their Detroit sample having been exposed to trauma over their lifetime, with a mean of 4.8 traumatic experiences per person, and 9.2% with a history of PTSD [2]. In civilian populations the lifetime prevalence for PTSD ranges between 7% and 12% and occurs twice as often in females [3–5]. The median time-to-recovery is between three and five years [4, 6]. Post-traumatic stress disorder shares high comorbidity with other psychiatric diagnoses (see Table 30.1). In comparison to unaffected individuals, there is a six-fold increased risk for major depression; about a four-fold increased risk for panic disorder or agoraphobia; a three-fold increased risk of alcoholism or substance abuse, and an estimated suicide attempt rate of approximately 20% [4, 7, 8]. Post-traumatic stress disorder is accompanied by functional and psychosocial disability [9, 10], physical symptoms, and health care utilization [8].

While PTSD is a more recent diagnostic term, initially appearing in 1980 in the DSM-III, the symptoms have been well known ever since wartime experiences were recorded. Terms such as "shell shock" and "war neurosis" were common after World War I to describe combat-related psychological disturbances. Following World Wars I and II, various symptoms currently attributed to PTSD occurred in the British veterans. These include clusters of symptoms attributed to a disability syndrome without psychological or cognitive symptoms, a somatic syndrome focused on the heart, and a neuropsychiatric syndrome with a range of somatic symptoms [11]. Medical labels include "disorders of the heart", "neurasthenia", "rheumatism", "effort syndrome", "psychoneurosis", and "non-ulcer dyspepsia". These labels are culturally determined in accordance to the prevailing health beliefs and concerns [11].

The Vietnam War fueled contemporary interest in post-combat psychological distress where over 15% of US men and 8.5% of US women were found to suffer from combat-induced PTSD [12]. Gulf War Syndrome has been another focus of concern where unexplained somatic symptoms predominate. In a

---

Sleep and Mental Illness, eds. S. R. Pandi-Perumal and M. Kramer. Published by Cambridge University Press.

Table 30.1 Psychiatric and medical comorbidities in PTSD

		Men (%)	Women (%)
Psychiatric comorbidity	Alcohol abuse/ dependence	51.9	27.9
	Drug abuse/ dependence	34.5	26.9
	Major depression	47.9	48.5
	GAD	16.8	15.0
	Panic disorder	7.3	12.6
	Agoraphobia	16.1	22.4
	Social phobia	27.6	28.4
	PTSD + one diagnosis	14.9	17.2
	PSTD + two diagnoses	14.4	18.2
	PSTD + three or more diagnoses	59.0	43.6

Source: Data from [4].

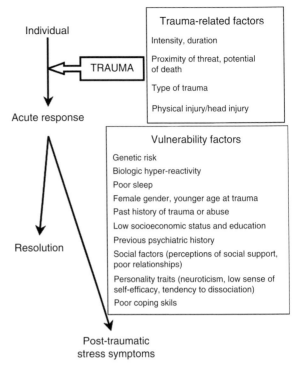

Figure 30.1 Individual and trauma-related vulnerability factors for PTSD.

study of PTSD and chronic fatigue syndrome (CFS), Gulf War veterans, compared with non-Gulf War veteran controls, reported significantly higher rates of PTSD and CFS. The prevalence of PTSD, but not CFS, was related to the intensity of deployment stress [13]. Recent research has employed anonymous survey questionnaires on mental health of US combat infantry units either before or after three or four months of being deployed in Iraq or in Afghanistan [14]. The data showed evidence for more symptoms of major depression, generalized anxiety, and PTSD in those who served in Iraq (15.6 to 17.1%) versus those who served in Afghanistan (11.2%) or those before deployment (9.3%). Specifically, symptoms of PTSD occurred in 12.9% of those who served in army units and 12.2% of marines who saw combat duty in Iraq. The rate of PTSD increased linearly depending upon the exposure to fire fights. Those military personnel who were wounded or injured were more likely to have PTSD.

There are many factors involved in determining the individual's response to a traumatic experience (Figure 30.1). Pre-existing mental health problems, an abusive or difficult childhood, or previous significant trauma have all been identified as risk factors for developing PTSD [15]. Premorbid sleep disturbance

has also been proposed as a risk factor, although the evidence is limited to a retrospective study of hurricane survivors [16]. One's cognitive–affective framework can also lead to maladaptive responses. Helplessness, a sense of loss of control, and catastrophic thinking are all characteristic dysfunctional cognitions post-trauma. Psychological defenses such as avoidance and denial are problematic, as are the maladaptive coping behaviors of drug and alcohol use.

Post-traumatic stress disorder tends to occur in families. Adult children of Holocaust survivors with PTSD are more likely to develop the disorder after trauma exposure than children of survivors without PTSD [17]. Both environmental and heritable factors are likely at play. Evidence for a heritable risk for PTSD has been demonstrated with both twin and molecular genetics studies [18]. Candidate genes include the D2 dopamine receptor (*DRD2*) and the serotonin transporter (*SLC6A4*). The low-expression variant polymorphism in the promoter of the *SLC6A4* gene has been found to be associated with development of PTSD in hurricane survivors, but only in combination with a high exposure level to the hurricane and low social support [19].

In keeping with a biological predisposition, one's risk of developing symptoms in response to trauma may be revealed by one's physiological reactions to stress. Characteristics such as greater startle reaction, heightened fear, slower habituation, and hyperactive sympathetic nervous system all predict development of PTSD symptoms on exposure to trauma [20].

After exposure to trauma, the neurobiological changes associated with PTSD include alterations in the limbic system, the hypothalamic–pituitary–adrenal (HPA) axis, and catecholamine responses. Decreased volume and activity of both the prefrontal cortex and the hippocampus, and hyper-responsivity of the amygdala, are notable findings in individuals with PTSD [21]. In terms of the HPA axis, there is evidence of dysregulation and sensitization of the hypothalamic responses by early-life adversity [22]. In individuals who develop PTSD, there is increased cortisol reactivity in the acute phase of their stress response producing stronger physiological response. In chronic PTSD, through protective negative feedback mechanisms, there is evidence of down-regulation of the HPA axis and hypocortisolism [23]. Persistent sympathetic nervous system activation and higher catecholamine levels are also characteristic of PTSD, which likely functions to increase alertness and produce a state of hyperarousal [24].

Sleep in PTSD: an overview

Sleep disturbance frequently occurs immediately following a traumatic experience. Difficulty initiating and maintaining sleep are the most common complaints, while nightmares are also frequently reported. As an example, in the six months following the Oklahoma bombing, 70% of survivors suffered from insomnia, and 55% from nightmares [25]. For the most part, sleep disturbance post-trauma is transient and improves with time [26]. However, when sleep problems persist – often in the form of nightmares, insomnia, and sleep avoidance – they portend the development of PTSD. Poor sleep impacts on ability to function, quality of life, and interpersonal relationships [27, 28] and is also a risk factor for the development of physical symptoms [29].

Persistent sleep impairment forms part of the DSM-IV diagnostic criteria for PTSD. Distressing dreams fall under the re-experiencing symptom cluster and difficulties falling or staying asleep form part of the hyperarousal symptoms [1]. In PTSD, a variety

of sleep changes have been reported (Figure 30.2). Sleep disturbance is thus widely accepted as a core feature of PTSD. Some studies have gone further and suggested that disruption of sleep physiology may in fact mediate the development of PTSD. One study found that the presence and severity of sleep disturbances in the immediate post-trauma period is associated with the persistence of post-traumatic stress symptoms and the development of PTSD (Figure 30.3) [30]. The role of sleep in the development of PTSD remains speculative, and the adaptation to traumatic experiences may involve several sleep-related mechanisms. One potential mechanism is the function of REM sleep in the consolidation and processing of traumatic memories [31]. Rapid eye movement sleep is also important in fear conditioning, as shown in animal experiments where REM deprivation impairs the normal extinction of conditioned fear responses [32].

Although research in the area of sleep and PTSD continues to advance, it is important to note some of the limitations in our current understanding. One challenge is the multiplicity of traumatic events that have been studied. These include Holocaust survivors, Vietnam veterans, and adult survivors of childhood sexual abuse, motor vehicle collision survivors, and survivors of natural disasters. Consequently the study populations are diverse in age, gender, mental health status, chronicity of illness, medical and psychiatric comorbidity, and medication use. The outcome is that many studies on sleep in PTSD offer inconsistent findings.

The issue of comorbidities is pivotal. A high proportion of individuals with PTSD are also diagnosed with a mood disorder (Table 30.1). Mood changes are clearly more than just a coincident phenomenon, and may be part of the causal pathway in producing post-traumatic symptoms. Many of the objective sleep changes seen in PTSD overlap with known sleep changes in depression, even where there is an attempt to exclude individuals with depression. The high coincidence of substance abuse, mood and anxiety disorders in individuals who have experienced trauma muddies the water, insomuch as it is difficult to assign observed sleep changes specifically to the effects of trauma and PTSD. Individuals with PTSD often have multiple unexplained physical symptoms leading to diagnosis with functional somatic syndromes such as fibromyalgia and chronic pain [33]. Medical problems both contribute to and are affected by sleep disturbance.

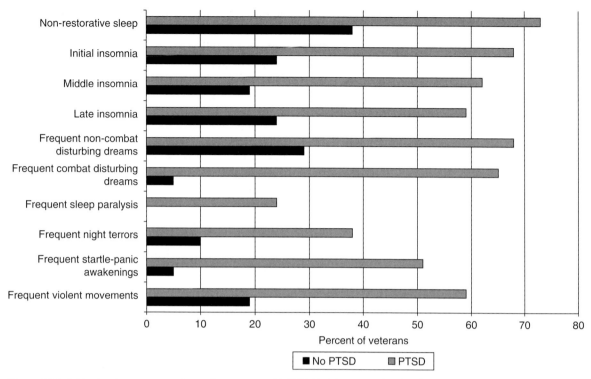

Figure 30.2 Subjective sleep symptoms in combat veterans with PTSD (dark bars; n = 37) and without PTSD (striped bars; n = 21). Data from [78].

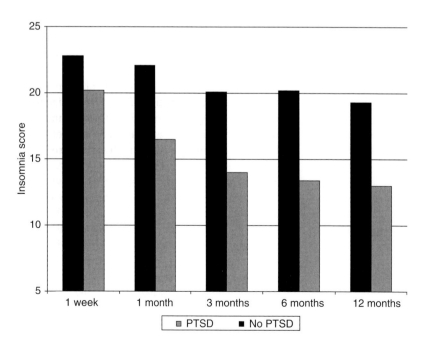

Figure 30.3 Self-reported insomnia severity at several points in the year following a motor vehicle accident, comparing those who met diagnostic criteria for PTSD at one year (dark bars; n = 26) to those who did not (striped bars; n = 76). Insomnia severity at one month post-accident is associated with PTSD diagnosis at one year. Data from [30].

Subjective sleep changes in PTSD
Sleep quality

Insomnia is the most common sleep complaint in PTSD, both in the acute and chronic phases. In a survey of Vietnam veterans 44% of combat veterans with PTSD had difficulty falling asleep, while difficulty staying asleep is reported by 91% of veterans [34]. Overall sleep disturbance is associated with increased PTSD severity, with mean Pittsburgh Sleep Quality Index (PSQI) scores from 10 for moderate PTSD to 13 for severe PTSD (out of a possible 21, with score >5 indicating significantly disturbed sleep) [35].

Insomnia in PTSD has features that distinguish it from idiopathic insomnia. Vietnam veterans with PTSD were compared to a group with insomnia but not PTSD. The PTSD group described more fear of sleep, more traumatic and disturbing thoughts when lying in bed, more tendencies to yell or talk in their sleep, and more restlessness and movement in bed [36]. This is further supported by sleep logs completed by Vietnam veterans when compared to sleep measurement by actigraphy. Veterans underestimate their sleep duration but also underestimate the total number of awakenings [37]. The veterans' experience of insufficient sleep results from sleep fragmentation rather than sleep restriction. The effect of trauma on disturbed sleep is durable. Holocaust survivors continue to describe insomnia decades after their internment [38].

Dreams and nightmares

In the immediate period post-trauma, individuals tend to report dreams of the specific events that they experienced, although this is not universal with many individuals either reporting no dreams or unrelated dreams [39, 40]. When the dreams evoke fear and anxiety and cause an awakening from sleep, they are labeled nightmares. These nightmares exist on a continuum, with dreams varying in the extent to which the traumatic event is represented directly or symbolically. The characteristic post-traumatic nightmare consists of exact replays of the traumatic events, coinciding with physiological activation, and at times, with movement and vocalization [41]. The significance of nightmares may be related to the processing of traumatic memory. Adaptive dreams involve the experience of traumatic memories with themes of mastery or survival. Maladaptive dreams of high emotional intensity and replay of traumatic events give way over time to anxious, trauma-themed, threatening, and aggressive dreams.

Dream content that is distressing and highly similar to the trauma has been found to be associated with the severity of PTSD in initial and follow-up assessments [39]. In an analysis of dream content from hurricane survivors 6 to 12 months after the disaster, all of those who had distressing hurricane-related dreams had the diagnosis of PTSD [42].

In studies of chronic PTSD, threatening dreams and nightmares are among the most persistent symptoms. In Vietnam veterans, nightmares were a quite specific predictor of the presence of PTSD, reported by 52% of veterans with PTSD compared to 5% without PTSD and 3% of civilians [34]. Over time, not all dreams in PTSD are specifically trauma-themed, but the content of dreams is typically threatening [43].

Disturbing dreams have been reported by individuals with PTSD on awakening from both REM and non-REM sleep [44–46]. One study found that "well adjusted" holocaust survivors had poor dream recall on awakening from REM compared to "less-adjusted" survivors and controls [47]. It is unclear whether poor dream recall was a protective lifelong trait of those well adjusted survivors, or if it developed as a mechanism to cope with their traumatic experiences.

Various theorists have proposed a psychodynamic understanding and approach to dreams. Freud's concept of a "repetition compulsion" defense mechanism where the dream provides a mental vehicle for re-experiencing the unsuccessfully repressed traumatic experience has been challenged by dream theorist Hartmann [48]. He proposes that the major ego deficit is thin or permeable boundaries. In his study of a small group of Vietnam War veterans with frequent repetitive nightmares, Hartmann found evidence of lifetime psychopathological vulnerability and that the stress of the war experience and their inherent thin ego defense boundaries increased their propensity to repetitive traumatic nightmares. In such people the nightmare becomes psychologically encapsulated but easily vulnerable to recurrence playback in their dreams following stressful experiences.

Another theoretical model of nightmares employs the concept of threat stimulation and rehearsal, with the function of improving biological survival. According to Revonsuo's evolutionary theory [49], when an individual is confronted by a major threat to survival there is an inherent automatic response whereby the traumatic dream provides a rehearsal function to improve skills in threat detection and response.

From a cognitive–behavioral perspective, nightmares can be understood as noxious stimuli that produce conditioned behaviors, such as waking up from the bad dream or avoiding sleep. Over time, these responses reinforce both the avoidance behavior and the distorted belief of being out of control and helpless in the face of the nightmares. This creates a sense of danger associated with the sleep environment and heightened arousal. In their cognitive model for re-experiencing symptoms, Ehlers and Clark [50] emphasize the importance of the negative appraisals of the nightmare (such as "I am going crazy") over the nightmare itself. However, the various psychological models that have been proposed to be the basis of repetitive nightmares do not adequately explain their etiology [41].

Objective sleep changes

For reasons outlined earlier, objective sleep research in PTSD is challenging. A lack of correlation between subjective sleep complaints and actigraphic or polysomnographic measures of sleep in several studies has been put forward as evidence that altered sleep perception is a central sleep issue in PTSD [51–53]. Interestingly, patients with PTSD often report better sleep in the laboratory than they obtain at home, possibly due to a sense of safety instilled by the clinical environment. Home polysomnography as an alternative to laboratory-based studies allows for an assessment of sleep in the context of a patient's habitual environment and behaviors [54].

Given the disparate populations studied – acute vs. chronic; combat vs. civilian; elderly vs. young – it is no surprise that consistent patterns can be difficult to discern. A recent review collected a selection of the best quality polysomnographic studies into a meta-analysis. They found an overall pattern of increased REM density, and a shift in sleep architecture with decreased slow-wave sleep and increased stage 1 sleep. These patterns were significant, with effect sizes in the small to medium range (0.24–0.43) [55]. This meta-analysis is consistent with the evidence to date, namely that changes in REM sleep and in the quality and continuity of sleep are the principal findings in PTSD.

Rapid eye movement sleep

Studies have found an increased rate of awakening from REM sleep [56–58]. Arousal from REM sleep may result from the intensity or fearfulness of dreams, or from intrinsic deficits in REM continuity. Chronic fragmentation of REM sleep may play a role in producing subtle memory or cognitive deficits.

Another interesting finding is that of increased REM density in PTSD [16, 59, 60]. Rapid eye movement density is a measure of the frequency of eye movements in REM sleep. Increased REM density is believed to signal increased intensity of the REM episode and has been found to be associated with depression.

Rapid eye movement sleep is characterized by a loss of muscle tone: a protective mechanism to prevent the acting out of dreams. In a few studies, individuals with PTSD were found to have an increase of motor activity in REM [46, 61, 62].

It remains unclear if these characteristics of REM sleep arise from trauma or rather are premorbid sleep traits that predispose an individual to develop symptoms post-trauma. Rapid eye movement sleep traits are known to occur in families. It is interesting to speculate that poor REM continuity and increased REM density may prevent the normal processing of trauma memories and dreams, leading to chronic nightmares and sleep impairment.

Arousal from sleep

There is some controversy about the role of hyperarousal in producing sleep changes in PTSD. A heightened state of arousal or hypervigilence is hypothesized to produce lighter, disruption-prone sleep. Some studies have indeed found that impaired sleep maintenance is a common sleep change in PTSD. Higher levels of arousal were found in hurricane survivors compared to an unexposed group [16]. Individuals with chronic combat-related PTSD have lower sleep efficiency and a higher number of awakenings even when compared to a depressed group [59]. Fragmented sleep has been also noted in a home polysomnography study [54]. One study comparing nightmare sufferers with and without PTSD found that those individuals with PTSD had more awakenings [63], suggesting that the nightmares were not primarily responsible for the arousals. These findings are challenged by a series of studies finding no evidence of more fragmented sleep in individuals with PTSD [56, 64–66].

The hyperarousal hypothesis has been tested by a series of arousal threshold experiments in chronic combat-related PTSD. Measures of EEG response to a series of tones increasing in loudness showed an elevated arousal threshold to both non-REM and REM sleep in chronic PTSD [66–68]. This unexpected finding has been explained as a compensatory measure to help preserve sleep continuity by actively suppressing awakening to external stimuli during sleep. Interestingly, when an above-threshold or startling stimulus was applied, the PTSD subjects had higher autonomic and movement responses, suggesting that an elevated startle response is present in sleep as it is in wake [67].

Autonomic responses in sleep

Sleep-related changes in autonomic function provide evidence of altered neuroendocrine functioning in individuals with PTSD. Through the measurement of heart rate variability in accident victims, Mellman et al. [69] identified a link between elevated sympathetic activation in REM sleep one month post-accident and the subsequent development of PTSD. Further evidence for inappropriate sympathetic activation in sleep is the finding of elevated nocturnal urine norephinephrine metabolite levels in individuals with PTSD [70]. Rapid eye movement heart rate variability decreased in a small group of cognitive behavioral therapy treatment responders [71].

Sleep breathing

The contribution of sleep-related breathing disorders to disrupted sleep in PTSD is largely unknown, although it appears that sleep apnea and PTSD frequently coexist. In one study, out of 12 veterans with a mean age of 31 years, five had apnea-hypopnea indices greater than ten per hour of sleep [66]. Krakow et al. [72] studied crime victims presenting to a nightmare and insomnia treatment program. Of this sample, 50% met criteria for a diagnosis of obstructive sleep apnea (OSA) and 90% had some degree of sleep-disordered breathing. Obstructive sleep apnea is also common in the older Veteran population. In the Veterans' health data base, nearly 3% have been diagnosed with sleep apnea, of which nearly 12% have the comorbid diagnosis of PTSD [73]. Those veterans with sleep apnea had significantly more mood and anxiety disorders, PTSD, psychosis, and dementia.

One of the links between PTSD and OSA is obesity, as there is an increased risk for obesity in both civilians and veterans with the diagnosis of PTSD [74, 75]. Substance-use disorders and the use of psychotropic medications also play a role. However, sleep apnea in patients with PTSD presents atypically: with fewer complaints of snoring and breathing problems, and more of insomnia, poor sleep quality, and cognitive–affective problems [76]. Underdiagnosis in this population is a significant concern, especially as treatment of sleep apnea may substantially improve sleep, nightmares, and PTSD symptoms [77].

Sleep movement

Periodic limb movement (PLM) is a sleep disorder diagnosed by polysomnography, with a prevalence starting at 2 to 5% in the general adult population and increasing with age. The limb movements occur in non-REM sleep and are often associated with brief arousals, poor quality sleep, and daytime fatigue. A few studies have identified higher frequency of limb movements in PTSD compared to controls [61, 78]. One study of 23 middle-aged veterans, of whom only 3 complained of leg kicking at night, found 76% had a PLM index greater than 5 [79]. When nightmare sufferers with and without PTSD were compared, both groups had increased movement in REM and non-REM sleep [63]. There is insufficient evidence to speculate about increased rates of PLMs in PTSD, but as in OSA, identification and treatment of any underlying primary sleep disorder will improve sleep complaints, daytime functioning, and may improve PTSD symptomatology.

Assessment of sleep problems in PTSD

Standardized assessment tools can help with the diagnosis of PTSD, the surveillance of symptoms over time, and the monitoring of treatment. A detailed clinical interview is required to make the diagnosis, and several structured interviews are available, including the commonly used Clinician Administered PTSD Scale (CAPS) [80]. Monitoring of symptom severity and frequency can be accomplished with a variety of adult self-report scales (Table 30.2).

Sleep logs are an important tool for the assessment of sleep in PTSD. The Pittsburgh Sleep Quality Index (PSQI) is also commonly used [81]. An addendum for assessing trauma-related sleep symptoms, the

Table 30.2 Commonly used self-report PTSD scales

	Number of items	Corresponds to DSM-IV criteria	Reference
Distressing Event Questionnaire (DEQ) (renamed PTSD Screening and Diagnostic Scale, PSDS)	35	Yes	[126]
Impact of Events Scale – Revised (IES-R)	22	Yes	[127]
Mississippi Scale for Combat-Related PTSD	17	No	[128]
Penn Inventory for Post-traumatic Stress Disorder	26	No	[129]
Trauma Symptom Inventory	100	Yes	[130]
Post-traumatic Stress Diagnostic Scale (PDS)	49	Yes	[131]
PTSD Checklist (PCL) – Civilian, Military, Specific Trauma	17	Yes	[132]

PSQI-A, has been developed although its validity has only been tested in women with PTSD [82]. Adequate screening for primary sleep disorders is essential, which can be accomplished through a good sleep history (including information from a bed partner) and physical exam, or through screening tools such as the sleep assessment questionnaire (SAQ) [83].

Dream and nightmare tracking can yield inconsistent results, particularly with retrospective reporting where nightmare frequency tends to be under-reported. Various nightmare logs and questionnaires have been developed, mainly for research purposes [84, 85]. The impact of disturbing dreams can be tracked using the Nightmare Effects Survey [86]. One study describes a PTSD dream content rating instrument although it has not been validated [43].

Management of sleep problems in PTSD

The goal of treatment in PTSD is the improvement of symptoms and enhancement of adaptive functioning. In traumatized individuals, improvement often takes the form of a restored sense of safety. Evidence and consensus-based practice guidelines for acute stress disorder and PTSD include both pharmacologic and psychotherapeutic interventions [87].

When suspected, primary sleep disorders should be investigated by polysomnography and treated according to guidelines. In addition, the prevention and treatment of comorbid psychiatric or medical problems, including substance abuse, should also be considered as part of the treatment for PTSD.

Pharmacology of sleep and PTSD

Drug trials in PTSD vary in their reporting of sleep symptoms, with many focusing on global effectiveness in PTSD symptom rather than improvement in individual symptom scales. Overall, selective serotonin reuptake inhibitor (SSRI) medications are considered first-line treatment in PTSD [88]. Where sleep is concerned, SSRIs are known to decrease REM sleep, increase REM latency, and decrease sleep continuity. Selective serotonin reuptake inhibitor medications are efficacious at reducing PTSD severity, but there are mixed results for sleep, with lingering sleep symptoms and nightmares, and in some cases, worsening of insomnia. In one randomized controlled trial (RCT) of sertraline, there was a 60% response rate to drug vs. 38% to placebo, but there was no improvement on the PSQI and an increase in insomnia from 22% to 35% [89]. Paroxetine trials have supported some efficacy in treating sleep symptoms, with somnolence a more common adverse effect [90, 91]. Fluoxetine, which is known to be disruptive to sleep, has not been found to significantly improve sleep or nightmares in PTSD [92]. Fluvoxamine, in an open-label study, was shown to improve sleep maintenance [93], but is poorly tolerated.

Other antidepressant medicines have been studied in PTSD, with inconclusive or varying evidence of benefit. There is limited data for tricyclic antidepressant and monoamine oxidase inhibitor medications. A series of open-label trials of nefazodone in PTSD found improved objective and subjective sleep quality and decreased nightmares [94, 95]. Nefazodone is known to have a positive effect upon sleep architecture in depression, but is no longer available because of reports of liver failure. Trazodone is in the same class as nefazodone. It has sedative properties, and less norepinephrine reuptake inhibition and more antihistamine properties than nefazodone. There are no controlled trials of trazodone in PTSD, with evidence limited to a survey of 72 PTSD patients where three quarters had improved nightmares and insomnia with a dose range of 50–200 mg nightly [96]. Mirtazapine is also known to have a favorable effect on sleep in depression. One trial comparing mirtazapine to sertraline in PTSD found their treatment effects to be equivalent, but did not comment specifically on sleep effects [97]. There is an anecdotal report of improved nightmares with mirtazapine [98].

Benzodiazepines are another class of drug commonly used to treat sleep disturbance in PTSD. However, such drugs have not been shown to be effective in improving PTSD symptoms in placebo-controlled trials [99, 100]. A few studies have suggested their use may in fact be detrimental [100, 101]. There are only case studies on the newer non-benzodiazepine hypnotics. Treatment guidelines do not support the use of benzodiazepines as monotherapy for acute stress or PTSD, citing concerns about addiction potential, withdrawal, and rebound effects [87].

Antipsychotic medications are used in PTSD when psychotic symptoms are present. In several small trials they have been studied in an "augmenting" role when first-line treatments are ineffective, although they are not approved for this indication. Sleep is one of the main symptoms targeted by adding an atypical antipsychotic, and a small placebo-controlled trial of olanzapine added to SSRI treatment did show a significant improvement in sleep as measured by the PSQI, but also a mean weight gain of 13 pounds over eight weeks [102]. Several open-label add-on studies have found improvement in sleep and PTSD symptoms with risperidone [103, 104], while one small RCT found improvement with risperidone monotherapy [105]. There have been similar findings in quetiapine add-on therapy open-label trials [106–109]. Atypical antipsychotics carry the risks of metabolic and extrapyramidal side effects, which may counter any possible benefits in PTSD.

Various anticonvulsant agents have drawn interest in PTSD, although there are no large, quality studies available. There is some evidence that the following agents help with the re-experiencing cluster of symptoms, and are also used at times in cases with

significant irritability or aggressivity. The effects of anticonvulsants on sleep have been studied, and gabapentin is known to improve slow-wave sleep. A retrospective chart review of gabapentin (as an add-on in patients on multiple medications) showed that 77% had moderate or marked improvement in their nightmares or insomnia [110]. Another GABAergic medication, tiagabine, significantly improved sleep, as measured by PSQI, from baseline in an open-label study [111]. Topiramate, as adjunctive treatment, has shown promising results in an open-label study. The response rate was over 70%, with 94% reporting a full cessation of nightmares [112]. However, in a recent placebo-controlled trial of topiramate as adjunctive treatment, the high drop-out rate due to CNS side effects precluded any conclusion about the effectiveness of treatment [113]. A placebo-controlled trial of lamotrigine had only 14 subjects, and provided anecdotal reports of improved sleep and nightmares [114].

Prazosin is a treatment that shows promise. It is a centrally and peripherally acting α1-adrenergic antagonist, first identified as a possible treatment for PTSD when veterans treated for benign prostatic hypertrophy reported reduction in trauma-related nightmares. Prazosin is all the more appealing for having a plausible mechanism of action: it is believed to target the increased CNS adrenergic activity in PTSD, in particular the hyper-responsiveness of α1-adrenergic receptors believed to play a part in the hyperarousal, the nightmares, and abnormal fear responses in PTSD. It is also now a relatively well studied drug in PTSD with several open-label studies and two small RCTs [115]. Doses in these studies ranged from 1 mg to 15 mg, with most in the region of 3 to 6 mg. The drug is quite well tolerated, with little effect on blood pressure when titrated gradually. A starting dose of 1 mg is suggested in order to avoid a rare idiosyncratic hypotensive reaction, with a 1 mg increase every few days to beneficial effect. The most common side effects are transient dizziness, nausea, and headache. One study found that a daytime dose of the medication also improved daytime PTSD symptoms, suggesting that it is more than a treatment for sleep and nightmares [116]. More recently, prazosin was studied as an adjunctive treatment in a small crossover RCT with home polysomnography [117]. Prazosin significantly increased total sleep time, REM sleep time, and REM episode duration, while decreasing REM latency. Prazosin also decreased nightmares and PTSD symptoms significantly more than placebo, with no difference in adverse events between groups. One limitation of these studies is that they have mainly involved the male combat veteran population, thus little is known about its use in women and civilians.

Psychotherapy interventions

Cognitive behavioral therapies (CBTs) are reported to be effective for the treatment of PTSD symptoms including sleep and nightmares. Various forms of CBT have been devised on the continuum of treatments from those that focus on cognitive processing to those that are primarily behavioral. The goal is to alter distorted threat appraisals, either through exposure and densensitization to triggers or through cognitive restructuring. A typical course of therapy involves education about the model and symptoms, relaxation techniques to improve tolerance of anxiety, a gradual exposure to memories of the traumatic experience, and in vivo exposures to anxiety triggers. Cognitive behavioral therapy for insomnia adds behavioral elements such as sleep hygiene education, stimulus control, and sleep restriction. Improvement of sleep and nightmares with CBT leads to improved daytime PTSD symptoms [118].

Exposure is the common thread through many of the psychotherapeutic interventions shown to be effective for nightmares in PSTD. Imagery rehearsal therapy is one example that has been shown to have a significant effect on decreasing nightmare frequency, increasing PSQI sleep scores, and decreasing PTSD symptoms. In the study by Krakow *et al.* [119], this was achieved with a three-session group intervention involving education about nightmares, instruction on imagery rehearsal, and then the recollection, rescripting, and rehearsing of a disturbing dream with a theme of mastery. A similar concept is employed in lucid dream therapy that teaches how to develop awareness of the dream content, while consciously manipulating it for a favorable outcome [120]. Therapy consists of exposure, mastery, and lucidity exercises and has been found effective in reducing nightmare frequency [121].

Eye movement desensitization and reprocessing (EMDR) is another therapy based upon brief exposure to traumatic material along with directed eye movements. Its proponents theorize that the eye movements stimulate neural mechanisms similar to those in REM sleep, and aim to induce processing of disturbing memories [122]. Eye movement desensitization and reprocessing has been found to be as effective as CBT, although the efficacy may be related to those components that are similar to CBT rather than the eye movements [123]. One polysomnography study found significantly higher sleep efficiencies after a brief course of EMDR [124].

Psychological debriefing is a controversial technique widely deployed in the immediate post-trauma period with the aim of preventing significant ASD or PTSD. There is no evidence showing efficacy for this intervention, and there is some concern it may have adverse effects [125].

Conclusion

In summary, abnormalities in sleep are a core feature of PTSD. The evidence supports the inclusion of recurrent nightmares and disturbances in sleep initiation and continuity as diagnostic features of this disorder. Persistent sleep disturbance after a traumatic experience may indeed herald the development of PTSD. While there has been considerable effort in attempting to understand the role of sleep, the reason for these sleep disturbances remains elusive. An important area of future research is premorbid sleep disturbance as a risk factor for PTSD.

Efforts at treating sleep problems in PTSD include psychological and behavioral therapies with some effect. Medication options aim to facilitate sleep, reduce arousals, and perhaps improve mood. The investigation and treatment of primary sleep disorders, when suspected, should be a main concern.

References

1. American Psychiatric Association. *Diagnostic and Statistical Manual of Mental Disorders (DSM-IV-TR)*. (Washington, DC: APA, 2000).

2. Breslau N, Kessler RC, Chilcoat HD, *et al.* Trauma and posttraumatic stress disorder in the community: the 1996 Detroit Area Survey of Trauma. *Arch Gen Psychiatry.* 1998;**55**:626–32.

3. Breslau N, Davis GC, Andreski P, *et al.* Traumatic events and posttraumatic stress disorder in an urban population of young adults. *Arch Gen Psychiatry.* 1991;**48**:216–22.

4. Kessler RC, Sonnega A, Bromet E, *et al.* Posttraumatic stress disorder in the National Comorbidity Survey. *Arch Gen Psychiatry.* 1995;**52**:1048–60.

5. Resnick HS, Kilpatrick DG, Dansky BS, *et al.* Prevalence of civilian trauma and posttraumatic stress disorder in a

representative national sample of women. *J Consult Clin Psychol.* 1993;**61**:984–91.

6. Breslau N, Davis GC. Posttraumatic stress disorder in an urban population of young adults: risk factors for chronicity. *Am J Psychiatry.* 1992;**149**:671–5.

7. Breslau N, Davis GC, Peterson EL, *et al.* Psychiatric sequelae of posttraumatic stress disorder in women. *Arch Gen Psychiatry.* 1997;**54**:81–7.

8. Davidson JR, Hughes D, Blazer DG, *et al.* Post-traumatic stress disorder in the community: an epidemiological study. *Psychol Med.* 1991;**21**:713–21.

9. Solomon SD, Davidson JR. Trauma: prevalence, impairment, service use, and cost. *J Clin Psychiatry.* 1997;**58** (Suppl 9):5–11.

10. Zatzick DF, Marmar CR, Weiss DS, *et al.* Posttraumatic stress disorder and functioning and quality of life outcomes in a nationally representative sample of male Vietnam veterans. *Am J Psychiatry.* 1997;**154**:1690–5.

11. Jones E, Hodgins-Vermaas R, McCartney H, *et al.* Post-combat syndromes from the Boer war to the Gulf war: a cluster analysis of their nature and attribution. *BMJ.* 2002;**324**:321–4.

12. Kulka RA, Schlenger WE, Fairbank JA, *et al.* Trauma and the Vietnam War generation: Report of findings from the National Vietnam Veterans Readjustment Study. (New York: Brunner/Mazel, 1990).

13. Kang HK, Natelson BH, Mahan CM, *et al.* Post-traumatic stress disorder and chronic fatigue syndrome-like illness among Gulf War veterans: a population-based survey of 30,000 veterans. *Am J Epidemiol.* 2003;**157**:141–8.

14. Hoge CW, Castro CA, Messer SC, *et al.* Combat duty in Iraq and Afghanistan, mental health problems, and barriers to care. *N Engl J Med.* 2004;**351**:13–22.

15. Brewin CR, Andrews B, Valentine JD. Meta-analysis of risk factors for posttraumatic stress disorder in trauma-exposed adults. *J Consult Clin Psychol.* 2000;**68**:748–66.

16. Mellman TA, David D, Kulick-Bell R, *et al.* Sleep disturbance and its relationship to psychiatric morbidity after Hurricane Andrew. *Am J Psychiatry.* 1995;**152**:1659–63.

17. Yehuda R, Halligan SL, Bierer LM. Relationship of parental trauma exposure and PTSD to PTSD, depressive and anxiety disorders in offspring. *J Psychiatr Res.* 2001;**35**:261–70.

18. Nugent NR, Amstadter AB, Koenen KC. Genetics of post-traumatic stress disorder: informing clinical conceptualizations and promoting future research. *Am J Med Genet C Semin Med Genet.* 2008;**148**:127–32.

19. Kilpatrick DG, Koenen KC, Ruggiero KJ, *et al.* The serotonin transporter genotype and social support and moderation of posttraumatic stress disorder and depression in hurricane-exposed adults. *Am J Psychiatry.* 2007;**164**:1693–9.

20. Pole N, Neylan TC, Otte C, *et al.* Prospective prediction of posttraumatic stress disorder symptoms using fear potentiated auditory startle responses. *Biol Psychiatry.* 2009;**65**(3):235–40.

21. Weiss SJ. Neurobiological alterations associated with traumatic stress. *Perspect Psychiatr Care.* 2007;**43**:114–22.

22. Gutman DA, Nemeroff CB. Persistent central nervous system effects of an adverse early environment: clinical and preclinical studies. *Physiol Behav.* 2003;**79**:471–8.

23. Bremner JD, Vythilingam M, Anderson G, *et al.* Assessment of the hypothalamic-pituitary-adrenal axis over a 24-hour diurnal period and in response to neuroendocrine challenges in women with and without childhood sexual abuse and posttraumatic stress disorder. *Biol Psychiatry.* 2003;**54**:710–18.

24. Breslau N. Neurobiological research on sleep and stress hormones in epidemiological samples. *Ann N Y Acad Sci.* 2006;**1071**:221–30.

25. North CS, Nixon SJ, Shariat S, *et al.* Psychiatric disorders among survivors of the Oklahoma City bombing. *JAMA.* 1999;**282**:755–62.

26. Lavie P. Sleep disturbances in the wake of traumatic events. *NEJM.* 2001;**345**:1825–32.

27. Norman SB, Stein MB, Davidson JR. Profiling posttraumatic functional impairment. *J Nerv Ment Dis.* 2007;**195**:48–53.

28. Goff BS, Crow JR, Reisbig AM, *et al.* The impact of individual trauma symptoms of deployed soldiers on relationship satisfaction. *J Fam Psychol.* 2007;**21**:344–53.

29. van den Berg B, Grievink L, van der Velden PG, *et al.* Risk factors for physical symptoms after a disaster: a longitudinal study. *Psychol Med.* 2008;**38**:499–510.

30. Koren D, Arnon I, Lavie P, *et al.* Sleep complaints as early predictors of posttraumatic stress disorder: a 1-year prospective study of injured survivors of motor vehicle accidents. *Am J Psychiatry.* 2002;**159**:855–7.

31. Holland P, Lewis PA. Emotional memory: selective enhancement by sleep. *Curr Biol.* 2007;**17**:R179–81.

32. Germain A, Buysse DJ, Nofzinger E. Sleep-specific mechanisms underlying posttraumatic stress disorder: integrative review and neurobiological hypotheses. *Sleep Med Rev.* 2008;**12**:185–95.

33. Schur EA, Afari N, Furberg H, *et al.* Feeling bad in more ways than one: comorbidity patterns of medically

unexplained and psychiatric conditions. *J Gen Intern Med.* 2007;**22**:818–21.

34. Neylan TC, Marmar CR, Metzler TJ, *et al.* Sleep disturbances in the Vietnam generation: findings from a nationally representative sample of male Vietnam veterans. *Am J Psychiatry.* 1998;**155**:929–33.

35. Germain A, Buysse DJ, Shear MK, *et al.* Clinical correlates of poor sleep quality in posttraumatic stress disorder. *J Trauma Stress.* 2004;**17**:477–84.

36. Inman DJ, Silver SM, Doghramji K. Sleep disturbance in post-traumatic stress disorder: a comparison with non-PTSD insomnia. *J Trauma Stress.* 1990;**3**:429–37.

37. Westermeyer J, Sutherland RJ, Freerks M, *et al.* Reliability of sleep log data versus actigraphy in veterans with sleep disturbance and PTSD. *J Anxiety Disord.* 2007;**21**:966–75.

38. Rosen J, Reynolds CF 3rd, Yeager AL, *et al.* Sleep disturbances in survivors of the Nazi Holocaust. *Am J Psychiatry.* 1991;**148**:62–6.

39. Mellman TA, David D, Bustamante V, *et al.* Dreams in the acute aftermath of trauma and their relationship to PTSD. *J Trauma Stress.* 2001;**14**:241.

40. Wood JM, Bootzin RR, Rosenhan D, *et al.* Effects of the 1989 San Francisco earthquake on frequency and content of nightmares. *J Abnorm Psychol.* 1992;**101**:219–24.

41. Phelps AJ, Forbes D, Creamer M. Understanding posttraumatic nightmares: an empirical and conceptual review. *Clin Psychol Rev.* 2008;**28**:338–55.

42. David D, Mellman TA. Dreams following Hurricane Andrew. *Dreaming.* 1997;**7**:209–14.

43. Esposito K, Benitez A, Barza L, *et al.* Evaluation of dream content in combat-related PTSD. *J Trauma Stress.* 1999;**12**:681–7.

44. van der Kolk B, Blitz R, Burr W, *et al.* Nightmares and trauma: a comparison of nightmares after combat with lifelong nightmares in veterans. *Am J Psychiatry.* 1984;**141**:187–90.

45. Kramer M, Schoen LS, Kinney L. Psychological and behavioral features of disturbed dreamers. *Psychiatr J Univ Ott.* 1984;**9**:102–6.

46. Hefez A, Metz L, Lavie P. Long-term effects of extreme situational stress on sleep and dreaming. *Am J Psychiatry.* 1987;**144**:344–7.

47. Kaminer H, Lavie P. Sleep and dreaming in Holocaust survivors. Dramatic decrease in dream recall in well-adjusted survivors. *J Nerv Ment Dis.* 1991;**179**:664–9.

48. Hartmann E. *The Nightmare: The Psychology and Biology of Terrifying Dreams.* (New York: Basic Books, 1984).

49. Revonsuo A. The reinterpretation of dreams: an evolutionary hypothesis of the function of dreaming. *Behav Brain Sci.* 2000;**23**:877–901.

50. Ehlers A, Clark DM. A cognitive model of posttraumatic stress disorder. *Behav Res Ther.* 2000;**38**:319–45.

51. Klein E, Koren D, Arnon I, *et al.* Sleep complaints are not corroborated by objective sleep measures in post-traumatic stress disorder: a 1-year prospective study in survivors of motor vehicle crashes. *J Sleep Res.* 2003;**12**:35–41.

52. Dagan Y, Zinger Y, Lavie P. Actigraphic sleep monitoring in posttraumatic stress disorder (PTSD) patients. *J Psychosom Res.* 1997;**42**:577–81.

53. Woodward SH, Bliwise DL, Friedman MJ, *et al.* Subjective versus objective sleep in Vietnam combat veterans hospitalized for PTSD. *J Trauma Stress.* 1996;**9**:137–43.

54. Germain A, Hall M, Katherine Shear M, *et al.* Ecological study of sleep disruption in PTSD: a pilot study. *Ann N Y Acad Sci.* 2006;**1071**:438–41.

55. Kobayashi I, Boarts JM, Delahanty DL. Polysomnographically measured sleep abnormalities in PTSD: a meta-analytic review. *Psychophysiology.* 2007;**44**:660–9.

56. Breslau N, Roth T, Burduvali E, *et al.* Sleep in lifetime posttraumatic stress disorder: a community-based polysomnographic study. *Arch Gen Psychiatry.* 2004;**61**:508–16.

57. Mellman TA, Bustamante V, Fins AI, *et al.* REM sleep and the early development of posttraumatic stress disorder. *Am J Psychiatry.* 2002;**159**:1696–701.

58. Habukawa M, Uchimura N, Maeda M, *et al.* Sleep findings in young adult patients with posttraumatic stress disorder. *Biol Psychiatry.* 2007;**62**:1179–82.

59. Mellman TA, Nolan B, Hebding J, *et al.* A polysomnographic comparison of veterans with combat-related PTSD, depressed men, and non-ill controls. *Sleep.* 1997;**20**:46–51.

60. Ross RJ, Ball WA, Dinges DF, *et al.* Rapid eye movement sleep disturbance in posttraumatic stress disorder. *Biol Psychiatry.* 1994;**35**:195–202.

61. Ross RJ, Ball WA, Dinges DF, *et al.* Motor dysfunction during sleep in posttraumatic stress disorder. *Sleep.* 1994;**17**:723–32.

62. Husain AM, Miller PP, Carwile ST. REM sleep behavior disorder: potential relationship to post-traumatic stress disorder. *J Clin Neurophysiol.* 2001; **18**:148–57.

63. Germain A, Nielsen TA. Sleep pathophysiology in posttraumatic stress disorder and idiopathic nightmare sufferers. *Biol Psychiatry.* 2003;**54**:1092–8.

64. Hurwitz TD, Mahowald MW, Kuskowski M, et al. Polysomnographic sleep is not clinically impaired in Vietnam combat veterans with chronic posttraumatic stress disorder. *Biol Psychiatry*. 1998;**44**:1066–73.

65. Engdahl BE, Eberly RE, Hurwitz TD, et al. Sleep in a community sample of elderly war veterans with and without posttraumatic stress disorder. *Biol Psychiatry*. 2000;**47**:520–5.

66. Lavie P, Katz N, Pillar G, et al. Elevated awaking thresholds during sleep: characteristics of chronic war-related posttraumatic stress disorder patients. *Biol Psychiatry*. 1998;**44**:1060–5.

67. Kramer M, Kinney L. Vigilance and avoidance during sleep in US Vietnam War veterans with posttraumatic stress disorder. *J Nerv Ment Dis*. 2003;**191**:685–7.

68. Dagan Y, Lavie P, Bleich A. Elevated awakening thresholds in sleep stage 3–4 in war-related post-traumatic stress disorder. *Biol Psychiatry*. 1991;**30**:618–22.

69. Mellman TA, Knorr BR, Pigeon WR, et al. Heart rate variability during sleep and the early development of posttraumatic stress disorder. *Biol Psychiatry*. 2004;**55**:953–6.

70. Mellman TA, Kumar A, Kulick-Bell R, et al. Nocturnal/daytime urine noradrenergic measures and sleep in combat-related PTSD. *Biol Psychiatry*. 1995;**38**:174–9.

71. Nishith P, Duntley SP, Domitrovich PP, et al. Effect of cognitive behavioral therapy on heart rate variability during REM sleep in female rape victims with PTSD. *J Trauma Stress*. 2003;**16**:247–50.

72. Krakow B, Melendrez D, Pedersen B, et al. Complex insomnia: insomnia and sleep-disordered breathing in a consecutive series of crime victims with nightmares and PTSD. *Biol Psychiatry*. 2001;**49**:948–53.

73. Sharafkhaneh A, Giray N, Richardson P, et al. Association of psychiatric disorders and sleep apnea in a large cohort. *Sleep*. 2005;**28**:1405–11.

74. Perkonigg A, Owashi T, Stein MB, et al. Posttraumatic stress disorder and obesity: evidence for a risk association. *Am J Prev Med*. 2009;**36**(1):1–8.

75. Vieweg WV, Julius DA, Bates J, et al. Posttraumatic stress disorder as a risk factor for obesity among male military veterans. *Acta Psychiatr Scand*. 2007;**116**:483–7.

76. Krakow B, Melendrez D, Warner TD, et al. Signs and symptoms of sleep-disordered breathing in trauma survivors: a matched comparison with classic sleep apnea patients. *J Nerv Ment Dis*. 2006;**194**:433–9.

77. Krakow B, Lowry C, Germain A, et al. A retrospective study on improvements in nightmares and post-traumatic stress disorder following treatment for co-morbid sleep-disordered breathing. *J Psychosom Res*. 2000;**49**:291–8.

78. Mellman TA, Kulick-Bell R, Ashlock LE, et al. Sleep events among veterans with combat-related posttraumatic stress disorder. *Am J Psychiatry*. 1995;**152**:110–15.

79. Brown TM, Boudewyns PA. Periodic limb movements of sleep in combat veterans with posttraumatic stress disorder. *J Trauma Stress*. 1996;**9**:129–36.

80. Weathers FW, Keane TM, Davidson JR. Clinician-administered PTSD scale: a review of the first ten years of research. *Depress Anxiety*. 2001;**13**:132–56.

81. Buysse DJ, Reynolds CF, Monk TH, et al. The Pittsburgh Sleep Quality Index: a new instrument for psychiatric practice and research. *Psychiatry Res*. 1989;**28**:193–213.

82. Germain A, Hall M, Krakow B, et al. A brief sleep scale for posttraumatic stress disorder: Pittsburgh Sleep Quality Index addendum for PTSD. *J Anxiety Disord*. 2005;**19**:233–44.

83. Unger ER, Nisenbaum R, Moldofsky H, et al. Sleep assessment in a population-based study of chronic fatigue syndrome. *BMC Neurol*. 2004;**4**:6.

84. Robert G, Zadra A. Measuring nightmare and bad dream frequency: impact of retrospective and prospective instruments. *J Sleep Res*. 2008;**17**:132–9.

85. Krakow B, Schrader R, Tandberg D, et al. Nightmare frequency in sexual assault survivors with PTSD. *J Anxiety Disord*. 2002;**16**:175–90.

86. Krakow B, Hollifield M, Schrader R, et al. A controlled study of imagery rehearsal for chronic nightmares in sexual assault survivors with PTSD: a preliminary report. *J Trauma Stress*. 2000;**13**:589–609.

87. Ursano RJ, Bell C, Eth S, et al. Practice guideline for the treatment of patients with acute stress disorder and posttraumatic stress disorder. *Am J Psychiatry*. 2004;**161**:3–31.

88. Stein DJ, Ipser JC, Seedat S. Pharmacotherapy for post traumatic stress disorder (PTSD). *Cochrane Database Syst Rev*. 2008;**3**:CD002795.

89. Davidson JR, Rothbaum BO, van der Kolk BA, et al. Multicenter, double-blind comparison of sertraline and placebo in the treatment of posttraumatic stress disorder. *Arch Gen Psychiatry*. 2001;**58**:485–92.

90. Stein DJ, Davidson J, Seedat S, et al. Paroxetine in the treatment of post-traumatic stress disorder: pooled analysis of placebo-controlled studies. *Expert Opin Pharmacother*. 2003;**4**:1829–38.

91. Tucker P, Zaninelli R, Yehuda R, et al. Paroxetine in the treatment of chronic posttraumatic stress disorder: results of a placebo-controlled, flexible-dosage trial. *J Clin Psychiatry*. 2001;**62**:860–8.

92. Meltzer-Brody S, Connor KM, Churchill E, *et al*. Symptom-specific effects of fluoxetine in post-traumatic stress disorder. *Int Clin Psychopharmacol*. 2000;**15**:227–31.

93. Neylan TC, Metzler TJ, Schoenfeld FB, *et al*. Fluvoxamine and sleep disturbances in posttraumatic stress disorder. *J Trauma Stress*. 2001;**14**:461–7.

94. Hidalgo R, Hertzberg MA, Mellman T, *et al*. Nefazodone in post-traumatic stress disorder: results from six open-label trials. *Int Clin Psychopharmacol*. 1999;**14**:61–8.

95. Neylan TC, Lenoci M, Maglione ML, *et al*. The effect of nefazodone on subjective and objective sleep quality in posttraumatic stress disorder. *J Clin Psychiatry*. 2003;**64**:445–50.

96. Warner MD, Dorn MR, Peabody CA. Survey on the usefulness of trazodone in patients with PTSD with insomnia or nightmares. *Pharmacopsychiatry*. 2001;**34**:128–31.

97. Chung MY, Min KH, Jun YJ, *et al*. Efficacy and tolerability of mirtazapine and sertraline in Korean veterans with posttraumatic stress disorder: a randomized open label trial. *Hum Psychopharmacol*. 2004;**19**:489–94.

98. Lewis JD. Mirtazapine for PTSD nightmares. *Am J Psychiatry*. 2002;**159**(11):1948–9.

99. Gelpin E, Bonne O, Peri T, *et al*. Treatment of recent trauma survivors with benzodiazepines: a prospective study. *J Clin Psychiatry*. 1996;**57**:390–4.

100. Braun P, Greenberg D, Dasberg H, *et al*. Core symptoms of posttraumatic stress disorder unimproved by alprazolam treatment. *J Clin Psychiatry*. 1990;**51**:236–8.

101. Mellman TA, Bustamante V, David D, *et al*. Hypnotic medication in the aftermath of trauma. *J Clin Psychiatry*. 2002;**63**:1183–4.

102. Stein MB, Kline NA, Matloff JL. Adjunctive olanzapine for SSRI-resistant combat-related PTSD: a double-blind, placebo-controlled study. *Am J Psychiatry*. 2002;**159**:1777–9.

103. David D, De Faria L, Mellman TA. Adjunctive risperidone treatment and sleep symptoms in combat veterans with chronic PTSD. *Depress Anxiety*. 2006;**23**:489–91.

104. Bartzokis G, Lu PH, Turner J, *et al*. Adjunctive risperidone in the treatment of chronic combat-related posttraumatic stress disorder. *Biol Psychiatry*. 2005;**57**:474–9.

105. Padala PR, Madison J, Monnahan M, *et al*. Risperidone monotherapy for post-traumatic stress disorder related to sexual assault and domestic abuse in women. *Int Clin Psychopharmacol*. 2006;**21**:275–80.

106. Ahearn EP, Mussey M, Johnson C, *et al*. Quetiapine as an adjunctive treatment for post-traumatic stress disorder: an 8-week open-label study. *Int Clin Psychopharmacol*. 2006;**21**:29–33.

107. Robert S, Hamner MB, Kose S, *et al*. Quetiapine improves sleep disturbances in combat veterans with PTSD: sleep data from a prospective, open-label study. *J Clin Psychopharmacol*. 2005;**25**:387–8.

108. Sokolski KN, Denson TF, Lee RT, *et al*. Quetiapine for treatment of refractory symptoms of combat-related post-traumatic stress disorder. *Mil Med*. 2003;**168**:486–9.

109. Hamner MB, Deitsch SE, Brodrick PS, *et al*. Quetiapine treatment in patients with posttraumatic stress disorder: an open trial of adjunctive therapy. *J Clin Psychopharmacol*. 2003;**23**:15–20.

110. Hamner MB, Brodrick PS, Labbate LA. Gabapentin in PTSD: a retrospective, clinical series of adjunctive therapy. *Ann Clin Psychiatry*. 2001;**13**:141–6.

111. Connor KM, Davidson JR, Weisler RH, *et al*. Tiagabine for posttraumatic stress disorder: effects of open-label and double-blind discontinuation treatment. *Psychopharmacology* (*Berl*). 2006;**184**:21–5.

112. Berlant JL. Prospective open-label study of add-on and monotherapy topiramate in civilians with chronic nonhallucinatory posttraumatic stress disorder. *BMC Psychiatry*. 2004;**4**:24.

113. Lindley SE, Carlson EB, Hill K. A randomized, double-blind, placebo-controlled trial of augmentation topiramate for chronic combat-related posttraumatic stress disorder. *J Clin Psychopharmacol*. 2007;**27**:677–81.

114. Hertzberg MA, Butterfield MI, Feldman ME, *et al*. A preliminary study of lamotrigine for the treatment of posttraumatic stress disorder. *Biol Psychiatry*. 1999;**45**:1226–9.

115. Taylor HR, Freeman MK, Cates ME. Prazosin for treatment of nightmares related to posttraumatic stress disorder. *Am J Health Syst Pharm*. 2008;**65**:716–22.

116. Taylor FB, Lowe K, Thompson C, *et al*. Daytime prazosin reduces psychological distress to trauma specific cues in civilian trauma posttraumatic stress disorder. *Biol Psychiatry*. 2006;**59**:577–81.

117. Taylor FB, Martin P, Thompson C, *et al*. Prazosin effects on objective sleep measures and clinical symptoms in civilian trauma posttraumatic stress disorder: a placebo-controlled study. *Biol Psychiatry*. 2008;**63**:629–32.

118. Krakow B, Johnston L, Melendrez D, *et al*. An open-label trial of evidence-based cognitive behavior therapy for nightmares and insomnia in crime victims with PTSD. *Am J Psychiatry*. 2001;**158**:2043–7.

119. Krakow B, Hollifield M, Johnston L, *et al.* Imagery rehearsal therapy for chronic nightmares in sexual assault survivors with posttraumatic stress disorder: a randomized controlled trial. *JAMA.* 2001;**286**:537–45.

120. Zadra AL, Pihl RO. Lucid dreaming as a treatment for recurrent nightmares. *Psychother Psychosom.* 1997;**66**:50–5.

121. Spoormaker VI, van den Bout J. Lucid dreaming treatment for nightmares: a pilot study. *Psychother Psychosom.* 2006;**75**:389–94.

122. Stickgold R. EMDR: a putative neurobiological mechanism of action. *J Clin Psychol.* 2002;**58**:61–75.

123. Seidler GH, Wagner FE. Comparing the efficacy of EMDR and trauma-focused cognitive-behavioral therapy in the treatment of PTSD: a meta-analytic study. *Psychol Med.* 2006;**36**:1515–22.

124. Raboni MR, Tufik S, Suchecki D. Treatment of PTSD by eye movement desensitization reprocessing (EMDR) improves sleep quality, quality of life, and perception of stress. *Ann N Y Acad Sci.* 2006;**1071**:508–13.

125. Rose S, Bisson J, Churchill R, *et al.* Psychological debriefing for preventing post traumatic stress disorder (PTSD). *Cochrane Database Syst Rev.* 2002; CD000560.

126. Kubany ES, Leisen MB, Kaplan AS, *et al.* Validation of a brief measure of posttraumatic stress disorder: the Distressing Event Questionnaire (DEQ). *Psychol Assess.* 2000;**12**:197–209.

127. Weiss DS, Marmar CR. The Impact of Event Scale: revised. In: Wilson J, Keane TM, eds. *Assessing Psychological Trauma and PTSD.* (New York: Guildford; 1996; 399–411).

128. Keane TM, Caddell JM, Taylor KL. Mississippi Scale for Combat-Related Posttraumatic Stress Disorder: three studies in reliability and validity. *J Consult Clin Psychol.* 1988;**56**:85–90.

129. Hammarberg M. Penn Inventory for posttraumatic stress disorder: psychometric properties. *Psychol Assess.* 1992;**4**:67–76.

130. Briere J. Psychometric review of Trauma Symptom Inventory (TSI). In: Stamm BH, ed. *Measurement of Stress, Trauma, and Adaptation.* (Lutherville, MD: Sidran Press, 1996; 381–3).

131. Foa E, Cashman L, Jaycox L, *et al.* The validation of a self-report measure of PTSD: The Posttraumatic Diagnostic Scale. *Psychol Assess.* 1997;**9**:445–51.

132. Blanchard EB, Jones-Alexander J, Buckley TC, *et al.* Psychometric properties of the PTSD Checklist (PCL). *Behav Res Ther.* 1996;**34**:669–73.

Sleep and substance use and abuse

Deirdre A. Conroy, J. Todd Arnedt, Kirk J. Brower, and Robert A. Zucker

Introduction

According to the National Institute of Drug Abuse, each year substance abuse and addiction costs the United States a half a trillion dollars [1] and contributes to more than half a million deaths [2]. Chronic substance use can lead to structural and chemical changes in the brain as well as a number of adverse behavioral outcomes. While there are numerous environmental factors that can increase the likelihood that an individual abuses drugs, identifying factors that may predispose the individual to drug use and abuse or that may prevent relapse is an area of increasing interest. Sleep disturbance can be a common complaint during the use of or withdrawal from substances of abuse, but may also predispose the individual to developing a substance use disorder (SUD) in the future. For example, a longitudinal epidemiological study showed that young adults with a prior history of insomnia at baseline were four times more likely to develop major depression, twice as likely to develop an alcohol-use disorder, seven times more likely to develop an illicit drug-use disorder, and twice as likely to develop nicotine dependence 3.5 years later [3]. Another study, by Wallander *et al.*, found that individuals who reported "insomnia," "hypersomnia," or "sleep disturbance" were two times more likely to consume excessive (>42 units/week) alcohol [4]. While in many cases sleep complaints in patients with SUDs are due to the use and abuse of the substance, in other cases sleep disturbance may pre-date the SUD and play a role in the pathophysiology of the addiction.

Patients with sleep disorders comorbid with SUDs may require special diagnostic and treatment considerations for several reasons. First, patients with idiopathic insomnia may be more likely to develop a substance use disorder as a method of coping with poor sleep or the impairment of daytime functioning that may result. Second, some sleep disorders, such as obstructive sleep apnea or periodic limb movement disorder, are known to occur more frequently in patients with substance use disorders than in other treatment populations. Third, most if not all substances can induce sleep disturbances that persist despite abstinence, and increase the risk for relapse [5]. For example, nightly use of alcohol may lead to difficulty falling asleep in the absence of the alcohol. Difficulty falling asleep may lead to resuming evening drinking in an attempt to self-medicate. Sleep disturbances that increase the risk for relapse may be a manifestation of protracted substance withdrawal, although persistent sleep disturbances may also stem from a primary sleep disorder that preceded the substance use disorder.

Evidence-based treatment in this population is limited. Patients with SUDs are often excluded from clinical trials of pharmacological and non-pharmacological treatments used to treat sleep disorders. Consequently, there is only sparse evidence upon which to base clinical practice. With one exception, all currently FDA-approved medications for treating insomnia are Schedule IV Controlled Substances that – while safe and effective for most treatment populations – are prone to abuse by patients with SUDs. Additional research on this patient population will further refine treatment strategies.

While nearly all substances carry some risk of sleep disruption, this chapter focuses primarily on substances of abuse. The evaluation and treatment of sleep disorders in patients with a current or past history of substance abuse will be also discussed in

Sleep and Mental Illness, eds. S. R. Pandi-Perumal and M. Kramer. Published by Cambridge University Press.
© Cambridge University Press 2010.

detail. We recognize that the majority of research has focused on alcohol-induced insomnia to the exclusion of other drugs, both licit and illicit. Much more research is needed on these other substances that can lead to chronic sleep difficulties. Sleep may provide a window into prevention and treatment of SUDs, which can be devastating for the individual, their family, and the community.

Substance-specific sleep disturbances

Alcohol

In healthy sleepers without a history of alcoholism, alcohol affects sleep differently in the first half compared to the second half of the night as alcohol is metabolized by the body. When alcohol is consumed close to bedtime, it shortens sleep onset latency (SOL) [6–8], prolongs rapid eye movement onset latency (ROL) [9], and increases slow-wave sleep (SWS) in the first half of the night [6, 7, 10]. Sleep quality worsens in the second half of the night. Stage 1 (S1) sleep, wakefulness, and the percentage of REM sleep increase [6], and SWS decreases [6, 7, 10].

Given alcohol's initial sedating properties, it is thought that adults with sleep problems may be more likely to turn to alcohol as a way to self-medicate. A laboratory study conducted by Roehrs et al. [11] suggests that subjects with insomnia drank alcohol for both its sleep and mood effects, particularly tension reduction. Moreover, in a forced choice paradigm across four nights in the sleep laboratory, when given the choice of color coded cups prior to bedtime, insomnia subjects chose the cups containing alcohol on 67% of the nights versus the non-insomniacs who chose the cups with alcohol on only 22% of the nights [11].

Sleep problems may also predispose an individual to developing an alcohol use disorder (AUD) or return to drinking alcohol [5, 12, 13] once abstinent. Our group reported on a longitudinal cohort of children at high risk for alcoholism, and found that mother-reported sleep difficulties in three- to five-year-old boys predicted earlier age of onset of drinking during early adolescence even after controlling for anxiety/depression, attention problems, and family history [14].

The onset measure is a robust indicator of problems with alcohol use in late adolescence, and it also is a strong predictor of AUD in adulthood (four-fold increase). More recent work with a larger sample of

the same cohort, and also including girls, replicated the male findings and also showed independent relationships of the early sleep difficulty to adolescent internalizing and externalizing problems [15]. This work suggests the predisposing factors tying sleep difficulties to later problem alcohol use are in place very early in life.

In an epidemiological study of more than 10,000 adults, the incidence of alcohol abuse over one year was twice as high in individuals with complaints of insomnia compared to those without insomnia complaints, after controlling for baseline psychiatric disorders [16]. Thus, both early-onset drinking [14] and new-onset alcohol abuse [16, 17] have been linked to a prior history of insomnia.

Insomnia is an extremely common sleep complaint in patients who are actively drinking alcohol as well as in patients who have stopped drinking. Across seven studies of 1,577 alcohol-dependent patients undergoing treatment, the average rate of self-reported insomnia was 58% (range = 36–91%) [18, 19], substantially higher than rates of insomnia among the general population. Alcohol-dependent patients with difficulty falling asleep may have abnormalities in their circadian rhythm, a critical sleep regulatory factor, that underlie the sleep complaint. One recent study, for example, revealed a delay in the onset of nocturnal melatonin secretion in alcohol-dependent patients compared to controls [20]. Another study suggested that, compared to healthy controls, alcohol-dependent individuals may have less homeostatic drive for sleep, a second factor necessary for sleep promotion, than healthy controls [21].

Sleep disordered breathing (SDB) has been shown to occur more frequently in alcohol-dependent patients, particularly in older males [22]. Moreover, results from an epidemiological investigation of the natural history of SDB show that men have a 25% greater chance of having mild SDB or worse SDB with every drink per day [23].

Movement disorders associated with sleep disruption, like restless legs syndrome [24] and periodic limb movements in sleep (PLMS), have been associated with individuals who consume ≥2 drinks/day. Aldrich and Shipley found that twice as many women who reported high alcohol use were diagnosed with periodic limb movement disorder compared to women reporting normal levels of alcohol consumption [25]. Recovering alcohol-dependent patients were also shown to have significantly more periodic limb movements associated with arousals from sleep (PLMA) than controls. Gann *et al.* found that PLMAs correctly predicted 80% of abstainers and 44% of relapsers after six months of abstinence [26].

In summary, both objective and subjective sleep problems may play a role in the development and course of AUDs, which has several implications for intervention. First, management of sleep problems in children may help prevent the early onset of alcohol use during young adolescence. Second, management of insomnia may help prevent AUDs from developing in adults. Finally, inquiry about sleep in patients with current AUD or a history of alcoholism may be an essential part of preventing relapse.

Nicotine

Most nicotine consumption occurs by smoking cigarettes, although the availability of nicotine replacement therapy to help people stop smoking is another important source with consequences for sleep. Nicotine increases catecholamines, vasopressin, growth hormone, adrenocorticotropic hormone, and endorphins in the brain, which can disturb sleep. The average cigarette contains 8 to 9 mg of nicotine, but the amount delivered varies because smokers can adjust dose by puffing volume, depth, rate, or intensity. Many studies, therefore, have employed the nicotine patch to regulate dose-dependent effects better [27].

Laboratory studies show that non-smokers with a nicotine patch took longer to fall asleep, had shorter TST, lower sleep efficiency (SE), and lower REM compared to participants with a placebo patch [28]. When a group of 62 light smokers were compared to 606 non-smokers, a greater percentage (39%) of light cigarette smokers (<15 cigarettes per day) reported chronic insomnia compared to non-smokers (31%) independent of health, demographics, behavioral, and psychological variables [29].

Depression history is associated with differences in REM sleep during nicotine exposure and withdrawal. A randomized controlled trial found that depressed non-smokers wearing nicotine patches showed increased REM sleep and short-term mood improvements compared to non-depressed non-smokers [30]. The increased REM sleep persisted during withdrawal in depressed patients, while REM sleep in non-depressed patients decreased [31].

Long-term studies have also found changes in sleep and mood disturbances for up to one year following smoking cessation. Heavy smokers (mean smoking history of 24 years) were studied across a smoking week and a withdrawal week. During the withdrawal week, smokers had more arousals, awakenings, and stage changes compared to the smoking week [32]. In the first long-term study across one year of abstinence, seven former chronic smokers (>20 cigarettes/day for at least ten years) who were not depressed underwent sleep studies at months 1, 2, 4, 6, 9, and 12. Rapid eye movement onset latency varied across the 12 months and then eventually decreased significantly from baseline. Interestingly, depression measures increased with abstinence and correlated with REM, ROL from sleep onset and S2, and stage shifts [33]. The authors posit that the increases in REM sleep and levels of depression may be due in part to an increased sensitivity of serotonergic neurons during withdrawal.

Other studies of sleep effects following smoking cessation have been reviewed elsewhere [34, 35]. Sleep disturbances during nicotine withdrawal have been shown to predict relapse to smoking cigarettes [36]. Finally, a developmental relationship between sleep problems in early childhood and early onset of occasional or regular smoking was also observed in the Michigan Longitudinal Study [14].

Marijuana

The vast majority of the research studies conducted on the effects of marijuana (MJ) on sleep indicate that sleep difficulties are present primarily during withdrawal. The few studies on bedtime administration of tetrahydrocannabinol (THC), the active ingredient in marijuana, have shown variable effects on sleep in normal volunteers, but study sample sizes have been universally small [37]. Marijuana taken at bedtime has been shown to increase (N = 7) [38], decrease (N = 2) [39] and to have no effect (N = 8) [40] on slow-wave sleep. Doses of 10, 20, and 30 mg of THC prior to sleep have decreased SOL after subjects reported achieving a "high" subjectively [41]. Studies are more conclusive with respect to sleep disruption during withdrawal from MJ. Among 1,735 frequent users of MJ (>21 occasions in a single year), 235 (13.5%) reported difficulty sleeping during withdrawal [42]. Another study reported that 33% of cannabis users had difficulty sleeping during withdrawal [43]. Difficulty falling asleep and decreased slow-wave sleep (SWS) percentage have also been documented by polysomnogram (PSG) during the first two nights of withdrawal [39], but no long-term sleep studies of previous MJ users have been conducted. Bolla *et al.* examined sleep of heavy MJ users (104 +/− 51 joints/week) in the three nights prior to and after MJ discontinuation. By the second night of withdrawal, MJ users demonstrated lower SE, shorter total sleep time (TST), longer SOL, and shorter ROL compared to controls [44], supporting the findings from previous studies that sleep is adversely affected during MJ withdrawal. Daytime consequences of MJ use prior to bedtime are reported only following higher doses of THC (15 mg THC plus 15 mg cannabidiol) and include increased sleepiness, mood changes, and impaired memory [40]. In summary, MJ may initially be associated with shorter latency to sleep in some individuals and can lead to sleep disruption across withdrawal. Here also, sleep problems in early childhood predicted early onset of MJ use in boys. A parallel relationship also was observed with early onset of other illicit drug use [14].

Cocaine and other stimulants

Self-administration of cocaine intranasally prior to sleep causes prolonged SOL, decreased SE, and decreased REM sleep [45]. Sleep problems have been shown to be the second most common complaint, behind depression, of patients during cocaine withdrawal. In one study, nearly three-quarters of a group of 75 active cocaine users complained of sleep disturbance during withdrawal [46]. During cocaine withdrawal, hypersomnia is typically observed, presumably compensation for extended sleep deprivation during binge use. Insomnia during withdrawal may also be observed, however, with a proportion of patients reporting poor quality sleep and prolonged latency to sleep [37]. One study found that specific complaints about sleep in abusers of smoked cocaine, who had been on a binge–abstinence cycle, did not surface until two weeks into withdrawal. These complaints became more intense thereafter [47].

The available data suggest that sleep complaints with amphetamine, metamphetamine, and methylphenidate abuse or dependence are similar to those reported with cocaine use disorders [48, 49]. The milder yet more widely used stimulant, caffeine, prolongs sleep onset latency and leads to complaints of insomnia due to its antagonist effects at adenosine receptors [50]. Some people are more sensitive to caffeine-induced insomnia than others, which may reflect genotypic differences [51, 52].

Opioids

Opioids can be used therapeutically for analgesic purposes or to assist medical detoxification of patients with addiction to illicit opioids such as heroin. Methadone and buprenorphine are also used for long-term maintenance treatment in opioid-dependent patients. Opioids with short half-lives (two to seven hours) are more prone to abuse than those with longer ones (with eight to twelve hours) [53]. Sleep laboratory studies suggest that opioids may affect sleep differently depending on whether or not the user is in pain and if the user is dependent on opioids. Opioids appear to have minimal impact on sleep continuity in healthy control subjects [54].

Subjective reports of opioid effects on sleep can vary. Many patients with pain report longer TST with opioids, presumably because of fewer pain-related arousals and awakenings [53]. Vella-Brincat *et al.* found an association between opioid use and reports of sleep disturbance, dreams, and nightmares in palliative care patients [55]. On the other hand, chronic pain patients with osteoarthritis reported sleeping better when their pain was relieved with tramadol [56]. Animal data suggest that sleep disruption may be a result of opioids decreasing GABA neurotransmission in the pontine reticular nucleus [57]. Opioids have also been associated with central sleep apnea in a dose-dependent fashion [58], occurring in about 30% of chronic users [59], a much higher rate than in the general population.

Objective sleep laboratory findings on methadone maintenance treatment (MMT) patients show that this group has more central sleep apnea, more frequent awakenings [60], lower SE, and lower SWS [61]. Subjective sleep quality is also impaired. Sleep assessments from 225 MMT patients showed that 84% reported clinically significant sleep disturbances as defined by a score on the Pittsburgh Sleep Quality Index (PSQI) of >5 (mean score [SD] = 10.64 [4.9]) [62]. A separate study also found elevated PSQI scores in a group of 101 MMT patients (mean [SD] = 9.4 [4.8]), which did not correlate with duration of MMT, gender, age, or abuse of opiates, cannabis, or cocaine [63]. Heroin-dependent patients detoxified with methadone reported even greater sleep problems than those maintained on methadone during the first months of heroin abstinence [64]. However, in an uncontrolled study, 57% of patients detoxified with a combination of buprenorphine and clonidine reported improved sleep [65].

Few studies have evaluated sleep across prolonged abstinence from opioids. Two early studies on male prisoners examined sleep across protracted methadone abstinence. Martin et al. found increased REM sleep and delta sleep after ten weeks of methadone withdrawal [66]. Kay found increased TST, decreased wake time, decreased REM sleep, and increased SWS across the 22-week study period of methadone abstinence [67].

In summary, similar to other substances of abuse discussed here, opioids can become deleterious to sleep with abuse or dependence. Early studies on prolonged methadone abstinence suggest that sleep may improve in MMT patients; however, studies longer than 22 weeks of abstinence are lacking.

Assessment

The clinical assessment of sleep complaints in patients with a current or past history of substance use disorder should include a thorough history of the sleep problem, particularly its chronicity with respect to the substance use. For patients with prominent complaints of insomnia, substances may not be the only cause. Usually, chronic insomnia has multiple perpetuating causes: other illnesses (i.e., psychiatric, medical, and sleep disorders), sleep-impairing medications (e.g., theophylline, activating antidepressants), inadequate sleep hygiene, and dysfunctional beliefs all need to be considered and addressed as appropriate. This issue is particularly relevant to patients with substance use disorders, who have high rates of co-occurring psychiatric and medical disorders. Nevertheless, substances are usually part of the problem, even if not necessarily the only cause of insomnia. Second, insomnia is a clinical diagnosis that does not typically require overnight sleep laboratory studies, including polysomnography, to make a diagnosis. According to the DSM-IV, insomnia is diagnosed when a patient has difficulty falling asleep, staying asleep, or feels that sleep is not refreshing for at least one month, and the sleep problem results in impairment in daytime functioning and/or clinically significant distress. A polysomnogram should be considered if there is high suspicion for other sleep disorders,

particularly sleep apnea and PLM disorder. This is particularly relevant to patients with a history of alcoholism, as it is known that rates of sleep apnea [22] and periodic limb movements [25] are higher in this population. A complete medication list should be considered when interpreting the results of the study. Treatment-resistant insomnia, when other causes are adequately treated, may also prompt an overnight sleep study. Third, assessment of sleep complaints is aided by asking patients to keep a sleep log for two weeks during early recovery after acute substance withdrawal symptoms have subsided. Sleep logs have several advantages, including an assessment of sleep patterns over time, documenting improvement with abstinence, and engaging the patient in the treatment process.

Treating sleep disorders in a substance-use population

Currently, insomnia is the most common sleep complaint managed by addiction medicine physicians. Other types of sleep complaints such as snoring or apnea are typically referred to a sleep disorders center. Physicians and other healthcare professionals working with patients who have a substance use disorder and insomnia are faced with unique challenges. They are often hesitant to prescribe a hypnotic for insomnia to a patient with a history of substance abuse or dependence because of the potential for abuse of that medication. This is especially true for the Schedule IV hypnotics (including benzodiazepine receptor agonists), which are first-line agents for insomnia in non-abusing patients with insomnia. Reticence may generalize to other commonly prescribed hypnotics and to over-the-counter agents, based on the rationale that any drug-induced sedation may reinforce an over-reliance on pills and/or provide a conditioned cue to trigger relapse to the substance of abuse. One study, for example, found that only 64% of 311 addiction treatment specialists reported prescribing a medication to improve sleep to a recovering alcoholic with insomnia during the first three months of detoxification [68]. Alternatively, other addiction physicians may assume that focusing on sleep disturbances in patients with substance use disorders is unnecessary because sleep complaints will likely remit when the substance use disorder has been adequately treated. Others may be less wary to prescribe Schedule IV hypnotics to patients with substance use disorders,

345

based on their efficacy and safety in other patient populations. Adjunctive patient contracts can sometimes be used in these cases. Lastly, limited awareness of other treatment options for insomnia may exist among the addiction community. Below, we outline the primary pharmacological and non-pharmacological treatments that are available for insomnia in patients with a history of substance use disorders.

Phamacological treatment options

Table 31.1 shows the most commonly used hypnotic agents for insomnia, their dose range, and pharmacokinetic profiles.

Benzodiazepines and benzodiazepine receptor agonists

Benzodiazepines and benzodiazepine receptor agonists (BzRAs) are safe and effective medications for the acute management of insomnia in non-substance abusing patients. However, because of the abuse liability of sedative-hypnotics in patients with a history of SUDs [69] and potential for overdose if mixed with alcohol or other CNS depressants, addiction specialists are appropriately reluctant to prescribe these agents to patients with a history of abuse.

Anticonvulsants

Selected anticonvulsants are commonly used in alcoholics for their sedative properties, in part because they do not lower the seizure threshold, an important issue given the risk of seizures in alcoholic-dependent patients. Gabapentin has a desirable hypnotic profile for this population because it has minimal known abuse potential, is not metabolized by the liver, does not interfere with the metabolism of other medications, and does not require blood monitoring for toxicity. In an open-label pilot study, alcohol-dependent patients with insomnia who were treated with gabapentin (mean dose [range] = 953 [200–1500] mg qhs), reported significantly improved sleep quality over a four- to six-week period [70]. When gabapentin (mean dose [range] = 888 [300–1800] mg qhs) was compared to trazodone (mean dose [range] = 105 [50–300] mg qhs) in another open pilot trial, both medications were associated with significantly improved scores on the Sleep Problems Questionnaire, but the gabapentin-treated group was less likely to feel tired upon awakening [71].

Furthermore, in a randomized double-blind trial of gabapentin in recently abstinent alcoholic patients with insomnia, the gabapentin group (median dose [range]=1,500 mg qhs [1,218–1,500 mg], had a delayed onset to heavy drinking across six weeks [72]. In summary, gabapentin has shown some promise as an effective medication to improve sleep in alcohol-dependent patients and may delay the return to drinking.

Antidepressants

Trazodone is the most commonly prescribed antidepressant medication for insomnia. Physicians tend to prescribe trazodone over other hypnotics because of its sedating side effect and low abuse potential. One randomized, double-blind trial among alcohol-dependent patients with insomnia showed that trazodone was associated with greater sleep improvements than placebo when measured via polysomnography [73]. Another study also showed superior sleep outcomes of trazodone vs. placebo over 12 weeks of treatment in alcohol-dependent patients, but indicated that problem drinking was *higher* in the trazodone-treated group compared to the placebo group [74]. The use of other sedating antidepressants, such as mirtazapine and doxepin, has not been studied in patients with substance use disorders.

Antipsychotics

Quetiapine is an atypical antipsychotic that is sometimes prescribed for sleep because of its sedating properties, likely due in part to antagonism of histamine, serotonin, and other CNS receptors [75] as well as reduction of nocturnal cortisol excretion [76]. In addition, several open-label pilot trials suggest that quetiapine may promote sleep and reduce relapse in substance-dependent patients [77–79].

Other hypnotics

Ramelteon, a melatonin receptor agonist approved for treatment of insomnia, may prove useful in alcohol-dependent patients, given the recent findings that melatonin levels are decreased in alcoholic patients [20], and because of its low abuse liability [69]. Studies in patients with substance use disorders are needed. Other over-the-counter remedies such as antihistamines, valerian, and melatonin have not been widely evaluated in substance abusing patients, although they are commonly used. Reasons

Table 31.1 Pharmacological options for insomnia in alcohol-dependent patients

Generic name	Trade name	Dose range (mg)	T_{MAX} (hr)[1]	$T_{1/2}$ (hr)[1]
FDA-approved medications to treat insomnia				
Benzodiazepine receptor agonists (with benzodiazepine chemical structures)				
Estazolam	ProSom	1–2	0.5–1.6	10–24
Flurazepam	Dalmane	15–30	3–6	50–100[2]
Quazepam	Doral	7.5–15	2	25–100[2]
Temazepam	Restoril	15–30	2–3	10–17
Triazolam	Halcion	0.125–0.5	1–2	1.5–5.5
Selective benzodiazepine receptor agonists (non-benzodiazepine structures)[3]				
Eszopiclone	Lunesta	1–3	1	~6
Zaleplon	Sonata	5–20	1	~1
Zolpidem	Ambien	5–10	1.6	2.5 (1.5–3.8)
Zolpidem CR	Ambien CR	6.25–12.5	1.5	2.8 (1.6–4)
Melatonin receptor agonist				
Ramelteon	Rozerem	8	0.5–1.5	1–2.6
FDA-approved medications for which insomnia treatment is off-label				
Sedating antidepressants				
Amitriptyline[4]	Elavil	25–150	2–8	5–45
Doxepin[4]	Sinequan	25–150	2–8	10–30
Mirtazapine	Remeron	7.5–45[5]	1–3	20–40
Nefazodone	Serzone	50–150	1	6–18[2]
Nortriptyline[4]	Pamelor	10–75[6]	2–8	20–55
Trazodone	Desyrel	25–300	1–2	3–9[7]
Sedating anticonvulsants				
Gabapentin	Neurontin	300–1,500	2–3	6–7
Sedating antipsychotics				
Quetiapine	Seroquel	25–100	1.5	6

Notes: All benzodiazepine receptor agonists are Schedule IV Controlled Substances, and should be used with caution, if at all, in alcohol-dependent patients.
[1]T_{MAX} = time to reach maximal plasma concentrations. $T_{1/2}$ = elimination half-life. All values are approximate for any given individual.
[2]Including active metabolites.
[3]Selective $GABA_A$ receptor agonists bind the alpha-1 protein subunit of $GABA_A$ receptors. Alpha-1 containing $GABA_A$ receptors are thought to mediate sedative and amnesic effects, but not anti-anxiety or muscle relaxant effects of the GABA system.
[4]Tricyclic antidepressants.
[5]Antihistaminergic effects predominate at low doses (7.5–15 mg).
[6]Can be titrated to a.m. level (50–150 mcg/ml) 12 hours after hs dose if no effect at lower doses.
[7]Major metabolite, mCPP, has 14-hour half-life.

for inconsistent findings with melatonin in healthy controls are unclear, but over-the-counter melatonin in the United States is not regulated by the FDA and the contents of any given product cannot be guaranteed.

Non-pharmacological treatment options

Cognitive behavioral therapy for insomnia (CBT-I) is a multicomponent treatment for insomnia that has been shown to have clinical efficacy for primary insomnia as well as insomnia that is comorbid with a number of different medical conditions. The goal of CBT-I is to address maladaptive behaviors used to cope with poor sleep and to counter dysfunctional beliefs and attitudes about sleep.

In a seminal study of older adults with insomnia but no history of addiction, CBT-I was superior to placebo and equally effective to a hypnotic alone (temazepam 7.5 and 30 mg) and to a hypnotic–CBT-I combination for reducing night-time wakefulness, increasing total sleep time, and increasing sleep efficiency. These initial treatment gains were maintained best in the group treated with CBT-I alone at two-year follow-up [80]. CBT-I has previously been viewed as contraindicated in patients with uncontrolled psychiatric disorders, but recent evidence suggests that higher remission rates can be achieved by combining CBT-I with a mood medication (escitalopram) compared to medication [81].

Cognitive behavioral therapy for insomnia encompasses several different treatment strategies for chronic insomnia. The most commonly used components of CBT-I are described below. Other components not discussed below may include progressive muscle relaxation, paradoxical intention, biofeedback, or light therapy.

Sleep restriction

Sleep restriction (SR) therapy addresses the common clinical finding that patients with insomnia spend an excessive amount of time in bed. The therapy temporarily restricts the time spent in bed and prohibits sleep at other times during the day. By restricting the allowable time for sleep over successive days, the homeostatic "sleep drive" or "pressure to sleep" presumably increases. The resulting mild sleep deprivation may promote consolidated sleep, leading to improvements in patient-reported sleep quality [82]. Once sleep is consolidated, sleep opportunity is gradually increased to relieve the daytime consequences associated with sleep deprivation, until optimal sleep quality and quantity is reached to maximize daytime functioning.

Stimulus control

Stimulus control (SC) helps patients with chronic insomnia who may develop habits that are incompatible with sleep (e.g., such as watching television in bed, talking on the phone in bed, or worrying about the fact that they are not sleeping while lying in bed). Over time, an association develops between the bed, the bedroom, and these sleep-incompatible activities. The goal of stimulus control is to alter this association by re-establishing the bed and bedroom with the pleasant experience of falling asleep and staying asleep [83].

Sleep hygiene

Sleep hygiene (SH) is an educational component of therapy that addresses behaviors that may help or hinder sleep. Patients with addiction may benefit from learning how drug use and withdrawal affects sleep or how substance use for sleep may exacerbate sleep problems. Other common recommendations include avoiding caffeine, nicotine, and exercise too close to bedtime, due to the stimulating effects of these behaviors. Sleep hygiene education should be only one facet of a multicomponent CBT-I treatment because SH in isolation is an insufficient treatment for insomnia [84–87].

Cognitive therapy

The goal of cognitive therapy in the context of CBT-I is to identify and explore dysfunctional attitudes and beliefs about sleep and to replace them with more appropriate self-statements that mitigate anxiety and worry about sleep problems and promote sleep-healthy behaviors. Common cognitive themes that are addressed include unrealistic sleep expectations, inability to control or predict sleep, and faulty beliefs about sleep-promoting practices. In patients with insomnia but no history of substance use disorders, improvements in sleep-related dysfunctional beliefs are positively associated with objective and subjective sleep improvements [88].

CBT-I for patients with addiction

Limited data exist on the effectiveness of CBT-I in patients with addiction. Two studies that have utilized this therapy with alcohol-dependent patients found improvements in subjective reports of sleep [89, 90]. Cognitive behavioral therapy for insomnia in alcohol-dependent patients also improved post-treatment scores on measures of anxiety and depression, fatigue, and some aspects of quality of life [89]. In a group setting, a six session CBT-I was used in 55 adolescents (aged 13 to 19) with insomnia complaints and a history of substance abuse. By the fourth session, subjective reports of sleep improved. By the final session (Session 6), adolescents reported decreased drug problems (as measured by the Substance Problem Index), which was maintained at one-year follow up [91]. In a small randomized study with 22 alcohol-dependent patients, patients who underwent ten, one-hour sessions of progressive muscle relaxation found greater improvement in sleep quality compared to a waiting list control. However, the study failed to use validated sleep measures [92].

Summary and conclusions

Insomnia and other sleep disturbances are exceedingly common during recovery in patients with addictions and may play a significant role in relapse. Pre-existing psychiatric conditions or the presence of a primary sleep disorder can predispose patients to developing insomnia. These factors must be elucidated as part of the chronology of the substance use disorder and insomnia. Although substance-induced sleep problems can improve with continued abstinence, persistent sleep problems may occur for at least two reasons. First, long-lasting alterations to the sleep centers of the brain may occur due to chronic drug exposure. Second, chronic sleep disturbance is typically associated with multiple perpetuating causes. Substance use may be just one of many reasons for sleep complaints. Assessment should consider the many causes of sleep disturbance. Pharmacological and non-pharmacological treatments exist to target insomnia associated with substance use disorders, but many are either inappropriate or have been inadequately tested in this specific patient population. More well controlled studies are needed to examine how sleep changes during recovery, to further explore the efficacy of the various treatment approaches in patients with addiction, and to evaluate the impact of such treatments on relapse and recovery.

References

1. Office of National Drug Policy. *The Economic Costs of Drug Abuse in the United States: 1992–2002.* (Washington, DC: Office of National Drug Policy, 2004).

2. Mokdad A, Marks J, Stroup D, Gerberding J. Actual causes of death in the United States, 2000. *JAMA.* 2004;**291**(10):1238–45.

3. Breslau N, Roth T, Rosenthal L, Andreski P. Sleep disturbance and psychiatric disorders: a longitudinal epidemiological study of young adults. *Biol Psychiatry.* 1996;**39**:411–18.

4. Wallander M, Johansson S, Ruigomez A, Garcia Rodriquez L, Jones R. Morbidity associated with sleep disorders in primary care: A longitudinal cohort study. *J Clin Psychiatry.* 2007;**9**:338–45.

5. Brower KJ. Insomnia, alcoholism and relapse. *Sleep Med Rev.* 2003;**7**(6):523–39.

6. MacLean A, Cairns J. Dose response effects on ethanol on the sleep of young men. *J Stud Alcohol.* 1982;**43**(5):434–44.

7. Williams D, MacLean A, Cairns J. Dose-response effects of ethanol on the sleep of young women. *J Stud Alcohol.* 1983;**44**(3):515–23.

8. Feige B, Gann H, Brueck R, *et al.* Effects of alcohol on polysomnographically recorded sleep in healthy subjects. *Alcohol Clin Exp Res.* 2006;**30**(9):1527–37.

9. Miyata S, Noda A, Atarashi M, *et al.* REM sleep is impaired by a small amount of alcohol in young women sensitive to alcohol. *Int Med.* 2004;**43**:679–84.

10. Allen R, Wagman A, Funderburk F. Slow wave sleep changes: alcohol tolerance and treatment implications *Adv Exp Med Biol.* 1977;**85A**:629–40.

11. Roehrs T, Papineau K, Rosenthal L, Roth T. Ethanol as a hypnotic in insomniacs: self administration and effects on sleep and mood. *Neuropsychopharmacology.* 1999;**20**(3):279–86.

12. Blumenthal S, Fine T. Sleep abnormalities associated with mental and addictive disorders: implications for research and clinical practice. *J Prac Psychiatry Behav Health.* 1996;**2**:67–79.

13. Brower KJ. Alcohol's effects on sleep in alcoholics. *Alcohol Res Health.* 2001;**25**:110–25.

14. Wong M, Brower KJ, Fitzgerald H, Zucker R. Sleep problems in early childhood and early onset of alcohol and other drug use in adolescence. *Alcohol Clin Exp Res.* 2004;**28**(4):578–87.

15. Wong M, Brower K, Zucker R. Childhood sleep problems, early onset of substance use, and behavioral problems in adolescence. *Sleep Med.* 2009;**10**(7):787–96.

16. Weissman MM, Greenwald S, Nino-Murcia G, Dement W. The morbidity of insomnia uncomplicated

by psychiatric disorders. *Gen Hosp Psychiatry.* 1997;**19**:245–50.

17. Ford D, Kamerow B. Epidemiologic study of sleep disturbances and psychiatric disorders. An opportunity for prevention? *JAMA.* 1989;**262**:1479–84.

18. Brower KJ, Aldrich M, Robinson EAR, Zucker RA, Greden JF. Insomnia, self-medication, and relapse to alcoholism. *Am J Psychiatry.* 2001;**158**:399–404.

19. Cohn T, Foster J, Peters T. Sequential studies of sleep disturbance and quality of life in abstaining alcoholics. *Addict Biol.* 2003;**8**:455–62.

20. Kühlwein E, Hauger RL, Irwin MR. Abnormal nocturnal melatonin secretion and disordered sleep in abstinent alcoholics. *Biol Psychiatry.* 2003;**54**:1437–43.

21. Irwin M, Gillin J, Dang J, *et al.* Sleep deprivation as a probe of homeostatic sleep regulation in primary alcoholics. *Biol Psychiatry.* 2002;**51**(8):632–41.

22. Aldrich MS, Brower KJ, Hall JM. Sleep-disordered breathing in alcoholics. *Alcohol Clin Exp Res.* 1999;**23**:134–40.

23. Peppard P, Austin D, Brown R. Association of alcohol consumption and sleep disordered breathing in men and women. *J Clin Sleep Med.* 2007;**3**(3):265–70.

24. Edinger J, Fins A, Sullivan R, *et al.* Sleep in the laboratory and sleep at home: Comparisons of older insomniacs and normal sleepers. *Sleep.* 1997;**20**(12):1119–26.

25. Aldrich M, Shipley J. Alcohol use and periodic limb movements of sleep. *Alcohol Clin Exp Res.* 1993;**17**(1):192–6.

26. Gann H, Feige B, van Calker D, Voderholzer U, Riemann D. Periodic limb movements during sleep in alcohol dependent patients. *Eur Arch Psychiatry Neurosci.* 2002;**252**:124–9.

27. Aubin H, Luthringer R, Demazieres A, Dupont C, Lagrue G. Comparison of the effects of a 24-hour nicotine patch and a 16-hour nicotine patch on smoking urges and sleep. *Nicotine Tob Res.* 2006;**8**:193–201.

28. Davila D, Hurt R, Offord K, Harris C, Shepard J. Acute effects of transdermal nicotine on sleep architecture, snoring, and sleep disordered breathing in nonsmokers. *Am J Respir Crit Care Med.* 1994;**150**:469–74.

29. Riedel B, Durrence H, Lichstein K, Taylor D. The relation between smoking and sleep: the influence of smoking level, health, and psychological variables. *Behav Sleep Med.* 2004;**2**(1):63–78.

30. Salin-Pascual R, de la Fuente J, Galicia-Polo L, Drucker-Colin R. Effects of transdermal nicotine on mood and sleep in nonsmoking major depressed patients. *Psychopharmacology (Berl).* 1995;**121**(4):476–9.

31. Wetter DW, Carmack C, Anderson C, *et al.* Tobacco withdrawal signs and symptoms among women with and without a history of depression. *Exp Clin Psychopharmacol.* 2000;**8**(1):88–96.

32. Prosise G, Bonnet M, Berry R, Dickel M. Effects of abstinence from smoking on sleep and daytime sleepiness. *Chest.* 1994;**105**(4):1136–41.

33. Moreno-Coutino A, Calderon-Ezquerro C, Drucker-Colin R. Long-term changes in sleep and depressive symptoms of smokers in abstinence. *Nicotine Tob Res.* 2007;**9**:389–96.

34. Colrain I, Trinder J, Swan G. The impact of smoking cessation on objective and subjective markers of sleep: review, synthesis, and recommendations. *Nicotine Tob Res.* 2004;**6**:913–25.

35. Hughes J. Effects of abstinence from tobacco: valid symptoms and time course. *Nicotine Tob Res.* 2007;**9**:315–27.

36. Boutou A, Tsiata E, Pataka A, *et al.* Smoking cessation in clinical practice: predictors of six-month continuous abstinence in a sample of Greek smokers. *Prim Care Respir J.* 2008;**17**:32–8.

37. Schierenbeck T, Riemann D, Berger M, Hornyak M. Effect of illicit recreational drugs upon sleep: cocaine, ecstasy, and marijuana. *Sleep Med Rev.* 2008;**12**(5):381–9.

38. Pivik R, Zarcone V, Dement W, Hollister L. Delta-9-tetrahydrocannabinol and synhexyl; effects on human sleep patterns. *Clin Pharmacol Ther.* 1972;**13**:426–35.

39. Freemon F. The effect of chronically administered delta-9-tetrahydrocannabinol upon the polygraphically monitored sleep of normal volunteers. *Drug Alcohol Depend.* 1982;**10**(4):345–53.

40. Nicholson A, Turner C, Stone B, Robson P. Effect of delta-9-tetrahydrocannabinol and cannabidiol on nocturnal sleep and early morning behavior in young adults *J Clin Psychopharmacol.* 2004;**24**(3):305–13.

41. Cousens K, Dimascio A. Delta-9-THC as an hypnotic. An experimental study of 3 dose levels. *Psychopharmacologia.* 1973;**33**(4)355–64.

42. Wiesbeck G, Schuckit M, Kalmijn J, *et al.* An evaluation of the history of marijuana withdrawal syndrome in a large population. *Addiction.* 1996;**91**(10):1469–78.

43. Copersino M, Boyd S, Tashkin D, *et al.* Cannabis withdrawal among non-treatment-seeking adult cannabis users. *Am J Addict.* 2006;**15**:8–14.

44. Bolla K, Lesage S, Gamaldo C, *et al.* Sleep disturbance in heavy marijuana users. *Sleep.* 2008;**31**(6):901–8.

45. Johanson C, Roehrs T, Schuh K, Warbasse L. The effects of cocaine on mood and sleep in cocaine-dependent males. *Exp Clin Psychopharmacol.* 1999;**7**(4):338–46.

46. Brower K, Maddahian E, Blow F, Beresford T. A comparison of self reported symptoms and DSM-III-R criteria for cocaine withdrawal. *Am J Drug Alcohol Abuse.* 1988;**14**(3):347–56.

47. Pace-Schott E, Stickgold R, Mazur A, *et al.* Sleep quality deteriorates over a binge-abstinence cycle in chronic smoked cocaine users. *Psychopharmacology.* 2005;**179**:873–83.

48. Gossop M, Bradley B, Brewis R. Amphetamine withdrawal and sleep disturbance. *Drug Alcohol Depend.* 1982;**10**:177–83.

49. McGregor C, Srisurapanont M, Jittiwutikarn J, *et al.* The nature, time course and severity of methamphetamine withdrawal. *Addiction.* 2005;**100**:1320–9.

50. Paterson L, Wilson S, Nutt D, Hutson P, Ivarsson M. Translational, caffeine-induced model of onset insomnia in rats and healthy volunteers. *Psychopharmacology.* 2007;**191**(4):943–50.

51. Retey J, Adam M, Khatami R, *et al.* A genetic variation in the adenosine A2A receptor gene (ADORA2A) contributes to individual sensitivity to caffeine effects on sleep. *Clin Pharmacol Ther.* 2007;**81**(5):692–8.

52. Luciano M, Zhu G, Kirk K, *et al.* "No thanks, it keeps me awake": the genetics of coffee-attributed sleep disturbance. *Sleep.* 2007;**30**:1378–86.

53. Gillin J, Drummond S, Clark C, Moore P. Medication and substance abuse. In: Kryger M, Roth T, Dement WC, eds. *Principles and Practice of Sleep Medicine,* 4th ed. (Philadelphia: Elsevier Saunders; 2005).

54. Dimsdale J, Norman D, DeJardin D, Wallace MS. The effect of opioids on sleep architecture. *J Clin Sleep Med.* 2007;**3**(1):33–6.

55. Vella-Brincat J, Macleod A. Adverse effects of opioids on the central nervous systems of palliative care patients. *J Pain Palliat Care Pharmacother.* 2007;**21**(1):15–25.

56. Kosinski M, Janagap C, Gajria K, Freedman J. Pain relief and pain related sleep disturbance with extended release tramadol in patients with osteoarthritis. *Curr Med Res Opin.* 2007;**23**(7):1615–26.

57. Watson C, Lydic R, Baghdoyan H. Sleep and GABA levels in the oral part of rat pontine reticular formation are decreased by local and systemic administration of morphine. *Neuroscience.* 2007;**144**(1):375–86.

58. Walker J, Farney R, Rhondeau S, *et al.* Chronic opioid use is a risk factor for the development of central sleep apnea and ataxic breathing. *J Clin Sleep Med.* 2007;**3**(5):455–61.

59. Teicher M, Wang D. Sleep disordered breathing with chronic opioid use. *Expert Opin Drug Saf.* 2007;**6**(6):641–9.

60. Staedt J, Wassmuth F, Stoppe G. Effects of chronic treatment with methadone and naltrexone on sleep in addicts. *Eur Arch Psychiatry Clin Neurosci.* 1996;**246**:305–9.

61. Teichtahl H, Prodromidis A, Miller B, Cherry G, Kronberg I. Sleep-disordered breathing in stable methadone programme patients: a pilot study. *Addiction.* 2001;**96**:395–403.

62. Stein M, Herman D, Bishop S, *et al.* Sleep disturbances among methadone maintained patients. *J Subst Abuse Treat.* 2004;**26**(3):175–80.

63. Peles E, Schreiber S, Adelson M. Variables associated with perceived sleep disorders in methadone maintenance treatment (MMT) patients. *Drug Alcohol Depend.* 2006;**82**(2):103–10.

64. Shi J, Zhao L, Epstein D, Zhang X, Lu L. Long-term methadone maintenance reduces protracted symptoms of heroin abstinence and cue-induced craving in Chinese heroin abusers. *Pharmacol Biochem Behav.* 2007;**87**(1):141–5.

65. Wallen M, Lorman W, Gosciniak J. Combined buprenorphine and chlonidine for short term opiate detoxification: patient perspectives. *J Addict Dis.* 2006;**25**(1):23–31.

66. Martin W, Jasinki D, Haertzen C, *et al.* Methadone: a reevaluation. *Arch Gen Psychiatry.* 1973;**28**(2):286–95.

67. Kay D. Human sleep and EEG through a cycle of methadone dependence. *Electroencephalogr Clin Neurophysiol.* 1975;**38**(1):35–43.

68. Friedmann P, Herman D, Freedman S, *et al.* Treatment of sleep disturbance in alcohol recovery: a national survey of addiction medicine physicians. *J Addict Dis.* 2003;**22**:91–103.

69. Griffiths RR, Johnson MW. Relative abuse liability of hypnotic drugs: a conceptual framework and algorithm for differentiating among compounds. *J Clin Psychiatry.* 2005;**66** (Suppl 9):31–41.

70. Karam-Hage M, Brower K. Gabapentin treatment for insomnia associated with alcohol dependence. *Psychiatry Clin Neurosci.* 2000;**157**:151.

71. Karam-Hage M, Brower K. Open pilot study of gabapentin versus trazodone to treat insomnia in alcoholic patients. *Psychiatry Clin Neurosci.* 2003;**57**:542–4.

72. Brower K, Kim HM, Strobbe S, *et al.* A randomized double-blind pilot trial of gabapentin versus placebo to

351

treat alcohol dependence and comorbid insomnia. *Alcohol Clin Exp Res.* 2008;**32**(8):1–10.

73. Le Bon O, Murphy J, Staner L, *et al.* Double-blind, placebo controlled study of the efficacy of trazodone in alcohol post-withdrawal sydrome: polysomnography and clinical evaluations. *J Clin Psychopharmacol.* 2003;**23**:377–83.

74. Friedmann P, Rose J, Swift R, *et al.* Trazodone for sleep disturbance after detoxification from alcohol dependence: a double-blind, placebo-controlled trial. *18th Annual Meeting and Symposium of the American Academy of Addiction Psychiatry*; 2007. (Coronado, CA: American Academy of Addiction Psychiatry, 2007).

75. Cohrs S, Pohlmann K, Guan Z, *et al.* Quetiapine reduces nocturnal urinary cortisol excretion in healthy subjects. *Psychopharmacologia.* 2004;**174**:414–20.

76. Cohrs S, Rodenbeck A, Guan Z, *et al.* Sleep-promoting properties of quetiapine in healthy subjects. *Psychopharmacol* 2004;**174**:421–9.

77. Croissant B, Klein O, Gehrlein L, *et al.* Quetiapine in relapse prevention in alcoholics suffering from craving and affective symptoms: a case series. *Eur Psychiatry.* 2006;**21**:570–3.

78. Monnelly E, Ciraulo D, Knapp C, LoCastro J, Sepulvda I. Quetiapine for treatment of alcohol dependence. *J Clin Psychopharmacol.* 2004;**24**:532–5.

79. Sattar SP, Bhatia S, Petty F. Potential benefit of quetiapine in the treatment of substance dependence disorders. *J Psychiatry Neurosci.* 2004;**29**(6):452–7.

80. Morin C, Colecchi C, Stone J, Sood R, Brink D. Behavioral and pharmacological therapies for late life insomnia: a randomized controlled trial. *JAMA.* 1999;**281**:991–9.

81. Manber R, Edinger J, Gress J, *et al.* Cognitive behavioral therapy for insomnia enhances depression outcome in patients with comorbid major depressive disorder and insomnia. *Sleep.* 2008;**31**(4):489–95.

82. Spielman A, Saskin P, Thorpy M. Treatment of chronic insomnia by restriction of time in bed. *Sleep.* 1987;**10**:45–56.

83. Bootzin R, Nicassio P. Behavioral treatments for insomnia. In: Hersen M, Eissler R, Miller P, eds. *Progress in Behavior Modification.* (New York, NY: Academic Press, 1978).

84. Edinger J, Sampson W. A primary care "friendly" cognitive behavioral insomnia therapy *Sleep.* 2003;**26**:177–82.

85. Engle-Friedman M, Bootzin R, Hazlewood L, Tsao C. An evaluation of behavioral treatments for insomnia in the older adult. *J Consult Clin Psychol.* 1992;**48**:77–90.

86. Friedman L, Benson K, Noda A. An actigraphic comparison of sleep restriction and sleep hygiene treatments for insomnia in older adults. *J Geriatric Psychiatry Neurol.* 2000;**13**:17–27.

87. Guilleminault C, Clerk A, Black J. Nondrug treatment trials in psychophysiological insomnia. *Arch Int Med.* 1995;**155**:838–44.

88. Edinger JD, Wohlgemuth WK, Radtke RA, Marsh GR, Quillian RE. Does cognitive-behavioral insomnia therapy alter dysfunctional beliefs about sleep? *Sleep.* 2001;**24**(5):591–9.

89. Arnedt J, Conroy D, Rutt J, *et al.* An open trial of cognitive-behavioral treatment for insomnia comorbid with alcohol dependence. *Sleep Med.* 2007;**8**(2):176–80.

90. Currie S, Clark S, Hodgins D, El-Guebaly N. Randomized controlled trial of brief cognitive-behavioural interventions for insomnia in recovering alcoholics. *Addiction.* 2004;**99**(9):1121–32.

91. Bootzin RR, Stevens SJ. Adolescents, substance abuse, and the treatment of insomnia and daytime sleepiness. *Clin Psychol Rev.* 2005;**25**:629–44.

92. Greeff A, Conradie W. Use of progressive relaxation training for chronic alcoholics with insomnia. *Psychol Rep.* 1998;**82**:407–12.

Chapter 32

Sleep following traumatic brain injury

Marie-Christine Ouellet, Simon Beaulieu-Bonneau, and Charles M. Morin

Introduction

Each year in the United States, it is estimated that more than 1.5 million individuals sustain a traumatic brain injury (TBI) ranging from minor to severe [1]. Often referred to as a silent epidemic, TBI can result in significant disability and major costs for patients, families, and society, even when the injury seems mild. Among the many residual and persistent sequelae of TBI, sleep complaints have been reported in proportions varying from 30 to 70% [2]. Despite their prevalence and early studies to point out their importance, it is only recently that a more vigorous scientific interest in sleep disturbances following TBI has grown. Rehabilitation clinicians have been more and more aware of the potential impacts of poor sleep on functional recovery after a brain injury. The presence of sleep–wake cycle disturbances has been linked to prolonged stays in the trauma as well as rehabilitation centers [3]. Indeed, although sleep disturbances may be perceived as secondary relative to more noticeable sequelae brought about by TBI such as cognitive impairments or physical limitations, problems sleeping at night and staying awake during the day can exacerbate other TBI-related symptoms such as pain, cognitive deficits, fatigue, or irritability. Sleep disturbances thus may actually compromise the rehabilitation process and significantly hinder TBI survivors' capacity to reintegrate social participative roles.

Overview of traumatic brain injury and its consequences

Epidemiological data on TBI are scarce and vary considerably across sources, in part because of the lack of a standard definition and a large proportion of TBI cases remaining unreported. In the United States, the annual incidence rate of TBI is estimated to be around 500 to 600 per 100,000 inhabitants [4, 5]. Of this number, approximately 75 to 80% require a visit to an emergency room, 15 to 20% lead to hospitalization, and 3 to 5% are fatal. The mechanism of brain lesion can be either open/penetrating or closed/blunt, the latter type being characteristic of more than 95% of all cases [6]. Brain injuries are also classified according to their severity, for which there are several approaches of classification, none being consensual. In this chapter, a three-level severity classification, including mild, moderate, and severe TBI, will be referred to most often. Several publications use the terms *concussion* or *minor TBI*, which can be included in the general category of mild injuries. The vast majority of TBI are mild (80%), 10% are moderate, and 10% are severe [1]. Traumatic brain injury severity is assessed shortly after the injury based on a set of criteria that usually include a combination of the following: duration of loss (coma) or alteration of consciousness, duration of post-traumatic amnesia, results of brain imagery (presence or absence of visible cerebral lesions), presence of neurological signs, and initial score on the Glasgow Coma Scale [7]. The Glasgow Coma Scale is a widely used assessment tool with a total score ranging from 3 to 15 (3–8: severe TBI; 9–12: moderate TBI; 13–15: mild TBI) summing up three components: eye, verbal, and motor response.

Falls and vehicle accidents are the most frequent causes of TBI, the latter yielding more serious injuries and increased mortality [5]. The age distribution of the incidence of TBI is characterized by higher frequency peaks among infants (<1 year old; most common mechanism: falls), adolescents and young adults (15–24 years old; vehicle accidents, aggressions,

Sleep and Mental Illness, eds. S. R. Pandi-Perumal and M. Kramer. Published by Cambridge University Press.
© Cambridge University Press 2010.

suicide attempts), and older adults (>75 years old; falls) [5, 8]. Other factors of increased risk of TBI include male gender (1.5 to 2.5:1 ratio compared to females), low socioeconomic status, low education level, unemployment, and alcohol and drug abuse [1, 8]. Brain injuries sustained in a military context (shell-shock or blast-related brain trauma) are also becoming the object of increasing attention.

The pathophysiological presentation of TBI is heterogeneous, depending on several factors such as the nature of the external forces engaged during the accident (i.e., direct impact, acceleration/deceleration, penetrating object, or blast waves) and the localization of lesions. Brain damage can be delineated in two stages [9, 10]. At the moment of impact, primary damage occurs, including focal lesions (i.e., contusions, lacerations, hematomas) and diffuse injuries to cerebral tissue (i.e., brain swelling, microscopic white matter lesions known as diffuse axonal injury). Secondary damage, evolving over hours and days following the impact as a result of primary damage, is characterized by cerebral ischemia and elevated intracranial pressure involving a cascade of interacting pathological processes (e.g., neurotransmitter release, inflammatory responses). There is also evidence that secondary damage may continue its course up to months or even years following the initial injury through the degeneration of neuronal fibers leading to long-term brain atrophy [11].

Outcome and prognosis after TBI are variable across individuals and influenced by a variety of factors (e.g., age, presence of injuries to other physiological systems, history of multiple TBI, personal and environmental resources), one of the most important being the severity of injury. Mild TBI is associated with a full functional recovery within 3 to 12 months post-injury for a large majority of individuals [12]. However, around 15% of people sustaining a mild TBI experience long-term consequences [13, 14]. There is evidence that even mild brain injury can cause structural damage to neurons, which may explain common persisting symptoms such as dizziness, headaches, cognitive impairments, depression, and sleep problems [15]. After moderate or severe TBI, about 85% of the recovery is thought to occur during the first six months, during which time most patients receive inpatient or outpatient rehabilitation services [9]. Subsequent permanent after effects are far more frequent and disabling than after mild TBI. Long-term changes can affect several domains, including cognition (e.g., attention, learning, or executive functioning), physical function (e.g., motor impairments), mental health (e.g., irritability, impulsivity, mood disorders), and functional/occupational capacities (e.g., unsuccessful return to work) [13].

Sleep disorders are also extremely common following TBI of all severities. While these problems have recently received increasing attention in the scientific literature, several researchers have stressed the importance of a better understanding of sleep disturbances and disorders and their correlates to improve early diagnosis and effective treatment of these conditions in individuals with TBI [16–19]. This is particularly relevant given that these sleep problems can be associated with or even hamper physical, cognitive, or functional consequences of TBI.

Etiology of sleep disturbances following TBI
Pathophysiological factors

The physiological processes leading to alterations in sleep following TBI remain poorly described. Via primary or secondary processes, damage to specific structures or systems involved in sleep regulation (e.g., suprachiasmatic nuclei of the hypothalamus, reticular activating system, pontine nuclei) or to connections between structures and systems may explain the appearance of sleep disorders following TBI.

Early animal studies indicate that the brainstem and reticular formation may be particularly vulnerable to experimentally provoked cerebral concussions because of converging forces in this area, particularly in mesencephalic–diencephalic structures [20–23]. In 1956, Strich did postmortem brain studies in individuals with dementia having survived several months after a head trauma. She noted numerous minute lesions in the brain stem as well as diffusely throughout the white matter and basal ganglia [24]. Some authors have suggested that trauma may induce premature aging of the brain stem structures, for example through a decrease in catecholamines [25].

It has been suggested that intracranial pressure control during sleep is altered by TBI. Regulated through circadian factors, intracranial pressure is normally higher during sleep compared to waking hours. This augmentation could be exaggerated in persons with TBI whose intracranial pressure is already heightened and these changes could affect sleep quality [26, 27].

Hormonal changes during nocturnal sleep have also been reported after TBI. Comparing TBI patients to healthy control subjects, Frieboes and colleagues noted alterations in the secretion of growth hormone and prolactin in the TBI group, possibly caused by diffuse lesions to the hypothalamus [28]. These hormonal secretion patterns were found to be similar to those observed in patients with remitted depression. The authors suggested three hypotheses to explain this resemblance: (1) similarly to depression, hormonal changes following TBI represent a biological scar resulting from anomalies that took place during the acute phase of the illness; (2) TBI is followed by intensive interventions that generate significant stress, thus provoking changes in the activity of certain hormones that play a role in depression; and (3) the frequent administration of corticosteroids to stabilize intracranial pressure after TBI may affect the secretion of growth hormone or prolactin, thus disturbing the continuity of sleep.

Recent data indicate that, similarly to patients suffering from narcolepsy, many patients with TBI have significantly decreased secretion of hypocretin-I – a hypothalamic neuropeptide involved in sleep–wake regulation – especially during the acute phase following trauma [29, 30]. This decrease in hypocretin seems more pronounced in moderate to severe TBI. This finding suggests that alterations in hypothalamic function may explain the development of disorders of the sleep–wake cycle after head trauma.

Other pathophysiological factors need to be investigated more fully to understand the etiology of sleep disorders after TBI. For example, the apolipoprotein E (*APOE*) genotype and more specifically its ϵ4 allele has been linked to adverse outcomes following TBI (mortality, vegetative state, disability) and could also be linked to sleep disorders after TBI. Indeed Sundström and colleagues recently found that post-TBI fatigue was especially pronounced for mild TBI patients who were carriers of the *APOE* ϵ4 allele [31]. The *APOE* ϵ4 allele is also known to be associated with obstructive sleep apnea [32].

Medications

The different pharmacological agents administered to patients who suffered a brain injury (e.g., corticosteroids, sedatives, analgesics, myorelaxants, anticonvulsants, antidepressants) can also alter the quality, quantity, and architecture of sleep as well as influence daytime levels of fatigue or sleepiness [33]. The mere timing of the administration of these medications can cause problems in sleep–wake patterns [33, 34]. Psychotropic medications, especially antidepressants – which are very frequently prescribed following TBI – have various impacts on sleep architecture. Some have been shown to increase REM sleep latency [35–37] as well as decrease stage 1 sleep [38, 39]. Other more energizing antidepressants (e.g., selective serotonin reuptake inhibitors) may also produce sleep disorders.

Pain

Pain can cause significant arousal thereby potentially affecting both sleep onset and sleep continuity. Pain has been associated with frequent intrusions of wakefulness into non-REM sleep, a condition referred to as alpha–delta sleep [40]. It has been suggested that approximately 60% to 80% of TBI survivors endure pain and that those with pain complaints also have significantly more insomnia complaints [41]. A recent systematic review indicates that 57.8% of TBI survivors suffer from chronic headaches. Other types of pain are also extremely common. Pain is also present – and sometimes even more frequent – in cases of mild injuries and it is not necessarily related to comorbid psychological problems (e.g., depression, post-traumatic stress disorder). Our team found that pain ratings significantly predicted the presence of insomnia in a cohort of mainly moderate to severe brain injury survivors [42].

Environmental factors

Hospital and rehabilitation environments may contribute to sleep problems following TBI. The sleep of patients treated for an illness or an injury in an intensive care unit is known to be significantly impaired due to multiple factors such as the illness of the patient, various and frequent therapeutic or diagnostic procedures, pain and anxiety produced by these procedures, the lack of zeitgebers, noise, etc. [43]. Polysomnographic studies of sleep in the intensive care unit (ICU) have found prolonged sleep latencies, fragmentation of sleep (arousals, decreased sleep efficiency), and significant decreases or even absence of stages 3, 4, and REM sleep [44, 45]. Following treatment in the ICU, during the hospital stay and the inpatient rehabilitation periods, sleep disturbances can also be brought about by environmental factors (e.g., noise, light, bed discomfort), as well as psychological and behavioral factors related to the environment (e.g., anxiety, loneliness) and sleep scheduling factors such as excessive time spent in bed. Cohen and colleagues reported that 81% of patients hospitalized for acquired brain injury complained of problems with either initiating or maintaining sleep, and 36% of them considered that the hospital environment was an important cause of their sleep problems [46].

Upon returning home or to another community location, TBI patients may again be faced with changes in their environment and sleep–wake routines. Maladjustment to these changes can thus also contribute to the development or maintenance of sleep problems. For example, many persons having suffered a brain injury are unable to return to work and therefore lack the routine associated with structured work schedules (e.g., fixed arising time, regular lunch time, regular bedtime). This may lead to excessive time spent in bed or more variable sleep–wake schedules.

Psychosocial stressors and comorbid psychopathology

Traumatic brain injury patients are likely to experience multiple psychosocial stressors such as major emotional adjustments to newly acquired cognitive and physical limitations, inability to return to work, problems with interpersonal relationships, and litigation. These stressors can translate into increased cognitive and emotional arousal at bedtime or during the night in the form of worrying, anxiety, rumination, or somatized tension [47]. Sleep problems can thus be set off by such psychosocial stressors at different times following an injury: in the acute period, during rehabilitation, upon returning home, upon reintegrating previous social roles, as well as many years post-injury if coping with permanent limitations is still stressful. If a person has difficulty coping effectively with such stressors, depression or anxiety may develop and exacerbate post-TBI sleep problems. Recent studies using standardized DSM-IV criteria have found prevalence rates of major depression following TBI varying between 17% and 61% [48–51]. Jorge and colleagues found that approximately 60% to 75% of the TBI patients who developed major depression also suffered from an anxiety disorder [50, 52]. Sleep disturbances in TBI may thus in part be due to comorbid psychopathology. In turn, sleep disturbances secondary to TBI could also be contributing to the development of depression, anxiety, and other psychological complications.

Polysomnographic studies of sleep following TBI

Until recently, there had been very few objective studies of sleep following TBI. The last few years, however, have seen a renewed interest in impacts of brain injury on sleep architecture, with a wave of studies published between 2006 and 2008. Although the early literature was limited by the lack of control groups in most studies and different methodologies to measure sleep, the most recent literature reflects attention towards the use of appropriate comparison groups, operationalized definitions of sleep disorders, and the use of standardized techniques such as polysomnography (PSG), actigraphy, and physiological measures of sleepiness.

Changes in sleep continuity

By far the most robust finding emerging from the growing literature on objective measures of sleep following TBI is that of increased fragmentation of sleep: at least seven studies reported increased time spent awake, more frequent awakenings, or decreased sleep efficiency in TBI patients [53–59]. These results corroborate the subjective complaints of sleep disturbances (i.e., symptoms of insomnia) reported by a large proportion of persons with TBI.

It is thus clear that a traumatic brain insult has general effects on sleep continuity and architecture (i.e., sleep stages), and this finding has been reported across the entire severity continuum, from minor/mild to severe TBI. This finding also seems to be consistent regardless of time since injury.

Changes in the macrostructure of sleep

Early studies in comatose patients indicate that sleep stages may be difficult to distinguish acurately following brain trauma, and that an absence of spontaneous sleep activity is more often associated with a poor prognosis such as a vegetative state or even death [60–62]. Conversely, EEG patterns resembling normal sleep are linked to a better prognosis and even improved cognitive recuperation [62–65]. Beyond the acute phase following brain injury, however, PSG measures of sleep seem to lose their prognostic value [62, 66].

Several studies have found increased percentages of either stage 1 [55, 58, 67] or stage 2 sleep [58, 67, 68]. In line with the view initially reported by George and colleagues [53], Schreiber and colleagues suggest that the increase in light sleep may be a "premature-like aging" process in TBI, whereby the sleep of these mainly young adults starts to resemble the sleep patterns seen in aging adults (45–50 years) where stages 1 and 2 become more prominent than slow-wave sleep [68]. Increased light sleep may account for more frequent subjective sleep complaints of difficulty falling asleep and feelings of fragmented or unrefreshing sleep in this population [55].

Most studies did not report significant changes in deep or slow-wave sleep in their samples of patients with TBI. However, one research team recently noted an increased proportion of slow-wave sleep and suggested possible mechanisms to explain this change: diffuse injuries may alter the homeostatic processes of sleep in TBI or EEG slow-wave activity may be increased due to neural reorganization or plasticity, which is thought to be intense in TBI patients due to continuous demands to adapt and relearn skills following an injury [56].

In a study examining sleep one to six months following severe TBI, Ron and colleagues were the first to document decreased REM sleep in these patients [62]. Another study with 16 young adults with severe injury corroborated this finding, but REM-sleep abnormalities had normalized by their 12-month follow-up [53]. Recently, Parcell and colleagues compared the sleep architecture of ten individuals with severe TBI to that of ten age- and sex-matched controls and confirmed that REM sleep is a vulnerable sleep stage following moderate to severe TBI [56]. Among 60 individuals with TBI reporting sleep complaints, Verma and colleagues found 24% of their sample to have reduced REM sleep percentage [58]. Reduced REM sleep was even found in adults having sustained minor TBI [68]. Other studies, either conducted with patients having sustained their injury at least six months before [55, 57], or with athletes having experienced multiple concussions/mild TBI [69], did not detect abnormalities in REM sleep. It thus remains unclear why REM sleep abnormalities persist in some individuals and not in others.

Ouellet and Morin found significantly shorter REM sleep latencies in a subgroup of non-medicated patients with mild to severe injuries [55]. They suggested that this may be related to generally increased depression symptoms characteristic of TBI. In the study by Verma and colleagues, shortened REM latencies were found in 13% of their sample [58]. Recently,

Williams and colleagues also found shorter REM sleep latencies in a group of nine mild TBI patients in part due to two of their patients entering REM sleep five minutes after sleep onset [59]. These authors suggest that this phenomenon may be characteristic of narcoleptic-like activity. This result fits well with reports of sleep onset REM periods (SOREMPs) in subsets of TBI patients during daytime sleep [30, 58, 68].

Changes in the microstructure of sleep

Few studies have examined the microstructure of sleep following TBI using power spectral analyses, and all were conducted following mild injuries. Parsons and colleagues studied eight adolescents with minor head injury within 72 hours of the impact, at six weeks and at twelve weeks post-injury [70]. They found that delta, theta, and alpha waveforms were all significantly elevated within 72 hours post-injury, but that all waveforms decreased thereafter, each according to an idiosyncratic sequence. Non-REM sleep underwent the most prominent changes seen over the twelve-week period. Theta activity was nonetheless found to intrude into the first REM cycle within six weeks, but this phenomenon decreased in the following weeks. Increases in alpha waveforms were the last to normalize. In a recent study by Williams and colleagues, nine patients with mild TBI (on average 30 months post-injury) were compared with nine healthy control participants on measures of sleep macrostructure and microstructure [59]. The timeframe of this study was thus very different than that used in the study by Parsons and colleagues [70]. The power spectral analyses did not reveal any significant differences between groups in mean power except in the beta band. However, the results indicate greater intra-subject variability for sigma, theta, and delta power in mild TBI patients compared to the control group during the sleep onset period. The authors suggest that these changes may be markers of a general disruption of the sleep onset process following mild TBI. Finally, a third study using spectral power analyses of REM and non-REM sleep revealed no significant differences between athletes with and without concussion [69]. However, increased delta activity and decreased alpha activity were observed in concussed athletes during wakefulness. The authors suggest that this finding may be related to intrusions of sleep EEG in the waking state.

Sleep disturbances following TBI

Insomnia

Insomnia is characterized by a variety of complaints reflecting dissatisfaction with the quality, duration, or efficiency of sleep. Individuals may report problems falling asleep, waking up several times or for prolonged periods during the night, waking up too early, or having unrefreshing sleep. Insomnia is often accompanied by reports of daytime fatigue, mood disturbances (e.g., irritability, dysphoria), and impairments of social and occupational functioning [47]. Criteria routinely used to operationalize insomnia symptoms in outcome research include a sleep-onset latency and/or wake after sleep onset greater than 30 minutes, associated with a sleep efficiency (ratio of total sleep time to time spent in bed) lower than 85%; these sleep difficulties have to be present at least three nights per week [71, 72]. Insomnia is thought to be chronic when it lasts more than one or six months, depending on the diagnostic system used.

Prevalence

Observations made by staff members (night nurses, rehabilitation professionals) in acute brain injury rehabilitation hospital units indicate that about 70% of patients have significant disturbances of their night-time sleep [3]. Beyond the acute period, the prevalence of self-reported symptoms of insomnia has ranged from 30 to 70% in various studies conducted from one month up to many years post-injury [2], suggesting that insomnia develops a chronic course in many individuals with TBI. To our knowledge, only two studies have examined the prevalence of insomnia *syndromes* (i.e., persons fulfilling diagnostic criteria for clinically significant insomnia). Fichtenberg and colleagues were the first to study post-TBI insomnia using the standardized DSM-IV criteria [73]. In a study of 50 patients consecutively admitted to a rehabilitation hospital and evaluated on average four months post-injury, they found a 30% prevalence rate of insomnia. Using a combination of the criteria of the DSM-IV [71] and the *International Classification of Diseases* [72], Ouellet and colleagues found that 29.4% of a sample of 452 patients with TBI for an average of eight years fulfilled the diagnostic criteria for an insomnia syndrome, and of these, 60% were not receiving any treatment for their sleep disturbances [42]. Taken together, these two studies suggest that insomnia that develops early following TBI persists over time and remains often untreated.

Factors associated with post-TBI insomnia

In the study by Ouellet and colleagues, the presence of an insomnia syndrome was associated with milder head injuries, and higher levels of pain, fatigue, and depression [42]. A study by Clinchot and colleagues found that older individuals and women with TBI were more likely to experience sleep difficulties [74]. Other factors related to insomnia in this study were the presence of headaches, alcohol abuse, and average or above-average memory and attention capacities. Conversely, individuals with more severe injuries and those working or going to school were less likely to have sleep disturbances. Fichtenberg and colleagues found that insomnia was associated with milder brain injuries and with the presence of depressive symptoms [75]. Age, gender, education, pain, or litigation status were not related to insomnia.

Insomnia and TBI severity

At least six studies have now documented an inverse relationship between the severity of the brain injury and the presence of sleep disorders following TBI [41, 42, 56, 74–76]. Sleep disturbances are thus more commonly reported by patients with milder injuries. Such milder injuries to the brain are accompanied by greater awareness of deficits when individuals are attempting to return to their pre-injury levels of functioning. The same phenomenon may explain why TBI survivors with milder injuries also report many symptoms of anxiety, depression, and pain.

Insomnia-related habits

Conditioning processes involved in the etiology of some forms of primary insomnia may also be at play in persons with TBI. Indeed, situational (bed/bedroom), temporal (bedtime), or behavioral (bedtime rituals) stimuli normally associated with sleep may become repeatedly associated with stress, anxiety, and emotional arousal due to difficulty falling or staying asleep. In addition, somatized tension and dysfunctional beliefs or attitudes about sleep that are characteristic of persons with primary insomnia may also contribute to post-TBI insomnia. Individuals with chronic insomnia tend to spend more time in bed, nap during the day, and have irregular sleep–wake schedules to compensate for sleep loss and fatigue [47]. Although these behaviors may be helpful in the short term, when used repeatedly, these strategies can lead to a desynchronization of the sleep–wake cycle and actually contribute to sleep problems. These behaviors are particularly frequent in TBI patients who are already prone to severe and chronic fatigue [77].

Excessive daytime sleepiness

Excessive daytime sleepiness (EDS), also referred to as hypersomnia or hypersomnolence, is also common after TBI. It is often confused with fatigue, which is experienced by the majority of TBI patients [77], and this confusion is present in both clinical practice and in the scientific literature. It is crucial to differentiate these two concepts as there is growing evidence that management and treatment strategies are different. While the presence of sleepiness is often associated with fatigue, a sensation of fatigue is not necessarily accompanied by sleepiness or sleep propensity. Fatigue is a subjective state that can be defined as weariness, weakness, or depleted energy. Sleepiness refers to sensations of physiological drowsiness, sleep propensity, or reduced alertness [78] and can be objectified with standardized assessment techniques such as daytime PSG recordings.

Excessive daytime sleepiness may present as a subjective complaint, as a physiological/objective sleep propensity, or as a core symptom of several sleep disorders (e.g., post-traumatic hypersomnia, sleep-related breathing disorders, narcolepsy). Subjective EDS refers to self- or informant-reported perception of the tendency to fall asleep or incapacity to maintain a desired alertness level. Depending on the instrument, EDS can be assessed as a trait (i.e., general perception of daytime sleepiness in recent times) or as a state (i.e., perception of daytime sleepiness at the moment of assessment). The Epworth Sleepiness Scale (ESS) [79] is one measure commonly used to evaluate trait sleepiness. The ESS includes eight daytime situations for which the respondent has to rate the probability to doze off or fall asleep in recent times.

Subjective EDS is reported by 14 to 55% of TBI patients [30, 58, 80–82]. The variability of the results can mostly be attributable to methodological discrepancies across studies, especially in terms of selection of patients (e.g., time elapsed between TBI and enrollment, recruitment setting, diagnostic criteria for TBI, presence of exclusion criteria), instruments used

(e.g., global symptoms questionnaires or checklists, sleepiness-focused measures such as the ESS), and definition of EDS (e.g., "sleeping more than usual", "tendency to nap at inappropriate times and places", exceeding a cut-off score on the ESS). When comparing the prevalence of sleepiness between TBI and control groups, some studies found a significantly higher prevalence among TBI patients [83], while others did not [41]. The absence of significant differences on mean ESS scores have also been reported, which has led some authors to suggest that the ESS may not be suitable to assess sleepiness in moderate to severe TBI because of the accompanying cognitive and self-awareness impairments [69, 81]. Excessive daytime sleepiness has been found to be significantly associated with time elapsed since injury, sleepiness being increasingly prevalent with time [46, 81]. Parcell and colleagues have also reported a significant correlation between higher self-reported EDS (assessed with ESS) and higher anxiety symptoms, as well as longer daytime naps for TBI patients compared to controls [81].

The Multiple Sleep Latency Test (MSLT) is the most commonly used method to assess physiological or objective sleepiness [84]. This test involves the assessment of sleep latency in the context of four to five 20-minute nap opportunities evaluated at two-hour intervals throughout the course of the day. The speed with which a person falls asleep provides an objective index of sleepiness. The Maintenance of Wakefulness Test (MWT) [84] is another objective test of sleepiness where the nap opportunities last 40 minutes (as opposed to 20 in the MSLT), and the instruction given to participants specifies to try to stay awake, as opposed to trying to fall asleep as quickly as possible in the MSLT. Because of its focus on trying to stay awake, the MWT has been suggested to be more relevant when the objective is to evaluate the level of daytime functioning (e.g., vigilance, cognitive function), while the MSLT remains the gold standard for the clinical diagnosis of sleep disorders associated with complaints of EDS [85]. The main outcome measure for both the MSLT and MWT is the mean sleep onset latency for all naps.

Recent investigations have reported that between 11 and 25% of TBI patients exceeded the criterion for EDS (defined as a mean sleep latency of less than five minutes on the MSLT) [30, 80]. In TBI samples presenting with subjective complaints of sleepiness or poor sleep, objective EDS is not a consistent finding.

Indeed, Verma and colleagues observed that 53% of their participants reached the objective MSLT criterion [58], while it was the case for only 28% in another study [86]. The weak or absence of an association between ESS scores and mean sleep latencies from MSLT is repeatedly documented and further reinforces the notion that subjective and objective EDS are different, perhaps even more so in the TBI population [30, 58, 80].

When documenting sleepiness in TBI, it is important to consider premorbid sleep history. In fact, it is possible that some patients had non-diagnosed sleep disorders involving EDS prior to their injury and that EDS may have contributed to the accident causing TBI [80, 87].

Sleep-related breathing disorders

The main presenting feature of sleep-related breathing disorders (SRBD) is altered respiration during sleep. Obstructive sleep apnea (OSA) is the most common disorder in this category, characterized by episodes of complete (apnea) or partial (hypopnea) upper airway obstruction occurring during sleep [88]. Typical symptoms include loud snoring, restless sleep, and daytime sleepiness. Central apnea, less frequently observed, is distinct from OSA as it does not implicate ventilatory effort. The diagnosis of a sleep apnea syndrome necessitates, among other criteria, at least five PSG-documented apneas or hypopneas per hour (apnea/hypopnea index [AHI] $\geq$ 5) [88]. Two studies on consecutive TBI patients evaluated the prevalence of an AHI equal to or greater than ten, and reported rates of 6% and 11%, respectively [89, 90]. This criterion was exceeded in 30% of a sample of TBI patients complaining of poor sleep, 74% of apneas/hypopneas being obstructive [58]. In TBI patients referred for a sleep evaluation because of complaints of daytime sleepiness, a diagnosis of SRBD was made in 30 to 40% of individuals [86, 91]. Among the potential contributing factors to the onset of SRBD following TBI, damage to the respiratory system following orofacial fractures has been proposed [86].

Narcolepsy

Narcolepsy is a sleep disorder characterized by the presence of EDS, cataplexy, hypnagogic hallucinations, and sleep paralysis. The diagnosis should be confirmed by nocturnal PSG to rule out other sleep disorders, followed by MSLT and at least two SOREMPs during MSLT naps [88]. Although the majority of narcolepsy cases are idiopathic and have a strong genetic basis, the disorder can be secondary to various conditions, including TBI. A recent paper reviewing 22 published cases of post-traumatic narcolepsy confirmed by PSG and MSLT concluded that the clinical presentation of this condition is far from uniform [92]. Symptom onset varies from a few hours to 18 months post-TBI; the presenting symptom can be EDS, cataplexy, or both; the development of a narcolepsy syndrome appears to be unrelated to the severity of injury, presence of loss of consciousness, or CT scan or MRI findings. The progressive nature of the disorder seems to be more consistent across patients [92]. Additional research is needed to explore potential etiologic factors of post-traumatic narcolepsy. Damage to the hypocretin system has been proposed as an explanation, given the fact that levels of this neuropeptide have been shown to be reduced in idiopathic narcolepsy [93, 94]. This hypothesis has been recently studied by Baumann and colleagues, with results showing that a hypocretin-1 deficiency was present in 95% of 31 patients with moderate to severe TBI acutely after the injury [29]. In a prospective study up to six months post-injury, low CSF hypocretin-1 levels were found in 4 out of 21 patients at six months compared to 25 out of 27 in the first days after TBI [30].

Post-traumatic hypersomnia

Post-traumatic hypersomnia (PTH), included in the diagnosis of hypersomnia due to medical condition according to the *International Classification of Sleep Disorders*, 2nd edition [88], is considered when a complaint of EDS is present almost daily following TBI. It is a diagnosis of exclusion, as other sleep disorders causing EDS have to be ruled out. It has been hypothesized that a large proportion of TBI patients may have this diagnosis, with complaints of sleepiness, fatigue, headaches, and cognitive impairments [19]. The prevalence of post-traumatic hypersomnia, defined with different criteria, varies from 10 to 30% across studies [30, 80, 87, 89].

Circadian rhythm sleep disorders

Circadian rhythm sleep disorders (CRSD) are characterized by a mismatch between the individual's sleep–wake rhythm and the 24-hour environment. In addition to the sleep–wake cycle, circadian rhythms of melatonin secretion and body temperature are often disturbed in CRSD. A few case studies of CRSD following TBI have been published [95–98]. These individuals mostly displayed delayed sleep phase disorder (DSPD), characterized by a prolonged delayed (usually more than two hours) in the sleep–wake episodes relative to conventional times. A more recent investigation reported data on fifteen mild TBI patients diagnosed with CRSD based on actigraphic recordings, eight of them having DSPD and seven having irregular sleep–wake rhythm disorder (i.e., high day-to-day variability in sleep onset and offset) [99]. In this study, melatonin and body temperature rhythms were also delayed in TBI compared to control participants. Additional research is warranted on sleep timing and CRSD after TBI, especially given that post-injury changes in bedtime and arising time are often reported [100].

Interaction between sleep disturbances and neuropsychiatric consequences of TBI

Depression and anxiety

There is extensive comorbidity between sleep disorders, particularly insomnia, and psychiatric disorders. Likewise, several studies have linked sleep disturbances to symptoms of anxiety and depression following TBI [42, 81]. Frieboes and colleagues hypothesized that the hormonal changes occurring following TBI mirror those seen in depression [28]. Recently, we found depression to be significantly associated with insomnia in TBI. Furthermore, shorter REM sleep latencies seen in some TBI participants resembled sleep abnormalities seen in depressive patients. Regarding anxiety, Rao and colleagues found that insomnia in the acute period following a brain injury (within three months) was closely tied to the appearance of anxiety features as evaluated with the structured clinical interview for DSM-IV [101]. The bidirectional relationship that often exists between sleep disturbances and depression or anxiety is most likely also at play following TBI. Because multiple comorbidities are frequent in this population (disorders of mood, anxiety, adjustment, substance abuse), a systemic approach with simultaneous attention to several dimensions of functioning is necessary (e.g., drug interactions, fatigue due to treatments exacerbating other problems).

Although its diagnosis is controversial in TBI because of possible loss or alteration of consciousness, post-traumatic stress disorder (PTSD) has been reported in 3 to 27% of patients with TBI [102]. It can be hypothesized that PTSD may bring about parasomnias (e.g., nightmares) into the spectrum of sleep disturbances following TBI, although these have not been reported to be particularly prevalent in this population. However, with the increasing numbers of soldiers coming back from combat zones with brain injury resulting from blasts, research results on the complex interactions between TBI, sleep problems, and PTSD may emerge.

Cognitive impairment

It is difficult to evaluate how sleep disorders may cause cognitive deficits or exacerbate impairments due to brain injury or associated psychopathology. Problems with EDS have been linked with cognitive deficits, although this literature is still very limited. Sleepy TBI individuals have been found to have slower average reaction times and more lapses in a vigilance measure, compared to non-sleepy counterparts [87]. Furthermore, in the general population, sleep apnea is well known to be associated with cognitive impairments, particularly in the attentional domain [103]. Only one study has investigated the impact of the presence of SRBD on cognitive functioning in TBI. Results indicated that TBI patients with OSA performed significantly worse than those without OSA on measures of sustained attention and episodic memory [104]. Given the high prevalence of disorders associated with EDS following TBI, it is imperative to study more closely the impacts of sleep–wake disturbances on cognitive functioning in these patients with already compromised cognition.

Very few studies have yet studied the impact of TBI-related sleep disturbances on cognitive function and it is difficult to tease apart the results. As shown earlier, there is an inverse relationship between TBI severity and frequency of sleep complaints, which confounds the impact of sleep on cognition in this population because milder injuries are associated with milder cognitive deficits. In fact, Mahmood and colleagues found that better executive functioning and speed of processing were associated with more sleep disturbances [76]. In order to more adequately evaluate whether insomnia symptoms have detrimental effects on cognition in TBI patients, future studies should use samples of patients of homogeneous severity. Furthermore, studies of pharmacological or non-pharmacological treatments of insomnia in TBI should include a careful cognitive assessment at pre- and post-treatment. In any event post-TBI insomnia may not cause specific exacerbation of cognitive problems but rather global consequences such as increased fatigue and mood disturbances, which may be more functionally detrimental.

The reductions in normal REM sleep following TBI may be an important research avenue to pursue because of the well known role of REM sleep in memory consolidation and because abnormalities in REM sleep have been shown to be associated with cognitive impairment.

Treatment of sleep disorders following TBI

Despite increasing awareness and scientific attention to post-TBI sleep disorders, treatment options specifically adapted to this population have not yet been appropriately examined. Clinicians must rely on evidence obtained in studies with non-brain injured individuals to guide their decisions pertaining to clinical management of TBI-related sleep–wake disturbances. Although this approach may be acceptable in several cases, the literature nonetheless points to concerns.

Insomnia

Cognitive behavioral therapy and benzodiazepine-receptor agonists are the only two treatment approaches with adequate research evidence for the management of persistent insomnia [105]. However, caution should be used when prescribing benzodiazepines to TBI patients, especially in the acute phase after the injury, as some animal studies have shown that these drugs might impair recovery [106, 107]. Flanagan and colleagues recommended against the use of benzodiazepines in TBI patients because of their adverse effects (including altered psychomotor skills, dizziness, and impaired memory), effects on normal sleep architecture, and potential for abuse [108]. The authors recommend the newer non-benzodiazepine sedative-hypnotics (e.g., zolpidem, zaleplon, zopiclone, and eszopiclone), which have been shown to have a lower risk for tolerance, to cause fewer effects upon withdrawal, and to produce fewer daytime cognitive effects. Similarly, Flanagan and colleagues suggest to avoid drugs with anticholinergic effects (e.g., tricyclic

antidepressants, diphenhydramine) in persons with TBI because of their effects on memory and attention, and because they have been shown to potentially lower the seizure threshold [108]. In an uncontrolled study, Li Pi Shan and Ashworth compared lorazepam and zopiclone administered for one week to patients with stroke and brain injury who complained of insomnia during their inpatient rehabilitation stay [109]. They found no difference between the two drugs in terms of subjective sleep measures including sleep duration, or in cognitive function as assessed with the Mini Mental State Examination. Research is definitely needed to make sure that the commonly used hypnotic medications are as effective in TBI patients and do not produce detrimental effects such as exacerbation of seizures, cognitive deficits, or alterations in mood.

Recently, Ouellet and Morin provided evidence for the efficacy of a cognitive behavioral intervention for insomnia associated with mild to severe TBI [110, 111]. This type of treatment has been shown to be effective in primary insomnia and in insomnia co-morbid with medical disorders [112]. With simple adaptations of the original treatment protocol [47] (e.g., shorter sessions, increased written material, involvement of significant others) and consideration of comorbid problems characteristic of TBI (e.g., depression symptoms, substance use, precarious psychosocial situations, decrease in motivation), treatment outcome was comparable to those found in primary insomnia with improvements seen in 73% of participants up to three months post-treatment. Treatment produced significant decreases in total wake time and significant increases in sleep efficiency. Non-pharmacological approaches, such as behavioral (e.g., restriction of time in bed, stimulus control), cognitive (e.g., cognitive restructuring) or environmental (e.g., bright-light therapy) interventions, offer promise to alleviate insomnia symptoms in the TBI population as they have been shown to be effective to various degrees in other populations with sleep disturbances.

Excessive daytime sleepiness

Data on treatment options for EDS after TBI are also scarce. For example, despite the relatively high prevalence of OSA in TBI, the only published report that we know of on the use of continuous positive airway pressure (CPAP) in TBI has been in the field of speech pathology, where CPAP was found to improve hypernasality and sentence intelligibility following TBI [113]. Although there is no reason to believe that CPAP would not be efficacious in TBI patients to treat sleep-related breathing disorders, issues relating to treatment adherence should perhaps be investigated in this population.

Stimulants (e.g., methylphenidate, dextroamphetamine) are frequently used to enhance cognitive functioning following TBI. Al-Adawi and colleagues retrospectively studied the effects of methylphenidate on the sleep–wake cycle by comparing 17 medicated and 13 non-medicated TBI patients [114]. They found no effect of methylphenidate on the number of hours slept during the night or the day. Francisco and Ivanhoe reported a case of a 27-year-old patient with post-TBI narcolepsy successfully treated with methylphenidate [115]. By six months, the patient was asymptomatic. Recently, Jha and colleagues published the results of a randomized controlled trial using a ten-week crossover protocol comparing the effects of modafinil and placebo on EDS and fatigue in 51 patients with mild to severe TBI [116]. Overall, modafinil did not appear to be beneficial: the only significant difference between modafinil and placebo was a greater decrease of sleepiness at week 4, which was not maintained at week 10. Moreover, modafinil was associated with more frequent complaints of insomnia compared to placebo. Clearly, additional research is warranted on treatment options for EDS in the TBI population.

Conclusion and directions for future research

A neglected field until recently, sleep is becoming an increasingly important issue in the rehabilitation of patients with TBI. Research has shown that large proportions of these patients report sleep disturbances of various nature (i.e., insomnia, sleepiness, disruption of the sleep–wake cycle), often persisting up to several years post-injury. These findings are consistent with clinical experience in sleep medicine practices where patients with TBI often present mixed complaints of difficulties sleeping at night combined with problems staying awake during the day and chronic fatigue. It is often difficult to determine the pathogenesis of these disorders because of the still poorly understood complex intertwining of neurophysiologic, psychological, behavioral, and environmental factors.

Although there have been several studies of sleep in the last few years, our understanding of sleep disorders after TBI is still fragmentary, thus holding back the development of treatments specifically tailored to this population with specific characteristics and needs. Future studies should of course use standardized sleep measurement techniques, operationalized diagnostic criteria and definitions of sleep disorders, and also strive to recruit larger samples of patients in order to evaluate the impact of several mediating factors (e.g., injury severity, time elapsed since injury, psychological symptoms, psychiatric comorbidity, cognitive deficits) on sleep patterns. Treatment studies are also needed in order to determine whether treatments typically used in the general population could be transposed or adapted to the TBI population. Finally, such studies could be invaluable to guide rehabilitation professionals in making appropriate choices of medications, behavioral therapies, psychotherapy, and other non-pharmacological interventions for TBI patients with sleep–wake disturbances. Indeed, sleep-disorders management can be challenging in this population because of the presence of cognitive deficits, psychomotor problems, comorbid psychiatric disturbances, and alterations in personality and behavior.

References

1. Kraus JF, Chu LD. Epidemiology. In: Silver JM, McAllister TW, Yudofsky SC, eds. *Textbook of Traumatic Brain Injury*. (Washington, DC, 2005; 3–26).

2. Ouellet MC, Savard J, Morin CM. Insomnia following traumatic brain injury: a review. *Neurorehabil Neural Repair.* 2004;**18**:187–98.

3. Makley MJ, English JB, Drubach DA, *et al.* Prevalence of sleep disturbance in closed head injury patients in a rehabilitation unit. *Neurorehabil Neural Repair.* 2008;**22**:341–7.

4. Langlois JA, Rutland-Brown W, Wald MM. The epidemiology and impact of traumatic brain injury: a brief overview. *J Head Trauma Rehabil.* 2006;**21**:375–8.

5. Rutland-Brown W, Langlois JA, Thomas KE, *et al.* Incidence of traumatic brain injury in the United States, 2003. *J Head Trauma Rehabil.* 2006;**21**:544–8.

6. Narayan RK, Michel ME, Ansell B, *et al.* Clinical trials in head injury. *J Neurotrauma.* 2002;**19**:503–57.

7. Teasdale G, Jennett B. Assessment of coma and impaired consciousness. A practical scale. *Lancet.* 1974;**2**:81–4.

8. Bruns J Jr., Hauser WA. The epidemiology of traumatic brain injury: A review. *Epilepsia.* 2003;**44** (Suppl 10):2–10.

9. Maas AI, Stocchetti N, Bullock R. Moderate and severe traumatic brain injury in adults. *Lancet Neurol.* 2008;**7**:728–41.

10. Werner C, Engelhard K. Pathophysiology of traumatic brain injury. *Br J Anaesth*. 2007;**99**:4–9.

11. Sidaros A, Skimminge A, Liptrot MG, *et al*. Long-term global and regional brain volume changes following severe traumatic brain injury: A longitudinal study with clinical correlates. *Neuroimage*. 2009;**44**:1–8.

12. Carroll LJ, Cassidy JD, Peloso PM, *et al*. Prognosis for mild traumatic brain injury: results of the WHO Collaborating Centre Task Force on Mild Traumatic Brain Injury. *J Rehabil Med*. 2004;**43** Suppl:84–105.

13. Ashman TA, Gordon WA, Cantor JB, *et al*. Neurobehavioral consequences of traumatic brain injury. *Mt Sinai J Med*. 2006;**73**:999–1005.

14. Holm L, Cassidy JD, Carroll LJ, *et al*. Summary of the WHO Collaborating Centre for Neurotrauma Task Force on Mild Traumatic Brain Injury. *J Rehabil Med*. 2005;**37**:137–41.

15. Troncoso JC, Gordon B. Neuropathology of closed head injury. In: Rizzo M, Tranel D, eds. *Head Injury and Postconsussive Syndrome*. (New York: Churchill Livingstone Inc., 1996).

16. Agrawal A, Cincu R, Joharapurkar SR. Traumatic brain injury and sleep disturbances. *J Clin Sleep Med*. 2008;**4**:177.

17. Castriotta RJ. Collaboration in research involving traumatic brain injury and sleep disorders. Response to Agrawal A. *et al*. Traumatic brain injury and sleep disorders. *J Clin Sleep Med*. 2008;**4**:178.

18. Verma NP. Importance of traumatic brain injury. Response to Agrawal A. *et al*. Traumatic brain injury and sleep disorders. *J Clin Sleep Med*. 2008;**4**:179.

19. Watson NF. Need for more traumatic brain injury research. Response to Agrawal A. *et al*. Traumatic brain injury and sleep disorders. *J Clin Sleep Med*. 2008;**4**:180–1.

20. Denny-Brown D, Russell WR. Experimental cerebral concussion. *J Physiol*. 1940;**99**:153.

21. Foltz EL, Jenkner FL, Ward AA Jr. Experimental cerebral concussion. *J Neurosurg*. 1953;**10**:342–52.

22. Foltz EL, Schmidt RP. The role of the reticular formation in the coma of head injury. *J Neurosurg*. 1956;**13**:145–54.

23. Ward AA. Physiological basis of concussion. *J Neurosurg*. 1958;**15**:129–34.

24. Strich SJ. Diffuse degeneration of the cerebral white matter in severe dementia following head injury. *J Neurol Neurosurg Psychiatry*. 1956;**19**:163–85.

25. George B, Landau-Ferey J, Benoit O, *et al*. [Night sleep disorders during recovery of severe head injuries]. *Neurochirurgie*. 1981;**27**:35–8.

26. Cooper R, Hulme A. Changes of the EEG, intracranial pressure and other variables during sleep in patients with intracranial lesions. *Electroencephalogr Clin Neurophysiol*. 1969;**27**:12–22.

27. Mahowald MW. Sleep in traumatic brain injury and other acquired CNS conditions. In: Culebras A, ed. *Sleep Disorders and Neurological Disease*. (New York: Dekker, 2000; 365–85).

28. Frieboes RM, Muller U, Murck H, *et al*. Nocturnal hormone secretion and the sleep EEG in patients several months after traumatic brain injury. *J Neuropsychiatry Clin Neurosci*. 1999;**11**:354–60.

29. Baumann CR, Stocker R, Imhof HG, *et al*. Hypocretin-1 (orexin A) deficiency in acute traumatic brain injury. *Neurology*. 2005;**65**:147–9.

30. Baumann CR, Werth E, Stocker R, *et al*. Sleep–wake disturbances 6 months after traumatic brain injury: a prospective study. *Brain*. 2007;**130**:1873–83.

31. Sundström A, Nilsson LG, Cruts M, *et al*. Fatigue before and after mild traumatic brain injury: pre- post-injury comparisons in relation to apolipoprotein E. *Brain Inj*. 2007;**21**:1049–54.

32. Gottlieb DJ, DeStefano AL, Foley DJ, *et al*. APOE epsilon4 is associated with obstructive sleep apnea/hypopnea: the Sleep Heart Health Study. *Neurology*. 2004;**63**:664–8.

33. Mahowald MW, Mahowald ML. Sleep disorders. In: Rizzo M, Tranel D, eds. *Head injury and Postconcussive Syndrome*. (New York: Churchill Livingstone, 1996; 285–304).

34. Kowatch RA. Sleep and head injury. *Psychiatr Med*. 1989;**7**:37–41.

35. Hubain PP, Castro P, Mesters P, *et al*. Alprazolam and amitriptyline in the treatment of major depressive disorder: a double-blind clinical and sleep EEG study. *J Affect Disord*. 1990;**18**:67–73.

36. Mouret J, Lemoine P, Minuit MP, *et al*. Effects of trazodone on the sleep of depressed subjects: a polygraphic study. *Psychopharmacology* (Berl). 1988;**95** Suppl:S37–43.

37. Ott GE, Rao U, Lin KM, *et al*. Effect of treatment with bupropion on EEG sleep: relationship to antidepressant response. *Int J Neuropsychopharmacol*. 2004;**7**:275–81.

38. Kaynak H, Kaynak D, Gozukirmizi E, *et al*. The effects of trazodone on sleep in patients treated with stimulant antidepressants. *Sleep Med*. 2004;**5**:15–20.

39. Yamadera H, Nakamura S, Suzuki H, *et al*. Effects of trazodone hydrochloride and imipramine on polysomnography in healthy subjects. *Psychiatry Clin Neurosci*. 1998;**52**:439–43.

40. Moldofsky H. Sleep influences on regional and diffuse pain syndromes associated with osteoarthritis. *Semin Arthritis Rheum.* 1989;**18**:18–21.

41. Beetar JT, Guilmette TJ, Sparadeo FR. Sleep and pain complaints in symptomatic traumatic brain injury and neurologic populations. *Arch Phys Med Rehabil.* 1996;**77**:1298–302.

42. Ouellet MC, Beaulieu-Bonneau S, Morin CM. Insomnia in patients with traumatic brain injury: frequency, characteristics, and risk factors. *J Head Trauma Rehabil.* 2006;**21**:199–212.

43. Friese RS. Sleep and recovery from critical illness and injury: a review of theory, current practice, and future directions. *Crit Care Med.* 2008;**36**:697–705.

44. Friese RS, Diaz-Arrastia R, McBride D, *et al.* Quantity and quality of sleep in the surgical intensive care unit: are our patients sleeping? *J Trauma.* 2007;**63**:1210–14.

45. Gabor JY, Cooper AB, Hanly PJ. Sleep disruption in the intensive care unit. *Curr Opin Crit Care.* 2001;**7**:21–7.

46. Cohen M, Oksenberg A, Snir D, *et al.* Temporally related changes of sleep complaints in traumatic brain injured patients. *J Neurol Neurosurg Psychiatry.* 1992;**55**:313–15.

47. Morin CM. *Insomnia: Psychological Assessment and Management.* (New York: Guilford, 1993).

48. Dikmen SS, Bombardier CH, Machamer JE, *et al.* Natural history of depression in traumatic brain injury. *Arch Phys Med Rehabil.* 2004;**85**:1457–64.

49. Hibbard MR, Uysal S, Sliwinski M, *et al.* Undiagnosed health issues in individuals with traumatic brain injury living in the community. *J Head Trauma Rehabil.* 1998;**13**:47–57.

50. Jorge RE, Robinson RG, Moser D, *et al.* Major depression following traumatic brain injury. *Arch Gen Psychiatry.* 2004;**61**:42–50.

51. Kreutzer JS, Seel RT, Gourley E. The prevalence and symptom rates of depression after traumatic brain injury: a comprehensive examination. *Brain Inj.* 2001;**15**:563–76.

52. Jorge RE, Robinson RG, Starkstein SE, *et al.* Depression and anxiety following traumatic brain injury. *J Neuropsychiatry Clin Neurosci.* 1993;**5**:369–74.

53. George B, Landau-Ferey J. Twelve months' follow-up by night sleep EEG after recovery from severe head trauma. *Neurochirurgia (Stuttg).* 1986;**29**:45–7.

54. Kaufman Y, Tzischinsky O, Epstein R, *et al.* Long-term sleep disturbances in adolescents after minor head injury. *Pediatr Neurol.* 2001;**24**:129–34.

55. Ouellet MC, Morin CM. Subjective and objective measures of insomnia in the context of traumatic brain injury: a preliminary study. *Sleep Med.* 2006;**7**:486–97.

56. Parcell DL, Ponsford JL, Redman JR, *et al.* Poor sleep quality and changes in objectively recorded sleep after traumatic brain injury: a preliminary study. *Arch Phys Med Rehabil.* 2008;**89**:843–50.

57. Prigatano GP, Stahl ML, Orr WC, *et al.* Sleep and dreaming disturbances in closed head injury patients. *J Neurol Neurosurg Psychiatry.* 1982;**45**:78–80.

58. Verma A, Anand V, Verma NP. Sleep disorders in chronic traumatic brain injury. *J Clin Sleep Med.* 2007;**3**:357–62.

59. Williams BR, Lazic SE, Ogilvie RD. Polysomnographic and quantitative EEG analysis of subjects with long-term insomnia complaints associated with mild traumatic brain injury. *Clin Neurophysiol.* 2008;**119**:429–38.

60. Evans BM, Bartlett JR. Prediction of outcome in severe head injury based on recognition of sleep related activity in the polygraphic electroencephalogram. *J Neurol Neurosurg Psychiatry.* 1995;**59**:17–25.

61. Laffont F. Les insomnies organiques. In: Billiard M, ed. *Le sommeil normal et pathologique: Troubles du sommeil et de l'éveil,* 2nd edn. (Paris: Masson, 1998; 178–88).

62. Ron S, Algom D, Hary D, *et al.* Time-related changes in the distribution of sleep stages in brain injured patients. *Electroencephalogr Clin Neurophysiol.* 1980;**48**:432–41.

63. Bergamasco B, Bergamini L, Doriguzzi T, *et al.* EEG sleep patterns as a prognostic criterion in post-traumatic coma. *Electroencephalogr Clin Neurophysiol.* 1968;**24**:374–7.

64. Bricolo A, Gentilomo A, Rosadini G, *et al.* Long-lasting post-traumatic unconsciousness. A study based on nocturnal EEG and polygraphic recording. *Acta Neurol Scand.* 1968;**44**:513–32.

65. Chatrian GE, White LE Jr., Daly D. Electroencephalographic patterns resembling those of sleep in certain comatose states after injuries to the head. *Electroencephalogr Clin Neurophysiol.* 1963;**15**:272–80.

66. Billiard M, Negri C, Baldy-Moulignier M, *et al.* Organisation du sommeil chz les sujets atteints d'inconscience post-traumatique chronique. *Rev Electroencephalogr Neurophysiol Clin.* 1979;**9**:149–52.

67. Lenard HG, Pennigstorff H. Alterations in the sleep patterns of infants and young children following acute head injuries. *Acta Paediatr Scand.* 1970;**59**:565–71.

68. Schreiber S, Barkai G, Gur-Hartman T, *et al.* Long-lasting sleep patterns of adult patients with minor traumatic brain injury (mTBI) and non-mTBI subjects. *Sleep Med.* 2008;**9**:481–7.

69. Gosselin N, Lassonde M, Petit D, *et al*. Sleep following sport-related concussions. *Sleep Med.* 2009;**10**(1):35–46.

70. Parsons LC, Crosby LJ, Perlis M, *et al*. Longitudinal sleep EEG power spectral analysis studies in adolescents with minor head injury. *J Neurotrauma.* 1997;**14**:549–59.

71. American Psychiatric Association. *Diagnostic and Statistical Manual of Mental Disorders*, 4th edn. (Washington, DC: American Psychiatric Association, 1994).

72. World Health Organization. *The International Classification of Diseases*, 10th edn. (Geneva, Switzerland: World Health Organization, 1992).

73. Fichtenberg NL, Zafonte RD, Putnam S, *et al*. Insomnia in a post-acute brain injury sample. *Brain Inj.* 2002;**16**:197–206.

74. Clinchot DM, Bogner J, Mysiw WJ, *et al*. Defining sleep disturbance after brain injury. *Am J Phys Med Rehabil.* 1998;**77**:291–5.

75. Fichtenberg NL, Millis SR, Mann NR, *et al*. Factors associated with insomnia among post-acute traumatic brain injury survivors. *Brain Inj.* 2000;**14**:659–67.

76. Mahmood O, Rapport LJ, Hanks RA, *et al*. Neuropsychological performance and sleep disturbance following traumatic brain injury. *J Head Trauma Rehabil.* 2004;**19**:378–90.

77. Ouellet MC, Morin CM. Fatigue following traumatic brain injury: Frequency, characteristics, and associated factors. *Rehabil Psychol.* 2006;**51**:140–9.

78. Pigeon WR, Sateia MJ, Ferguson RJ. Distinguishing between excessive daytime sleepiness and fatigue: toward improved detection and treatment. *J Psychosom Res.* 2003;**54**:61–9.

79. Johns MW. A new method for measuring daytime sleepiness: the Epworth sleepiness scale. *Sleep.* 1991;**14**:540–5.

80. Castriotta RJ, Wilde MC, Lai JM, *et al*. Prevalence and consequences of sleep disorders in traumatic brain injury. *J Clin Sleep Med.* 2007;**3**:349–56.

81. Parcell DL, Ponsford JL, Rajaratnam SM, *et al*. Self-reported changes to nighttime sleep after traumatic brain injury. *Arch Phys Med Rehabil.* 2006;**87**:278–85.

82. Watson NF, Dikmen S, Machamer J, *et al*. Hypersomnia following traumatic brain injury. *J Clin Sleep Med.* 2007;**3**:363–8.

83. Perlis ML, Artiola L, Giles DE. Sleep complaints in chronic postconcussion syndrome. *Percept Mot Skills.* 1997;**84**:595–9.

84. Littner MR, Kushida C, Wise M, *et al*. Practice parameters for clinical use of the multiple sleep latency test and the maintenance of wakefulness test. *Sleep.* 2005;**28**:113–21.

85. Arand D, Bonnet M, Hurwitz T, *et al*. The clinical use of the MSLT and MWT. *Sleep.* 2005;**28**:123–44.

86. Guilleminault C, Yuen KM, Gulevich MG, *et al*. Hypersomnia after head-neck trauma: A medicolegal dilemma. *Neurology.* 2000;**54**:653–9.

87. Castriotta RJ, Lai JM. Sleep disorders associated with traumatic brain injury. *Arch Phys Med Rehabil.* 2001;**82**:1403–6.

88. American Academy of Sleep Medicine. *The International Classification of Sleep Disorders*, 2nd edn. (Westchester, IL: American Academy of Sleep Medicine, 2005).

89. Masel BE, Scheibel RS, Kimbark T, *et al*. Excessive daytime sleepiness in adults with brain injuries. *Arch Phys Med Rehabil.* 2001;**82**:1526–32.

90. Webster JB, Bell KR, Hussey JD, *et al*. Sleep apnea in adults with traumatic brain injury: a preliminary investigation. *Arch Phys Med Rehabil.* 2001;**82**:316–21.

91. Guilleminault C, Faull KF, Miles L, *et al*. Posttraumatic excessive daytime sleepiness: a review of 20 patients. *Neurology.* 1983;**33**:1584–9.

92. Ebrahim IO, Peacock KW, Williams AJ. Posttraumatic narcolepsy – two case reports and a mini review. *J Clin Sleep Med.* 2005;**1**:153–6.

93. Dauvilliers Y, Baumann CR, Carlander B, *et al*. CSF hypocretin-1 levels in narcolepsy, Kleine-Levin syndrome, and other hypersomnias and neurological conditions. *J Neurol Neurosurg Psychiatry.* 2003;**74**:1667–73.

94. Nishino S, Ripley B, Overeem S, *et al*. Hypocretin (orexin) deficiency in human narcolepsy. *Lancet.* 2000;**355**:39–40.

95. Boivin DB, Caliyurt O, James FO, *et al*. Association between delayed sleep phase and hypernyctohemeral syndromes: a case study. *Sleep.* 2004;**27**:417–21.

96. Nagtegaal JE, Kerkhof GA, Smits MG, *et al*. Traumatic brain injury-associated delayed sleep phase syndrome. *Funct Neurol.* 1997;**12**:345–8.

97. Patten SB, Lauderdale WM. Delayed sleep phase disorder after traumatic brain injury. *J Am Acad Child Adolesc Psychiatry.* 1992;**31**:100–2.

98. Quinto C, Gellido C, Chokroverty S, *et al*. Posttraumatic delayed sleep phase syndrome. *Neurology.* 2000;**54**:250–2.

99. Ayalon L, Borodkin K, Dishon L, *et al*. Circadian rhythm sleep disorders following mild traumatic brain injury. *Neurology.* 2007;**68**:1136–40.

100. Steele DL, Rajaratnam SM, Redman JR, *et al.* The effect of traumatic brain injury on the timing of sleep. *Chronobiol Int.* 2005;**22**:89–105.

101. Rao V, Spiro J, Vaishnavi S, *et al.* Prevalence and types of sleep disturbances acutely after traumatic brain injury. *Brain Inj.* 2008;**22**:381–6.

102. Ashman TA, Spielman LA, Hibbard MR, *et al.* Psychiatric challenges in the first 6 years after traumatic brain injury: Cross-sequential analyses of Axis I disorders. *Arch Phys Med Rehabil.* 2004;**85**:S36–42.

103. Aloia MS, Arnedt JT, Davis JD, *et al.* Neuropsychological sequelae of obstructive sleep apnea-hypopnea syndrome: a critical review. *J Int Neuropsychol Soc.* 2004;**10**:772–85.

104. Wilde MC, Castriotta RJ, Lai JM, *et al.* Cognitive impairment in patients with traumatic brain injury and obstructive sleep apnea. *Arch Phys Med Rehabil.* 2007;**88**:1284–8.

105. National Institutes of Health. NIH State of the Science Conference statement on Manifestations and Management of Chronic Insomnia in Adults statement. *J Clin Sleep Med.* 2005;**1**:412–21.

106. Goldstein LB. Prescribing of potentially harmful drugs to patients admitted to hospital after head injury. *J Neurol Neurosurg Psychiatry.* 1995;**58**:753–5.

107. Schallert T, Hernandez TD, Barth TM. Recovery of function after brain damage: severe and chronic disruption by diazepam. *Brain Res.* 1986;**379**:104–11.

108. Flanagan SR, Greenwald B, Wieber S. Pharmacological treatment of insomnia for individuals with brain injury. *J Head Trauma Rehabil.* 2007;**22**:67–70.

109. Li Pi Shan RS, Ashworth NL. Comparison of lorazepam and zopiclone for insomnia in patients with stroke and brain injury: a randomized, crossover, double-blinded trial. *Am J Phys Med Rehabil.* 2004;**83**:421–7.

110. Ouellet MC, Morin CM. Cognitive behavioral therapy for insomnia associated with traumatic brain injury: a single-case study. *Arch Phys Med Rehabil.* 2004;**85**:1298–302.

111. Ouellet MC, Morin CM. Efficacy of cognitive-behavioral therapy for insomnia associated with traumatic brain injury: a single-case experimental design. *Arch Phys Med Rehabil.* 2007;**88**:1581–92.

112. Morin CM, Bootzin RR, Buysse DJ, *et al.* Psychological and behavioral treatment of insomnia: update of the recent evidence (1998–2004). *Sleep.* 2006;**29**:1398–414.

113. Cahill LM, Turner AB, Stabler PA, *et al.* An evaluation of continuous positive airway pressure (CPAP) therapy in the treatment of hypernasality following traumatic brain injury: a report of 3 cases. *J Head Trauma Rehabil.* 2004;**19**:241–53.

114. Al-Adawi S, Burke DT, Dorvlo AS. The effect of methylphenidate on the sleep–wake cycle of brain-injured patients undergoing rehabilitation. *Sleep Med.* 2006;7:287–91.

115. Francisco GE, Ivanhoe CB. Successful treatment of post-traumatic narcolepsy with methylphenidate: a case report. *Am J Phys Med Rehabil.* 1996;**75**:63–5.

116. Jha A, Weintraub A, Allshouse A, *et al.* A randomized trial of modafinil for the treatment of fatigue and excessive daytime sleepiness in individuals with chronic traumatic brain injury. *J Head Trauma Rehabil.* 2008;**23**:52–63.

Chapter 33

Sleep in borderline personality disorder

José Manuel de la Fuente

Borderline personality disorder (BPD) is a well characterized syndrome that is now detectable with some diagnostic tools such as the Diagnostic Interview for Borderline patients (DIB) [1] or the DSM-IV [2]. Borderline personality disorder, which is the most frequently diagnosed personality disorder [3], is characterized by brief episodes of affective manifestations, brief psychotic episodes, emotional instability, impulsive and unpredictable behavior, frequent self-mutilations, and altered interpersonal relations. Sleep complaints are very frequent and objective sleep-EEG (S-EEG) abnormalities have been reported.

The link between BPD and the affective disorders is unclear [4–12]. Opinions proposing an affective nature of BPD [13, 14] are contrasted with others that suggest BPD and affective disorders to be independent [8–11, 15, 16]. These authors suggest that the depressive state associated with BPD could be distinct from non-borderline depression in terms of quality and duration of symptoms [5, 6, 17]. Emptiness, loneliness, labile affect [17], behavioral dysregulation, anger and tension [5], self-condemnation, abandonment fears, self-destructiveness and hopelessness [6] appear to be specific clusters of borderline affective symptoms. Moreover, some authors including ourselves have proposed the depressive symptoms in BPD to have a distinct biological substrate from those in the non-borderline depression [4, 8–11, 12, 18, 19]. Pharmacological studies have shown differences in treatment responses between BPD and major depression (MD). Conventional antidepressants have exhibited poor response and even worsening in BPD [15, 20].

As BPD patients have an extremely poor quality of life, high risk of suicide and self-destructiveness, and a very poor response to treatments, the knowledge of the nature of the depressive symptoms in BPD appears to be fundamental as it could imply key therapeutic strategies or suggest new research directions in this field, which are substantially needed for these patients.

To clarify the biological nature of the depressive symptoms in BPD, different methodologies such as the endocrinology tests dexamethasone suppression test (DST) and thyrotropin-releasing hormone stimulation test (TRH-ST) have been studied in BPD [4, 8, 10, 11, 18, 21–31]. In some of these studies the DST and TRH-ST findings seem to be related to a concomitant diagnosis of major depression rather than to BPD itself [18, 32]. In others, the results have been obtained from BPD patients without MD [8, 10, 11] and have claimed against the existence of a biological link between BPD and MD. Recently functional positron emission studies have found arguments to differentiate BPD from affective disorders. Soloff et al. [33] showed that 5-HT(2A) receptor binding was increased in the hippocampus of BPD subjects independent of their depressed mood whereas the 5-HT(2A) receptor binding appears to be decreased in major depression [34].

Sleep-EEG studies have been found to show utility in the characterization of the affective disorders and of other psychiatric syndromes [35]. In an attempt to clarify the pathophysiology of BPD, at least 17 studies on S-EEG have been carried-out, to date.

In an opening period, the sleep studies were done with the largely assumed idea that BPD patients would belong to the affective–depressive disorders spectrum. In line with this belief, the samples of patients were extremely heterogeneous and most studies included borderline patients with major depression and other Axis I and/or Axis II diagnoses. Bell et al. [36] studied the effect of a pre-existing diagnosis of borderline personality disorder on clinical and S-EEG correlates of depression, i.e., the sleep in major depressives with an Axis II diagnosis of BPD. The sample for this pioneer study, attempting to "delineate the relationship between BPD and affective disorders," was composed of 15 inpatients with a DSM-III major depressive disorder and with "predominantly borderline personality disorders" and 18 Research Diagnostic Criteria (RDC) major depressive disorder not BPD patients. A comparison of S-EEG between major depressives with BPD and primary major depressives without BPD revealed no significant differences between the two groups. The main finding of this study was that a pre-existing diagnosis of BPD in major depression patients did not alter the "characteristic" short latency of REM sleep and the sleep continuity disturbances reported in major depression. A surprising finding of this study was the fact that the depressed BPD had a very similar rate of suicidal ideation and behavior to the non-BPD major depressives.

In McNamara et al. [37] the sleep of ten DIB, borderline women patients (six of them with an RDC diagnosis of major depression), ten patients with primary non-delusional RDC depression (seven of them were women) and ten female controls were compared. The two patient groups showed more sleep continuity disturbances, less slow sleep, and greater REM activity and density (particularly during the first REM period) than normal controls. First-night REM latencies were more variable in the borderline than in the depressed group, but by the second night both groups showed shorter REM latencies than the controls. The authors affirmed that the similarities in S-EEG suggest a relationship between borderline disorder and the affective spectrum and cast doubt on the definition of the borderline disorder as a pure character type divorced from the affective spectrum.

In a quite clear illustration of diagnostic heterogeneity, Reynolds and associates [38] studied the S-EEG in a group of depressed BPD patients. They compared 20, retrospective and prospective, DIB BPD patients (17 women with mean HDRS scores of 19 and 17.4 respectively) to ten non-BPD major depressives (seven women, mean HDRS = 19) and to ten female controls. The BPD sample had many other SADS-L diagnoses (5: intermittent depression; 2: "primary" major depressive disorder; 2: bipolar II major depression; 3: labile personality; 5: alcohol abuse; 4: schizotypal features; 1: antisocial personality;

1: ciclothymia; and 7: drug abuse). In this miscellaneous BPD and major depression sample, the authors described similar reduced (less than 65 minutes) REM latencies in major depressives (85%) and BPD patients (70%) compared to controls (35%). Despite the fact that the mean HDRS were not statistically different between the patient groups (indicating that they were comparing two groups of chiefly depressed patients with equal intensities in their major depressive disorders), they concluded that their results supported the concept of a close relationship between BPD and affective illness.

Akiskal et al. [39] attempted to clarify the nosologic status of BPD. They compared 24 DSM-III "non-schizotypal" BPD outpatients without an acute major depression, mania, or schizophreniform disorder to 16 patients with other DSM-III personality disorders, 30 major depressives without BPD, and to 14 controls. They found almost exactly equal REM latencies in the BPD and the major depression groups (slightly shortened to 63 minutes) while the other personality and the control groups had much longer REM latencies. The authors cast doubts on the nosologic existence of BPD as a unitary entity. The, at least troublesome, flaw in this study was that the BPD group, which was diagnosed as not having major depression, scored significantly higher on the Beck Depression Inventory than the non-BPD major depression group (BPD = 17 vs. MD = 11; $p < 0.02$) indicating that in fact, the intensity of the depressive symptoms was higher in the BPD group than in the "primary affective group". The authors explain this fact by the possibility that BPD would have a tendency to overendorse subjective affective complaints. This explanation would have appeared sound to explain simply high scores on the depression scales in BPD without current major depression but it seems somewhat weak to explain higher scores in BPD without major depression than in major depressives. So the possibility arises that in this study, actually two groups of major depression patients showed identical REM latencies.

In a work studying different biological markers, Lahmeyer et al. [31] compared 17 DSM-III and DIB, BPD patients who also met multiple Axis I diagnoses including affective and drug/alcohol dependence disorders, to 20 major depressives without BPD but who were not assessed for other Axis I diagnoses. There were no significant differences in S-EEG parameters between the two groups. Once again, the HRDS scores in the BPD and the major depression group were not different (24.29 vs. 26.34; $p =$ ns).

Benson and colleagues [16] compared S-EEG patterns of 18 DSM-III borderline patients with and without a history of affective disorder. The groups were compared to each other and to controls. Eight BPD patients met RDC criteria for present or past major depression, 14 for present or past alcohol abuse, and 13 for present or past drug abuse. The three groups could not be distinguished in terms of REM latency. The two BPD groups (with and without past or present RCD major depression) could not be distinguished in any S-EEG parameter. Borderlines had less total sleep, more stage 1 sleep, and less stage 4 sleep than controls. The authors conclude that, if one assumes that REM latency is a biological marker for mood disorder (which they did not necessarily believe), then BPD would not be a variant of affective illness.

In 1993, from an initial group of 57 borderlines, Battaglia et al. [40] recorded ambulatory polysomnographies of ten "never-depressed" DSM-IIIR BPD patients and compared them to controls. They excluded from the study all subjects with "current or past evidence of major depression, bipolar disorder, cyclothymia and dysthymia as revealed in the DIS-R interview". The patients had several other lifetime Axis I and II diagnoses. Borderline subjects had a significantly shorter REM latency (mean = 63.9 minutes) than controls and normal S-EEG architectures. Although the authors do not describe the follow-up of those "never-depressed" BPD patients (therefore making the reader not able to know whether one or more of the patients subsequently developed an affective disorder or not) they conclude that reduced REM latency can be a trait indicator of liability to depression, present before the clinical appearance of the disorder. The same team [41] in 1999 studied again "never-depressed subjects with borderline personality disorder" and compared them by continuous 48-hour ambulatory electroencephalographic monitoring to controls. The BPD group had significantly higher REM density during the first REM period and one man with BPD who later committed suicide had REM density values exceeding the mean value of his group by 2 SD. Regardless of the fact that they studied "never depressed" subjects, the authors astonishingly concluded that REM density in the first REM period could be a marker of liability to mood disorders.

In an Egyptian sample of 20 ICD-10 BPD patients without comorbid depression Asaad and coworkers [14] compared their patients to 20 patients with major depression and to 20 controls. The two patient groups differed significantly from controls especially in sleep continuity measures. The BPD group had more sleep latency, less slow sleep, higher REM% and shorter REM latency than controls. Borderline personality disorder patients had longer REM latency (mean = 58.35) than major depressives (mean = 54.05). The authors concluded that, as they found great similarity in EEG sleep profile between BPD and major depression patients, this would suggest a common biological origin for both conditions, with the differences being quantitative rather than qualitative. However, they found more reduced REM latencies in MD than in BPD patients but, appropriately, the authors mentioned the meta-analysis by Benca et al. [35], not then available to Akiskal et al. [39], which suggested that REM latency is not useful in distinguishing mood disorders from other disorders, including BPD.

In a new attempt to clarify the link between BPD and the affective disorders De la Fuente et al. [9] compared 20 off-medication BPD inpatients without coexisting major depression to 20 MD patients without BPD and to 20 controls. The aim of the study was to examine the relationships between BPD and MD from the perspective of the S-EEG and to contribute to the characterization of the S-EEG in BPD. Both BPD and MD patients had less total sleep time, more prolonged sleep onset latency, and a greater percentage of wakefulness than control subjects. Borderline personality disorder patients and control subjects had more stage 2 sleep than MD patients. Borderline personality disorder patients had a longer duration of REM sleep, and less stage 3, stage 4, and slow-wave sleep than MD patients and control subjects. Rapid eye movement latency did not differentiate the three groups. Thus, BPD and MD patients shared sleep-continuity characteristics, but sleep architecture differentiated the two patient groups. The authors also compared the BPD patients with (N = 9) and without (N = 11) lifetime prevalence of MD. Borderline personality disorder patients with a past history of MD had more wakefulness and less slow-wave sleep than BPD patients without a history of MD; other sleep parameters, age, sex, and HDRS scores were not statistically different in the two BPD subgroups. The authors conclude that although BPD and MD may coexist, their study offers arguments favoring the concept that they are not biologically linked and that BPD patients with depressive symptoms often experience an affective syndrome different from that in MD patients without BPD, in terms of quality and duration of symptoms and of the biological substrate.

The same team [10, 11] tested the effects of the anti-epileptic and thymo-regulator drug carbamazepine (CBZ) on dexamethasone suppression and sleep electroencephalography in BPD. Even though CBZ had shown contradictory results in BPD and in a previous study the authors had found CBZ not to be useful in the treatment of BPD [7], this study was performed as the authors assumed that, even if the "epilepsy hypothesis to BPD" seemed difficult to sustain, the scientific evidence showed mounting evidence of brain dysfunction without focal abnormality in this syndrome. The effect of a drug such as CBZ on the S-EEG, which has a preferential action in limbic structures and a beneficial action in aggressive behavior, appeared interesting to study in BPD. So the authors investigated the effects of CBZ versus placebo on S-EEG in a sample of 20 DSM-IIIR and DIB, BPD patients without concomitant major depression. Carbamazepine given at doses that are therapeutic for epilepsy and affective disorders increased slow-wave sleep, which had been shown to be significantly decreased in BPD compared to major depressives and controls in their 2001 study.

Lindberg et al. [42] in a work that studied S-EEG in human impulsive aggression, compared 16 DSM-IV antisocial males charged with highly violent offences, six of whom also met the criteria for BPD to 11 controls. The antisocial patients with BPD had significantly more awakenings and lower sleep efficiency than the subjects with only antisocial personality disorder. These results resemble the results from De la Fuente et al. [9]. Interestingly Lindberg et al. [42] also found that subjects with severe conduct disorder in childhood anamnesis (only two of them were BPD) had a higher amount of slow-sleep compared with males with only mild or moderate conduct disorder (BPD = 4). For the authors their results gave further support to the growing evidence of the fact that brain dysfunction predisposes to severe aggressive behavior.

Assuming that BPD and MD may coexist but that they are not biologically linked and that BPD patients with depressive symptoms often experience an affective syndrome different from that in MD patients without BPD, in terms of quality and duration of symptoms and of biological substrate, De la Fuente et al. [12] performed an S-EEG study aimed to verify whether the BPD-associated depressive symptoms could be biologically linked to recurrent brief depression (RBD) or if, alternatively, they constituted a separate (idiosyncratic) affective disorder. They examined S-EEG characteristics in 20 BPD, 20 RBD, 20 MD patients, and 20 controls. Among the BPD patients, 12 were also diagnosed as having clinical RBD. Borderline personality disorder patients showed differences in sleep continuity and especially in sleep architecture compared with RBD, MD, and controls. Borderline personality disorder patients with or without clinical RBD did not show significant differences in any sleep parameter. Interestingly, BPD patients with or without clinical RBD had less slow-wave sleep activity not only than MD but also than non-borderline RBD patients. The authors proposed that although BPD patients can have concomitant MD, they often exhibit a specific BPD-associated affective syndrome that is different from both MD and non-borderline RBD in the quality and duration of symptoms and in the biological substrate.

Philipsen et al. [43], in a work aimed to study whether the subjective ratings of sleep disturbances in BPD patients were associated with objective S-EEG findings and whether alterations of the S-EEG spectral power could be observed in non-depressed BPD patients when compared with controls, and that also implicitly tested whether the sleep of BPD patients showed depression-like abnormalities (as had been previously described), performed S-EEG and spectral EEG analysis in 20 unmedicated female DSM-IV BPD patients without a current comorbid major depression but with other Axis I diagnoses and compared them to 20 controls. Borderline personality disorder patients showed significantly decreased stage 2 compared to controls. They found a marked discrepancy between objective and subjective sleep measurements. Spectral EEG analysis showed increased delta power in total (REM and non-REM) sleep in BPD. The authors did not find the previously reported similarities in S-EEG between BPD and major depression. Probably this study would have been more robust in this aspect if it had been performed with a third group of major depression patients without BPD.

Semiz et al. [44] compared 88 DSM-IIIR BPD patients without other Axis II diagnoses and without "any psychotic or mood disorder, acute and post-traumatic stress disorder or an organic condition during the past 1 year" but with other Axis I diagnoses (including substance abuse) to 100 controls.

The authors designed the study to examine the rate of nightmare disorder (ND) and to determine the levels of dream anxiety and subjective sleep quality in patients with BPD. Another aim was to determine whether dream anxiety was associated with childhood trauma, dissociative experiences, and subjective sleep disturbance in BPD patients. The hypothesis as to whether BPD patients with ND exhibited a more severe clinical profile than those without ND was also tested. Borderline personality disorder patients experienced a significantly greater rate of nightmares (49%), elevated levels of dream anxiety, and disturbed sleep (95.5%) than controls. In the BPD group, dream anxiety was correlated with rates of early traumatic experiences, dissociative symptoms, and impaired subjective sleep quality. As measured clinically, BPD patients with ND exhibited a more severe clinical profile than those without ND.

In the same year Hornung et al. [45] compared the S-EEG, during one night, in 15 DSM-IV female BPD patients versus 15 female controls in order to study the declarative and procedural memory consolidation during sleep in BPD. They assumed that the neuro-cognitive deficits exhibited by BPD patients could possibly interact with processes of sleep-related memory and (as recent findings point to the importance of sleep in memory consolidation in healthy young adults) that "declarative memory benefits from early nocturnal sleep, when slow-wave sleep predominates, whereas procedural memory is enhanced through late nocturnal sleep, when REM sleep prevails". Patients stopped the treatments only three days before the sleep study. Three patients had concomitant major depression and nine had received antidepressant medication prior to study participation. Nothing was said about other Axis I or II concomitant diagnoses. Before and after the study night, declarative and procedural memory performances were tested. Subjective sleep quality was assessed by a sleep questionnaire and objective sleep quality was measured by a portable sleep-recording device. Despite the fact that they did not find any difference between groups in any S-EEG objective measure, more specifically there were no significant differences between patients and controls in total REM sleep or in slow-wave sleep, the authors described that during the study night, the restorative value of sleep was significantly reduced in BPD patients. No significant differences were found regarding overnight performance improvement in

the declarative and procedural memory tasks. The authors conclude that their findings suggest that declarative and procedural memory consolidation during sleep is intact in BPD patients.

Finally and also in 2008, Bastien et al. [46] have compared S-EEG and subjective reports in 12 DSM-IV BPD patients to 30 chronic primary insomniacs (15 "psychophysiological" insomnia and 15 "paradoxical" insomnia) and to 15 "good sleepers" (GS: people having no subjective complaints of sleep difficulties and reporting sleep efficiency >85%). They found the subjectivity of BPD and GS sleep to be similar. Insomniacs took longer to fall asleep, were awake longer after sleep onset, and during the night slept less and had lower sleep efficiency than both GS and BPD patients. Objectively, (S-EEG) BPD and insomniacs had longer sleep onset, shorter sleep time, and lower sleep efficiency than GS. Furthermore, BPD patients had more stage 4 sleep than "paradoxical" insomniacs. The authors conclude that BPD patients suffer from insomnia and that while BPD patients reported feeling less refreshed upon awakening, they spent more time in stage 4 sleep than other individuals.

As closing remarks it can be said that the study of sleep and more precisely of the S-EEG has made several important contributions to the knowledge of the pathophysiology of BPD. In a first period, S-EEG demonstrated sleep alterations, which resembled, in some studies, the findings made in the affective disorders but this was not the case in other studies. The samples in this first period had a tendency to be heterogeneous and the authors were somewhat predisposed to work with the assumed hypothesis that BPD was a form of affective disorder.

In the second period, the samples began to be more homogeneous and in some studies the comorbidity with affective disorders were seriously taken into account. The diminished total sleep time, increased sleep onset latency, very diminished slow-wave sleep (even more reduced than in major depression); normal REM latencies and increased REM duration began to appear as characteristics of non-major depression–BPD patients. Nevertheless, it must be said that these findings are far from being definite and that they need further research in order to establish the appropriate sensitivity and specificity for each parameter in BPD.

Finally, the most recent S-EEG studies on BPD have clearly opened the door to demonstrate biologically the possibility proposed by different authors [5, 6, 8–12, 17, 18, 19, 28] that BPD patients often exhibit a specific BPD-associated affective syndrome that could be different from both MD and the non-BPD recurrent brief depression in the quality and duration of symptoms and the biological substrate. The S-EEG profile of this idiosyncratic BPD-affective disorder could be characterized by continuity and architecture sleep disturbances such as a diminished total sleep time with increased sleep onset latency and wakefulness, extremely reduced slow-wave sleep, and increased REM duration with normal REM latencies. Further studies in large homogeneous samples of BPD patients, without present Axis-I comorbidity, are warranted.

References

1. Gunderson JG, Kolb JE, Austin V. The diagnostic interview for borderline patients. *Am J Psychiatry.* 1981;**138**(7):896–903.

2. American Psychiatric Association. *Diagnostic and Statistical Manual of Mental Disorders*, 4th edn. (Washington, DC: American Psychiatric Press, 1994).

3. Gunderson JG, Zanarini MC. Current overview of the borderline diagnosis. *J Clin Psychiatry.* 1987;**48** Suppl:5–14.

4. Korzekwa M, Links P, Steiner M. Biological markers in borderline personality disorder: new perspectives. *Can J Psychiatry.* 1993;**38** Suppl 1:S11–5.

5. Coid JW. An affective syndrome in psychopaths with borderline personality disorder? *Br J Psychiatry.* 1993;**162**:641–50.

6. Rogers JH, Widiger TA, Krupp A. Aspects of depression associated with borderline personality disorder. *Am J Psychiatry.* 1995;**152**(2):268–70.

7. De la Fuente JM, Lotstra F. A trial of carbamazepine in borderline personality disorder. *Eur Neuropsychopharmacol.* 1994;**4**(4):479–86.

8. De la Fuente JM, Mendlewicz J. TRH stimulation and dexamethasone suppression in borderline personality disorder. *Biol Psychiatry.* 1996;**40**(5):412–18.

9. De la Fuente JM, Bobes J, Vizuete C, Mendlewicz J. Sleep-EEG in borderline patients without concomitant major depression: a comparison with major depressives and normal control subjects. *Psychiatry Res.* 2001;**105**(1–2):87–95.

10. De la Fuente JM, Bobes J, Vizuete C, Mendlewicz J. Effects of carbamazepine on dexamethasone suppression and sleep electroencephalography in borderline personality disorder. *Neuropsychobiology.* 2002;**45**(3):113–19.

11. De la Fuente JM, Bobes J, Vizuete C, Mendlewicz J. Biological nature of depressive symptoms in borderline personality disorder: endocrine comparison to recurrent brief and major depression. *J Psychiatr Res.* 2002;**36**(3):137–45. Erratum in: *J Psychiatr Res* 2002;**36**(4):267–8.

12. De la Fuente JM, Bobes J, Morlán I, et al. Is the biological nature of depressive symptoms in borderline patients without concomitant Axis I pathology idiosyncratic? Sleep EEG comparison with recurrent brief, major depression and control subjects. *Psychiatry Res.* 2004;**129**(1):65–73.

13. Schultz PM, Soloff PH, Kelly T, et al. A family study of borderline subtypes. *J Pers Disord.* 1989;**3**:217–29.

14. Asaad T, Okasha T, Okasha A. Sleep EEG findings in ICD-10 borderline personality disorder in Egypt. *J Affect Disord.* 2002;**71**(1–3):11–18.

15. Soloff PH, George A, Nathan S, et al. Amitriptyline versus haloperidol in borderlines: final outcomes and predictors of response. *J Clin Psychopharmacol.* 1989;**9**(4):238–46.

16. Benson KL, King R, Gordon D, Silva JA, Zarcone VP Jr. Sleep patterns in borderline personality disorder. *J Affect Disord.* 1990;**18**(4):267–73.

17. Westen D, Moses J, Silk KR, et al. Quality of depressive experience in borderline personality disorder and major depression: when depression is not just depression. *J Person Disord.* 1992;**6**:382–93.

18. Krishnan RR, Davidson JRT, Rayasam K, Shope F. The dexamethasone suppression test in borderline personality disorder. *Biol Psychiatry.* 1984;**19**:1149–53.

19. Kavoussi RJ, Coccaro EF, Klar H, Lesser J, Siever LJ. The TRH stimulation test in DSM-III personality disorder. *Biol Psychiatry.* 1993;**34**:234–9.

20. Cole JO, Salomon M, Gunderson J. Drug therapy in borderline patients. *Comp Psychiatry.* 1984;**25**:249–54.

21. Carroll BJ, Greden J, Feinberg M, et al. Neuroendocrine evaluation of depression in borderline patients. *Psychiatr Clin North Am.* 1981;**4**:67–75.

22. Soloff PH, George A, Nathan RS. The dexamethasone suppression test in patients with borderline personality disorder. *Am J Psychiatry.* 1982;**139**:1621–3.

23. Sternbach HA, Fleming J, Extein I, Pottash ALC, Gold MS. The dexamethasone suppression and thyrotropin-releasing hormone test in depressed borderline patients. *Psychoneuroendocrinology.* 1983;**8**:459–62.

24. Baxter L, Edell W, Gerner R, Fairbanks Z, Gwirtsman H. Dexamethasone suppression test and Axis-I diagnoses of inpatients with DSM-III borderline personality disorder. *J Clin Psychiatry.* 1984;**45**:150–301.

25. Beeber AR, Kline MDD, Pie RW, Manning JM. Dexamethasone suppression test in hospitalised depressed patients with borderline personality disorder. *J Nerv Ment Dis.* 1984;**172**:301–3.

26. Val E, Gaviria FM, Lahmeyer HW, *et al.* Affective disorders and borderline personality. In: Pichot P, Berner P, eds. *Psychiatry: the State of the Art, Vol. 2. Biological Psychiatry.* (New York: Plenum Press, 1985; 171–6).

27. Silk KR, Lohr NE, Cornell DG, *et al.* The dexamethasone suppression test in borderline and non borderline affective patients. In: McGlashan TH, ed. *The Borderline: Current Empirical Research.* (Washington, DC: American Psychiatric Press, 1985; 99–116).

28. Siever LH, Coccaro EF, Klar H, *et al.* Biological markers in borderline and related personality disorders. In: Shagass C, Josiassen RG, Wagner BH, *et al.* eds. *Biological Psychiatry: Proceedings of the IVth World Congress of Biological Psychiatry.* (New York: Elsevier, 1986; 566–8).

29. Nathan SR, Soloff PH, George A, Peters J, McCarthy T. DST and TRH tests in borderline personality disorders. In: Shagass C, Josiassen RC, eds. *Biological Psychiatry – 1985.* (New York: Elsevier Science Publishing, 1985, 566–8).

30. Kontaxakis V, Markianos M, Vaslamatzis G, *et al.* Multiple neuroendocrinological responses in borderline personality disorder patients. *Acta Psychiatr Scand.* 1987;**76**(5):593–7.

31. Lahmeyer HW, Val E, Gaviria FM, *et al.* EEG sleep, lithium transport, dexamethasone suppression, and monoamine oxidase activity in borderline personality disorder. *Psychiatry Res.* 1988;**25**(1):19–30.

32. Soloff PH, Cornelius J, George A. The depressed borderline: one disorder or two? Relationship between Axis I and Axis II disorders: implications for treatment. *Psychopharmacol Bull.* 1991;**27**:23–30.

33. Soloff PH, Price JC, Meltzer CC, *et al.* 5HT2A receptor binding is increased in borderline personality disorder. *Biol Psychiatry.* 2007;**62**(6):580–7.

34. Mintun MA, Sheline YI, Moerlein SM, *et al.* Decreased hippocampal 5-HT2A receptor binding in major depressive disorder: in vivo measurement with [18F] altanserin positron emission tomography. *Biol Psychiatry.* 2004;**55**(3):217–24.

35. Benca RM, Obermeyer WH, Thisted RA, Gillin JC. Sleep and psychiatric disorders. A meta-analysis. *Arch Gen Psychiatry.* 1992;**49**(8):651–68.

36. Bell J, Lycaki H, Jones D, Kelwala S, Sitaram N. Effect of preexisting borderline personality disorder on clinical and EEG sleep correlates of depression. *Psychiatry Res.* 1983;**9**(2):115–23.

37. McNamara E, Reynolds CF 3rd, Soloff PH, *et al.* EEG sleep evaluation of depression in borderline patients. *Am J Psychiatry.* 1984;**141**(2):182–6.

38. Reynolds CF 3rd, Soloff PH, Kupfer DJ, *et al.* Depression in borderline patients: a prospective EEG sleep study. *Psychiatry Res.* 1985;**14**(1):1–15.

39. Akiskal HS, Yerevanian BI, Davis GC, King D, Lemmi H. The nosologic status of borderline personality: clinical and polysomnographic study. *Am J Psychiatry.* 1985;**142**(2):192–8.

40. Battaglia M, Ferini-Strambi L, Smirne S, Bernardeschi L, Bellodi L. Ambulatory polysomnography of never-depressed borderline subjects: a high-risk approach to rapid eye movement latency. *Biol Psychiatry.* 1993;**33**(5):326–34.

41. Battaglia M, Ferini Strambi L, Bertella S, Bajo S, Bellodi L. First-cycle REM density in never-depressed subjects with borderline personality disorder. *Biol Psychiatry.* 1999;**45**(8):1056–8.

42. Lindberg N, Tani P, Appelberg B, *et al.* Human impulsive aggression: a sleep research perspective. *J Psychiatr Res.* 2003;**37**(4):313–24.

43. Philipsen A, Feige B, Al-Shajlawi A, *et al.* Increased delta power and discrepancies in objective and subjective sleep measurements in borderline personality disorder. *J Psychiatr Res.* 2005;**39**(5):489–98.

44. Semiz UB, Basoglu C, Ebrinc S, Cetin M. Nightmare disorder, dream anxiety, and subjective sleep quality in patients with borderline personality disorder. *J Psychiatr Res.* 2008;**42**(8):653–8.

45. Hornung OP, Regen F, Warnstedt C, *et al.* Declarative and procedural memory consolidation during sleep in patients with borderline personality disorder. *J Psychiatr Res.* 2008;**42**(8):653–8.

46. Bastien CH, Guimond S, St-Jean G, Lemelin S. Signs of insomnia in borderline personality disorder individuals. *J Clin Sleep Med.* 2008;**4**(5):462–70.

Chapter 34

Dream differences in psychiatric patients

Milton Kramer

There has been a vigorous search for the biological differences that are presumed to exist among the various psychiatric entities [1]. Much of the present volume is an exposition of the differences in the biological and physiological organization and structure of sleep that are found in various psychiatric illnesses. Freud [2] shared this view of the fundamental nature of biological explanations as he stated in the *Interpretation of Dreams*, "Even when investigation shows that the primary exciting cause of a phenomenon is psychical [mental], deeper research will one day trace the path further and discover an organic basis for the mental event". However, he encouraged that the exploration of the mental continue. "But if at the moment we cannot see beyond the mental, that is no reason for denying its existence" [2] and, I would add, its importance.

The analogy between dreaming and psychosis was observed in the eighteenth century if not before [3]. Kant [4] (1764) observed, "The madman is a waking dreamer." Schopenhauer [5] (1862) calls "dreams a brief madness and madness a long dream." And Jung [6] said that if we "let the dreamer walk about and act like a person awake . . . we [would] have the clinical picture of dementia praecox [schizophrenia]." J Hughlings Jackson's [7] view was "if we could find out about dreams, we would find out about insanity." Freud [8] was of the opinion that as we better understand dreams, it will enhance our understanding of psychosis. Hartmann [9] (1981) is of a similar opinion. And long before Hobson's speculation [10] (1997), Hagen [11] (1846) describes delirium as similar to dreaming. Freud [12] observes that "Very little research has hitherto been carried out into the modifications occurring in dream-life during chronic psychoses." This has certainly continued to be the case. Ramsey [13] reviewing the pre-REM literature

found only 20 articles from six psychiatric patient groups. Nuhic and I [14] reviewed the English language literature from 1966 to 2005 and found 94 articles from the six psychiatric groups of interest that contained a total of 98 studies. Roth and I [15] had earlier reported a more extensive literature search, which identified 71 different articles, which contained 75 studies from 7 diagnostic groups.

There is implicit in our search for dream content differences among psychiatric illnesses that with a change in the state of the dreamer there is a change in dream content. Even within an individual a state change is related to dream content [16]. Kramer and Roth [17] as well as Cartwright *et al.* [18] have provided evidence that the alteration of affective state from night to morning is related to the content of the intervening night's dreams. And how you feel on awakening in the morning is a major predictor of psychomotor performance in the morning [19]. Dream content changes with effective antidepressant medication treatment [20] so if one changes the dreamer's state their dream content changes. Most patients beginning long-term psychotherapy have a negative affective tone to their initial dream and in those who improve in treatment, the last dream reported has a positive affective tone [21]. It is apparent then that the content of your dreams reflects your current state, affects your waking performance, and that changes in your waking condition from illness to recovery are reflected in changes in your dream experience.

Method

The present chapter is an update of the review I published with Nuhic in 2007 [14]. I hoped to extend the data by examining the articles found in

Medline from 2005 to 2008 for dreams that had been previously reported [15] in the seven diagnostic categories, namely schizophrenia, depression, post-traumatic stress disorder [PTSD], eating disorders, organic brain disorders, mental retardation, and alcoholism and drug abuse.

I obtained 90 articles from my 2005 to 2008 Medline search: 5 for schizophrenia, 24 for depression, 48 for PTSD, 5 for eating disorders, 1 for brain damage, none for mental retardation, and 7 for alcohol and drug abuse. Only those articles that described a dream content study in one of the illness categories could be selected for study. Unfortunately, none of the articles found by the search met the illness and content criteria. The results to be reported are a summary of those found in the 1978 [15] and 2007 [14] reviews. Parenthetically the absence of dream content studies in psychiatric illnesses in the past three years reflects the decreased interest in the mental compared to the biological aspects of psychiatric illness.

I combined the results of the two prior reviews [14, 15] to achieve an overview of the studies on dream content in the major mental illnesses. This overview will assess both the methodological adequacy and dream content found in these studies covering the period from Ramsey's review in 1953 [13] through 2008.

Results

Methodological aspects of the studies

Combining the results of the two previous reviews [14, 15] allows me to report on dream content in a fairly large number of studies: 38 for schizophrenia, 34 for depression, 63 for PTSD, 11 for eating disorders, 11 for organic brain disease, 4 for mental retardation, and 12 for alcoholism and drug abuse for a total of 173 studies. We have increased from the 20 studies of dreams in mental illness that Ramsey reported in his review in 1953 [13], hopefully the quality has improved as well.

Type, nature, and site of the studies

Almost three quarters of the reports are studies (72%), while case reports make up approximately a quarter of the reports (28%). Both types of reports, if systematically utilized, may be of value in delineating the dream experience in psychopathologic groups. Clues about potentially interesting or important areas to pursue in studying the dreams of a particular illness group may be suggested by a case study that then may be explored in appropriate follow-up studies.

The studies are mainly descriptive in nature (55%) with separate group studies making up about a third of the studies (37%) and repeated measure designs accounting for less than a tenth of the studies (8%). The descriptive studies, lacking a comparison group, do not allow an inference that the dream reports are related to the mental illness from which the dreamer is suffering. The one third or so separate group studies have a control group for comparison, assuming that group differences are found opens the possibility that the dream content differences that are found may be attributable to the illness that the patient group is said to have. The repeated measure studies addresses the question of whether the dream content difference between the illness group and the control group is a state or trait aspect of the patients' dreams. If it were a state function it would change with a change in the illness, and if it did not then it might be a trait function of the dreamer perhaps related to a predisposition to the illness being studied.

In all separate group studies the appropriateness of the controls is of concern, e.g., that all potentially confounding variables are matched but the variable in question, the illness under study. Half of the control groups (50%) are of patients with a different illness than the one under study. This illness control increases the possibility that any differences that are found are due to the illness of the group and not to just being ill. Of the separate group studies controls, 30% were a comparison to a non-ill group so that any differences that were found may be related to a sick–well difference between groups and not to the particular illness being studied. Interestingly 20% of the separate group studies controls include both a well and a sick group comparison.

The discovery of REM sleep [22], during which much but not all of dreaming occurs, opened the possibility of recovering more of a night's dreaming experience than could be recovered from post-sleep waking recall. However, almost three quarters of the reviewed studies (71%) were from dreams collected by spontaneous recall outside of a sleep laboratory, the remainder (29%) were from sleep laboratory awakenings during REM sleep. A more comprehensive dream collection is achieved from laboratory-collected dreams. The availability to dream investigators of sleep laboratories is restricted and may account for only 29% of studies reporting on laboratory-collected dreams.

The adequacy of the description of the patient sample

Sample size

There were 51 laboratory studies with 891 subjects and 122 non-laboratory studies with 19,221 subjects. The average laboratory study had 17 subjects while the average non-laboratory study had 158 subjects. The laboratory studies had a minimally acceptable number of subjects while the non-laboratory studies appear to have on average an acceptable number of subjects. These comments on sample size would be more meaningful if power analyses had been done in the studies but this was not the case. The limited ecomomic support for dream researchers contributes to the large discrepancy in sample size between laboratory and non-laboratory studies.

Patient selection

The basis for the selection of patients (45%), the basis for diagnostic classification (47%), the specificity of diagnostic subtype assignment (34%), and whether the patients were taking medication or receiving physical treatments (31%) were reported in only a third to a half of the studies. The ability to replicate a study would be sorely limited given the scant information given about selection, diagnosis, and medication that these studies provide. The content of dreams is highly likely to be affected by all of them.

Information about demographic variables was commonly provided in the studies for variables such as the subjects' sex (87%) and age (68%) but inadequately for marital status (29%), race (26%), education (25%), general health (18%), and social class (18%), all of which have been shown to affect dream content [23]. Inadequate subject characterization could well contribute to replication failures in a field where, unfortunately, replication generally has been rarely done.

The setting in which the dream is experienced and reported may well affect the content of the dream obtained. The hospital was the setting in 39% of the studies, an outpatient setting, generally the patient's home, was the setting for 48% of the studies, both hospital and home was the setting for 10%, and no setting was reported in 2% of the reports. Differences found in dream content, for example, in depressed patients studied while in the hospital may be different from those obtained from depressed patients sleeping

at home because of the setting difference as well as factors such as the intensity of the depression and the medication the patient may be taking.

The adequacy of the description of the control sample (separate groups only)

Sample size

The separate group studies require a control group that must be carefully chosen to match the illness group in all the factors that may influence the dream experience except the illness variable. There were 64 studies: 20 done in the sleep laboratory and 44 were non-laboratory studies. The average sample size for the laboratory studies was 17 and for the non-laboratory control group was 65. The numbers appear adequate but as noted above in describing the study sample a power analysis would allow a more precise statement about the adequacy of the control sample.

Control sample selection

The basis for selection (55%) and diagnosis (45%) was given in about half the studies, similar to what was found in the patient sample. The specificity of diagnosis (35%) and whether the subject was on medication or receiving physical treatment (26%) was reported in about a third of cases or less, similar to the inadequate levels found in the description of patient sample.

The demographic variables' frequency was well reported in the control subjects for sex (83%) and fairly well for age (66%) and education (48%), and too infrequently for race (22%), social class (20%), general health (20%), and marital status (18%). The demographic variables are reported with about the same frequency for the control patients as they were for the study sample.

The setting in which the dream is experienced and reported is essentially the same for the control and target subjects as one might have expected. The control subjects had 35% of their dreams in the hospital, 51% out of the hospital, and 14% involved collection both in and out of the hospital.

The method of dream content collection

Dream content collection appears to be a very straightforward undertaking, yet there are a number of factors in the collection process that could affect the results of a dream content study [24]. The number of nights or days of dream collection will, of course, influence the outcome of any study and this variable is reported in only 44% of studies. Similarly, the number of dreams collected needs to be specified as it reflects the pool of dreams for study and it was reported in almost two thirds (59%) of the studies. In order to report a dream it must be recalled and too low a recall rate could well contribute to a distortion in what dreams are reported and examined. Unfortunately, only 28% of studies reported the recall rates of their subjects. This low recall reporting makes it difficult to assess the sampling adequacy of most of the studies that are being reviewed.

The interpersonal aspects of the reporting process can influence what dreams are experienced and reported [25, 26]. This should encourage reporting by whom and when the dream reports were collected. These two variables, by whom and when, were reported in 55% and 53% of the studies respectively. The mode of awakening in the sleep laboratory has been shown to alter the likely of recall but is only reported in 25% of the laboratory studies, an unacceptably low rate. The manner or protocol for eliciting the report of the dream experience is rarely reported (17%) while the method of recording the dream (53%) is more commonly described. The questions asked clearly will influence the material obtained. Asking, "what were you dreaming?" does not give the same result as asking, "what was going through your mind before I awakened you?" The mode of recording may also alter the report obtained, e.g., being in the room using a tape recorder or doing an interview through an intercom or having a subject write out his dream may not yield the same result. The dream collection protocol may inquire about associations to the dream report and this should be specified as it was in some of these studies (35%).

The method of scoring dream content

Generally, the actual dream report is reworked in some manner to remove redundancies in the report or to remove explanations or clarifications that are not descriptions of the dream experience [24]. The rules governing these protocol preparations are essential if a replication of the study is to be undertaken, but they are rarely reported (16%). To establish the replicability of the scoring process, which sets the limits on the validity that it is possible to obtain in any study, the use of more than one scorer, "blind" to the hypothesis and data source of the dream report being scored, is essential. Only 17% of the studies

under review reported scoring by two or more scorers. Startling was the finding that 35% of the studies made no mention of the number of raters and 48% used only one rater. Only one study reported recalibrating the reliability of the scorers periodically during the scoring process [27].

The type of dream scoring scale utilized was thematic in about a third of the studies (37%), item scoring in about a quarter (27%), and not reported in a third (36%). The scale source was ad hoc in almost half the studies (46%), not reported in about a third (35%), and not given in about a third (35%). The value of using a standard scale, and there are many, is that data about the scale's reliability and validity are available. Often combining aspects of a standard scoring system can be done to examine a unique property of a dream report that is of interest [28].

Attention to the manner in which the dream report is prepared and scored is essential to developing a body of knowledge about the dream life of the mentally ill or any other scientific exploration of dreaming. A common measurement tool is essential in building a body of knowledge; none has been agreed upon in dream research.

The nature of the statistical analysis

Statistical tests could have been reported by the 77 separate groups and repeated measure studies of the total 173 studies (45%) as the case reports and the descriptive studies would not be expected to have any statistical analysis. Of those studies that might have had a statistical analysis, 82% actually reported a statistical analysis of their data and of those, 86% reported the number of tests done. The statistics applied were appropriate to the design in 81% of the studies with statistical analysis and 63% were preplanned and 37% were post hoc. Three quarters (76%) of the studies with statistical analysis reported significant results. Thirty-nine studies is a relatively small number of studies to characterize the seven mental illnesses that are the basis for this review of dreaming in psychiatric illness.

Dream content results

The 63 studies that had a statistical analysis of their dream content were reduced to 48 (76%) that had positive findings [14, 15]. Since Ramsey's 1953 [13] summary of the pre-REM studies of dreams in psychiatric illness, only 48 acceptable studies have been added in 55 years, a very meager output. A summary of the content reports from all the studies for each of the diagnostic entities will be presented in what follows.

Schizophrenia

The dream reports of schizophrenics compared to other groups are less complex and more direct, sexual, anxious, negative, and hostile. The hostility is primarily directed at the dreamer although the patient is less likely to be the focus of the dream. Their dream reports are more bizarre and implausible and they have more interest in their dreams. With increasing anxiety, motion and anxiety in the dream report increases. Strangers were their most frequent dream character and there were more males and groups of characters in their dreams. Waking hallucinations and dream content were similar as was the degree of paranoia, which is contrary to Freud's view that they would be compensatory. Judges were able to sort one patient's dreams from another and one night's dreaming from another. The ability to sort their dreams by subject and by nights for a subject underlines the individuality of the schizophrenic patient [29]. Lobotomized schizophrenics had a lower recall rate in the sleep laboratory than a non-lobotomized group. The most consistent findings in the dreams of schizophrenics are that hostility is more common in their dreams, that reflections of a thought disorder, e.g., implausibility and bizarreness, occurred more often and that there is more anxiety in their dreams.

Depression

Depressed patients dream as frequently as the non-depressed, but their dream reports were shorter and had less traumatic or depressive content even after the depression has remitted. This suggests a compensatory relationship between the waking and dreaming state in depression. Family members were more frequent in their dreams. If hostility was present in the dreams it was as likely to be directed at the dreamer as away from the dreamer. Anxiety and hostility are not prominent affects in the dreams of the depressed. Their dreams had more friendly interactions and fewer aggressive interactions than those of schizophrenics but more failures and misfortunes. With clinical improvement, hostility decreased while intimacy, motility, and heterosexuality increased. There is an increase in death themes in depressed suicidal

patients and in bipolar patients before becoming manic.

Masochism in the dreams of the depressed is more common in women and is more likely a trait than a state characteristic, as its frequency does not change when the depression lifts. A past focus is not universal in the dreams of the depressed nor is it unique to the depressed state. The content of their dreams may have prognostic significance for both response to treatment and spontaneous recovery. The affective state of the dreamer covaries with the content of the dream. It has been noted that changes in dreams across the night may contribute to the coping capacity of the dreamer. A failure to self-regulate mood is associated with a suicidal tendency. Those dreamers reporting negative dreams earlier in the night are more likely to be in remission after one year. Mood regulation processes may have an implication for the treatment of depression. The only independently verified findings in the dreams of the depressed are that their dreams are shorter and that characters with family roles appear with increased frequency. Masochism has not been found to occur with increased frequency in the dreams of the depressed.

Post-traumatic stress disorder [PTSD]

Interest in PTSD patients and their dreams was stimulated by the high incidence of the disorder in veterans of the Vietnam War and sustained by the effect on soldiers who served subsequently in the Gulf and Iraq. The condition became part of the American psychiatric nomenclature in 1980 although it had been described in the English language literature for over a hundred years.

Ross and his colleagues have taken the position that a sleep disturbance is the essence of PTSD. They have characterized the dreams of PTSD patients as vivid, affect laden, disturbing, outside the realm of current waking experience, but representative of earlier life experience, repetitive, stereotyped, and easy to recall. The dream disturbance is relatively specific to the disorder, and PTSD may be fundamentally a disorder of the REM sleep mechanism. They grant that non-REM sleep may be involved as well, as the dream disturbance occurs early in the night and has movement associated with it.

Others have suggested that the special aspect of PTSD is the intrusive imagery and recurrent dreams and nightmares that have challenged the view of dreaming described by Ross. Not all dreaming in

PTSD is a recapitulation of the trauma. Trauma sufferers can have disturbing arousals out of both REM and non-REM sleep. There can be different types of nightmares in PTSD and the traumatic dream can change across time, reflect classical Freudian dream work mechanisms, and is not a meaningless re-enactment of the trauma.

It is generally accepted that the dream experience is disturbing, but this may be more a reaction to the dream than in the dream itself. The affect-laden nature of the disturbing dream has not been confirmed. The disturbing dream can be reactivated later in life. The vividness of the dream has been addressed and the dream is not easily recalled. Dream recall in patients with active PTSD is lower than in normal individuals but higher than in well adjusted former PTSD patients.

A consensus has emerged suggesting that the hallmark of PTSD is a disturbance in psychological dreaming and possibly non-REM sleep early in the night. Disturbed dreaming covaries with combat exposure and torture, not with the complaint of a sleep disturbance. The disturbing dream tends to occur early during sleep, as do increases in movement, spontaneous awakenings, autonomic discharge, elevated arousal threshold, and a heightened startle response. The disturbing dream is not sleep-stage bound. Stereotypical dream content is not typical of the disturbing dream. Failure or avoidance of recall may be an adaptational strategy.

An excellent review of dreaming in PTSD is provided by Wittman and colleagues [30] and Levin and Nielsen [31] provide a challenging neurocognitive model for disturbed dreaming, PTSD, and affect distress.

Eating disorders

Anorexics and bulimics both report dreaming and their dreams have been shown to be useful in psychotherapy in contradiction to what has been described as the lack of accessibility to the inner lives of alexythymics. A similar finding of dream reporting has been described for asthmatics [32], which also has been considered an alexythymic condition.

For eating disorder patients, the rate of dream recall is low on self-report questionnaires but normal in the sleep laboratory. This discrepancy may reflect the degree of interest that these patients have in their inner life and/or a desire to avoid it, which we have suggested (see above) may be an adaptational strategy in PTSD.

Dreaming about food is high in eating disorder patients, more so in bulimics than anorexics. Aggressive dreams are less common in these patients than normal individuals and may reflect a passive, avoidant approach to life.

Brain damaged

There is a decrease in dream reporting associated with aging and with dementia. Dreams of lost resources are common in the aged and minimally to moderately demented. The more severely brain damaged had more characters in their dream reports than the less severely damaged. A questionnaire study found no relationship between dream report frequency and the degree of atrophy on computerized tomography scans. Repetitive visual imagery in the brain damaged was not found to be REM bound. The dream content of right-hemispherectomized patients is the same as controls suggesting that the left hemisphere plays a critical role in dream generation. Other anatomic bases for dreaming using brain lesion data [33] suggest that the basis for dreaming is bilateral, involving the bilateral medio-basal prefrontal cortex and the inferior parietal area of both sides of the brain. Exploring the dreams of brain-damaged patients in psychotherapy has been found to be useful in the rehabilitative process.

Mental retardation

The dreams of patients with mental retardation are simple, contain day residues, are primarily visual, but with little color, variety, or vividness. The theme of being at home is very common in the institutionalized mentally retarded. The contents of their thematic apperception responses and their dreams are very similar. There is a sex difference in their dreams, similar to that of normal subjects. Male retardates have more aggressive dreams and dream more about sports, finding money, and eating. Female patients with mental retardation have more color in their dreams and dream more about falling and being chased.

Alcoholism and drug abuse

Alcoholics have more dreams of oral incorporation, see themselves more often in dreams as the object of aggression than non-alcoholics, and have fewer sexual interactions. Judges can discriminate the dreams of alcoholics from non-alcoholics. Detoxifying alcoholics who dream about drinking are more likely to abstain longer from drinking than those who do not. The implication of dreaming about drinking or drug use as a predictor of abstinence remains unclear. It does raise the possibility of dreaming having adaptive significance.

Conclusions

The causes of the various mental illnesses have not been revealed by the study of their dream content. The small number of studies in many of the entities of interest and the general lack of scientific rigor continues to limit any potential value in the study of dreams. The shift from a psychological to a biological emphasis in the study of mental illness has only served to further a diminished interest in the study of dreams. However, we know more about the dream in PTSD and depression than we had known before. The studies on PTSD point to the central role of dreaming rather than REM sleep in this condition and the stabilizing role of non-recall in maintaining adaptation in these patients. The impairment of the role of dreaming in affect regulation may be central to understanding the mood changes in depression.

It appears from this review that what one does or does not dream about may contribute to the waking adaptational process. The change in dream content with a change in the state of the dreamer is highly suggestive of a possible adaptational role. Whether it's the avoidance of the trauma experience by the decreased recall of dreaming seen in PTSD patients or the continued experience of drinking in the dreams of alcoholics, or failures in mood regulation in the depressed, examining the dream in patients with mental illness may facilitate our understanding of the adaptational process.

The study of the process of dream construction in normal individuals as well as the mentally ill, utilizing the dream manipulation techniques suggested by Tart [34], and the available analytic techniques, has not been undertaken and could well enhance our understanding of the cognitive process in dreaming.

References

1. Benca R. Sleep in psychiatric disorders. *Neurol Clin.* 1996;**14**:739–64.

2. Freud S. *The Interpretation of Dreams.* Volumes IV and V of The Standard Edition. (London: Hogarth Press, 1953; 41–2).

3. Aristotle. *On Dreams.* Translated by J. Beane. (eworks@Adelaide, 2007).

4. Kant I. Cited In: Freud S. *The Interpretation of Dreams.* Volumes IV and V of The Standard Edition. (London: Hogarth Press, 1953; 90).

5. Schopenhauer A. Cited In: Freud S. *The Interpretation of Dreams.* Volumes IV and V of The Standard Edition. (London: Hogarth Press, 1953; 90).

6. Jung C. *The Psychology of Dementia Praecox.* (London: Princeton University Press, 1960; 86).

7. Jackson JH. In: J. Taylor, ed. *Selected Writings of John Hughlings Jackson,* Volume 2. (New York: Basic Books, 1958; 45).

8. Freud S. *The Interpretation of Dreams.* Volumes IV and V of The Standard Edition. (London: Hogarth Press, 1953).

9. Hartmann, E. *The Nightmare: The Psychology and Biology of Terrifying Dreams.* (New York: Basic Books 1984).

10. Hobson J. Dreaming as delirium: a mental status analysis of our nightly madness. *Semin Neurol.* 1997;**17**:121–8.

11. Hagen F. Cited In: Freud S. *The Interpretation of Dreams.* Volumes IV and V of The Standard Edition. (London: Hogarth Press, 1953; 90).

12. Freud S. *The Interpretation of Dreams.* Volumes IV and V of The Standard Edition. (London: Hogarth Press, 1953; 89).

13. Ramsey G. Studies of dreaming. *Psychol Bull.* 1953;**50**:432–55.

14. Kramer M, Nuhic Z. A review of dreaming by psychiatric patients: an update. In: Pandi-Perumal SR, Ruoti R, Kramer M, eds. *Sleep and Psychosomatic Medicine.* (Boca Raton, FL: Taylor and Francis, 2007; 137–55).

15. Kramer M, Roth T. Dreams in psychopathological groups: a critical review. In: Williams R, Karacan I, eds. *Sleep Disorders: Diagnosis and Treatment.* (New York: John Wiley, 1978; 323–49).

16. Kramer, M. The selective mood regulatory function of dreaming: an update and revision. In: Moffitt A, Kramer M, Hoffmann R, eds. *The Functions of Dreaming.* (Albany, NY: State University of New York Press, 1993; 139–96).

17. Kramer M, Roth T. The relationship of dream content to night-morning mood. In: Popoviciu L, Asigian B, Bain G, eds. *Sleep.* (Basel: S. Karger, 1980; 622–4).

18. Cartwright R, Luten A, Young M, Mercer P, Bears M. Role of REM sleep and dream affect in over-night mood regulation: a study of normal volunteers. *Psychiatric Res.* 1998;**81**:1–8.

19. Johnson L, Spinweber C, Gomez S, Matteson L. Daytime sleepiness, performance, mood, nocturnal

sleep: the effect of benzodiazepines and caffeine on their relationship *Sleep.* 1990;13:121–35.

20. Kramer M, Whitman R, Baldridge B, Ornstein P. Drugs and dreams III: the effects of imipramine on the dreams of the depressed. *Amer J Psychiat.* 1968;**124**:1385–92.

21. Kramer M, Glucksman M. Changes in dream affect during psychoanalytic therapy. *J Am Acad Psychoanal Dyn Psychotherapy.* 2006;**34**:249–60.

22. Aserinsky E, Kleitman N. Regularly occurring periods of eye motility, and concomitant phenomena, during sleep. *Science.* 1953;**118**:273–4.

23. Winget C, Kramer M, Whitman R. Dreams and demography. *Can Psychiatr Assoc J.* 1972;**17** (Suppl 2): SS203–208.

24. Winget C, Kramer M. *Dimensions of Dreams.* (Gainesville: University Presses of Florida, 1979).

25. Whitman R, Kramer M, Baldridge B. Which dream does the patient tell? *Arch Gen Psychiatry.* 1963;**8**:277–82.

26. Fox R, Kramer M, Baldridge B, Whitman R, Ornstein P. The experimenter variable in dream research. *Dis Nerv Syst.* 1968;**29**:698–701.

27. Kramer M, Roth T, Palmer T. The psychological nature of the REM dream report and T.A.T. stories. *Psychiatric J Univ Ottawa.* 1976;**1**:128–35.

28. Kramer M, Trinder J, Whitman R, Baldridge B. The incidence of masochistic dreams in the night collected dreams of depressed subjects. *Psychophysiology.* 1969;**6**:250.

29. Kramer M, Hlasny R, Jacobs G, Roth T. Do dreams have meaning? An empirical inquiry. *Am J Psychiatry.* 1976;**133**:778–81.

30. Wittmann L, Schredl M, Kramer M. Dreaming in posttraumatic stress disorder: a critical review of phenomenology, psychophysiology and treatment. *Psychother Psychosom.* 2007;**76**:25–39.

31. Levin R, Nielsen T. Disturbed dreaming, posttraumatic stress disorder, and affect distress: a review and neurocognitive model. *Psychol Bull.* 2007;**133**:482–526.

32. Hirsch N, Kinney L, Kramer M. Specificity of dream content and dream recall in asthma sufferers *Sleep Res.* 1981;**10**:164.

33. Solms M. *The Neuropsychology of Dreams: a Clinico-Anatomical Study.* (Mahwah, NJ: L. Erlbaum Associates, 1997).

34. Tart C. From spontaneous event to lucidity: a review of attempts to consciously control nocturnal dreaming. In: Wolman B, ed. *Handbook of Dreams.* (New York: Van Nostrand Reinhold, 1979).

Chapter 35

Forensic issues of sleep in psychiatric patients

Irshaad Ebrahim and Peter B. Fenwick

Introduction

And I see men become mad and demented from no manifest cause and at the same time doing many things out of place, and I have known many persons in sleep groaning and crying out, some in a state of suffocation, some jumping up and fleeing out of doors, and deprived of their reason till they awaken and afterwards becoming well and rational as before, although they be pale and weak.

Hippocrates, 400 BC

Psychiatrists are often called upon to provide expert testimony or reports in forensic cases that involve behavior that may have arisen from sleep or during the sleep period. Knowledge of the various sleep disorders that are associated with behavioral manifestations is thus important and essential if a psychiatrist is to be involved in the forensic assessment of a person accused of a sleep-related crime. The interface between psychiatric diagnosis, sleep disorders, and psychotropic medication is a complex and little understood area. This becomes more complex when the spectre of apparent sleep-related violence, murder, sexual assault, or other apparent sleep-related criminal activity intervenes. This chapter seeks to provide the practicing psychiatrist, fellow medical professionals, and students, basic knowledge of and access to essential references of the medical, psychiatric, and legal issues that arise when sleep disorders are implicated in the forensic arena.

Automatism and the law

"An automatism is an involuntary piece of behaviour over which an individual has no control. The behaviour is usually inappropriate to the circumstances, and may be out of character for the individual. It can be complex, co-ordinated and apparently purposeful and directed, though lacking in judgment. Afterwards the individual may have no recollection or only a partial and confused memory for his actions. In organic automatisms there must be some disturbance of brain function sufficient to give rise to the above features." [1]

In the UK and the USA and those jurisdictions based on UK law, for a person to be convicted of a crime, the law requires that the defendant has committed a criminal act (*actus reus*) and that he had a knowing intent to commit that act (*mens rea*). It is this element that must be shown to be lacking when a defence of automatism is used [2–5].

The legal definition of automatism is based on the doctrine of *mens rea*, the fundamental basis of English law. Everyone who has reached the age of discretion is, unless the contrary is proved, presumed at law to be sane and accountable for his actions. "*Actus non fecit reus mens sit rea*," the deed does not make a man guilty unless his mind is guilty. Unless the offence is a statutory one that carries an absolute liability (e.g., driving with a raised blood alcohol level), the doctrine of *mens rea*, or the presence of a guilty mind, can only be negated by certain considerations.

Legally, automatisms are divided into two categories, *sane* (or *non-insane* in the UK) arising from an *external cause* (e.g., a blow to the head or a bee sting) and *insane* (arising from *an internal factor* such as a brain disorder e.g., a stroke or epilepsy).

These categories arose following the Denning judgement in the case of *Attorney General* v. *Bratty*, where Lord Denning wanted to make certain that those individuals who were habitually violent due to a medical condition would be detained in hospital. He said "It seems to me that any mental disorder which has manifested itself in violence and is prone to recur is a disease of the mind. At any rate, it is the sort of disease

Sleep and Mental Illness, eds. S. R. Pandi-Perumal and M. Kramer. Published by Cambridge University Press.
© Cambridge University Press 2010.

for which a person should be detained in hospital rather than being given an unqualified acquittal."

There have been a number of developments of this principle. Possibly most important is the Canadian and Australian view. "The law had developed two main tests to establish whether or not automatism stemmed from a mental disorder: the internal cause theory, set up by Martin JA in *Raby* vs. *The Queen* (1977) 17 OR (2D) 1, and continuing danger theory referred to by La Forest, J. in *R* vs. *Parkes* (1992) SCR 87. This was modified in *R* vs. *Stone's* case (1999 2 SCR 290 at 396–398) where Vastarache J found that both approaches are relevant factors in determining into which category a condition falls and other policy factors may also be taken into account to provide a holistic approach." [6, 7]

The medical concept of automatism – complex behavior in the absence of conscious awareness or volitional intent – is straightforward; the legal concept is quite different. It is sometimes easy, medically, to distinguish these two categories. For example, an attack by a swarm of bees resulting in a reflex turning of the steering wheel of a car is clearly a sane automatism. An epileptic fit arising from a damaged brain and leading to a violent killing is clearly an insane automatism. But between these two extremes the medical and legal grounds do not coalesce happily. From a medical point of view any abnormality of brain function, which has led to a disorder of behavior, will usually contain components of both sane and insane automatism. For example, the blow to the head (external) only produces the automatism because it disrupts the functioning of the neurons in the brain (internal). It makes little sense to say that an offence committed in a confusional state following the injection of insulin is sane, while a similar state from too much insulin secreted by the pancreas is insanity.

It is important to remember that the law is not concerned with the medical diagnosis, but only with the state of mind at the time the act was committed. This was highlighted in the case of *R* vs. *Kemp*, where Mr. Justice Devlin discussed the difference between the medical diagnosis and the important legal criterion of a disordered mind. He said: "It does not matter for the purpose of the law whether the defect of reason is due to degeneration of the brain or to some other form of mental derangement. That may be a matter of importance medically, but it is of no importance to the law, which merely has to consider the state of mind in which the accused is, not how he got there."

A further clarification of automatism following the above principle is provided by Yeo [5] in discussing the Canadian case of *R* vs. *Stone*:

- Automatism comprises involuntary conduct involving a complete lack of capacity to contain one's conduct.

- Unconsciousness or impaired consciousness is not essential for a state of automatism to exist. Evidence of unconsciousness or impaired consciousness is relevant, not because it is essential to a finding of automatism, but to show that the defendant's conduct was involuntary.

- Expert evidence should be directed to showing whether the defendant's conduct was involuntary rather than to showing whether s/he was unconscious or semi-unconscious at the time of the alleged offence.

- To help decide whether a defendant was suffering from mental disorder automatism or non-mental disorder automatism, the triers of fact should consider whether the cause of the automatic state was due to an internal or external cause, and also whether the defendant poses a continuing danger to the community.

- When considering these factors, the triers of fact should not regard them as conclusive of the issue nor as mutually exclusive factors. Rather, they should take a holistic approach with the overarching concern being whether societal protection requires the defendant to undergo medical treatment. If so, the finding should be one of mental disorder automatism.

- Expert evidence should be directed to showing whether or not the defendant continued to be a danger to society and in need of medical treatment.

- In cases of mental disorder automatism, expert evidence should concentrate on showing whether the defendant's conduct was involuntary and not whether s/he did not appreciate the nature and quality of her/his act or know that it was wrong.

- Upon a finding that the defendant suffered from mental disorder automatism, the court should concentrate on the special verdict of not responsible on account of mental disorder, without being required to determine further whether the defendant did not appreciate the nature and quality of her/his act or did not know that it was wrong. [So not following the McNaughten Rules]

Physicians giving expert testimony must remember that a medical diagnosis is not a defense. Thus having epilepsy, a cerebral tumor, or a sleep disorder is not a defense on its own. It is only the state of mind at the time the offence was carried out that is significant, e.g., that an automatism was present at that time. Neither does the legal categorization take into account the severity of the offence. A severe and prolonged attack in a confusional state following a head injury is a sane automatism; walking naked through a crowded hotel bar in a sleepwalking episode is insanity.

The legal definition does not contain any reference to time. This arose again from the case of *R* vs. *Kemp*. In discussing the cerebral arteriosclerosis that was said to have caused the automatism at the time of the offence, Lord Justice Devlin said: "In my judgement the condition of the brain is irrelevant. So is the question of whether the condition of the mind is curable or incurable, transitory or permanent. ... Temporary insanity is sufficient to satisfy them [the McNaughten rules]." Thus the law is not concerned with time. A minor flick of the hand in a brief epileptic myoclonic jerk – a matter of half a second – which knocks a vase off a shelf and injures a passer-by is insanity, as is a cerebral tumor leading to automatic confusional states lasting for months [8].

There has been recent discussion within both the legal and medical professions mainly in Canada and Australia of the value of keeping a *mens rea* automatism defence. It was argued in the 1989 Crimes Bill in New Zealand that the *mens rea* test of automatism may at times be difficult to define, and thus "the real test is one of involuntariness. If the accused was not wholly unconscious but nevertheless acted involuntarily, he or she would be protected from criminal responsibility." This shifts the emphasis from the *mens rea* to the *actus reus* [9].

The categorization of sane (non-insane) and insane automatism as applied to sleepwalking has also divided the medico-legal community, for in Canada sleepwalking is held to be sane automatism and in the UK and USA sleepwalking is held to be insanity. However, we can expect the legal view to continue towards the enhancement of the *actus reus* with a diminishing emphasis on the *mens rea*.

The Criminal Procedure (Insanity and Fitness to Plead) Act 1991 (in England and Wales) does in fact allow the judge to dispose of the case sensibly on a special verdict. He or she can give an absolute discharge or a treatment order, except in the case of a mandatory sentence (murder) when he must send the defendant to hospital (this would now be a medium secure psychiatric unit) with or without a restriction order. It is likely that the assessment would only be for long enough to assess dangerousness and public safety. But that still leaves the emotional question of the label of insanity and the "quagmire of automatism." In the USA, the approach to automatism varies from state to state leaving inconsistencies in the assessment of crimes related to medical causes of automatic behavior [10].

The causes of sleep-related automatism are wide and varied and some of the more commonly implicated disorders are listed in Table 35.1. It is therefore important, in the assessment of a person presenting with an apparent automatism, to systematically investigate for all these possibilities.

The parasomnias

The American Academy of Sleep Medicine (AASM), after extensive consultation, published the 2nd edition of *The International Classification of Sleep Disorders* (ICSD-2) in 2005. The ICSD-2 provided, for the first time, a thorough diagnostic and coding manual for sleep disorders based on scientific and clinical evidence [11].

Parasomnias are defined in the ICSD-2 as "undesirable physical events or experiences that occur during entry into sleep, within sleep, or during arousals from sleep. These events are manifestations of central nervous system activation transmitted into skeletal muscle and autonomic nervous system channels, often with experiential concomitants." Parasomnias are classified as clinical disorders "because of the resulting injuries, sleep disruption, adverse health effects and untoward psychosocial effects."

Parasomnias are classified into three broad categories:

- Disorders of arousal (from non-REM sleep)
- Parasomnias usually associated with REM sleep
- Other parasomnias (including those due to drug or substance)

For the purposes of this chapter, we will concentrate on those parasomnia most commonly implicated in sleep and psychiatry namely:

- The disorders of arousal
- REM sleep behavior disorder
- Parasomnia due to drug or substance

Table 35.1 The differential diagnosis of sleep related automatisms

Organic medical and neurologic disorders

A. Vascular

   1. Transient global amnesia (including migraine)

B. Mass lesions

   1. Increased intracranial pressure

   2. Deep midline structural lesions

C. Toxic/metabolic

   1. Endocrine

   2. Hypoxia/carbon monoxide poisoning

   3. Drugs/alcohol (intoxication/withdrawal)

   4. Thiamine deficiency (Wernicke–Korsakoff syndrome)

D. Infectious (limbic encephalitis)

E. Central nervous system (CNS) trauma

F. Seizures

   1. Siezure disorders e.g., complex partial seizures.

   2. Nocturnal siezure disorder e.g., nocturnal frontal lobe epilepsy

Sleep disorders

A. Disorders of arousal (confusional arousals [sleep drunkenness], sleepwalking, sleep terrors)

B. Rapid eye movement (REM) sleep behavior disorder

C. Nocturnal seizures

D. Automatic behavior

E. Narcolepsy and idiopathic CNS hypersomnia

F. Sleep apnea

G. Sleep deprivation

H. Sleep schedule/circadian rhythm disorder (including jet-lag)

Psychogenic disorders

A. Dissociative states that may arise directly from sleep

   1. Fugues

   2. Multiple personality disorder

   3. Psychogenic amnesia

B. Post-traumatic stress disorder

C. Malingering

D. Munchausen by proxy

Disorders of arousal

The ICSD-2 classifies the disorders of arousal (DOA) into three types: confusional arousals, sleepwalking, and sleep terrors. It provides detailed descriptions of each diagnostic category including: essential features, associated features, demographics, predisposing and precipitating factors, familial patterns, onset course and complications, pathology and pathophysiology. In addition, the ICSD-2 provides the polysomnographic and other objective findings to help confirm the diagnosis.

Confusional arousal disorders

These disorders occur in both sleepwalkers and in individuals without a previous history of sleepwalking. They occur in response to a sudden disturbance (noise, touch, physical proximity) during the deep phase of sleep (stages 3 and 4). The subject awakens into a confusional state, which can lead to violence or aggressive outbursts [11, 12].

In this state there is disturbance of cognition, emotion, and attention. The subject's behavior is confused and may be very complex. The episode lasts for a few minutes before both consciousness and clarity return. However, following a sudden arousal the subject rarely may alert into serious stereotyped pervasive anger when he may attack usually the first person he encounters, often the arouser, without any provocation causing serious wounds or even death. When serious violence occurs from sleep in someone without a history of sleepwalking, the diagnosis of a confusional arousal should be considered.

These episodes may be potentiated by alcohol or the taking of sedative/psychotropic medication and are more likely to occur if the subject is sleep deprived. The episodes may be more complex and last longer if the subject is a sleepwalker because they will arouse into a state similar to the non-sleepwalker but intermixed with sleepwalking behavior and EEG changes i.e., the confusional arousal leads into a sleepwalking episode [11–14].

The diagnosis of confusional arousals depends on the circumstances of the offence.

- The subject must have been asleep for a sufficient length of time to reach deep sleep (stage 3 or 4).
- The stimulus must be sufficient to induce an awakening.

- The abnormal behavior must start immediately on arousal.
- Usually the episode is short, a matter of a few minutes, but with alcohol this may be lengthened.

These episodes at first glance appear to be due to an external factor (the arousing stimulus) and thus fall within the rubric of sane automatism (as defined in *R* vs. *Quick*). However, if the aroused sleeper is also a sleepwalker, then they may well arouse into a sleepwalking episode and the legal classification will be one of insanity. The mind controlling the hand that plunges in the knife is thus considered by the law to be both sane (non-insane) and insane although it is likely insanity will be accepted by the court [3, 15–17].

Sleepwalking

Sleepwalking is classified as a disorder of arousal as it involves the incomplete arousal of a person from a state of deep sleep (usually stage 3 or 4 NREM sleep). Thus many sleepwalking episodes occur within one to two hours after sleep onset – the period within which we have the majority of our deep NREM sleep. Although this is the usual pattern of sleepwalking onset, sleepwalking episodes can occur in the transition from stage 2 sleep (a lighter stage of slow-wave sleep) to REM (dreaming) sleep, and so may occur in the later part of the night. Sleepwalking runs in families and is thought to be a genetic disorder [18–20].

Sleepwalking usually appears in childhood, continues through adolescence and often stops in adulthood. Rarely, it can appear for the first time in adulthood, frequently in relation to medication, alcohol, or physical illness, or in the presence of other psychiatric or neurological illness. Between 2 and 4% of the adult population have reported sleepwalking at some time [14, 20–23].

The behavior in a sleepwalking episode can be extremely variable and may be very complex. It can vary from sitting up in bed through hitting or putting your hands round your partner's neck or getting up and wandering around the room, to very complex episodes when the sleepwalker may exit the house, and even drive cars. Classically, most sleepwalking episodes last from five to fifteen minutes and usually consist of wandering around the house, sometimes urinating in cupboards and usually returning to bed. In cases where severe violence has been reported

during sleepwalking, the episode may last up to an hour. There is usually no memory of the episode on waking [23].

The diagnosis of sleepwalking and related disorders remains largely based on clinical history. Sleepwalking and related disorders rarely occur during standard diagnostic sleep laboratory studies and if they do occur, particularly in the forensic context, a high index of suspicion should be raised for possible malingering. The ICSD-2 criteria for sleepwalking are the most comprehensive in any diagnostic or coding manual.

The ICSD-2 diagnostic criteria for sleepwalking are as follows:

a. Ambulation occurs during sleep
b. Persistence of sleep, an altered state of consciousness, or impaired judgment during ambulation is demonstrated by at least one of the following:

   i. Difficulty in arousing the person
   ii. Mental confusion when awakened from an episode
   iii. Amnesia (complete or partial) for the episode
   iv. Routine behaviours that occur at inappropriate times
   v. Inappropriate or nonsensical behaviours
   vi. Dangerous or potentially dangerous behaviours

c. The disturbance is not better explained by another sleep disorder, medical or neurological disorder, mental disorder, medication use, or substance use disorder.

In the forensic context, where there is an increased likelihood of malingering and manipulation, a multidisciplinary and more encompassing approach is also required. These criteria, therefore, need to be viewed within the context of the specific events reported (i.e., the alleged crime) and taken into consideration with the full medical psychiatric, forensic, and family history of the defendant and the events of the alleged crime.

Parasomnias usually associated with REM sleep: REM sleep behavior disorder (RBD)

Rapid eye movement (REM) sleep behavior disorder (RBD) is an REM-stage parasomnia characterized by a history of excessive nocturnal motor activity, usually the violent enactment of dreams, associated with the absence of muscle atonia during REM sleep. The exact prevalence of RBD is unclear, but almost 90% of patients are men aged between 52 and 61 years at the time of presentation, and in about a quarter of these patients there is a history of sleeptalking, shouting, limbs twitching or jerking without complex behaviors, which may have preceded the development of RBD by many years with a mean of 22 years (range: 2 to 48 years). Psychiatric disorders and/or their treatment have been causally associated with RBD onset in approximately 10% of patients. While transient (acute) RBD can be seen after taking certain drugs or during drug withdrawal, the chronic type is usually idiopathic or associated with an underlying degenerative neurological condition. Rapid eye movement sleep behavior disorder may manifest as a subclinical (asymptomatic) entity and be a chance finding on polysomnography (PSG). Characteristic PSG findings include the loss of normal REM atonia and/or increased phasic electromyographic (EMG) activity during REM sleep. The literature suggests that RBD is effectively treated with clonazepam in the majority of cases [24–29].

The commonest psychiatric associations are with alcohol withdrawal, stimulant abuse, and treatment with psychotropic medication (fluoxetine, venlafaxine, and tricyclic antidepressants) and an association with major stressful events. The tricyclic antidepressants, selective serotonin reuptake inhibitors (SSRIs), and monoamine oxidase inhibitors can trigger or exacerbate RBD. The role of serotonin in the pathophysiology of RBD is not fully understood but may relate to the actions of serotonin and possibly noradrenalin on the striatal dopamine transporter. The effects of psychiatric medication on sleep and in particular, the potential of some psychotropic agents to precipitate RBD, is of daily clinical relevance to psychiatrists. A clear demonstration of a temporal relationship between the onset of symptoms and addition of or a change in the dosage of medication usually makes the diagnosis obvious. Improvement in a patient's symptoms after removal of the medication points to an iatrogenic cause for the RBD [30–34].

The classification and causes of RBD are shown in Table 35.2.

Sexsomnia

There is a long documented history of sexual behavior during sleep and the first forensic case was published in 1897, where Motet describes an example

Table 35.2 Causes of REM sleep behavior disorder (RBD)

Acute RBD	Etiology
Withdrawal	Alcohol
	Meprobamate
	Pentazocine
	Nitrazepam
	Rapid withdrawal of tricyclic antidepressants
Intoxication	Biperiden
	Tricyclic antidepressants
	Monoamine oxidase inhibitors
	Caffeine
	Mirtazapine
Chronic RBD	
Idiopathic	
Traumatic	
Toxic-metabolic	Tricyclic antidepressants
	Fluoxetine
	Venlafaxine
	Selegeline
	Anticholinergics
Vascular	Subarachnoid hemorrhage
	Vasculitis
	Ischemic
Tumors	Acoustic neuroma
	Pontine neoplasms
Infectious, post-infectious	Guillain–Barré syndrome
Degenerative	Parkinson's disease (PD)
	Multiple system atrophy (MSA)
	Dementia with Lewy bodies (DLB)
	Progressive supranuclear palsy
	Shy–Drager syndrome
	Olivopontocerebellar degeneration (OPCD)
	Amyotrophic lateral sclerosis
	Anterior/dorsomedial thalamic syndrome (fatal familial insomnia)

Table 35.2 (cont.)

Acute RBD	Etiology
	Dementia (including Alzheimer's disease and corticobasal degeneration)
	Normal pressure hydrocephalus
	Multiple sclerosis and demyelinating disorders
Developmental, congenital, familial	Familial/congenital RBD
	Narcolepsy
	Tourette's syndrome
	Group A xeroderma pigmentosum
	Mitochondrial encephalomyopathy

of somnambulism and exhibitionism. In October 1880, D. was arrested outside a public urinal in Rue Saint-Celie. He remained in the urinal for more than half an hour where he attempted to entice a policeman by exposing his genitals. Following his arrest and up to the time of his committal to the state prison three days later, he was in a state of half stupor. When he emerged from this state he claimed to remember nothing of the events surrounding his conviction and sentence of three months' imprisonment. Dr. Motet was alerted and a successful appeal was lodged on the basis that the offence against public decency occurred in a state of nocturnal somnambulism.

Sexual behavior during sleep is rarely reported in the literature and generally it is not mentioned when violence during sleep is reported. In 1986, Wong [35] reported the case of a 34-year-old man with episodes of nocturnal masturbation that he considered "somnambulism variant." Further reports were obtained of individuals who engaged in sleep-related sexual behavior, all of whom had prior histories of parasomnia. A comprehensive account of sexual behavior in the forensic context was provided by Fenwick in a landmark paper in 1996 [4]. Subsequently, a case report was published suggesting an overlap between the syndromes of RBD and somnambulism. In 1998, a further forensic case of somnambulistic sexual behavior was reported, that of a 45-year-old man with a history of sleepwalking being accused of fondling his daughter's friend. More recently two case series were

published independently by two leading experts in the field. All of the patients were identified as having an underlying sleep disorder with automatic behavior. These disorders included (1) disorders of arousal (non-REM parasomnias) that include confusional arousal, sleep terror, and sleepwalking; (2) REM sleep behavior disorder (RBD); (3) nocturnal partial complex seizures; and (4) obstructive sleep apnea (OSA).

Sexual offences and their relationship to sleep can be divided into two categories. The first category is the condition in which the perpetrator of the offence is asleep and during his sleep carries out behavior that is interpreted as being sexual and criminal. The second category is one in which the victim is asleep and the perpetrator is awake and commits the offence on the sleeping partner.

Somnambulistic sexual behavior (also called sexsomnia, sleep sex) is considered a variant of sleepwalking disorder as the overwhelming majority of people with sexsomnia have a history of sleepwalking and/or a family history of sleepwalking. The behavior can vary from explicit sexual vocalizations, to violent masturbation, to complex sexual acts including anal, oral, and vaginal penetration. There is usually no memory of the episode on waking. The sexual behavior can be either simple or complex and will typically last for a few minutes. In the simple cases the sleepwalker may caress or stroke their partner's body; these movements may sometimes apparently be more sexually directed, with groping or caressing of the partner's genitals. In the more complex cases a sleepwalker will leave their bed and if there are other sleepers in the house they may get into bed with them or they may interact in a sexual way with other members of the household. Sometimes the behavior may appear sexual though it is simply a byproduct of the sleepwalking episode. Many people sleep in the nude and so may sleepwalk naked in public. This cannot be interpreted as exhibitionism, although it may offend public decency [4, 35–40].

The difficulty in interpreting the significance of behavior during sleepwalking episodes is that it is not possible to gain access to subjective mental content. It is thus not possible to know whether, when a sleepwalker caresses the genitals of his partner, he is carrying out a sexual act or whether his behavior is simply an automatism that is devoid of explicit sexual meaning. This difficulty can never be resolved. A sexual interpretation of the behavior could be made

389

more easily if the sleepwalker were sexually aroused. However, sexual (genital) arousal in slow-wave sleep is uncommon and thus no conclusions can be drawn from its absence, although its presence would suggest sexual arousal with the possibility of subjective sexual intent.

In 1944, Ohlmeyer and coworkers discovered the occurrence of penile erection cycles during sleep in adult males. Such sleep-related erections (SRE) appeared at 85-minute intervals and episodes had an average duration of 25 minutes. As a result of this initial study, Oswald in 1962 noted that erection accompanied some REM periods, but subsequent investigations of Fisher in 1965 and Karacan in 1966 demonstrated a strong temporal association between the occurrence of erection and REM. Erectile episodes were found to dovetail with over 95% of REM periods while erection was entirely absent during non rapid eye movement (NREM) sleep, except immediately before and after REM periods. Karacan reported that 80% of REM periods displayed this phenomenon although there were also occasional instances of erection during NREM sleep. Somnambulistic episodes occur or arise out of stage 3 and 4 of NREM sleep, and the presence of an erection is thus not considered an exclusion criterion for sleepwalking [41–43].

Two recent and comprehensive reviews on the topic are strongly recommended for the reader-practitioner who may be involved in a forensic case involving sex and sleep [44, 45].

Parasomnia due to drug or substance

The medical literature contains numerous case reports and case series of sleepwalking and nocturnal wandering episodes following ingestion of a wide variety and combination of medications and substances. Medications reported to be associated with sleepwalking/nocturnal wandering fall into almost all psychotropic and hypnotic classes of medication.

The ICSD-2 classifies these behaviors under the section "Parasomnia due to drug or substance" and lists the following characteristics:

i. The essential feature of this diagnosis is the close temporal relationship between exposure to a drug, medication, or biological substance and the onset of parasomnia signs and symptoms.

ii. The emergent parasomnia can be a de novo parasomnia, the aggravation of a chronic

intermittent parasomnia, or the reactivation of a previous parasomnia.

iii. The parasomnias most predictably associated with medications or biological substances are the disorders of arousal (DOA), sleep related eating disorder (SRED), REM sleep behavior disorder (RBD) and parasomnia overlap disorder.

Zolpidem

Zolpidem tartrate (Ambien) is the single most prescribed short-term sleep aid in the United States and as a consequence it has become the most studied of all hypnotic medications. As early as 1999, it was reported to initiate sleepwalking, which ceased when the medication was stopped [46, 47]. The Food and Drug Administration requires the manufacturers of zolpidem to provide an educational guide for each prescription recipient. The guide informs patients about the potential risks of zolpidem, which include unusual sleep-related behaviors such as driving while not fully awake with accompanying amnesia, and making telephone calls and eating while "asleep." [48]

Zolpidem-associated amnesia and somnambulism

There have been multiple case reports of somnambulism associated with Zolpidem use [46, 48–57]. Zolpidem has also been associated with the development of amnesia and visual hallucinations and compulsive behaviors including eating [50, 58–60]. There are two published clinical trials of zolpidem-induced anterograde amnesia/somnambulism [61, 62] The first study in 93 surgical patients reported that both midazolam 15 mg and zolpidem 20 mg produced significantly more anterograde amnesia (i.e., 45% of patients) than placebo (7%) [61]. In a large series of patients with insomnia in Switzerland, the adverse effects of anterograde amnesia/somnambulism were observed in 1.1% of those using zolpidem [62]. More recently, in a well designed study, the prevalence of somnambulism and amnesia in patients taking zolpidem for longer than six months was found to be 5.1%, which is considerably higher that the 2 to 4% accepted prevalence for sleepwalking in the general population [63]. There is a single case report of zaleplon (Sonata) associated somnambulism.

Zolpidem and sleep-related eating disorder (SRED)

Zolpidem has also been associated with complex behaviors, in particular nocturnal eating behaviors.

Sleep-related eating syndromes comprise a spectrum of abnormal behaviors combining features of sleep and eating disorders. First described in 1955 as "night-eating syndrome" (NES), more recently it has been provided a unique diagnostic category in the ICSD-2 as sleep-related eating disorder (SRED) [52, 59, 60].

One of the first case series of zolpidem-associated SRED was provided in 2002 in a well documented series of five patients [52]. Sleep-related eating disorder has also been associated with somnambulism [64, 65]. Winkelman noted that 11 of 23 (48%) patients had multiple abrupt awakenings from slow-wave sleep consistent with a diagnosis of somnambulism [64]. Schenk et al. reported that 84% of their patients with SRED had somnambulism [65]. Two of the five patients in the Mayo Clinic series exhibited nocturnal wanderings without eating only after zolpidem ingestion and while they did not have ambulation during polysomnography, both had multiple arousals from slow-wave sleep [52]. There have been further case reports and case series describing three female patients who, while taking zolpidem, experienced anterograde amnesia and "compulsive activities," which were reported as cleaning, shopping, and eating. These complex behaviors abruptly stopped with the discontinuation of zolpidem [47, 60]. Most patients with SRED appear to have underlying intrinsic sleep disorders. Schenck et al. have noted association with somnambulism (70%), RLS/PLMD (13%), sleep apnea (10%), and narcolepsy. The onset of this syndrome has also been reported after withdrawal from alcohol, tobacco products, opiates, and cocaine, and also with triazolam use. Traditional benzodiazepine medications (in particular triazolam and temazepam) have also been previously associated with amnesic nocturnal SRED [65–67]. Table 35.3 provides a comprehensive list of relevant publications regarding zolpidem and amnesic sleep and other related behaviors.

Benzodiazepines

Episodes of amnesic nocturnal wandering have been reported with benzodiazepines and other hypnotic medications. An interesting case series from France describes four forensic cases in which patients' unusual behaviors (not all sleep related) were attributed to hypnotic medications. The behaviors included two cases of robbery and one attempted murder while under the influence of a benzodiazepine hypnotic. The fourth case involved a female rape victim who was on a benzodiazepine who claimed amnesia for the assault. Table 35.4 provides an overview of the relevant publications and descriptions of reported sleep behaviors in patients on benzodiazepines [68–70].

Lithium and other psychotropic medications

There have been several case reports of somnambulism precipitated by a variety of medications including lithium, sodium valproate, paroxetine, tricyclic antidepressants, bupropion, olanzapine, topiramate, etc. These case reports have often involved patients who were on combination treatment, had undiagnosed or previously diagnosed epilepsy, and in several cases the relationship between treatment and/or dose adjustment and onset of sleep behaviors is poorly recorded. Tables 35.5 and 35.6 contain a detailed list of reports and publications of sleep-related behaviors that have been associated with lithium, antidepressant, and psychotropic medications [47].

The role of medications in priming or precipitating somnambulism requires careful and thorough evaluation particularly in the forensic context. There are, though, many documented cases of hypnotic and psychotropic medications where there is a clear temporal relationship between the introduction of the medicine and the onset of the behaviors and a reduction or cessation of the behaviors when the medications were stopped.

Malingering

The DSM-IV-TR defines malingering as "the intentional production of false or grossly exaggerated physical or psychological symptoms, motivated by external incentives such as avoiding military duty, avoiding work, obtaining financial compensation, evading criminal prosecution, or obtaining drugs."

In a survey of forensic practitioners Rogers found 16% of malingerers in forensic cases and about 8% in non-forensic cases. In a further study 15 to 17% of malingerers were found in forensic examinees and 7 to 8% in non-forensic [71, 72]. Pollock, using the MMPI-2 and the SIRS Interview Schedules, in 60 consecutive referrals from prison to a regional secure unit found 32% to be either fabricating or exaggerating their symptoms. More interesting is malingering in civil cases of head injury, when rates as high as 40% were found [73, 74].

Table 35.3 Zolpidem and sleep-related behaviors

Reference	Type of study/report	Concomitant medication	Patient demographic and medical history	Behavior and relationship to medication
Tsai et al. (2009) [63]	Retrospective study with patient and family interviews.	The majority of patients were taking psychotropic medications at the time of evaluation.	5.1% reported incidence of somnambulism or amnesic sleep-related behavioural problems subsequent to starting zolpidem.	The behavioral problems included three patients who watched television, five who used the telephone, one who walked to her boyfriend's house, and four for mixed behaviors (i.e., watching television, telephone use, eating, or talking with his/her family) all with amnesia for the episodes.
	Sample size of 255 patients with psychiatric diagnoses and insomnia. Psychiatric patients treated with zolpidem for insomnia for more than six months.		Of the thirteen, six were male and seven were female. The average age was 42.5 years and the average dosage of zolpidem was 10.0 mg per day. Their diagnosed diseases were as follows: schizophrenia (2), affective disorders (3), anxiety disorders (3), sleep disorders (3), and adjustment disorders (2).	The dosages of zolpidem in patients with an incidence of somnambulism and anterograde amnesia were lower than those of patients without these behaviors.
Sansone et al. (2008) [48]	Single case report	Simvastatin, Metformin Hydrochlorothiazide Sumatriptan Citalopram	51-year-old female with multiple medical diagnoses including hyperlipidemia, diabetes mellitus, hypertension, carpal tunnel syndrome, restless legs syndrome, migraine, and depression. Stable on medication for more than one year. Zolpidem prescribed for insomnia.	Nocturnal behaviors commenced after starting zolpidem, she had experienced two episodes of somnambulism with amnesia. The patient had no prior history of somnambulism. During these episodes, she walked down the steps from her second story bedroom to the kitchen and ingested normal amounts of food. The following morning, the patient queried her husband, the only other household inhabitant, about the empty food-packaging materials on the counter top. They concluded that she had been sleepwalking and eating in her sleep.
Tsai et al. (2007) [60]	Case series – three patients	N/A	Three female patients being treated for insomnia.	Three women experienced anterograde amnesia and compulsive repetitive behaviors after zolpidem use. These activities consisted of cleaning, shopping, and eating. These behaviors stopped after discontinuation of the zolpidem.

Study	Study type	Drug(s)	Patient/sample	Outcome
Yang et al. (2005) [56]	Single case report	N/A	50-year-old male rehabilitation inpatient with prior history of alcoholism and head trauma who had recently undergone hip surgery.	Walked in sleep on first two nights after taking zolpidem for the first time. Episodes ceased when zolpidem discontinued.
Sharma et al. (2005) [55]	Single case report	Aripiprazole Venlafaxine Quetiapine	19-year-old male patient with schizoaffective disorder and associated impulse control disorder.	Zolpidem added for insomnia. Within a few days walked into parents' room in "middle of night" with subsequent amnesia.
Harazin et al. (1999) [46]	Single case report	N/A	46-year-old male army officer with complaint of insomnia.	On the fourth night and subsequent to this for several nights arose two to three hours after bedtime and went to kitchen where he prepared and ate food. Refused to interact with family members and claimed amnesia for episodes. All episodes ceased when zolpidem discontinued.
Lange (2005) [54]	Single case report	Venlafaxine	13-year-old girl with major depression. Treated for depression successfully with venlafaxine, but insomnia persisted.	Parent tried to help her up to her bedroom 30 minutes after sleep onset following first dose. She started to walk around aimlessly. Parents woke her up. She was briefly confused. Had amnesia for episode. Medication was changed to citolapram with no repetition of behavior.
Mendelson (1994) [49]	Single case report	N/A	20-year-old male participating in sleep research study of effects of hypnotics on perception of sleep and wakefulness. Tones were administered to determine auditory threshold.	During a sleep study after one week of zolpidem use he was noted to get out of bed and start walking around after an auditory tone was present during stage 4 sleep. He was confused and had amnesia for the episode.
Sauvanet et al. (1988)	Outpatient retrospective study. Sample size = 96 patients	N/A	96 outpatients with complaints of insomnia. Mean age of 56.8 + 1.6 years.	A single episode of sleepwalking was noted in this group over two months of treatment.
Satter et al. (2003)	Single case report	Citalopram Sodium valproate	47-year-old man with bipolar affective disorder, manic.	Episodes of sleepwalking started two days after commencement of sodium valproate. When this was stopped sleepwalking ceased. When reintroduced, sleepwalking returned. When zolpidem stopped sleepwalking continued.

Table 35.3 (cont.)

Reference	Type of study/report	Concomitant medication	Patient demographic and medical history	Behavior and relationship to medication
Yanes Baonaza et al. (2003)	Single case report		66-year-old man with ischemic cardiomyopathy, diabetes type II and insomnia.	After being on lormetazepam 2 mg/day for a year switched to zolpidem. About four weeks later the patient presented with four episodes of complex behavior in his sleep including one episode where he left his home and returned later. Episodes stopped when zolpidem stopped.
Schenck et al. (2005) [65]	Case series of 19 patients	Various antidepressants	19 patients being treated for insomnia. 16 females, 3 males with mean age of 47.4 + 13.4 yrs. 84% had current or recent diagnosis of major depression or other psychiatric disorders.	When zolpidem was added to treatment for insomnia complaints, all patients developed sleep-related eating disorder. Multiple episodes occurred nightly including consumption of high caloric foods and also included cooking and two episodes of sleep driving to buy food. Several injuries were noted as well as two small fires. All episodes stopped when zolpidem stopped.
Morgenthaler & Silber et al. (2002) [52]	Case series of five patients	D	Five patients (three males and two females) with a mean age of 55.4 years. Placed on zolpidem for complaint of insomnia.	Sleep-related eating disorder began with zolpidem treatment in four of the patients and increased in severity for the fifth. All episodes ceased with discontinuation of zolpidem.

Table 35.4 Benzodiazepines and sleep-related behaviors

Reference	Type of study/report	Medication	Concomitant medication	Patient demographic and medical history	Behavior and relationship to medication
Poitras (1980) [69]	Case series of three patients	Triazolam	Oxazepam Trimipramine	37-year-old obese male	Sleep eating. Amnesia.
		Triazolam	Chlordiazepoxide Diazepam Maprotiline	49-year-old male	Sleep eating. Amnesia.
		Triazolam	Trifluorperazine Amitriptyline	47-year-old female	Sleep eating. Amnesia.
Menkes (1992)	Single case report	Triazolam	N/A	53-year-old obese female	Sleep eating. Amnesia from time of initial prescription.
Regenstein et al. (1985)	Case report – two patients	Triazolam	N/A	29-year-old woman with severe insomnia, headaches, crying spells	Dressed self in middle of night. Amnesia.
		Temazepam	N/A	30-year-old man with sleep onset insomnia and undergoing caffeine withdrawal	Screaming, naked, breaking dishes, unresponsive to others. With amnesia in the morning.
Laurema (1991) [70]	Single case report	Triazolam alternating with midazolam	N/A	53-year-old male with RLS and PLMS with complaints of severe insomnia	At least nine episodes of wandering the house including sleep eating. Found shoe polish in refrigerator. Alternated triazolam and midazolam and episodes occurred on the same night.
Lemoine et al. (1997)	Single case report	Triazolam	Temazepam Clorazepate	19-year-old woman	Aroused during night and stabbed woman in her care 35 times.
Goulle & Anger (2004) [68]	Case reports – two patients	Bromazepam	N/A	A 30-year-old woman was victim of a rape she did not remember	Amnesia and sexual assault. Bromazepam detected in her urine.
		Flunitrazepam	N/A	A 45-year-old woman was the perpetrator of a murder attempt on her boyfriend with a rifle. The shot went through his thorax	Automatism, amnesia, and murder attempt.

Malingering in a forensic sleep setting is a special case. Usually the malingerer is suggesting that his behavior at the time of the crime was due to a sleep disorder and was not carried out in full consciousness. History, and repeated history taking, are important tools. It is also essential to study the defendant's first account, given to the police, as this often reveals a much greater knowledge of the offence than is subsequently claimed. Suspicion of malingering should be raised if the defendant claims to have sleepwalked for the first time during the offence. A clear history, and family history if possible, of a parasomnia should be

Table 35.5 Antidepressants and sleep-related behaviors

Reference	Type of study/report	Medication	Concomitant medication	Patient demographic and medical history	Behavior and relationship to medication
Kawashima et al. (2003)	Single case report	Paroxetine	N/A	61-year-old female with mixed anxiety and depressive disorder.	Started on paroxetine 10 mg and increased to 20 mg two weeks later. One week after increased dose began to sleepwalk on a nightly basis. Episodes occurred in first few hours after sleep onset lasting 15 minutes. Behaviors included wandering about the house and attempting to leave the house. When paroxetine was discontinued all episodes stopped.
Alao et al. (1999)	Single case report	Paroxetine then sertraline	N/A	34-year-old woman with major depression and HIV positive.	Paroxetine was started at 10 mg and gradually increased to 20 mg. After several days at 20 mg, three days after the dose was increased, sleepwalking episodes occurred up to three times nightly. She would awaken in other rooms of the house without any memory. On occasion she awakened breathing rapidly and frightened. All episodes disappeared when dose decreased to 10 mg and reappeared when increased again to 20 mg. Paroxetine was replaced with sertraline 50 mg. When increased to 100 mg sleepwalking episodes returned as before.
Ferrandiz-Santos et al. (2000)	Single case report	Amitriptyline	N/A	50-year-old female with four-month history of anxiety, depression and insomnia.	When dose reached 150 mg began to arise from bed nightly in the first two hours of sleep and walked through house. Amnesic.
Khazall et al. (2003)	Single case report	Bupropion	N/A	33-year-old male undergoing smoking cessation treatment.	14 days after treatment started, he stopped smoking. Three days later telephone friend two hours after sleep onset for 15 minutes. Amnesic for episode. Experienced additional episodes including sleep eating over next two weeks.

sought with corroborative evidence from a partner or family members. Support for a parasomnia should also be sought from polysomnogram investigations. These may point in the direction of either possible sleepwalking or REM behavior disorder or an underlying nocturnal epileptiform disorder. Ongoing longer term observational assessment may be necessary in rarer instances – here in the prison hospital setting it may be possible to observe the defendant over a number of weeks. If this is a sleepwalking case, then the defendant is under significant pressure to produce sleepwalking episodes to bolster his or her defense.

Table 35.6 Lithium and neuroleptics and sleep-related behaviors

Reference	Type of study/report	Medication	Concomitant medication	Patient demographic and medical history	Behavior and relationship to medication
Scott (1988)	Single case report	Thioridazine	N/A	44-year-old male	Initially presented with clear case of stress related somnambulism. Misdiagnosed with epilepsy and "stress related psychosis". Treated with thioridazine. Episodes increased in severity. Attempted to strangle wife during episode.
Nadel (1981)	Single case report	Methyprylon	Chlorpromazine Amitriptyline	35-year-old female treated for ten years for schizoaffective disorder. Obese on a 1,200 calorie diet	Following addition of the methypryon to treat her insomnia, episodes of sleep eating began within days.
Charney et al. (1979)	Case series of 11 patients	Thioridazine	Lithium	28-year-old female with bipolar disorder, manic, alcoholic	Sleepwalking episodes started after two days after initiation of thioridazine and continued nightly for several nights and thereafter once per week. Episodes stopped when drug discontinued. Return of episodes when these medications were reinstated.
		Lithium	Perphenazine	21-year-old woman with schizoaffective disorder	Two weeks after start of lithium approximately two hours after sleep onset sleepwalking episode observed. Upon awakening that morning a generalized tonic/clonic seizure was noted.
		Perphenazine	Lithium	41-year-old female with schizoaffective disorder and numerous psychiatric hospitalizations. Possible seizure disorder	After two days of combined treatment patient found sleepwalking in hallway. Two more episodes were noted later that same week. Following the last episode an apparent seizure was noted after awakening in the morning. Sleepwalking ceased with decrease in perphenazine and an increase in lithium.
		Chlorpromazine Lithium		19-year-old male bipolar, manic	Behaviors commenced two days after lithium dose increased. Sleepwalking ceased when chlorpromazine changed for perphenazine and lithium decreased.

Table 35.6 (cont.)

Reference	Type of study/report	Medication	Concomitant medication	Patient demographic and medical history	Behavior and relationship to medication
		Perphenazine	Lithium	28-year-old male bipolar, manic	Sleepwalking episodes commenced three days after perphenazine introduced and ceased when perphenazine decreased.
		Chlorpromazine	Lithium	26-year-old female with schizoaffective disorder	Sleepwalking episodes commenced within a week of introduction of chlorpromazine and ceased when this was switched to thioridazine with addition of diazepam.
		Lithium	Thioridazine	34-year-old female schizoaffective	Behaviors commenced within four days of lithium initiation.
		Lithium	Haloperidol	34-year-old female bipolar, manic	Behaviors commenced within five days of lithium initiation.
		Lithium	Thioxanthine	15-year-old female schizoaffective, depressed	Behaviors commenced within three days of lithium initiation. No details provided.
		Lithium	Prolixin	49-year-old female bipolar, depressed	Behaviors commenced within three days of lithium initiation. No details provided.
Paquet et al. (2002)	Single case report	Olanzapine	Lithium	52-year-old man with bipolar disorder. Treated with lithium on ongoing basis. Following a hypomanic episode olanzapine added	Sleepwalking and sleep eating started several days after starting olanzapine. Noted to walk through apartment to kitchen and eat large quantities of sweets.
Kolivakis et al. (2001)	Case report – two patients	Olanzapine	N/A	63-year-old man with 41-year history of schizophrenia	Wandering about house and occasionally injuring self commenced seven days after Olanzapine increased from 10 mg to 20 mg.
		Olanzapine	N/A	62-year-old woman with 35-year history of schizophrenia	Not specified other than sleepwalking commenced after dose increased to 20 mg.
Glassman et al. (1986)	Single case report	Benztropine	Lithium Chlorpromazine Triazolam	39-year-old male with multiple admissions for schizoaffective disorder	Noted by room mates to arise and wander without purpose around room two nights after benztropine added.
Landry et al. (1999)	Case series of 27 patients on lithium	Lithium	Various combinations	27 of 389 patients (6.9%) attending lithium clinic reported sleepwalking	

Reference	Study type	Drug	Drug	Patient	Clinical description
Huapaya (1979)	Case series of seven patients	Chlorprothixene	Perphenazine	30-year-old woman with schizoaffective psychosis	Had two episodes of sleepwalking. When chlorprothixene was reduced sleepwalking did not recur.
		Methaqualone	Amobarbital Secobarbital Diphenhydramine	54-year-old woman with major depression	Had repeated episodes of sleepwalking while taking these medications. When methaqualone was discontinued no further episodes of sleepwalking were noted.
		Methaqualone Diphenhydramine	Thioridazine	49-year-old woman with chronic generalized anxiety disorder	Three episodes of sleepwalking noted. She was noted by husband to attempt to pour hot tea into a glass, left house and tried to open car door and attempted to open door to house. When methaqualone and diphenhydramine replaced with another compound sleepwalking episodes ceased.
		Methaqualone	N/A	29-year-old woman with major reactive depression	During episodes of sleepwalking gave her baby neuroleptic medication requiring the baby's hospitalization. A change in medications resulted in no further episodes.
		Methylphenidate	Alcohol	48-year-old man with depression, alcohol dependence and drug abuse	Awoke in bathroom to find himself drinking from a bottle of acetone.
		Perphenazine Lithium	Oxazepam Maprotiline	40-year-old man with major depressive disorder	Several episodes of sleepwalking including one in which he left the house and later awakened in the street at night. After many changes in medication given flurazepam resulting in cessation of sleepwalking episodes.
		Amitriptyline	Alcohol	50-year-old man with major depression and alcohol dependence syndrome	Noted by wife to arise at 2 a.m. and start shaving.
Luchins et al. (1978)		Thioridazine Trichloroethanol	N/A	44-year-old woman with paranoid schizophrenia	After taking 100 mg thioridazine and a double dose of trichloroethanol aroused from bed, entered daughter's room and stabbed her to death. Found to be in a floridly psychotic state the next morning.
Varkey et al. (2003)		Topiramate	N/A	27-year-old male with severe, intractable migraines	Two episodes in which he awakened from sleep, undressed and walked out of his room with amnesia for episodes. Within two weeks of commencing topiramate. Amnesia.

It is important that nursing and paramedical staff are made aware of this possibility and that intervention with the sleepwalking defendant is carried out and, more importantly, a full mental state of the defendant's memory for the episode is taken next morning.

In summary, a detailed history and comparison with the account given by the defendant will usually reveal an attempt to malinger. Otherwise standard tests of repeated history taking and examination of the details of the offence should make detection of malingering possible. Finally, the examining physician should bear in mind that lying is always a possibility.

Clinical assessment in forensic sleep medicine

The history must include detailed description of the event and the degree of amnesia, current and past medical, as well as family, history. Moreover, it should elicit presence of previously mentioned potential risk factors such as alcohol, drug or medication intake, sleep deprivation, stressful life event, or anxiety, prior to the episode. It is also recommended that social habits, employment records, and determination of the frequency of violence and its stereotypic nature are investigated. A complementary history with the spouse, bed partner, or family member is essential. The clinician should establish how soon after sleep onset these events have occurred, whether they were dreaming at the time, and the degree of amnesia for the events. Psychiatric examination to determine whether there is or was before the event a current psychiatric diagnosis of anxiety or mood disorder may be helpful. Information about the circumstances of the person's life prior to the episode is essential as most of the documented episodes have occurred during periods of increased life stress. Periods of poor sleep are common, due either to a sleep-related breathing disorder, or insomnia related to anxiety. A history of disrupted sleep, followed by a "crash" into recovery sleep is also supportive of the diagnosis. Deep (delta) sleep rebound after deprivation may well trigger a sleepwalking episode in a person with the inherited sleepwalking pathology and consequent difficulty switching from deep sleep to REM sleep.

A personality pattern that is within normal limits is usual. Subtle signs of overcontrol of emotion and excessive conformity have been found especially in people who do not express feelings easily and are likely to "go it alone" when in trouble [20]. An assessment of any history of violence is important for determining dangerousness.

A neurological examination, MRI, and EEG testing to help rule out a seizure disorder or other neurological pathology should be standard practise. A drug screen should precede sleep studies.

Sleepwalking/automatism cases usually come to the attention of sleep experts because the defendant has no memory of the events of the night. It is thus important, as a clinician, to look at all the factors that might have led to this loss of memory. These may have organic or behavioral causes. Behaviorally, the defendant may simply be lying, and have a perfect memory. This must be put forward to the court as a possibility. Second, there may be psychological suppression of memory, the factors looking at the exact nature of the memory loss will allow the clinician to say on the balance of probability this is likely to have been the cause. Next, organic factors such as epilepsy, dementia, etc., should all be considered and the relevant tests carried out, all with the aim of determining the integrity of the defendant's memory at the time of the tests and then inferring from the patient's history whether these factors could have been present at the time of the offense.

Under present law in the UK and USA, the defense used by those who have offended during a sleep-related episode is either sane (non-insane) or insane automatism. Non-insane automatism is appropriate in cases of sudden arousal from sleep in a non-sleepwalker, where it is considered that an external factor (which is unlikely to recur) was the stimulus for the episode. Insane automatism is used in cases of sleepwalking, as a tendency to sleepwalk is considered an internal factor. This distinction makes little medical sense as in many cases, particularly if the evoked behavior is complex, the sudden arousal may trigger a sleepwalking episode.

The following criteria are a suggested minimum for the clinical diagnosis of sleepwalking in the forensic context:

Predisposing factors

i. Family history. A family history of sleepwalking is usually found in people who sleepwalk;

ii. Childhood sleepwalking. It is common for the onset of sleepwalking to be in childhood;

iii. Adolescent sleepwalking. Although most sleepwalkers start sleepwalking in childhood, a few begin in adolescence. However, most adolescent sleepwalkers will also have a childhood history of sleepwalking;

iv. Late onset sleepwalking is rare, and usually only occurs after a precipitating cause, for example head injury. Sleep experts generally regard with suspicion any episode of sleepwalking which is said to be the first episode in an adult, and on which a legal defense is to be based.

Specific factors

i. Sleep stage. Episodes will occur out of deep stage 3 and/or 4 NREM sleep and thus are most likely to occur within two hours of sleep onset, but may occur from stage 2 sleep. The nature and quality of the previous sleep mentation must be that of stage 2, 3 or 4 sleep. It is helpful if on awakening the mentation is non-narrative, and non-dream-like with only a vague visual content, and consists mostly of thoughts and feelings.

ii. There should be disorientation on awakening. A straight arousal into clear consciousness is unlikely to occur on awakening from a somnambulistic automatism.

iii. Confusional behavior should occur. Any witness to the entire event should report inappropriate automatic behavior, preferably with an element of confusion.

iv. There is usually complete amnesia for the event. Memories are poorly recorded during stage 3 and 4 sleep and equally poorly recalled. It is, however, possible for fragments of distorted memory to be retained.

v. *Trigger or precipitating factors* are important such as the presence of an underlying sleep disorder such as sleep disordered breathing (SDB) and periodic limb movements (PLMs). The presence of noise and touch due to proximity may also trigger sleepwalking.

vi. *Modulating or priming factors* including the use of alcohol, drugs (prescribed and recreational), caffeine, prior sleep deprivation, or the presence of recent stressful life event(s) have been reported to be associated with sleepwalking episodes.

vii. Concealment. There should be no attempt at concealment. Attempts to conceal the incident suggest the presence of consciousness and intent.

viii. Out of character behavior. The behavior is almost always out of character for the individual. Thus violence in a sleepwalking episode can occur in individuals who have never or seldom previously shown violent behavior.

If a patient fulfils all or most of the criteria listed above, the diagnosis is often straightforward. Sleep laboratory studies will add value by excluding or identifying possible trigger factors or other organic causes for the behavior, e.g., sleep-disordered breathing, periodic limb movements of sleep, or epilepsy.

Nocturnal polysomnography (PSG) involves the detailed study of the overnight sleep patterns of an individual. The PSG measures a variety of physiological parameters (hence poly) including brain waves (electro-encephalogram or EEG), muscle tone and movement (electromyogram or EMG), eye movements (electro-oculogram or EOG), cardiovascular rhythms (electro-cardiogram or ECG), respiratory parameters such as air flow, chest and abdominal movements, arterial oxygen saturation, and body position. The data gathered from the study are then analyzed using internationally accepted criteria.

Witnessing a sleepwalking episode during the PSG study is rare and in the forensic context a witnessed sleepwalking episode should alert one to the possibility of malingering. The primary reason for undertaking PSG is to exclude the presence of an underlying precipitating factor such as sleep disordered breathing (SDB) or periodic limb movements of sleep. The ICSD-2 lists the PSG features for both sleepwalking and confusional arousal disorder. In the forensic context, while their presence may assist in the diagnosis, they can in no way be used to indicate that the person was actually sleepwalking or had a confusional arousal at the time in question. In addition, these PSG features, although suggestive (when combined with a clinical history) can only be used to assist with establishing a diagnosis but are not diagnostic on their own. A normal PSG does not exclude the diagnosis of sleepwalking [10–12, 16, 17, 20, 75].

It must be emphasized that as in the diagnosis of any medical condition the diagnosis does not rest purely on the results of investigations, but rather on the analysis of all data including the history, physical examination, mental state, cognitive state, and the results of tests and investigations. Very important are the facts of the case and the behavior during the "event" all of which must fit that of a sleepwalking episode.

References

1. Fenwick P. Automatism, medicine and the law. *Psychol Med Monogr.* 1990; Suppl **17**:1–27.

2. Fenwick P. Somnambulism and the law: a review. *Behav Sci Law.* 1987;**5**:343–57.

3. Fenwick P. Automatism and the law. *Lancet.* 1989;**2**:753–4.

4. Fenwick P. Sleep and sexual offending. *Med Sci Law.* 1996;**36**:122–34.

5. Yeo S. Clarifying automatism. *Int J Law Psychiatry.* 2002;**25**:445–58.

6. Bratty v Attorney General for Northern Ireland 1961b: *Northern Ireland Law Reports.* pp. 78–110 (103–4).

7. McSherry B. Men behaving badly: current issues and provocation, automatism, mental impairment and criminal responsibility. *Psychiatry Psychology Law* 2005;**12**:15–22.

8. R v Kemp. Weekly Law Reports. *1 Queens Bench.* pp. 407. 1957.

9. Government, Crimes Bill 1989, introduced in May 1989, xxvii, 156p., See on Clause 19, "Involuntary acts" pp. iv–v and 14.

10. McCall Smith A, Shapiro CM. *Forensic Aspects of Sleep.* (John Wiley and Sons, 1997).

11. American Academy of Sleep Medicine. *International Classification of Sleep Disorders. Diagnostic and Coding Manual (ICSD-2)*, 2nd edn. (Westchester, IL: AASM, 2005).

12. Mahowald M, Cramer Bornemann MA. NREM sleep-arousal parasomnias. In: Kryger MH, Roth T, Dement WC, eds. *Principles and Practice of Sleep Medicine*, 4th edn. (Philadelphia, PA: Elsevier Saunders, 2005; 892–925).

13. Broughton RJ, Shimizu T. Dangerous behaviour at night. In: Shapiro C, McColl Smith A, eds. *Forensic Aspects of Sleep.* (Chichester: Wiley, 1997; 65–83).

14. Moldofsky H, Gilbert R, Lue FA, MacLean AW. Forensic sleep medicine: violence, sleep, nocturnal wandering: sleep-related violence. *Sleep.* 1995;**18**(9):731–9.

15. Fenwick PB. Automatism. In: Bluglass R, Bowden P, eds. *Principles and Practice of Forensic Psychiatry.* (Edinburgh and New York: Churchill Livingstone, 1990; xxi, 10, 53, 84, 271–85, 1405).

16. Ebrahim IO, Wilson W, Marks R, Peacock KW, Fenwick P. Violence, sleepwalking and the criminal law: (1) The medical aspects. *Criminal Law Review.* 2005;601–13.

17. Wilson W, Ebrahim IO, Fenwick P, Marks R. Violence, sleepwalking and the criminal law: (2) The legal aspects. *Criminal Law Review.* 2005;614–23.

18. Broughton RJ. Sleep disorders: disorders of arousal? Enuresis, somnambulism, and nightmares occur in confusional states of arousal, not in dreaming sleep. *Science.* 1968;**159**:1070–8.

19. Hublin C, Kaprio J, Partinen M, *et al.* Prevalence and genetics of sleepwalking: a population based twin study. *Neurology.* 1997;**48**(1):177–81.

20. Cartwright R. Sleepwalking violence: a sleep disorder, a legal dilemma, and a psychological challenge. *Am J Psychiatry.* 2004;**161**:1149–58.

21. Bixler EO, Kales A, Soldatos CR, *et al.* Prevalence of sleep disorders in the Los Angeles metropolitan area. *Am J Psychiatry.* 1979;**136**(10):1257–62.

22. Ohayon MM, Guilleminault C, Priest RG. Night terrors, sleepwalking, and confusional arousals in the general population: their frequency and relationship to other sleep and mental disorders. *J Clin Psychiatr.* 1999;**60**(4):268–76.

23. Broughton R. NREM arousal parasomnias. In: Kryger MH, Roth T, Dement WC, eds. *Principles and Practice of Sleep Medicine*, 3rd edn. (Philadelphia, PA: W.B. Saunders, 2000; 693–706).

24. Schenck CH, Bundlie SR, Mahowald MW. Human REM sleep chronic behaviour disorders: a new category of parasomnia. *J Sleep Res.* 1985;**14**:208.

25. Mahowald MW, Schenck CH. REM sleep parasomnias. In: Kryger MH, Roth T, Dement WC, eds. *Principles and Practice of Sleep Medicine*, 3rd edn. (Philadelphia, PA: W.B. Saunders, 2005).

26. Olson EJ, Boeve BF, Silber MH. REM sleep behaviour disorder: demographic, clinical and laboratory findings in 93 cases. *Brain.* 2000;**23**(2):331–9.

27. Boeve BF, Silber MH, Ferman TJ, *et al.* Association of REM sleep behavior disorder and neurodegenerative disease may reflect an underlying synucleinopathy. *Mov Disord.* 2001;**16**(4):622–30.

28. Schenck CH, Mahowald MW. REM sleep behavior disorder: clinical, developmental and neuroscience perspectives 16 years after its formal identification in Sleep. *Sleep.* 2002;**25**(2):120–38.

29. Sforza E, Krieger J, Petiau C. REM sleep behavior disorder: clinical and physiopathological findings. *Sleep Med Rev.* 1997;**1**:57–69.

30. Schenck CH, Hurwitz TD, Mahowald MW. REM sleep behavior disorder: a report on a series of 96 consecutive cases and a review of the literature. *J Sleep Res.* 1993, **2**:224–31.

31. Nightingale S, Orgill JC, Ebrahim IO, *et al.* The association between narcolepsy and REM behaviour disorder (RBD). *Sleep Med.* 2005;**6**(3):253–8.

32. Boeve BF, Silber MH, Saper CB, *et al.* Pathophysiology of REM sleep behaviour disorder and relevance

to neurodegenerative disease. *Brain.* 2007;**130**(11): 2770–88.

33. Learned-Coughlin SM, Bergström M, Savitcheva I, *et al.* In vivo activity of bupropion at the human dopamine transporter as measured by positron emission tomography. *Biol Psychiatry.* 2003;**54**(8):800–5.

34. Ebrahim IO, Peacock KW. REM sleep behavior disorder – psychiatric presentations: a case series from the United Kingdom. *J Clin Sleep Med.* 2005;**1**(1):43–7.

35. Wong KE. Masturbation during sleep: a somnambulistic variant? *Singapore Med J.* 1986;**27**:542–8.

36. Hurwitz TD, Mahowald MW, Schluter JL. Sleep-related sexual abuse of children. *Sleep Res.* 1989;**18**:246.

37. Shapiro CM, Fedoroff JP, Trajanovic NN. Sexual behavior in sleep, a newly described parasomnia. *Sleep Res.* 1996;**25**:367.

38. Alves R, Aloe F, Tavares S. Sexual behavior in sleep, sleepwalking and possible REM behavior disorder: a case report. *Sleep Res Online.* 1999;**2**:71–2.

39. Rosenfeld DA, Elhajar AJ. Sleep sex: a variant of sleepwalking. *Arch Sex Behav.* 1998;**27**:269–78.

40. Guilleminault C, Moscovitch A, Yuen K, Poyares D. Atypical sexual behavior during sleep. *Psychosom Med.* 2002;**64**:328–36.

41. Shapiro CM, Fedoroff JP, Trajanovic NN. Sexual behavior in sleep: a newly described parasomnia. *Sleep Res.* 1996;**25**:367.

42. Shapiro CM, Trajanovic NN, Fedoroff JP. Sexsomnia: a new parasomnia, *Can J Psychiat.* 2003;**48**:311–17.

43. Ebrahim IO. Somnambulistic sexual behaviour (sexsomnia). *J Clin Forensic Med.* 2006;**13**:219–24.

44. Andersen ML, Rosana DP, Alves SC, *et al.* Sexsomnia: abnormal sexual behavior during sleep. *Brain Res Rev.* 2007;**56**(2):271–82.

45. Schenck CH, Arnulf I, Mahowald MW. Sleep and sex: what can go wrong? A review of the literature on sleep related disorders and abnormal sexual behaviors and experiences. *Sleep.* 2007;**30**(6):683–702.

46. Harazin J, Berigan TR. Zolpidem tartrate and somnambulism. *Mil Med.* 1999;**164**:669–70.

47. Hughes JR. A review of sleepwalking (somnambulism): the enigma of neurophysiology and polysomnography with differential diagnosis of complex partial seizures. *Epilepsy Behav.* 2007;**11**(4):483–91.

48. Sansone RA, Sansone LA. Zolpidem, somnambulism, and nocturnal eating – Letter to the Editor. *Gen Hosp Psychiatry.* 2008;**30**:90–1.

49. Mendelson WB. Sleepwalking associated with zolpidem. *J Clin Psychopharmacol.* 1994;**14**:150.

50. Canaday BR. Amnesia possibly associated with zolpidem administration. *Pharmacotherapy.* 1996;**16**:687–9.

51. van Puijenbroek EP, Egberts AC, Krom HJ. Visual hallucinations and amnesia associated with the use of zolpidem. *Int J Clin Pharmacol Ther.* 1996;**34**:318.

52. Morgenthaler TI, Silber MH. Amnestic sleep-related eating disorder associated with zolpidem. *Sleep Med.* 2002;**3**:323–7.

53. Sattar SP, Ramaswamy S, Bhatia SC, Petty F. Somnambulism due to probable interaction of valproic acid and zolpidem. *Ann. Pharmacother.* 2003;**37**:1429–33.

54. Lange CL. Medication-associated somnambulism. *J Am Acad Child Adolesc Psych.* 2005;**44**:211–12.

55. Sharma A, Dewan VK. A case report of zolpidem-induced somnambulism. *Prim Care Companion J Clin Psychiat.* 2005;**7**:74.

56. Yang W, Dollear M, Muthukrishnan SR. One rare side effect of zolpidem – sleepwalking: a case report. *Arch Phys Med Rehabil.* 2005;**86**:1265–6.

57. Barrett, J, Underwood A. Perchance to … eat? *Newsweek.* 2006;**147**:54.

58. Kito S, Koga Y. Visual hallucinations and amnesia associated with zolpidem triggered by fluvoxamine: a possible interaction. *Int Psychogeriatr.* 2006; **18**:749–51.

59. Najjar M. Zolpidem and amnestic sleep related eating disorder. *J Clin Sleep Med.* 2007;**3**,637–8.

60. Tsai MJ, Tsai YH, Huang YB. Compulsive activity and anterograde amnesia after zolpidem use. *Clin Toxicol (Phila).* 2007;**45**:179–81.

61. Praplam-Pahud J, Forster A, Gamulin Z, *et al.* Pre-operative sedation before regional anaesthesia: comparison between zolpidem, midazolam and placebo. *Br J Anaesth.* 1990;**64**:670–4.

62. Ganzoni E, Santoni JP, Chevillard V, *et al.* Zolpidem in insomnia: a 3-year post-marketing surveillance study in Switzerland. *J Int Med Res.* 1995;**23**:61–73.

63. Tsai JH, Yang P, Chen CC, *et al.* Zolpidem-induced amnesia and somnambulism: Rare occurrences? *Eur Neuropsychopharmacology.* 2009;**19**(1):74–6.

64. Winkelman JW. Clinical and polysomnographic features of sleep related eating disorder. *J Clin Psychiatry.* 1998;**59**(1):14–19.

65. Schenck CH, Connoy DA, Castellanos M, *et al.* Zolpidem-induced sleep-related eating disorder (SRED) in 19 patients. *Sleep.* 2005;**28**:A259.

66. Winkelman JW. Sleep-related eating disorder and night eating syndrome: sleep disorders, eating disorders, or both? *Sleep.* 2006;**29**:949–54.

67. Howell MJ, Schenck CH, Crow SJ. A review of nighttime eating disorders. *Sleep Med Rev.* 2009;**13**(1):23–34.

68. Goulle J-P, Anger J-P. Drug-facilitated robbery or sexual assault. Problems associated with amnesia. *Ther Drug Monit.* 2004;**26**:206–10.

69. Poitras R. A propos d'episodes d'amnesies anterogrades associes a l'utilisation du triazolam. *Union Med Can.* 1980;**109**(3):427–9.

70. Laurema H. Nocturnal wandering caused by restless legs and short-acting benzodiazepines. *Act Psychiatr Scand.* 1991;**83**:492–3.

71. Rogers R, Sewell K, Morey LC, Ustad KL. Detection of feigned mental disorders on the personality assessment inventory: a discriminant analysis. *J Pers Assess.* 1996;**67**(3):629–40.

72. Bagby RM, Rogers R, Buis T, *et al.* Detecting feigned depression and schizophrenia on the MMPI-2. *J Pers Assess.* 1968;**3**:650–64.

73. Pollock PH, Quigley B, Worley KO. Feigned mental disorder in prisoners referred to forensic mental health services. *J Psychiatr Ment Health Nurs.* 1997;**4**(1):9–15.

74. Mittenberg W, Patton C, Canyock EM, Condit DC. Base rates of malingering and symptom exaggeration. *J Clin Exp Neuropsychol.* 2002;**24**(8):1094–102.

75. Kayumov L, Pandi-Perumal SR, Fedoroff P, Shapiro CM. Diagnostic values of polysomnography in forensic medicine. *J Forensic Sci.* 2000;**45**(1):191–4.

Chapter 36

Sleep abnormalities and Prader–Willi syndrome

Joseph Barbera, Inna Voloh, Glenn Berall, and Colin M. Shapiro

Introduction

Prader–Willi syndrome (PWS) is a complex, multi-system genetic disorder with an estimated prevalence of 1/15,000 to 1/30,000. Characteristic features include neonatal hypotonia, short stature, facial dysmorphia, hypogonadism, hyperphagia with morbid obesity, failure of satiety, developmental delay with mild to moderate retardation, and a number of behavioral and psychiatric disturbances (including maladaptive behaviors pertaining to food, temper tantrums, obsessive–compulsive tendencies, and other symptoms consistent with an autism spectrum disorder). This constellation of symptoms is highly suggestive of the presence of hypothalamic dysfunction in such individuals. The genetics of PWS are complex, but in general PWS is the result of an absence of the normally active paternally derived genes in the chromosome 15q11–13 region. In approximately 70% of cases, this is the result of deletion of the paternally derived 15q11–13 region. Approximately 25% of PWS cases are due to maternal disomy of chromosome 15 (two maternal copies of the maternal chromosome 15). The remainder of cases result from translocations involving chromosome 15 or microdeletions of the imprinting center within 15q11–q13 [1–6].

Sleep disturbances, in the form of excessive daytime sleepiness (EDS), and sleep apnea, were initially listed as a minor diagnostic criterion in the diagnosis of PWS, based on earlier case reports [6]. However, in the last two decades the prominence of excessive daytime sleepiness in PWS patients has become increasingly recognized, and a number of investigators have looked at the correlates and potential causes of the sleepiness associated with this condition. This chapter will review this literature, beginning with a review of the prevalence and extent of sleepiness in PWS, the potential contribution of sleep-disordered breathing to this sleepiness, and finally evidence suggesting the presence of a primary hypersomnolence in patients with PWS. What is evident from such a review is that the cause of sleepiness in PWS is not a straightforward matter. While sleepiness in the PWS patient poses particular challenges to the treating physician, it may also provide significant insights into the basic mechanism regulating sleep and wakefulness.

Sleepiness and Prader–Willi syndrome: prevalence, extent, and correlates

In a large survey given to caregivers of adult PWS patients (N = 232), Greenswag [7] found that such patients were commonly rated as being "sleepy." Such sleepiness moreover was correlated with patient weight. In a similar survey (N = 61), Clarke et al. [8] found that adult PWS patients were frequently rated as experiencing excessive daytime sleepiness as well as increased nocturnal sleep. Such sleepiness, however, did not seem to correlate with patient weight, nor did it correlate with a number of behavioral abnormalities surveyed. Richdale et al. [9] in a survey of 29 pediatric and adult subjects with PWS found the presence of subjective daytime sleepiness in ten subjects, in comparison with no subjects in a control group. The PWS group also scored significantly higher on the Epworth Sleepiness Scale (ESS) than the control group. The authors did not find a correlation between excessive daytime sleepiness and body mass index (BMI) or weight in the PWS group. They did find, in the PWS group, a correlation between daytime sleepiness as measured by the ESS and a number of behavioral disturbances on the Developmental Behaviour Checklist

Sleep and Mental Illness, eds. S. R. Pandi-Perumal and M. Kramer. Published by Cambridge University Press.
© Cambridge University Press 2010.

(DBC). In a sleep questionnaire study, Cotton and Richdale [10] found excessive daytime sleepiness to be commonly described in children with PWS, but rarely in other intellectual disability groups including autism and Down Syndrome. Hass et al. [11] found ratings of sleepiness in a scatter plot analysis of seven PWS adult patients to be more common during periods when there were no scheduled activities, confirming anecdotal reports that PWS patients tend to fall asleep during passive, unengaging activities.

A number of other studies conducted in sleep laboratories have also corroborated the presence of subjective or caregiver reported excessive daytime sleepiness in patients with PWS, although such studies generally involve patients being referred to a sleep laboratory for various reasons and may be prone to selection bias. Vela-Bueno et al. [12] reported the presence of symptomatic excessive daytime sleepiness in eight out of nine pediatric and adult patients with PWS referred to their study. Kaplan et al. [13] reported the experience of hypersomnolence in all five patients investigated in their study. Clift et al. [14] found that 12 out of 17 PWS patients exhibited daytime sleepiness based on either caregiver ratings, the ESS, or the MSLT. Subjective ratings of alertness, on the other hand, were normal. Richards et al. [15] found evidence of excessive daytime sleepiness in 8 out of 14 adult PWS patients based on caregiver ratings and on the Epworth Sleepiness Scale (ESS > 9). Manni et al. [16] reported that all 14 adult and pediatric PWS patients they studied (unselected for sleep disorders) were reported by caregivers as being sleepy during the day. Williams et al. [17] reported that 20 out of 30 pediatric PWS patients were given a score by their caregivers of ≥10 on the ESS, indicating significant daytime sleepiness.

A number of studies have also looked at the presence of objective sleepiness in patients with PWS, although again, these studies were conducted on patients referred to a sleep clinic and as such are prone to selection bias. Harris et al. [18] demonstrated moderate to severe sleepiness in four out of four PWS patients, two with what would be considered severe or pathological sleepiness (mean sleep latency <5 minutes) with each patient exhibiting one SOREM nap. Hertz et al. [19] conducted MSLTs on fourteen adult patients with PWS and found that ten patients exhibited daytime sleepiness on MSLT testing (MSLT <10 minutes), with six exhibiting severe sleepiness (mean sleep latency <5 minutes). Helbing-Zwanenburg

et al. [20] found evidence of excessive daytime sleepiness in 20 out of 21 randomly chosen adult PWS patients (95%) based on 24-hour ambulatory recording, in comparison to 2 out of 19 controls (10%). Clift et al. [14] found 7 out of 14 PWS patients exhibited pathological sleepiness on the MSLT. Richards et al. [15] reported pathological sleepiness on the MSLT in four out of ten patients. Vgontzas et al. [21] reported moderate to severe sleepiness in five out of eight PWS subjects based on a modified MSLT protocol. Hiroe et al. [22] reported moderate to severe sleepiness in all three PWS cases they subjected to the MSLT. Manni et al. [16] reported abnormal MSLT values in eight out of ten PWS subjects they investigated (even taking into account Tanner staging for adolescent patients). Priano et al. [23] reported moderate to severe sleepiness on the MSLT in 11 out of 18 adult PWS patients studied. Williams et al. [17] reported a mean MSLT of nine minutes in 20 pediatric PWS patients with five patients exhibiting an MSLT score consistent with narcolepsy, with two SOREMP and an average mean sleep latency in this subgroup of 5.9 minutes.

In summary, patients with PWS frequently experience significant excessive daytime sleepiness, based on subjective and objective criteria such as the MSLT. This sleepiness seems to be predominantly in passive, unengaging situations, but there is a paucity of data with respect to characterizing alertness in such patients, including performance on the Maintenance of Wakefulness Test (MWT). Mixed results have been found with respect to correlating excessive daytime sleepiness in PWS with weight. Finally, some studies have suggested that the sleepiness experienced by PWS patients may account for some of the behavioral disturbances observed in such patients, arguing for the effective assessment and management of such sleepiness in the overall care of PWS patients.

Sleep-disordered breathing and Prader–Willi syndrome

One obvious explanation for the presence of sleepiness in patients with PWS would be sleep-related breathing disorders, which patients with PWS may be at risk for. Specifically, this population may be at risk for the development of obstructive sleep apnea/ hypopnea syndrome because of obesity, hypotonia, viscous secretions, cranio-facial dysmorphism, and alveolar hypoventilation due to an increased presence of restrictive lung disease and absent or reduced ventilator responses to hypercapnia and hypoxia [24]. As a result, a number of studies have investigated the presence and nature of sleep-disordered breathing in PWS.

Prevalence of sleep disordered breathing in Prader–Willi syndrome

A number of studies have indeed confirmed the presence of sleep-disordered breathing in PWS, whether in the form of sleep apnea or hypoventilation. Freidman et al. [25] found significant sleep apnea in four out of nine pediatric and adult patients with PWS, while another two exhibited prominent oxygen desaturations in sleep in the absence of apneic events, and another two exhibited mild central apnea. Harris et al. [18] reported significant apneas and REM related hypoxia in three out of four PWS patients. Clift et al. [14] found that 16 out of 24 PWS patients exhibited significant REM-related oxygen desaturations in REM sleep. Seven patients were deemed to have significant sleep apnea with desaturations worthy of treatment with continuous positive airway pressure (CPAP). Richards et al. [15] found significant sleep apnea (AHI > 10) in 12 of 14 adult PWS patients.

O'Donaghue et al. [26] found significant sleep apnea (AHI > 10/hour) in 9 of 13 (69%) "unselected" PWS subjects. Four subjects also exhibited pathological rises in $TcCO_2$ (>10 mm Hg) with two meeting the criteria for obesity hypoventilation syndrome. Furthermore, they demonstrated that increased age-adjusted BMIs were associated with more severe hypoxia (minimum SaO_2) during the night and more sleep disturbances (high arousal index and low sleep efficiency). Subjective daytime inactivity/sleepiness was associated with higher AHIs, lower minimum SaO_2, and higher BMIs. They also found that higher impulsivity was associated with lower minimum SaO_2, an increased arousal index and higher BMIs.

Priano et al. [23] found significant sleep apnea (AHI ≥ 5) in 6 out of 22 PWS patients studied, although 15 patients in their study had prolonged periods of oxygen desaturation, commonly in REM sleep.

Festen et al. [27] found a median AHI of 5.1 in 53 pediatric patients with PWS participating in a randomized controlled trial of growth hormone. Most of the events, however, were central in nature. No correlation was found between AHI and BMI. However, the authors also reported that 4 out of 45 (9%) non-obese patients exhibited obstructive sleep apnea as

defined by an obstructive apnea index >1, while 4 out of 8 (50%) obese patients did likewise. In a subgroup of these patients (n = 35) a follow-up PSG, done after six months of growth hormone (GH) treatment, resulted in a non-significant decline in the AHI.

Yee et al. [28] found significant sleep apnea (defined as a Respiratory Disturbance Index (RDI) >5 events/hour) in 18 out of 19 (95%) PWS patients referred consecutively from a PWS clinic. The mean total RDI for the PWS group, however, was not significantly different from an obese control group, although the PWS group exhibited more significant nocturnal hypoxia. Nine of the PWS patients also fulfilled the criteria for obesity hypoventilation syndrome, based on BMI and arterial blood gases.

Lin et al. [29] found a mean RDI of 5.8 ± 3.7/hr in a group of 30 PWS subjects (not selected for complaints of sleep problems). A roughly equal proportion of central and obstructive apneas were observed. An RDI of >2 was observed in 28 out of 30 (93%) subjects and an RDI of >10 in 5 subjects (17%). The authors also noted a desaturation index (DI) (desaturations >4%) of 8.1 ± in the group. Age-adjusted BMIs were associated with more severe hypoxemia in sleep (based on a number of measures) and more sleep disturbance (based on the arousal index). The authors did not find a correlation between any sleep variable and genotype.

Festen et al. [30] found evidence of sleep-disordered breathing in 22 PWS infants entered into their study, with a median AHI of 6.1 events per hour, with the majority of events recorded being central in nature. Overall AHI did not correlate with psychomotor development as measured by the Bayley Scales of Infant Development – II, although four infants who had obstructive sleep apnea syndrome exhibited more severely delayed mental development.

Williams et al. [17] reported that in a retrospective review of 37 pediatric patients referred to their clinic with suspected sleep disordered breathing, 70% demonstrated an elevated AHI (≥1/hour), 86% showed significant hypoxemia (oxygen desaturation <93%), and 62% having significant hypercarbia (end tidal CO_2 > 50 mmHg). All 37 patients demonstrated significant sleep-disordered breathing in one of these three forms. The authors found a positive correlation between AHI and adjusted BMI. A similar association between BMI and AHI, as well as measures of oxygen desaturation, were described by Hertz et al. [31].

On the other hand a number of studies have failed to demonstrate the expected increased prevalence of sleep-disordered breathing in PWS. In an early study, Vela-Bueno et al. [12] studied nine pediatric and adult patients with PWS with two to four consecutive overnight studies. Despite the fact that all the patients complained of excessive daytime sleepiness, only one exhibited the presence of obstructive sleep apnea. One patient was noted to have severe hypoventilation in REM sleep.

Kaplan et al. [13] reported a mildly elevated AHI in only one of five pediatric and adult PWS patients studied, despite all five patients experiencing daytime hypersomnolence and having morbid obesity. Two patients in their sample exhibited significant oxygen desaturations attributed to hypoventilation in REM or NREM sleep. Helbing-Zwanenburg et al. [20] did not find significant sleep apnea in any of 13 cases investigated for this. Hertz et al. [19] investigated 24 adult and pediatric patients for sleep apnea. Despite a high prevalence of morbid obesity and MSLT-confirmed daytime sleepiness in the sample, only three patients exhibited significant sleep apnea (AHI > 10/hour). Nine patients in their sample exhibited significant nocturnal oxygen desaturations, generally during REM sleep. Moreover basal SaO_2 and lowest SaO_2 correlated with BMI. The authors noted that nocturnal desaturation and AHI correlated with daytime sleepiness as measured by the MSLT, although a number of patients exhibited significant daytime sleepiness in the absence of sleep-disordered breathing. Vgontzas et al. [21] did not find significant sleep-disordered breathing or hypoventilation in any of eight PWS subjects studied. Hiroe et al. [22] found mild sleep apnea syndrome in only one of three PWS cases studied (employing esophageal monometry), despite the presence of daytime sleepiness based on the MSLT in all three cases. Manni et al. [16] found an elevated respiratory distress index (RDI) in four out of fourteen PWS subjects, with three exhibiting significant oxygen desaturations during the night, despite the presence of daytime sleepiness in all subjects. Voloh et al. [32] found significant sleep apnea in only 1 of 14 pediatric and adult PWS patients studied.

As discussed by Nixon and Brouillette [24], studies on the presence of sleep-disordered breathing in PWS (including sleep apnea and hypoventilation) have given prevalence estimates in the range of 0 to 100%, with the most obvious influencing factor being variable inclusion criteria used in such studies. Other potential criticisms of such studies include small sample sizes, mixed pediatric and adult sample groups, and variable methods for recording and defining respiratory events (including the use of adult criteria for pediatric patients).

Overall, however, it does seem reasonable to conclude that patients with PWS are at increased risk for sleep-disordered breathing, in particular obstructive sleep apnea and hypoventilation, with weight being a prominent risk factor. However, it is also apparent that sleep-disordered breathing alone cannot fully account for the sleepiness experienced by patients with PWS. At both the individual and group level we see patients with PWS and significant daytime sleepiness who do not have any sleep-disordered breathing, or in whom sleep-disordered breathing is disproportionate to the degree of daytime sleepiness present.

Prader–Willi syndrome and abnormal ventilatory response

A number of studies have suggested that there may be more to sleep-disordered breathing in Prader–Willi syndrome than obstructive phenomena. As noted, several studies have documented an increased prevalence of central events in PWS [27, 29, 33]. Several studies have also demonstrated that PWS patients have abnormal ventilatory control during wakefulness, including abnormal ventilatory responses to hyperoxia, hypoxia, and hypercarbia [34–36]. A number of studies have also demonstrated abnormalities in ventilatory control during sleep. Livingston et al. [37] found a significantly elevated central apnea index (1.5 ± 0.4/hour) in ten PWS patients studied, in comparison with nine controls (0.1 ± 0.1/hour), in addition to a significantly higher baseline and peak end tidal CO_2 levels. Moreover the authors found that the PWS group exhibited a significantly higher arousal threshold in response to a hypercapnic challenge during slow-wave sleep. No differences were found between the groups in terms of obstructive events or hypoxemia. Arens et al. [38] reported a decreased arousal and cardiorespiratory response to a hypoxic challenge during slow-wave sleep in 13 adult PWS patients. Schlüter et al. [39] investigated eight pediatric PWS patients (including infants) in comparison with matched controls. The PWS group did not exhibit an increased incidence of obstructive apneas but did exhibit an increased number of all apneas >2 seconds duration per hour of sleep, as well as decreased nadir of oxygen desaturation and decreased respiratory response to hypercapnia.

In summary several studies have documented blunted hypoxic and hypercarbic responses in PWS, suggesting potential deficiencies in peripheral chemoreceptors or even central respiratory mechanisms in PWS (see below regarding the relevance of this to the use of growth hormone treatment in PWS), which may impact on all forms of sleep-disordered breathing.

Treatment of sleep-disordered breathing and PWS

Few studies have looked at the treatment of sleep apnea in PWS, but those studies that have reported such treatment provide further insights into the presence of sleep apnea in PWS, and its relationship to excessive daytime sleepiness in such patients. Friedman et al. [25] reported one PWS patient with obstructive sleep apnea undergoing tonsillectomy and adenoidectomy with his symptoms improving "somewhat." Harris et al. [18] reported a dramatic improvement in sleep apnea in one PWS patient with weight loss, improvement on the MSLT, but persistent daytime sleepiness. In another study, Harris et al. [40] also reported persistent daytime sleepiness in a group of PWS patients despite a resolution of their sleep-disordered breathing following weight loss. Sforaza et al. [41] reported the case of a 20-year-old patient with moderate sleep apnea successfully treated with CPAP. Hertz et al. [19] reported two pediatric patients who experienced significant improvement in their sleep apnea with tonsillectomy and adenoidectomy. Hiroe et al. [22] reported continued sleepiness in a 15-year-old boy with PWS, despite resolution of his mild sleep apnea with a uvulopalatopharyngoplasty (UPPP). This case emphasizes that there may be more than one cause of EDS in patients with PWS and treatment of sleep apnea may be necessary but not sufficient to remove EDS in PWS. Pavone et al. [42] demonstrated a significant improvement in both the median AHI and median oxygen desaturation index (ODI) in five pediatric PWS patients undergoing adenotonsillectomy. Clift et al. [14] treated seven PWS patients with CPAP, with most respiratory events being abolished. Of the five patients who were compliant with treatment over six months, three experienced an improvement in daytime sleepiness. Vgontzas et al. [43] reported a case of severe obstructive sleep apnea in a 21-year-old female with PWS, which was successfully treated with CPAP, but with continued sleepiness as exhibited by the MSLT. A repeat study after significant weight loss revealed an absence of sleep apnea, but with persistent sleepiness and REM abnormalities on daytime napping. Esnault-Lavandier and Mabin [44] employed clomipramine (20 mg/day) in the treatment of an 11-year-old boy with PWS, with elimination of his excessive daytime sleepiness, as measured by the MSLT, despite persistence of severe obstructive sleep apnea syndrome.

In summary, treatments proposed for the sleep-disordered breathing associated with PWS run the full range of treatment options available to non-PWS patients, and include surgery, CPAP, and conservative measures such as weight loss. Such treatments do seem to be generally successful in alleviating sleep-disordered breathing in PWS patients. However, cases where the treatment of sleep-disordered breathing in PWS does not alleviate daytime sleepiness [14, 18, 22, 25, 40, 43] further reinforce the hypothesis that sleep-disordered breathing alone cannot account for the presence of daytime sleepiness in this population.

Sleep-disordered breathing: Prader–Willi syndrome and growth hormone therapy

In the last decade, growth hormone (GH) has become an approved treatment in PWS, having been shown to improve linear growth, lean-to-fat ratio, mobility, behavior, and quality of life in PWS [45]. However, concerns have been raised with regards to the use of GH in PWS following a number of case reports detailing sudden death in PWS shortly after the initiation of GH treatment. A number of the reported cases involved respiratory failure, and included cases associated with sleep-disordered breathing [45, 46]. Mechanisms by which GH may lead to respiratory failure in PWS patients include an increase in the size of lymphoid and soft tissues in the upper respiratory tract with GH therapy, an increase in metabolic rate with increased oxygen demand and ventilator load, and a normalization of previously decreased hydration, which increases volume load [45].

Beyond case descriptions, studies to date have failed to definitively demonstrate an exacerbation of sleep-disordered breathing with GH, and some have even shown an improvement in respiratory function. In a double-blind, placebo-controlled cross-over study in 12 PWS patients, Haqq et al. [47] found a significant improvement in a number of pulmonary function measures (peak flow, percentage vital capacity, forced expiratory rate) after six months of GH treatment. Moreover, GH treatment was associated with a decrease in the number of apneas and hypopneas exhibited by patients on polysomnography, although this decrease was not statistically significant. Festen et al. [27] found a non-significant decrease in the AHI in 35 PWS patients after six months of GH treatment. Williams et al. [17] did not find a significant difference between measures of sleep-disordered breathing in 16 PWS patients on GH treatment and those not on such treatment. Miller et al. [48] examined 25 PWS patients both before and after six weeks of GH treatment. Growth hormone treatment was associated with a reduction in the AHI in 19 patients (in particular with regards to central events) but a worsening in 6 patients. The authors hypothesized that a sub-group of PWS patients may be at risk for a worsening of sleep-disordered breathing with GH treatment. Lindgren et al. [49] demonstrated improved resting ventilation, central inspiratory drive, and ventilator response to CO_2 during wakefulness in nine PWS patients after six to nine months of GH treatment.

Given the ongoing concerns around GH treatment and sleep-disordered breathing, it has been recommended that all children with PWS for whom GH is being proposed undergo overnight polysomnography as well as an otorhinolaryngologic examination, and that any sleep-disordered breathing identified be aggressively treated prior to initiating GH therapy [45, 46]. One group has also recommended repeat polysomnography after six weeks of GH therapy [48].

Summary

Patients with Prader–Willi syndrome do seem to have a higher prevalence of sleep-disordered breathing, in the form of obstructive sleep apnea or hypoventilation, with weight being a prominent risk factor. Moreover an increased prevalence of central events and blunted hypoxic and hypercarbic responses suggest the presence of deficiencies in peripheral chemoreceptors or central respiratory mechanisms in PWS patients, which may further contribute to the sleep-disordered breathing in this population. However, it is also apparent that sleep-disordered breathing alone does not fully account for the presence of excessive daytime sleepiness in PWS patients. Patients with PWS have exhibited an absence of sleep-disordered breathing, or a level of sleep-disordered breathing disproportionate to the degree of daytime sleepiness present. Moreover the treatment of sleep-disordered breathing in this population does not necessarily lead to a complete alleviation of sleep-disordered breathing. Clearly the excessive sleepiness in this population is multifactorial in origin with sleep-disordered breathing representing only one contributory factor.

The above considerations aside, sleep-disordered breathing in PWS has been show in many cases to be a significant contributor to the daytime sleepiness associated with PWS patients and has been associated with an increased risk of death in such patients, both with and without GH therapy [45]. Sleep-disordered breathing may also contribute to the cognitive and behavioral deficits in PWS patients, as it does in the non-PWS population [50]. As such, clinicians should have a high suspicion of sleep-disordered breathing in patients with PWS and a low threshold for proceeding with appropriate investigations (including polysomnography). Treatment options, based on case reports, include the full range of typical treatments for sleep-disordered breathing in non-PWS patients with sleep-disordered breathing, and include weight loss, CPAP therapy, and surgery.

Primary hypersomnolence and Prader–Willi syndrome

As noted above, a number of studies looking at the presence of sleep-disordered breathing in PWS have led to the general consensus that the sleep-disordered breathing alone cannot account for the significant excessive daytime sleepiness experienced by PWS patients. This fact, in addition to an absence of any other identifiable sleep disorders, has led to the conclusion that the sleepiness of PWS may also be due to a primary, idiopathic or "narcolepsy-like" sleepiness, with hypothalamic dysfunction playing a putative role. The evidence for this comes primarily from the presence of REM abnormalities in PWS patients, and more recently studies on hypocretin/orexin.

REM sleep abnormalities and Prader–Willi syndrome

Vela-Bueno et al. [12] were the first to note an increased prevalence of REM abnormalities in PWS. In their study of nine pediatric and adult patients with PWS, five were noted to have a SOREM in at least one of two to four overnight sleep studies. These REM abnormalities were notably in the absence of significant obstructive sleep apnea. Harris et al. [18]

reported moderately shortened REM latencies in two out of four PWS patient during overnight polysomnography with all four patients exhibiting one SOREM nap on MSLT testing, although three of these patients exhibited significant sleep apnea. Kaplan et al. [13] noted normal sleep architecture and REM onset latency in the overnight polysomnography of five patients studied. Helbing-Zwanenburg et al. [20] noted SOREM episodes in the overnight studies of 7 out of 21 PWS patients studied, with 7 PWS patients also exhibiting SOREM episodes during daytime naps (vs. none in a control group). Hertz et al. [19] found that 13 out of 24 adult and pediatric PWS patients exhibited shortened REM latency on polysomnography. Five patients exhibited at least one SOREM episode on the MSLT. Rapid eye movement parameters did not correlate with nocturnal oxygen desaturation nor daytime sleepiness as measured by the MSLT. Clift et al. [14] found normal REM latency without any clear SOREM episodes in 17 pediatric and adult PWS patients. Livington et al. [37] reported sleep onset REM during overnight polysomnography in seven out of ten PWS patients studied. Vgontzas et al. [21] reported three out of eight subjects having shortened REM latency on overnight polysomnography, and four subjects experiencing at least one SOREM episode during two daytime naps. Prader–Willi syndrome patients with EDS also had a higher number of REM periods and shorter REM intervals in comparison with their non-EDS counterparts, as well as normal, narcoleptic, and obese control groups. Manni et al. [16] found REM sleep onset in three out of fourteen PWS subjects during overnight polysomnography, and five out of ten subjects experiencing at least two SOREMPs on the MSLT. Yee et al. [28] found the mean REM latency during overnight polysomnography to be significantly shorter in a group of 19 adult PWS patients in comparison to an obese control group, despite comparable mean total RDI scores (although the PWS group did exhibit significantly more nocturnal hypoxemia). Lin et al. [29] found a shortened mean REM latency of 67.4 ± 30 minutes in a group of 30 pediatric PWS patients. Williams et al. [17] reported a normal mean REM latency in 37 pediatric PWS patients of 84 ± 57 minutes, although the large variability in this result is notable.

Sforza [41] reported a case of a 20-year-old patient with PWS with a SOREMP on overnight polysomnography and SOREMP on four out of six naps on a modified MSLT, in addition to moderate sleep apnea. Treatment with CPAP resulted in elimination of sleep apnea, but with a persistent SOREMP on the first night of treatment. Vgontzas et al. [43] reported a patient with persistent shortened REM latency and SOREM episodes on daytime sleepiness following successful treatment of severe sleep apnea with weight loss.

In summary, a number of studies have documented the presence of significant REM sleep dysregulation in PWS in the form of shortened REM latency, and increased prevalence of SOREMPs on overnight polysomnography or the MSLT. In general this REM dysregulation does not seem to be accounted for by the increased prevalence of sleep-disordered breathing in this population, nor any other obvious sleep disorders. Such REM dysregulation implies a disruption in the circadian rhythms of PWS patients or a dysfunction in fundamental sleep–wake mechanisms (or both). These observations also suggest the presence of a primary hypersomnolence akin to narcolepsy, which is itself associated with excessive daytime sleepiness and REM sleep dysregulation. Finally such REM dysregulation may be linked with the abnormal thermoregulation observed in PWS, pointing to hypothalamic dysfunction as the cause of such dysregulation [12]. This in turn has some implications with respect to treatment strategies for PWS patients (see below).

Prader–Willi syndrome and narcolepsy

The presence of REM abnormalities and excessive daytime sleepiness not otherwise explained suggests the presence not only of a narcolepsy-like syndrome in patients with Prader–Willi syndrome, but narcolepsy itself. The majority of studies, however, have not reported the presence of narcolepsy symptoms in their PWS samples, including cataplexy, hypnagogic/hypnopompic hallucinations, and sleep paralysis. Some exceptions include Helbing-Zwanenburg et al. [20], who reported that the presence of cataplexy in 6 of 21 patients with PWS and EDS was "very likely," but commented that cataplexy was even more difficult to prove in the PWS population than in narcolepsy. Clift et al. [14] described three out of 17 PWS patients with a loss of muscle tone triggered by laughter, but felt that this was unlikely to be true cataplexy with REM sleep atonia, but rather an exaggerated physiological response in patients with pre-existing hypotonia. A number of small studies conducting HLA bloodtyping in PWS patients have not found a pattern consistent with a narcoleptic population [16, 19, 20]. Vgontzas *et al.* [21] reported significant differences in the sleep and REM patterns of a PWS group in comparison with a group of patients with narcolepsy. They hypothesized that PWS was associated with a "generalized hypoarousal" with REM abnormalities appearing as a compensatory mechanism.

Overall, while the hypersomnolence associated with PWS appears to be primary in nature and associated with dysregulation of REM sleep, features shared by the condition known as narcolepsy, it does not seem to be due to narcolepsy itself. However, the presence of cataplexy in some patients suggests an increased prevalence of narcolepsy in the PWS population. Alternatively, the putative role of the hypothalamus in both narcolepsy (see below) and PWS point to overlapping pathophysiological mechanisms, and hence shared symptomology. Of note another primary hypersomnia, which is hypothesized to involve hypothalamic involvement, is Klein–Levin syndrome, and at least two cases with both PWS and Klein–Levin syndrome have been reported [51, 52].

Hypocretin/orexin and Prader–Willi syndrome

Hypocretin (known synonymously as orexin) is a peptide neurotransmitter found in the dorsal and lateral hypothalamus. Soon after its discovery, disturbances in the hypocretin system were identified as playing a pathophysiological role in narcolepsy. Narcolepsy in humans has been associated with decreased hypocretin CSF levels and degeneration of hypocretin neurons. In addition to its role in sleep regulation, hypocretin/orexin has been associated with a number of other effects including appetite regulation, autonomic and endocrine function, and pleasure/reward pathways [53].

In keeping with the proposed role of hypothalamic dysfunction in the etiology of the primary hypersomnolence associated with PWS, a number of studies have reported decreased CSF hypocretin levels in patients with PWS. In a large study of CSF hypocretin-1 levels in patients with hypersomnolence, Mignot *et al.* [54] identified a 16-year-old with PWS with low levels (≤ 110 pg/ml by direct radioimmunoassay) of CSF hypocretin comparable to that of narcolepsy. In a similar study in children with a variety of neurological disorders, Arri *et al.* [55] identified a neonate with PWS with intermediate (≥ 110 to ≤ 200 pg/ml) levels of CSF hypocretin-1. Dauvilliers *et al.* [52] reported the

case of a 21-year-old male with both PWS and Klein–Levin syndrome who exhibited a nearly twofold decrease in CSF hypocretin-1 during an episode of hypersomnia (111 pg/ml) in comparison with levels taken when asymptomatic (221 pg/ml). Nevsimalova *et al.* [56] reported the findings of low and intermediate levels of CSF hypocretin-1 in two cases of PWS, who exhibited severe and moderate levels of daytime sleepiness on the MSLT respectively. Another two cases, without daytime sleepiness, exhibited normal CSF hypocretin-1 levels.

Finally, Fronczek *et al.* [57] studied the postmortem hypothalami of seven PWS patients and found no significant difference in the number of hypocretin neurons between the PWS group and a group of controls.

Overall, the findings noted above, albeit limited, support the notion of hypothalamic dysfunction as the cause of excessive daytime sleepiness seen in PWS syndrome. Based on the limited evidence it seems that the sleepiness in PWS is associated with a deficiency of hypocretin/orexin in the hypothalamus, but not necessarily a degeneration of hypocretin neurons as is seen in narcolepsy.

Treatment of primary sleepiness in Prader–Willi syndrome

Treatment of the primary sleepiness in PWS has been severely limited. Behavioral measures, such as extended nocturnal sleep, have been proposed. A limited number of case reports have reported a beneficial impact of stimulants in the excessive daytime sleepiness associated with PWS, but concerns have been raised about the adverse effects such medications can have on appetite and behavior [24]. One potentially beneficial, but as yet untested, treatment for primary sleepiness associated with PWS is the wakefulness agent modafinil [58]. We have used the amino acid tryptophan in doses up to 4.5 g in children and adults with PWS showing hypersomnolence. This has usually been in the context of showing fragmented sleep in polysomnographic recordings. We have had dramatic resolution of hypersomnia in some patients and, in a couple of cases, we have had the spontaneous comment that previous hypothermia has been simultaneously improved.

Conclusion

Excessive daytime sleepiness is a frequent and significant symptom of patients with Prader–Willi

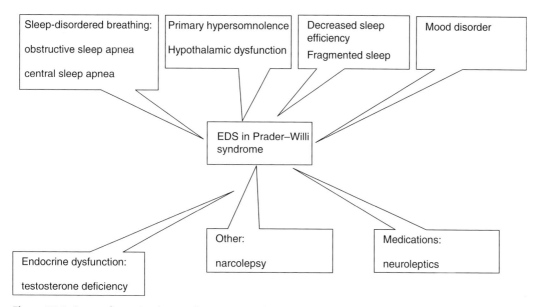

Figure 36.1 Causes of excessive daytime sleepiness in Prader–Willi syndrome.

syndrome. Patients with PWS possess a number of risk factors that predispose them to sleep-disordered breathing, but sleep-disordered breathing in itself, in many cases, cannot account for all of the daytime sleepiness experienced by such patients. A number of studies have suggested the presence of a primary hypersomnolence in PWS as evidenced by significant REM sleep dysregulation and more recently studies involving CSF hypocretin-1. Hypothalamic dysfunction is implicated in a number of symptoms characteristic of PWS, and such dysfunction likely underscores the primary hypersomnolence observed in these patients.

It is important for both the treating physician and those designing further studies to keep in mind that a number of factors have been implicated beyond those already identified (summarized in Figure 36.1). Patients with PWS, for example, are frequently put on sedating psychotropic agents for a variety of psychiatric or behavioral disturbances [23]. Prader–Willi syndrome patients may have disruptions in sleep architecture in the form of decreased sleep efficiency [19] or fragmented sleep in the form of multiple arousals or the cyclic alternating pattern (CAP). Prader–Willi syndrome is characterized by a number of endocrine abnormalities, and one author (JB) has seen at least one case where a substantial improvement in daytime sleepiness occurred in a patient with PWS

following testosterone supplementation. No studies have systematically examined the effect of growth hormone deficiency itself as a cause of sleepiness.

The excessive daytime sleepiness associated with PWS is likely to be multifactorial in origin with a number of factors contributing to its expression. The complexity of hypersomnolence in PWS provides a challenge to both the treating physician and researchers, but also provides a unique insight into basic sleep–wake mechanisms.

References

1. Bittel DC, Butler MG. Prader-Willi syndrome: clinical genetics, cytogenetics and molecular biology. *Expert Rev Mol Med.* 2005;**7**(14):1–20.

2. Cassidy SB, Driscoll DJ. Prader-Willi syndrome. *Eur J Hum Genet.* 2009;**17**(1):3–13.

3. Chen C, Visootsak J, Dills S, Graham JM, Jr. Prader-Willi syndrome: an update and review for the primary pediatrician. *Clin Pediatr (Phila).* 2007;**46**(7):580–91.

4. Goldstone AP, Holland AJ, Hauffa BP, Hokken-Koelega AC, Tauber M. Recommendations for the diagnosis and management of Prader-Willi syndrome. *J Clin Endocrinol Metab.* 2008;**93**(11):4183–97.

5. Gunay-Aygun M, Schwartz S, Heeger S, O'Riordan MA, Cassidy SB. The changing purpose of Prader-Willi syndrome clinical diagnostic criteria and proposed revised criteria. *Pediatrics.* 2001;**108**(5):E92.

6. Holm VA, Cassidy SB, Butler MG, *et al.* Prader-Willi syndrome: consensus diagnostic criteria. *Pediatrics.* 1993;**91**(2):398–402.

7. Greenswag LR. Adults with Prader-Willi syndrome: a survey of 232 cases. *Dev Med Child Neurol.* 1987; **29**(2):145–52.

8. Clarke DJ, Waters J, Corbett JA. Adults with Prader-Willi syndrome: abnormalities of sleep and behaviour. *J R Soc Med.* 1989;**82**(1):21–4.

9. Richdale AL, Cotton S, Hibbit K. Sleep and behaviour disturbance in Prader-Willi syndrome: a questionnaire study. *J Intellect Disabil Res.* 1999;**43**(5):380–92.

10. Cotton S, Richdale A. Brief report: parental descriptions of sleep problems in children with autism, Down syndrome, and Prader-Willi syndrome. *Res Dev Disabil.* 2006;**27**(2):151–61.

11. Maas AP, Didden R, Bouts L, Smits MG, Curfs LM. Scatter plot analysis of excessive daytime sleepiness and severe disruptive behavior in adults with Prader-Willi syndrome: a pilot study. *Res Dev Disabil.* 2009;**30**(3):529–37.

12. Vela-Bueno A, Kales A, Soldatos CR, *et al.* Sleep in the Prader-Willi syndrome. Clinical and polygraphic findings. *Arch Neurol.* 1984;**41**(3):294–6.

13. Kaplan J, Fredrickson PA, Richardson JW. Sleep and breathing in patients with the Prader-Willi syndrome. *Mayo Clin Proc.* 1991;**66**(11):1124–6.

14. Clift S, Dahlitz M, Parkes JD. Sleep apnoea in the Prader-Willi syndrome. *J Sleep Res.* 1994;**3**(2):121–6.

15. Richards A, Quaghebeur G, Clift S, *et al.* The upper airway and sleep apnoea in the Prader-Willi syndrome. *Clin Otolaryngol Allied Sci.* 1994;**19**(3):193–7.

16. Manni R, Politini L, Nobili L, *et al.* Hypersomnia in the Prader-Willi syndrome: clinical-electrophysiological features and underlying factors. *Clin Neurophysiol.* 2001;**112**(5):800–5.

17. Williams K, Scheimann A, Sutton V, Hayslett E, Glaze DG. Sleepiness and sleep disordered breathing in Prader-Willi syndrome: relationship to genotype, growth hormone therapy, and body composition. *J Clin Sleep Med.* 2008;**4**(2):111–18.

18. Harris JC, Allen RP. Sleep disordered breathing and circadian disturbance of REM sleep in Prader-Willi syndrome. *Sleep Res.* 1985;**14**:235.

19. Hertz G, Cataletto M, Feinsilver SH, Angulo M. Sleep and breathing patterns in patients with Prader Willi syndrome (PWS): effects of age and gender. *Sleep.* 1993;**16**(4):366–71.

20. Helbing-Zwanenburg B, Kamphuisen HA, Mourtazaev MS. The origin of excessive daytime sleepiness in the Prader-Willi syndrome. *J Intellect Disabil Res.* 1993;**37**(6):533–41.

21. Vgontzas AN, Bixler EO, Kales A, *et al.* Daytime sleepiness and REM abnormalities in Prader-Willi syndrome: evidence of generalized hypoarousal. *Int J Neurosci.* 1996;**87**(3–4):127–39.

22. Hiroe Y, Inoue Y, Higami S, Suto Y, Kawahara R. Relationship between hypersomnia and respiratory disorder during sleep in Prader-Willi syndrome. *Psychiatry Clin Neurosci.* 2000;**54**(3):323–5.

23. Priano L, Grugni G, Miscio G, *et al.* Sleep cycling alternating pattern (CAP) expression is associated with hypersomnia and GH secretory pattern in Prader-Willi syndrome. *Sleep Med.* 2006;**7**(8):627–33.

24. Nixon GM, Brouillette RT. Sleep and breathing in Prader-Willi syndrome. *Pediatr Pulmonol.* 2002;**34**(3):209–17.

25. Friedman E, Ferber R, Wharton R, Dietz W. Sleep apnea in the Prader-Willi syndrome. *Sleep Res.* 1984;**13**:142.

26. O'Donoghue FJ, Camfferman D, Kennedy JD, *et al.* Sleep-disordered breathing in Prader-Willi syndrome and its association with neurobehavioral abnormalities. *J Pediatr.* 2005;**147**(6):823–9.

27. Festen DA, de Weerd AW, van den Bossche RA, *et al.* Sleep-related breathing disorders in prepubertal children with Prader-Willi syndrome and effects of growth hormone treatment. *J Clin Endocrinol Metab.* 2006;**91**(12):4911–15.

28. Yee BJ, Buchanan PR, Mahadev S, *et al.* Assessment of sleep and breathing in adults with Prader-Willi syndrome: a case control series. *J Clin Sleep Med.* 2007;**3**(7):713–18.

29. Lin HY, Lin SP, Lin CC, *et al.* Polysomnographic characteristics in patients with Prader-Willi syndrome. *Pediatr Pulmonol.* 2007;**42**(10):881–7.

30. Festen DA, Wevers M, de Weerd AW, *et al.* Psychomotor development in infants with Prader-Willi syndrome and associations with sleep-related breathing disorders. *Pediatr Res.* 2007;**62**(2):221–4.

31. Hertz G, Cataletto M, Feinsilver SH, Angulo M. Developmental trends of sleep-disordered breathing in Prader-Willi syndrome: the role of obesity. *Am J Med Genet.* 1995;**56**(2):188–90.

32. Voloh I, Chung SA, Kayumov L, Berall G, Shapiro CM. Sleep patterns in Prader-Willi patients on and off medications. *Sleep.* 2002;**25**:A259.

33. Festen DA, Wevers M, de Weerd AW, *et al.* Psychomotor development in infants with Prader-Willi syndrome and associations with sleep-related breathing disorders. *Pediatr Res.* 2007;**62**(2):221–4.

34. Arens R, Gozal D, Omlin KJ, *et al.* Hypoxic and hypercapnic ventilatory responses in Prader-Willi syndrome. *J Appl Physiol.* 1994;**77**(5):2224–30.

35. Gozal D, Arens R, Omlin KJ, Ward SL, Keens TG. Absent peripheral chemosensitivity in Prader-Willi syndrome. *J Appl Physiol.* 1994;**77**(5):2231–6.

36. Menendez AA. Abnormal ventilatory responses in patients with Prader-Willi syndrome. *Eur J Pediatr.* 1999;**158**(11):941–2.

37. Livingston FR, Arens R, Bailey SL, Keens TG, Ward SL. Hypercapnic arousal responses in Prader-Willi syndrome. *Chest.* 1995;**108**(6):1627–31.

38. Arens R, Gozal D, Burrell BC, *et al.* Arousal and cardiorespiratory responses to hypoxia in Prader-Willi syndrome. *Am J Respir Crit Care Med.* 1996;**153**(1):283–7.

39. Schluter B, Buschatz D, Trowitzsch E, Aksu F, Andler W. Respiratory control in children with Prader-Willi syndrome. *Eur J Pediatr.* 1997;**156**(1):65–8.

40. Harris JC, Allen RP. Is excessive daytime sleepiness characteristic of Prader-Willi syndrome? The effects of weight change. *Arch Pediatr Adolesc Med.* 1996;**150**(12):1288–93.

41. Sforza E, Krieger J, Geisert J, Kurtz D. Sleep and breathing abnormalities in a case of Prader-Willi syndrome. The effects of acute continuous positive airway pressure treatment. *Acta Paediatr Scand.* 1991;**80**(1):80–5.

42. Pavone M, Paglietti MG, Petrone A, *et al.* Adenotonsillectomy for obstructive sleep apnea in children with Prader-Willi syndrome. *Pediatr Pulmonol.* 2006;**41**(1):74–9.

43. Vgontzas AN, Bixler EO, Kales A, Vela-Bueno A. Prader-Willi syndrome: effects of weight loss on sleep-disordered breathing, daytime sleepiness and REM sleep disturbance. *Acta Paediatr.* 1995;**84**(7):813–14.

44. Esnault-Lavandier S, Mabin D. The effects of clomipramine on diurnal sleepiness and respiratory parameters in a case of Prader-Willi syndrome. *Neurophysiol Clin.* 1998;**28**(6):521–5.

45. Stafler P, Wallis C. Prader-Willi syndrome: who can have growth hormone? *Arch Dis Child.* 2008;**93**(4):341–5.

46. Eiholzer U. Deaths in children with Prader-Willi syndrome. A contribution to the debate about the safety of growth hormone treatment in children with PWS. *Horm Res.* 2005;**63**(1):33–9.

47. Haqq AM, Stadler DD, Jackson RH, *et al.* Effects of growth hormone on pulmonary function, sleep quality, behavior, cognition, growth velocity, body

composition, and resting energy expenditure in Prader-Willi syndrome. *J Clin Endocrinol Metab.* 2003;**88**(5):2206–12.

48. Miller J, Silverstein J, Shuster J, Driscoll DJ, Wagner M. Short-term effects of growth hormone on sleep abnormalities in Prader-Willi syndrome. *J Clin Endocrinol Metab.* 2006;**91**(2):413–17.

49. Lindgren AC, Hellstrom LG, Ritzen EM, Milerad J. Growth hormone treatment increases CO_2 response, ventilation and central inspiratory drive in children with Prader-Willi syndrome. *Eur J Pediatr.* 1999;**158**(11):936–40.

50. Camfferman D, Lushington K, O'Donoghue F, Doug MR. Obstructive sleep apnea syndrome in Prader-Willi syndrome: an unrecognized and untreated cause of cognitive and behavioral deficits? *Neuropsychol Rev.* 2006;**16**(3):123–9.

51. Gau SF, Soong WT, Liu HM, *et al.* Kleine-Levin syndrome in a boy with Prader-Willi syndrome. *Sleep.* 1996;**19**(1):13–17.

52. Dauvilliers Y, Baumann CR, Carlander B, *et al.* CSF hypocretin-1 levels in narcolepsy, Kleine-Levin syndrome, and other hypersomnias and neurological conditions. *J Neurol Neurosurg Psychiatry.* 2003;**74**(12):1667–73.

53. Ganjavi H, Shapiro CM. Hypocretin/orexin: a molecular link between sleep, energy regulation, and pleasure. *J Neuropsychiatry Clin Neurosci.* 2007;**19**(4):413–19.

54. Mignot E, Lammers GJ, Ripley B, *et al.* The role of cerebrospinal fluid hypocretin measurement in the diagnosis of narcolepsy and other hypersomnias. *Arch Neurol.* 2002;**59**(10):1553–62.

55. Arri J, Kanbayashi T, Tanabe Y, *et al.* CSF hypocretin-1 (orexin-A) levels in childhood narcolepsy and neurologic disorders. *Neurology.* 2004;**63**:2440–2.

56. Nevsimalova S, Vankova J, Stepanova I, *et al.* Hypocretin deficiency in Prader-Willi syndrome. *Eur J Neurol.* 2005;**12**(1):70–2.

57. Fronczek R, Lammers GJ, Balesar R, Unmehopa UA, Swaab DF. The number of hypothalamic hypocretin (orexin) neurons is not affected in Prader-Willi syndrome. *J Clin Endocrinol Metab.* 2005;**90**(9):5466–70.

58. Camfferman D, McEvoy RD, O'Donoghue F, Lushington K. Prader Willi syndrome and excessive daytime sleepiness. *Sleep Med Rev.* 2008;**12**(1):65–75.

Index